8th Edition

Medical Terminology
An Illustrated Guide

医学术语图解指南

— 第 8 版 —

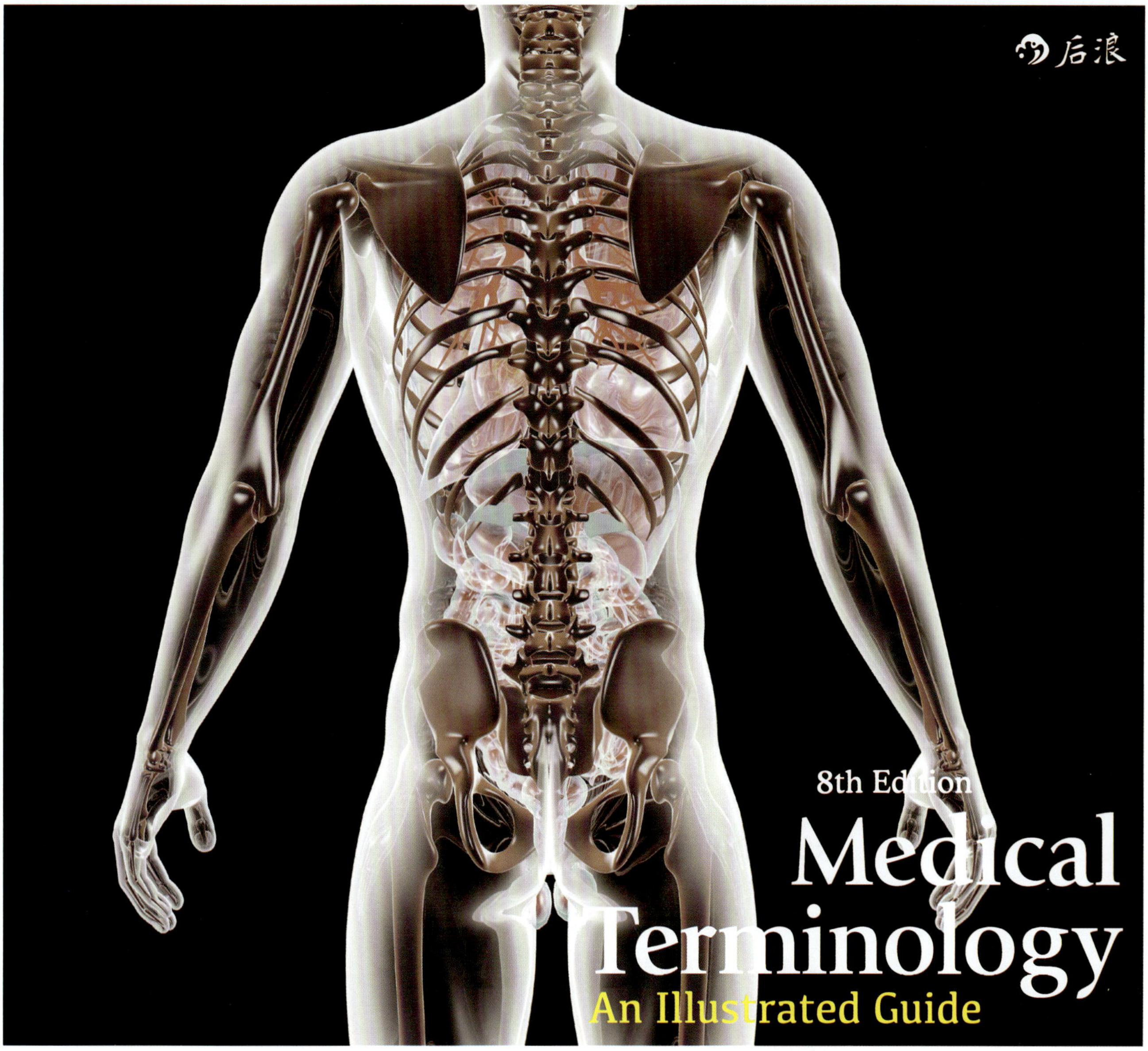
后浪
8th Edition
Medical Terminology
An Illustrated Guide

医学术语图解指南

— 第 8 版 —

[美] 芭芭拉·詹森·科恩　安·德佩特里＿著
龚 辉 刘 皓 王文法＿译

Barbara Janson Cohen
Ann DePetris

北京联合出版公司
Beijing United Publishing Co.,Ltd.

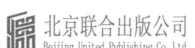

图书在版编目（CIP）数据

医学术语图解指南：第 8 版 /（美）芭芭拉·詹森·科恩等著；龚辉，刘皓，王文法译. -- 北京：北京联合出版公司，2018.7

ISBN 978-7-5596-2069-9

Ⅰ.①医… Ⅱ.①芭… ②龚… ③刘… ④王… Ⅲ.①临床医学—名词术语—指南 Ⅳ.① R4-61

中国版本图书馆 CIP 数据核字 (2018) 第 086440 号

This is a translation of Medical Terminology An illustrated Guide, 8th Edition. Wolters Kluwer Health did not participate in the translation of this title and therefore it does not take any responsibility for the inaccuracy or errors of this translation.

这本书中提到了药物适应证、不良反应和用法用量，但它们有可能是有变化的。敦促读者审查所提到的药品制造商的包装信息和数据。作者、编辑、出版商或分销商对该出版物的信息错误、遗漏不负责任，对出版物的内容不作任何保证、表示或暗示。作者、编辑、出版商和分销商对该出版物所产生的人身或财产的伤害和（或）损害不承担任何责任。

Published by arrangement with Wolters Kluwer Health Inc., USA

医学术语图解指南：第 8 版

著　　者：[美] 芭芭拉·詹森·科恩 等
译　　者：龚　辉　刘　皓　王文法
选题策划：后浪出版公司
出版统筹：吴兴元
特约编辑：曹秋月
责任编辑：李　伟
营销推广：ONEBOOK
装帧制造：墨白空间·张莹

北京联合出版公司出版
（北京市西城区德外大街 83 号楼 9 层　100088）
北京盛通印刷股份有限公司印刷　新华书店经销
字数 1300 千字　889 毫米 × 1194 毫米　1/16　44.5 印张
2018 年 7 月第 1 版　2018 年 7 月第 1 次印刷
ISBN 978-7-5596-2069-9
定价：298.00 元

后浪出版咨询(北京)有限责任公司 常年法律顾问：北京大成律师事务所　周天晖 copyright@hinabook.com
未经许可，不得以任何方式复制或抄袭本书部分或全部内容
版权所有，侵权必究
本书若有质量问题，请与本公司图书销售中心联系调换。电话：010-64010019

译者名单

主　译　　龚　辉　刘　皓　王文法
副主译　　胡　军　蔡贵榕　张睿娟　李正伟

译者委员会名单（以姓氏笔画为序）

王文红　　天津市儿童医院
王文法　　楚雄彝族自治州人民医院
王永刚　　解放军第 302 医院
王　艇　　大连明医汇美容管理有限公司
王　颐　　解放军第 309 医院
毛　宁　　安徽省太和县人民医院
刘　皓　　中山大学孙逸仙纪念医院
李正伟　　吉林大学第二医院
张荣强　　陕西中医药大学
张勇军　　遵义医学院第五附属（珠海）医院
张睿娟　　山西医科大学第二医院
郝春艳　　山西医科大学第一医院
胡　军　　江苏省人民医院
段虎斌　　山西医科大学第一医院
钱亚龙　　北京大学人民医院
龚　辉　　复旦大学附属金山医院
廉秋芳　　延安大学咸阳医院
蔡贵榕　　成都市金牛区妇幼保健院

内容简介

本书是一本图文并茂的指南，分别介绍了医学术语的基本组成、疾病与治疗，及人体各个系统。每个章节中的预测试可评估阅读前的知识水平，练习题可巩固所学内容，复习资料能够强化记忆。案例研究采用中英文对照的方式将病历报告的主诉、检查与临床病程完整地呈现，使读者在学习病历报告的书写方法的同时规范医学术语的应用。本书全彩印刷，使用大量表格与图示为医学生提供方便、快捷的术语查询，是医学、护理、检验等相关专业人员学习专业英语的必备参考、应试书。

前　言

在广泛的医疗保健领域，医学术语是基本知识。本书旨在满足健康领域从业实践中所需的基本学习要求。在您的培训和未来的职业生涯中，您需要学习数千个新术语，如果没有学会将单词分解的技能，这个工作可能会把您压垮。这些词根、后缀和前缀在不同的术语中重复出现，但含义相同，了解这些含义将帮助您定义和记住一大堆词，这个过程就像使用一组构建块来组装不同的结构，用更科学的例子来形容，就像使用DNA中的四个碱基来编码制造蛋白质所需的所有氨基酸。

在简介部分之后，每章都从一个具体人体系统图解概述开始，其中包含与该系统相关的关键术语的定义，随后是单词组成部分表和相应的练习。再转到人体系统的异常情况，包括关于疾病和治疗的部分，随后是相关关键术语的定义。补充术语部分包括如果时间允许或者某人对该专业特别感兴趣的"知道更好"的词和短语。系统章节的顺序与传统解剖学和生理学书籍中的顺序略有不同，本书的构架强调其临床重要性，从心血管、呼吸和消化系统开始，后续介绍了需要在更专业的领域进行治疗的系统，如泌尿、生殖和肌肉骨骼系统。

我们试图使这本书使用简单，并与临床实践相结合。本书还包括许多语音发音，当它们被说出时您可以识别并熟练地应用这些专业术语，在线学生学习资源提供了许多额外的活动和音频词汇表。每一章都有一个简短的开放案例研究，开始可能有一些不熟悉的词和缩写。书内的案例是为了激发您对章节内容的兴趣，并给您一种对医疗状况和语言的感觉。如果您不完全理解也不要担心，在学习本章后，再回看是否更容易理解。

您可能是在开始一个漫长的事业旅程，我们希望这本书能够帮助您，为您的事业生涯打下坚实的基础，早日获得成功。

—Barbara Cohen
—Ann DePetris

译者前言

学习医学英语术语是一项艰巨的任务，对母语是英语的人而言如是，对母语不是英语的人则更是。医学英语术语大多源自于拉丁语和希腊语，单词很长，发音困难，而且处于不断发展变化之中，难以学习并掌握。但这也不是一件不可完成的任务，有很多方法可以帮助学习医学英语术语，本书提供的图解方式即是一种颇为有效的方法。通过精美、详解的图片，将需要学习的医学术语形象地表现出来，大大有助于增强记忆，提高效率。同时，本书中还将医学术语的词根、前缀、后缀作为重点进行说明介绍，并通过简洁、科学的文字说明，将大量的医学术语展现给读者，还提供了一些非常有益的练习和复习题，使读者可以在学习的同时自我测评，通过重复记忆加强对所学医学术语的掌握。另外，书中还附有一些案例研究，为读者在英语语境中学习医学术语提供了良好的机会。

在本书的翻译过程中，每个医学术语第一次出现时，都在译文中保留了英语原文。同时为了能够在英语语境中学习，案例研究部分都是双语表述。出于同样的目的，练习和复习部分基本保留了英语，以促进读者用英语思考、学习。图片中的文字也保留了英语，以便读者直接对照记忆。另外，本书对几乎所有医学术语都提供了一种所谓"音形一致"的音标，但考虑到国内读者在学习英语时接触的都是国际音标，临时改变反而会造成不适，所以在翻译中我们将音标都替换为国际音标，以方便读者练习发音。

由于译者水平有限，翻译中出现错误之处在所难免。另外，由于多个译者共同翻译，可能会出现个别术语前后不一致的现象，虽经反复审校，但难以保证杜绝，敬请读者见谅。

编者的话

随着市场的开放，外版书引入中国，医生、医学生走出国门深造的机会越来越多，掌握医学英语是对外交流学习的基本要求。众所周知，学医是很苦的，学习医学英语就更难，《医学术语图解指南（第8版）》这本书正是为大家解决学习医学英语难记、难懂、量大的问题，阅读后会有茅塞顿开之感，死记硬背的方法会被一扫而光，在不知不觉中掌握学习方法，此书确实为大家打开了一扇通往医学世界的大门。

《医学术语图解指南（第8版）》能帮您解决英语词汇量不足、不懂如何学习英语的问题，帮您改变死记硬背的"拙方法"。这本书图文并茂的特点，并不会让您感觉学习医学英语的枯燥乏味，反而能激发您学习英语的兴趣。

《医学术语图解指南（第8版）》是一本图文并茂的指南，第一部分介绍了医学词汇的基本组成，第二部分介绍了身体结构、疾病的种类和治疗方法，第三部分介绍的是全身系统疾病。

本书长年畅销不衰，以下特点是其他教科书不能替代的：

- 每章节以预测试题开始，可以帮助您评估阅读本章节前的医学英语专业知识水平。
- 学习目标部分给出阅读本章节时的重点、难点，起到了很好的指导作用。
- 中英文对照的案例研究自然而完整的将一份病历报告应有的主诉、检查与临床病程展现给读者，在反复的学习与思考中，病历报告的书写思路与方法伴随着医学术语逐渐渗透，这在其他书中是很少见到的。
- 词根、前缀、后缀是构成词汇的基石，也是词形变化的关键所在，对于记忆和理解词汇有着重要作用。
- 书中每章节的练习约占全书的四分之一，专项练习针对性强，形式多样，可以边学边练，加强记忆，起到融会贯通的作用，从而在自然中掌握学习方法。

一个单词的关联词和衍生词往往会被混淆、难记、更难应用于工作中，这是学习医学英语的最难点，本书会帮您走出谜团，教您如何记忆、理解和应用，强化思维能力，达到事半功倍的效果。本书对医生、医学生、护士是难得的重要的参考书，相信阅读后会有意想不到的收获和终身受益之效果。

阅读指南

《医学术语图解指南（第 8 版）》被创建和开发是为了帮助您掌握医学的语言，正文中提供的工具和功能将帮助您处理书中呈现的内容，请花一点时间浏览本用户指南，它将向您介绍能够增强学习效果的功能。

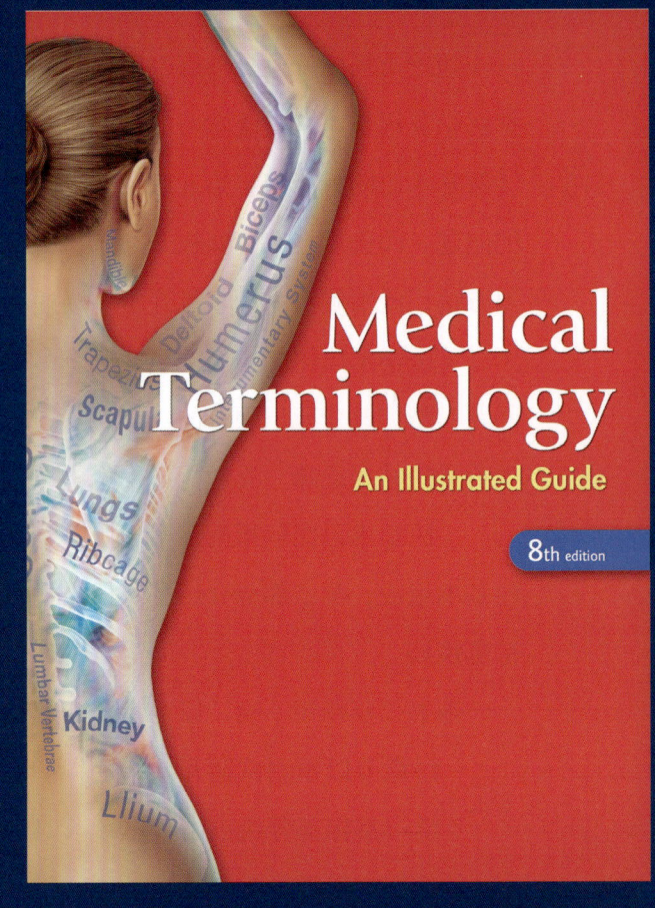

章节内容、学习目标和预测试

章节开头的案例研究和学习目标会帮助您确定学习目的，并使自己熟悉本章涵盖的内容。章节预测试在每章的开头检测学生对以前知识的掌握情况。学生应该在章节开始之前完成每个章节预测试，并在章节完成后再次进行测试，以便考量学习效果。

详细的插图

插图：详细的全彩插图和照片是每一章节的亮点，其中包括临床照片和组织显微照片，许多插图被放大并添加了注释，特别有助于视觉学习者。

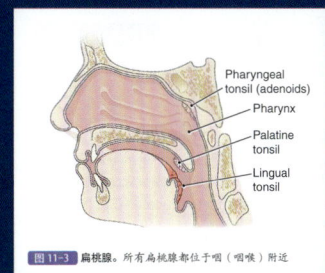

图 11-3 扁桃腺。所有扁桃腺都位于咽（咽喉）附近。

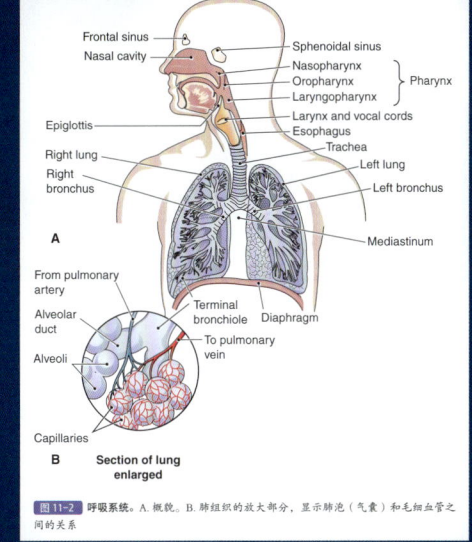

图 11-2 呼吸系统。A. 概貌。B. 肺组织的放大部分，显示肺泡（气囊）和毛细血管之间的关系

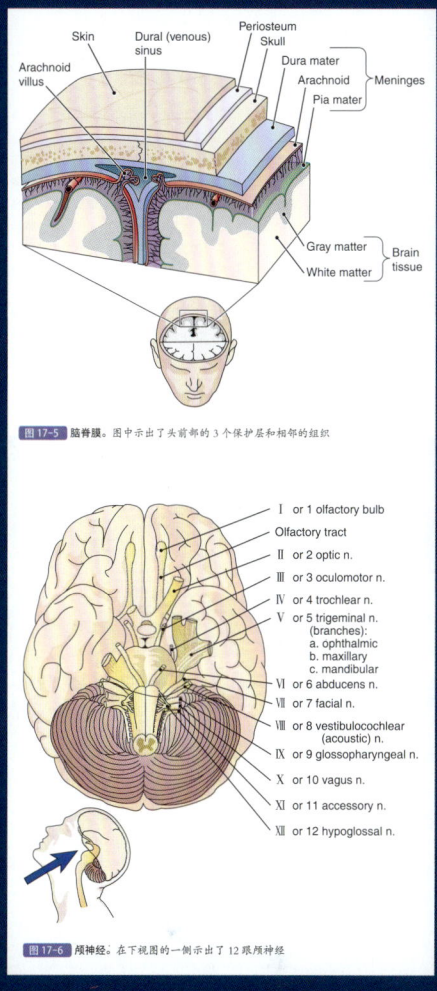

图 17-5 脑骨膜。图中示出了头前部的3个保护层和相邻的组织

图 17-6 颅神经。在下视图的一侧示出了12对颅神经

功能框

功能框强调重要信息

聚焦单词框为章节中选定的术语提供历史来源或其他有趣的信息。

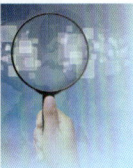

聚焦单词 框 10-2
首字母缩写

首字母缩写（acronym）是使用名称或短语中每个单词的第一个字母的缩写。因为在技术术语的数量和复杂性增加时节省时间和空间，它们变得非常受欢迎。适用于血液研究的一些示例是 CBC（全血细胞计数，complete blood count）以及 RBC（red blood cell）和 WBC（white blood cell）。一些其他常见的首字母缩略词包括 CNS（中枢神经系统，central nervous system 或临床护理专家 clinical nurse specialist）、ECG（心电图，electrocardiogram）、NIH（国立卫生研究院，National Institutes of Health）和 STI（性传播感染，sexually transmitted infection）等。

如果首字母缩写具有元音并且适合发音，它本身可以用作一个词，例如 AIDS（获得性免疫缺陷综合征，acquired immunodeficiency syndrome）、ELISA（酶联免疫吸附测定，enzyme-linked immunosorbent assay）、JAMA（美国医学协会杂志，Journal of the American Medical Association）、NSAID［ensed］（非甾体抗炎药，nonsteroidal antiinflammatory drug）和 CABG（冠状动脉旁路移植术，coronary artery bypass graft），这不可避免地变成"卷心菜（cabbage）"。很少有人知道 LASER（激光）是首字母缩写，意思是"受激辐射的发射光放大 light amplification by stimulated emission of radiation"。

首字母缩略词通常是短语在文章中第一次出现时被引入，然后在没有解释的情况下使用。如果您要花费时间在一篇文章中沮丧地搜索一个首字母缩写的含义，你可能希望像其他读者一样，所有的首字母缩略词及其含义将会被列在每篇文章的开头。

临床观点
眼睛手术：高技术一瞥 框 18-3

白内障（cataracts）、青光眼（glaucoma）和屈光不正是常见的眼睛疾病。在过去，白内障和青光眼的治疗集中在控制疾病。屈光不正使用眼镜和新近的隐形眼镜矫正。现在，使用激光和微手术技术，眼科医生能够切除白内障，减轻青光眼，并使屈光不正的人们摆脱眼镜和隐形眼镜。这些高技术方法包括：

· 准分子激光原位角膜磨镶术（laser in situ keratomileusis, LASIK）矫正屈光不正。在这种方法中，医生使用激光改造角膜，以便使光线直接折射到视网膜，而不是折射到视网膜之前或之后。用微型角膜刀（microkeratome）在角膜的外层切下一个皮片，在用计算机控制的激光雕刻角膜的中层，然后再将切下的皮片放回原处。这个过程只需几分钟，患者能够快速恢复视力，通常只有很小的术后疼痛。

· 超声乳化白内障吸出术（Phacoemulsification）消除白内障。在这种方法中，医生通过巩膜在接近角膜外边缘处做一个小切口（约 3mm），将超声波探头从这个切口插入晶状体中心。探头使用声波乳化晶状体的中心核，然后将其吸出。再将一个人工晶状体永久植入到晶状体囊中（图 18-15）。这种方法通常是无痛的，患者在术后一两天中可能会感觉不适。

· 激光小梁成形术（laser trabeculoplasty）治疗青光眼。这种方法使用激光帮助将液体排出眼睛，降低眼压。激光瞄准位于角膜和虹膜之间的排泄通道，通过烧灼打开通道，改善液体排出。这种方法通常也是无痛的，只需要几分钟即可。

临床观点框专注于人体治疗过程以及在临床环境中使用的技术。

健康职业
放射技术人员 框 5-1

放射技术人员（radiologic technologist）通过对身体的 X 线图像（radiograph）帮助诊断医学疾病。他们还使用 CT 扫描和其他成像技术对患者进行检查，以帮助医生诊断。根据机构的患者安全移动程序，他们必须使患者为放射学检查做好准备，将患者置于适当的位置；然后将设备调整到正确的角度和高度，并调整用于拍摄 X 线或其他诊断图像的设置。他们必须正确地定位图像受体，并在曝光后取出并处理图像。他们还要保存患者记录和维护设备。放射技术人员必须通过使用保护装置和发射最低可能的辐射量，为自身和患者尽可能降低辐射危害。他们佩戴徽章来监测辐射水平，并记录他们的暴露情况。

放射技术人员可以专门从事特定的成像技术，如骨密度测定（bone densitometry）、心血管介入放射成像（cardiovascular-interventional radiography）、计算机断层扫描（computed tomography）、乳腺 X 线照相术（mammography）、磁共振成像（magnetic resonance imaging）、核医学（nuclear medicine）和质量管理。其中一些将在后面的章节中描述。

大多数放射技术人员在医院工作，但也能在医生办公室、诊断成像中心（例如，做乳腺 X 线照相术）和门诊护理中心工作。放射技术人员最低必须具有副学士学位才有资格获得专业认证，监督或教学职位需要更高的学位。放射学技术教育联合审查委员会（Joint Review Committee on Education in Radiologic Technology）负责认可大多数教育项目。美国放射技术员注册处（American Registry of Radiologic Technologists，ARRT）在放射学以及其他成像技术（CT、核磁共振、核医学等）领域提供国家认证考试。在美国大多数州作为放射技术人员就业，都要求 ARRT 认证。目前，这个领域的工作机会良好。美国放射技术人员协会（American Society of Radiologic Technologists）在 www.asrt.org 网站上有关于这个职业的信息。

健康职业框专注于各种健康职业，展示如何将医学术语的知识应用于现实世界的职业生涯中。

供你参考
血液细胞 框 10-1

细胞种类	每毫升数量	说明	功能
erythrocyte 红细胞（red blood cell）	500 万	极小（直径 7μm），没有核的双面凹盘	携带绑定在血蛋白上的氧气，也运送二氧化碳并缓冲血液
leukocyte 白细胞（white blood cell）	5 000~10 000	比红细胞大，有明显的分段的（粒性）或不分段的（无颗粒）核，根据染色特性分类	免疫。抵抗病原体并摧毁外来物质和碎片。存在于血液、组织和淋巴系统
platelet 血小板（thrombocyte）	150 000~450 000	大细胞（巨核细胞）的分段	止血。形成血小板堵塞并开始凝血

供您参考框为章节中的术语提供补充信息。

单词组成部分表

细节表

以易于参考的格式（包括在医学术语中使用的实例）给出每章介绍的词根、前缀和后缀。单词组成部分有助于学习和理解常用术语。

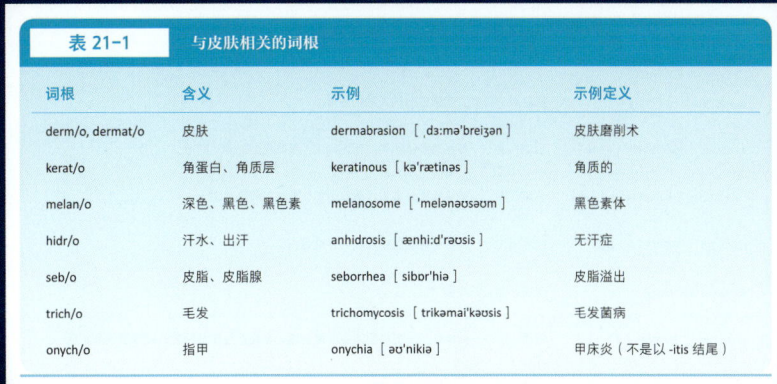

练习

练习的目的是测试您此前所学的知识，然后再进入下一个学习主题。

术语表

关键术语包括最常用的术语。

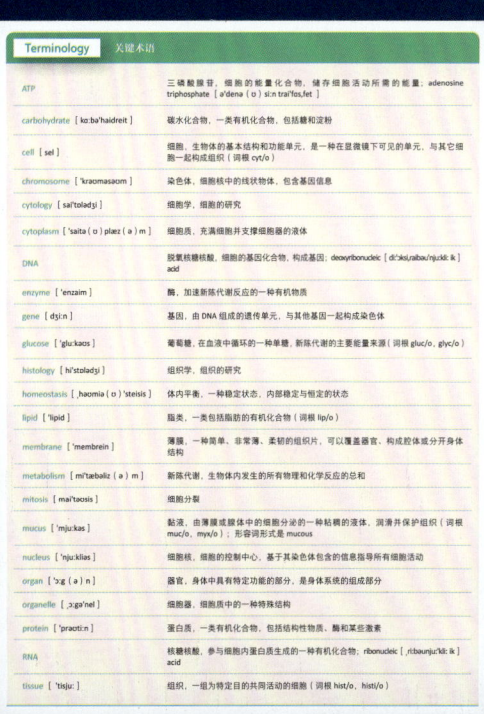

Terminology 补充术语

amino acids [əˈmiːnəʊ]		氨基酸，能够生成蛋白质的含氮化合物
anabolism [əˈnæbəlɪz(ə)m]		合成代谢，一种制造身体物质的新陈代谢；新陈代谢的建立阶段
catabolism [kəˈtæbəlɪz(ə)m]		分解代谢，一种将物质分解成能量和简单化合物的新陈代谢
collagen [ˈkɒlədʒ(ə)n]		胶原蛋白，一种在结缔组织中发现的纤维蛋白
cortex [ˈkɔːteks]		皮质，器官的外层
glycogen [ˈglaɪkədʒ(ə)n]		糖原，肝糖一种储存在肝脏和肌肉中的复合糖化合物，当需要能量时被分解为葡萄糖
interstitial [ˌɪntəˈstɪʃ(ə)l]		细胞间隙，组织内细胞之间的空隙
parenchyma [pəˈreŋkɪmə]		软组织，器官中的功能性组织
parietal [pəˈraɪɪt(ə)l]		腔壁的，与腔体壁相关的，用于描述体腔内部的薄膜
soma [ˈsəʊmə]		躯体，身体
stem cell		干细胞，一种能够发育成任意不同类型细胞的未成熟细胞，一种前体细胞
visceral [ˈvɪs(ə)r(ə)l]		内脏的，与体内器官相关的，用于描述器官表面的薄膜

补充术语列出了更专业的术语

Terminology 缩略语

AF	Acid fast	抗酸
CA, Ca	Cancer	癌症
CIS	Carcinoma in situ	原位癌
FUO	Fever of unknown origin	不明原因的发热
Gm⁺	Gram-positive	革兰氏阳性
Gm⁻	Gram-negative	革兰氏阴性
MRSA	Methicillin-resistant Staphylococcus aureus	耐甲氧西林的金黄色葡萄球菌
Staph	Staphylococcus	葡萄球菌
Strep	Streptococcus	链球菌
VRSA	Vancomycin-resistant Staphylococcus aureus	耐万古霉素的金黄色葡萄球菌

缩略语按常见术语列出

章节复习练习

章节复习练习旨在测试您对章节内容的了解，位置在每章的结尾。

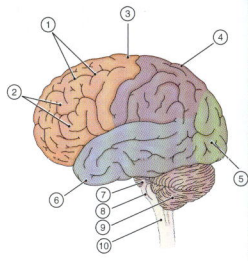

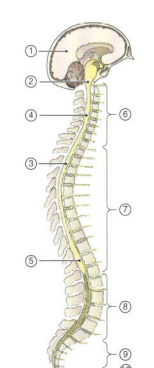

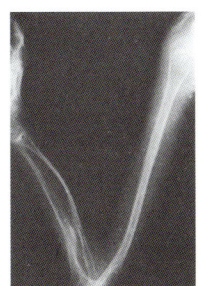

案例研究和案例研究问题

案例研究和每章结尾的案例研究问题在医疗报告的背景下呈现术语，这是一个很好的复习工具，它们能够测试您医学术语的积累量，并将术语应用于临床。

目 录

PART 1　医学术语简介　1

1. 医学术语的概念　2
2. 后缀　16
3. 前缀　32
4. 细胞、组织和器官　50
5. 身体结构　70

PART 2　疾病与治疗　91

6. 疾病　92
7. 诊断、治疗与手术　114
8. 药物　144

PART 3　人体系统　171

9. 循环：心血管与淋巴系统　172
10. 血液与免疫　216
11. 呼吸系统　250
12. 消化系统　284
13. 泌尿系统　320
14. 男性生殖系统　348
15. 女性生殖系统、妊娠与分娩　372
16. 内分泌系统　418
17. 神经系统和行为障碍　442
18. 感觉系统　486
19. 骨骼系统　520
20. 肌肉系统　558
21. 皮肤　584

附录 1　610
附录 2　611
附录 3　634
附录 4　644
附录 5　655
附录 6　662
附录 7　664
附录 8　666
附录 9　667

答案　668

PART 1 医学术语简介

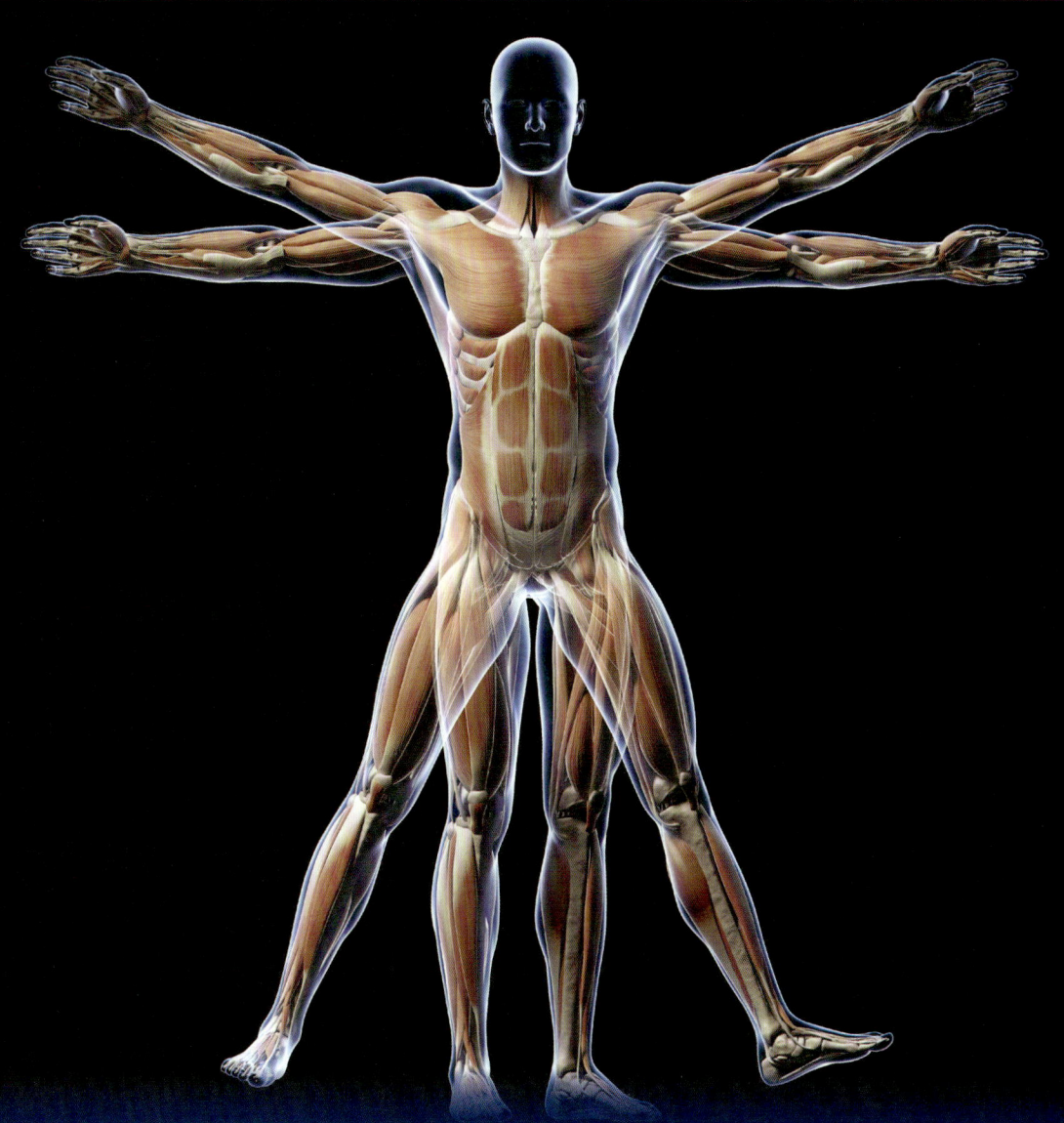

Chapter 1 ▶ Concepts of Medical Terminology
第 1 章　医学术语的概念

Chapter 2 ▶ Suffixes
第 2 章　后缀

Chapter 3 ▶ Prefixes
第 3 章　前缀

Chapter 4 ▶ Cells, Tissues, and Organs
第 4 章　细胞、组织和器官

Chapter 5 ▶ Body Structure
第 5 章　身体结构

CHAPTER 1

医学术语的概念

预测试

多项选择。选择最佳答案，并在每个数字的左边写上您选择的字母。

____1. The main part of a word is called the
   a. origin
   b. prefix
   c. root
   d. extension

____2. A word part at the beginning of a word is a
   a. prefix
   b. combining form
   c. preview
   d. root

____3. A word part at the end of a word is the
   a. vowel
   b. adjective
   c. insertion
   d. suffix

____4. The adjective form of cervix, meaning "neck," is
   a. cervical
   b. cervixal
   c. cervous
   d. cerval

____5. The ch in the word chemical is pronounced like the letter
   a. s
   b. h
   c. k
   d. f

____6. The ps in the word psychology is pronounced like the letter
   a. p
   b. s
   c. j
   d. k

____7. The word below that has a hard g is
   a. grip
   b. page
   c. gem
   d. judge

____8. The symbol ↓ means
   a. start
   b. turn
   c. decrease
   d. left

学习目标

学完本章后，应该能够：

1 ▶ 解释医学术语的用途。
2 ▶ 给出大多数医学单词的组成部分所源于的语言。
3 ▶ 定义词根、后缀和前缀。
4 ▶ 解释什么是组合形式以及为什么要使用它们。

5 ▶ 根据正文给出的音标读出单词。
6 ▶ 列出医学词典的三个功能。
7 ▶ 确定案例研究中的医学单词和缩略语，复习医学术语的概念。

Case Study: J. V. 's Digestive Problems
案例研究：J. V. 的消化问题

Chief Complaint
J. V., a 22-year-old（y/o）college student, visited the university health clinic and stated he had a four-month history of a burning pain in the middle of his chest. He notices it more at night and has difficulty sleeping because of the pain. He also states that the pain seems to occur more frequently following late-night college gatherings where pizza, spicy chicken wings, and beer are served.

主诉
J. V. 是一名 22 岁（y/o）的大学生，到学校的健康门诊说近四个月中在胸部中间有烧灼痛。他注意到晚上疼痛加重，且因为疼痛造成睡眠问题。他还说在夜晚聚会吃过匹萨饼、辣鸡翅和啤酒后疼痛发作得更频繁。

Examination
A well-nourished 22-year-old male complaining of（c/o）epigastric（upper abdominal）pain no longer relieved by antacids; orthopnea—currently sleeping with three pillows to aid in breathing; occasional swallowing problems, or dysphagia; ETOH（alcohol）consumption is six to eight beers per week; nonsmoker; no neurologic, musculoskeletal, genitourinary, or respiratory deficits. Referred to a gastroenterologist for ↑ acid production and gastroesophageal reflux disease（GERD）.

检查
一名营养良好的 22 岁男性主诉（complain c/o）上腹部（epigastric）疼痛，不能再通过抗酸剂缓解，端坐呼吸——枕三个枕头睡眠以协助呼吸；偶尔有吞咽问题，或吞咽困难（dysphagia）；酒精（alcohol，ETOH）消耗量为每周 6～8 瓶啤酒；不吸烟；无神经（neurologic）、肌肉骨骼（musculoskeletal）、泌尿生殖（genitourinary）或呼吸（respiratory）功能障碍。后请消化科医生（gastroenterologist）检查酸的生产上升和胃食管反流病（gastroesophageal reflux disease，GERD）。

Clinical Course
The gastroenterologist saw J. V. and ordered an x-ray study of his upper gastrointestinal（GI）system. Results demonstrated reflux disease, and J.V. underwent an esophageal gastroduodenoscopy（EGD）to visually examine his digestive organs from his esophagus to his small intestine. Results showed no evidence of bleeding, ulcerations, or strictures. The student was given educational material on GERD, including dietary recommendations. He was started on Prevacid and will be reevaluated in six months.

In this chapter, you learn about how medical words are constructed and also learn about the use of abbreviations and other types of shorthand in medical writing. Later in the chapter, we revisit J. V. and see how he is progressing under treatment.

临床病程
消化科医生检查了 J. V.，并要求对他的上消化道（GI）系统进行 X 线检查。结果显示回流病，并且 J.V. 做了食管胃十二指肠镜检查（esophageal gastroduodenoscopy，EGD）以视觉检查他从食管（esophagus）到小肠（small intestine）的消化器官（digestive organ）。结果显示没有出血（bleeding）、溃疡（ulceration）或狭窄（stricture）的证据。该学生获得了关于 GERD 的教育材料，包括膳食建议。他开始服用兰索拉唑（prevacid），将在 6 个月内复诊。

在本章中，你将学习如何构建医学词汇，并了解医学写作中缩略词和其他类型速记的使用。在本章的后面，我们再来看一下 J. V. 在治疗过程中的进展。

简介

医学英语术语是用于医学专业人员有效、准确交流的特殊术语,每个医学相关领域都需要对所有医学术语的认知和了解。由于主要来源于希腊语和拉丁语,医学术语在全世界都是一致不变的。医学术语的表达很有效率,尽管有些词汇很长,它们通常会把一整个句子缩短为一个单词。例如 gastroduodenostomy[ˈgæstrəˌdjuːədəˈnɒstəmi](胃十二指肠吻合术),表示"胃与小肠最初部分的联系"(图1-1)。gastro 表示胃;duoden 表示十二指肠,小肠的起始部分;ostomy 表示吻合术。

医学术语量很大,学习它就好像学习整个一门外语的词汇。不过,与所有不断发展的领域中的行话一样,医学术语也总是在不断扩展。想一想我们的词汇表随着计算机的发展所增加的词汇,例如软件、搜索引擎、电子邮件、聊天室和博客等。虽然任务看起来难以完成,但有一些方法能够帮助学习和记忆这些单词,甚至帮助猜测那些不熟悉的单词的意思。大多数医学单词能够被分为几个部分——词根、前缀和后缀——无论在哪里出现,它们的含义都不会改变。通过学习这些词根、前缀和后缀,你就能够分析并记住很多单词。

医学英语单词构成

单词通常由三个部分构成:

1. 词根是每个医学单词的基础单元,它建立了单词的基本含义,其他修饰部分都是加在其上的。

2. 后缀加在词根之后的一个或几个短的组成成分,用于修饰词根的含义。后缀通常用在其前面的一个短线表示,例如 -itis(发炎)。

3. 前缀是加在词根之前的一个短的组成部分,

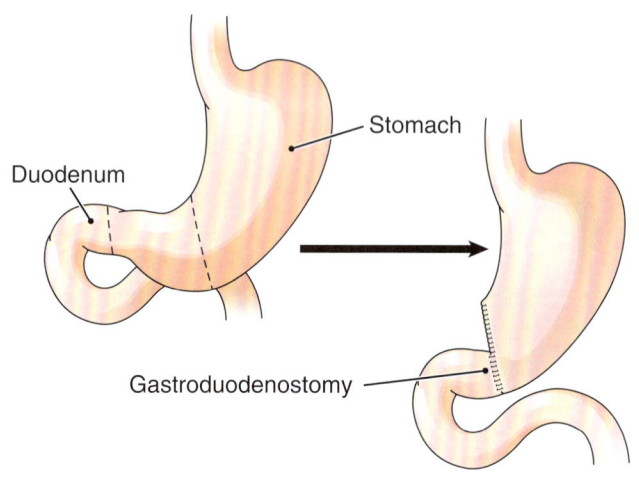

图 1-1 胃十二指肠吻合术(gastroduodenostomy)。胃(gastro)和小肠的第一部分或十二指肠(duoden)之间的吻合术(ostomy)

框 1-1

健康职业
健康信息技术人员

患者的医疗记录被用作所有医疗护理提供的基础。每次患者接受治疗时,将信息添加到患者的医疗记录中,其中包括病史、关于症状的数据、测试结果、诊断、治疗和随访护理。健康信息技术员(health information technician,HIT)组织和管理这些记录,并与医生、护士和其他卫生专业人员密切合作,以确保他们为优质的患者护理提供完整和准确的基础。

准确的医疗记录对于行政管理、第三方付款人和研究人员至关重要。健康信息技术人员为患者接受的每个诊断和治疗过程分配一个代码,并且该信息用于准确的患者计费。此外,健康信息技术人员分析医疗记录以揭示健康和疾病的趋势。这项研究可以用于改善患者护理,降低管理成本,并协助建立新的医学治疗。

为了阅读和解释医疗记录,健康信息技术人员需要有医学术语的完整背景。计划从事此职业的学生可以获得健康信息技术证书或在社区学院完成健康信息技术副学士学位课程。那些想要进入行政管理角色的人可以完成高级研究和在大学获得健康信息学学士学位。要被认证为注册卫生信息技术员(RHIT),需要参加认证考试。许多机构倾向于雇佣获得专业认证的个人。

大多数卫生信息技术人员在医院和护理机构长期工作。另一些人可能在医疗诊所、政府机构、保险公司和咨询公司工作。由于对医疗护理的需求不断增长,预计健康信息技术将成为美国增长最快的职业之一。

关于该职业的更多信息请登录 www.ahima.org,与美国健康信息管理协会(American Health Information Management Association)联系。

用于修饰词根的含义。通常用在其后面的一个短线表示，例如 pre-（之前）。

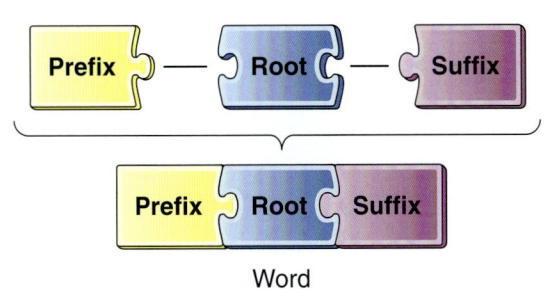

单词由词根、后缀和前缀组成

我们用单词 learn（学习）作为一个词根来做说明。如果我们加上后缀 -er 组成 learner，就有了"学习的人"。如果我们加上前缀 re- 组成 relearn，就有了"再次学习"。词根不一定是完整的单词，实际上大多数医学词根都来自于其他语言，为的就是在组合中使用。例如希腊单词 kardia 意为"心脏"，为我们提供了词根 cardi。拉丁单词 pulmo 意为"肺"，提供了词根 pulm。在一些情况下，希腊和拉丁词根被用于相同的身体结构。例如希腊词根 nephr 和拉丁词根 ren 都被用于与 kidney（肾）有关的单词（图 1-2）。

请注意，同一个词根在不同的研究领域可能有不同的含义，就像单词 spam（罐头猪肉）、menu（菜单）、browser（食青饲料的动物）、surfing（冲浪）、cookie（小甜饼）在日常用语中有着与计算机领域不同的含义一样。词根 myel 意为"髓"，可用于骨髓或脊髓。词根 scler 意为"硬"，但也可以用于白眼球。cyst 意为"一个充满的囊或袋"，但也可以指膀胱。在确定一个单词的含义时，有时需要考虑其上下文。

组合单词包含不止一个词根，例如单词 eyeball（眼球）、bedpan（便盆）、frostbite（冻疮）和 wheelchair（轮椅）。医学组合单词的例子有 cardiovascular（心血管的）、urogenital（泌尿与生殖系统的）和 lymphocyte（淋巴细胞）等。

组合形式

当一个后缀或另一个以辅音开头的词根被加到一个词根上，在该词根与后面的组成部分之间要插入一个元音，以方便发音。这个组合元音通常是 o，

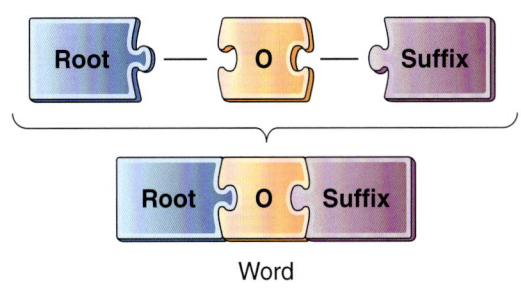

一个组合元音可以加在一个词根与一个单词组成部分之间

就像前面的示例 gastroduodenostomy 那样，但有时可能会是 a、e 或 i。

因此，当后缀 -logy（研究）被加到词根 neur（神经或神经系统）时，要插入一个组合元音：

neur + o + logy = neurology（神经系统的研究，神经病学）

与组合元音一起出现的词根被称为组合形式。

本书中给出的词根都与其最常见的组合元音一起，二者之间加一斜线，表示他们是词根，如 neur/o。

如果与词根组合的部分以元音打头，组合元音

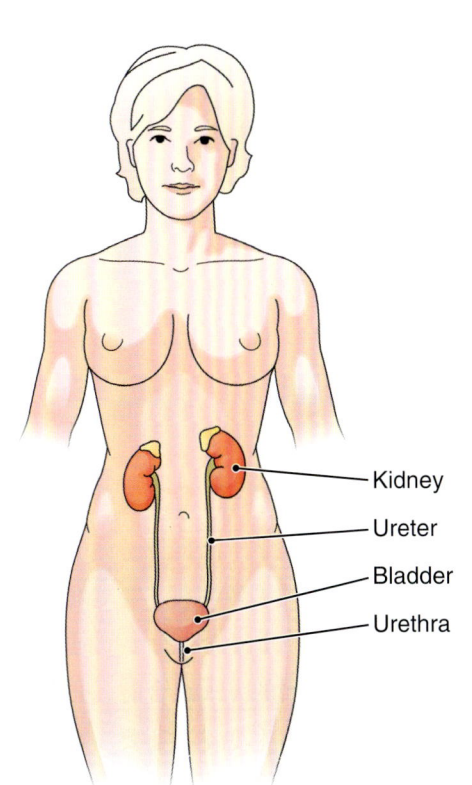

图 1-2 以多个词根命名的结构。在医学术语中，希腊语词根 nephr 和拉丁语词根 ren 都指泌尿系统的器官肾

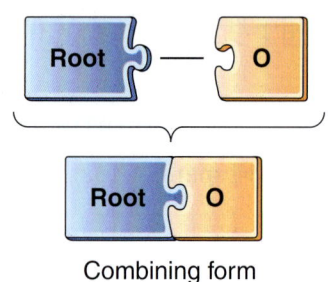

一个词根与组合元音一起被称为组合形式

通常就不会出现。例如，词根 nuer 与后缀 -itis（意为炎症）组合：

neur + itis = neuritis（神经炎症）

这一规则也有例外，特别是在他们影响发音或含义的时候，后面你会观察到这一点。

单词词源

上面说过，大多数医学词汇来自希腊语（G.）和拉丁语（L.）。本书中偶尔也会涉及原始单词的含义，它们很有趣，还可能有助于学习。例如，muscle（肌肉）来自于一个意为"老鼠"的拉丁单词，因为肌肉在皮肤之下的运动被认为像是一只老鼠在蹦蹦跳跳。coccyx（脊骨的尾端）是用布谷鸟命名的，因为其形状像布谷鸟的鸟喙（图 1-3）。一本好的医学词典会提供这些有趣的医学单词词源信息。

以 x 结尾的单词

当在以 x 结尾的单词上加后缀时，x 要变为 g 或 c。如果在 x 前是辅音，例如 yx 或 nx，x 要变为 g。例如，pharynx（咽喉）要变为 pharyngeal［fəˈrindʒiəl］，意为"与咽喉相关"；coccyx（脊骨的末段）要变为 coccygeal［kɔkˈsidʒiəl］，意为"与尾骨相关"。

如果 x 前是元音，例如 ax 或 ix，x 要变为 c。因此，thorax（胸）要变为 thoracic［θɔːˈræsik］，意为"与胸相关"；cervix（颈）要变为 cervical［ˈsɜːvikl］，意为"与颈相关"。

以 rh 打头的后缀

当在一个词根后加上以 rh 打头的后缀时，r 要

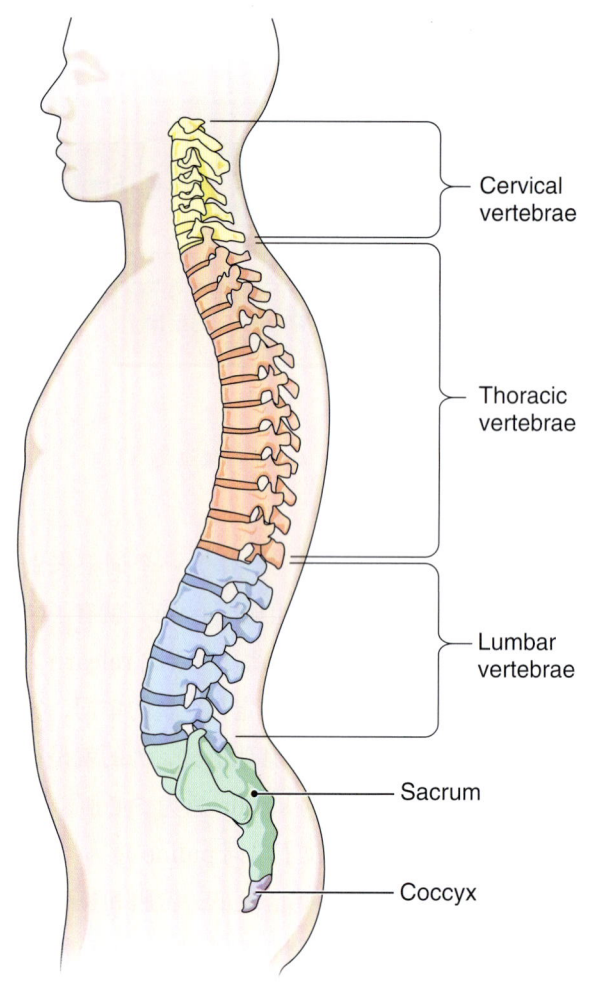

图 1-3　单词来源。coccyx（脊骨的尾端）是用布谷鸟命名的，因为其形状像布谷鸟的鸟喙

双写。例如：

hem/o（血液）+ -rhage（逆出）= hemorrhage（逆出的血液，出血）

men/o（月经）+ -rhea（流动、排出）= menorrhea（月经排出）

发音

本书为所出现的医学术语提供了标准音标，在网络资源中，有一个大的语音词典，要很好地利用这一帮助。在学习时要大声重复念出每个单词的发音。

请留意，在以不同的方式组合时，同一个单词组成部分的发音可能会发生变化。还要注意，被接受的发音可能因地而异。本书中每个单词只会给出一个发音，但要为发音差异做好准备，如框 1-2 所示。

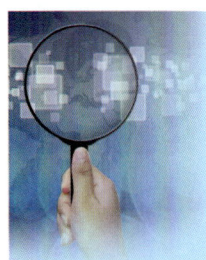

聚焦单词
发音

正文中的发音，有时会难以决定使用一个术语的哪个发音。每个国家，甚至一个国家的不同地区的发音都有所不同，想想美国南方口音与中西部或东北部口音的差别有多大吧。一般的规则是使用最常用的发音，或者在给出多个发音时把最常用的放在前面。

单词 gynecology 在美国的发音中会带有硬 g，但在其他许多地方会使用软 g，如［ˌdʒaini'kɒlədʒi］。与大脑（cerebrum）相关的单词会有不同的重音节，形容词发音通常第二个音节是重音，但在 cerebrum［'seri:brəm］和 cerebrospinal［ˌseribrəʊ'spainəl］中，重音节是不一样的。

十二指肠（duodenum）通常发音为［ˌdjuːə'diːnəm］，但［ˌdjuː 'ədiːnəm］也可以接受。肚脐（navel）的科学术语 umbilicus 通常发音的重音在第二音节，但有时也在第三音节。有时一些替代性发音听起来像外语。

软的和硬的 c 和 g

软 c，如在 racer 中，发音［s］

硬 c，如在 candy 中，发音［k］

软 g，如在 page 中，发音［dʒ］

硬 g，如在 grow 中，发音［g］

不发音的字母和不寻常的发音

不发音的字母和不寻常的发音可能会在查词典时造成麻烦，特别是它们出现在单词开头。框 1-3 中有一些示例。

当框 1-3 中的组合出现在一个单词中时，可能发音不同。例如 diagnosis［ˌdaiəɡ'nəusis］，意为诊断，其中的 g 要发音；apnea［æp'niə］，意为呼吸暂停，其中的 p 要发音；nephroptosis［ˌnefrɒp'təusis］，意为肾下垂，其中的 p 也要发音。

学习风格

术语学习模式描述了人们学习时最依赖的感官上的差异。视觉学习者想要看到印刷的文字，他们喜欢图形、图表和图片。听觉学习者需要听到词的发音，他们喜欢谈论学到的知识，并从课程中听到的记录受益。触觉学习者使用触摸，例如写出答案或重新键入注释，他们喜欢跟随示范学习新的技能。当然，在某种程度上我们使用所有的感官，并且使用的渠道越多，我们越有可能吸收和记住新的信息。希望本书的读者使用多种感官来帮助学习，阅读书中的新单词，写出练习答案，并大声朗读所学的术语。与使用香水广告销售产品的时尚杂志不同，嗅觉还没有被纳入教科书。也许有一天本书的资源中将有一个气味的功能！

缩略词

缩短的单词或词首字母能够节省书写体格检查报告和病历的时间。我们通常用 TV 表示 television（电视），Jr. 表示 junior（年少的），C 表示摄氏温度读数，UV 表示 ultraviolet（紫外线），Dr. 表示 doctor（医生）。还有一些缩写词如 ml，表示 milliliter（毫升）；dB 表示 decibels（分贝），声强的单位；CA 表示 cancer（癌症）；hgb 表示 hemoglobin（血红蛋白）；ECG 表示 electrocardiogram（心电图）。

短语缩写

首字母缩写是短语的每个单词的第一个字母构成的缩写形式。日常的首字母缩写有 ASAP（as soon as possible，尽快）、ATM（automated teller machine，自动柜员机）和计算机的 RAM（random access memory，随机存储器）等。由于在命名物体、组织和程序时节省时间和空间，首字母缩写很流行。它们被广泛应用于政府机构：FDA（Food and Drug Administration，食品和药物管理局）、USDA（United States Department of Agriculture，美国农业部）和 NIH（National Institutes of Health，美国国立卫生研究院）。一些医学术语的首字母缩写有表示 blood pressure（血压）的 BP，表示 magnetic resonance imaging（磁共振成像）的 MRI，表示 acquired

> **供你参考** 框1-3
> **不发音的字母和不寻常的发音**

字母	发音	示例	示例定义
ch	k	chemical ['kemikl]	化学（词根 chem/o 意为"化学"）
dys	dis	dysfunction [dis'fʌŋ(k)ʃn]	功能障碍（dys-）
eu	u	euphoria [juːˈfɔːriə]	欣快症（eu- 意为"真实或良好"）
gn	n	gnathic ['næθik]	颌的（gnath/o）
ph	f	phantom ['fæntəm]	幻影
pn	n	pneumonia [njuːˈməʊniə]	肺炎（pneumon/o）
ps	s	pseudonym ['sjuːdənim]	化名（-nym）
pt	t	ptosis ['təʊsis]	下垂，向下位移
rh	r	rhinoplasty ['rainə(ʊ),plæsti]	鼻整形术（rhin/o）
x	z	xiphoid ['zifɒid]	剑突（来源于希腊语 xiphos, 意为"剑"）

immunodeficiency syndrome（获得性免疫缺陷综合征，即艾滋病）的 AIDS，表示 central nervous system（中枢神经系统）的 CNS 和表示 registered nurse（注册护士）的 NR 等。

符号

符号在病历中常被用于速记。例如Ⓛ和Ⓡ分别代表左和右，↑和↓代表增加和减少。

符号和缩写词能够节省时间，但如果他们不是众所周知的话，可能会引起混乱。在不同的机构中用法各异，同一个缩写词在不同的领域会有不同的含义。例如，CFR 可能意为 chronic renal failure（慢性肾衰竭）或 case report form（病例报告表），MS 能够表示 mitral stenosis（二尖瓣狭窄）或 multiple sclerosis（多发性硬化症）。就像词根会有多个含义一样，如果首字母缩写没有明确定义，其解释取决于上下文。

医学词典

对与医学领域相关的每个人而言，医学词典都是非常有价值的参考资源。这不仅包括那些完整未删减的版本，也包括那些易于携带的袖珍版和医学缩略语词典。许多词典在互联网上都有，很多还做成了智能手机上的 APP。词典会给出单词的含义、发音、同义词、词源和相关名词。那些针对护理和专职医疗人员的词典还给出了完整的临床信息，包括一些患者护理的注意事项。

除了每个词条和短语的信息外，医学词典包含一些有用的附录，包括计量、临床试验、药品、身体结构和信息资源等。

Terminology 关键术语

acronym	[ˈækrənim]	首字母缩写，以短语中每个单词的第一个字母构成的缩略语
combining form		组合形式，一个词根与一个将该词根与另一个单词组成部分，例如一个后缀或另一个词根，相连接的元音字母的组合。组合形式用词根与元音字母之间的斜线表示，例如 neur/o
compound word		复合单词，包含多于一个词根的单词
prefix	[ˈpri:fiks]	前缀，加在词根之前以修饰其含义的单词组成部分
root	[ru:t]	词根，单词的基础单元
suffix	[ˈsʌfiks]	后缀，加在词根之后以修饰其含义的单词组成部分

Case Study Revisited 案例研究再访

J. V.'s Case Study Follow-Up

J. V. was scheduled for an esophageal gastroduodenoscopy as an outpatient procedure. The gastroenterologist was able to visualize the esophagus and the inside of the stomach. The area around the esophageal sphincter was a normal pink in color and showed no signs of esophagitis or ulceration. J.V. was started on a proton pump inhibitor to reduce stomach acid and was advised to limit his intake of spicy foods and alcohol. At his follow-up appointment, he reported no repeat episodes of epigastric pain.

J. V. 案例研究跟进

J. V. 被安排进行作为门诊流程的食管胃十二指肠镜检查。胃肠科医生能够看到食管和胃的内部，食管括约肌周围的区域是正常的粉红色，并且没有显示食管炎（esophagitis）或溃疡的迹象。J.V. 开始使用质子泵抑制剂（proton pump inhibitor）以减少胃酸，并建议他限制摄入辛辣食物和酒精。在他的随访中，他报告没有上腹部疼痛的重复发作。

CHAPTER 1 复习

填空

1. A word part that always comes after a root is a（n） _____.

2. A root with a vowel added to aid in pronunciation is called a（n） _____.

3. Combine the word parts dia, meaning "through," and rhea, meaning "flow," to form a word meaning "passage of fluid stool" _____.

4. The abbreviation ETOH means（refer to Appendix 2） _____.

5. Use Appendix 3 to find that the suffix in gastroduodenoscopy, seen in J.V.'s opening case study, means _____.

6. Combine the root cardi, meaning "heart," with the suffix -logy, meaning "study of," to form a word meaning "study of the heart" _____.

7. Use Appendix 6 at the back of the book to find that the suffix -al, as in esophageal, seen in J.V.'s case study follow-up means _____.

8. Appendix 1 shows that the symbol ↑ means _____.

多项选择

选择最佳答案，并在每个数字的左边写上您选择的字母。

____ 9. Epi- in the term epigastric is a
   a. word root
   b. prefix
   c. suffix
   d. combining form

____ 10. The oid in the term xiphoid is a
   a. root
   b. prefix
   c. derivation
   d. suffix

____ 11. The term musculoskeletal is a（n）
   a. abbreviation
   b. word root
   c. combining form
   d. compound word

____ 12. The adjective for larynx is
   a. larynxic
   b. laryngeal
   c. larynal
   d. largeal

____ 13. The combining form for thorax（chest）is
   a. thorax/o
   b. thor/o
   c. thorac/o
   d. thori/o

____ 14. In J.V.'s case study, the term GERD represents a（n）
   a. combining form
   b. acronym
   c. prefix
   d. suffix

____ 15. In the case study, the ph in dysphagia is pronounced as
   a. f
   b. p
   c. h
   d. s

读出下列单词

16. dyslexia _____

17. rheumatism _____

18. pneumatic _____

19. chemist _____

20. pharmacy _____

根据音标写出它们代表的单词

21. ［ˈkɑːdiæk］ _____

22. ［ˈhaidrədʒən］ _____

23. ［ˈɒkjələ（r）］ _____

24. ［ˈintəfeis］ _____

25. ［rʊˈmætik］ _____

单词构建

根据下列定义使用所提供的单词组成部分写出单词。要加上组合元音，每个单词组成部分可以多次使用。

> -itis   -logy   -ptosis   nephr   -o   -gastr   cardi   neur

26. Inflammation of the stomach _____

27. Study of the nervous system _____

28. Dropping of the kidney _____

29. Study of the kidney _____

30. Inflammation of a nerve _____

31. Downward displacement of the heart _____

单词分析

定义下列单词，给出每个单词组成部分的含义。如果需要，可以使用词典。

32. dysmenorrhea_____
    a. dys_____
    b. men/o_____
    c. –rhea_____

33. cardiologist_____
    a. cardi/o_____
    b. -log/o_____
    c. –ist_____

34. nephritis_____
    a. nephr/o_____
    b. –it is_____

35. renogastric_____
    a. ren/o_____
    b. gastr/o_____
    c. –ic_____

Additional Case Studies
补充案例研究

Case Study: D. S.'s Arthritic Knees
案例研究

Chief Complaint
D. S., a 68 y/o male, presents to his family doctor c/o bilateral knee discomfort that worsens prior to a heavy rainstorm. He states that his "arthritis" is not getting any better. He has been taking NSAIDs but is not obtaining relief at this point. His family physician referred him to an orthopedic surgeon for further evaluation.

Past Medical History
D.S. was active in sports in high school and college. He tore his ACL while playing soccer during his junior year in college, at which time he retired from intercollegiate athletics. His only other physical complaint involves stiffness in his right shoulder, which he attributes to pitching while playing baseball in high school. Current Medications NSAIDs prn for arthritic pain; Lipitor 10 mg for mild hyperlipidemia.

X-Rays
Bilateral knee x-rays revealed moderate degenerative changes with joint space narrowing in the left knee; severe degenerative changes and joint space narrowing in the right knee.

主诉
D. S. 是一名68岁的男性，向他的家庭医生主诉双侧膝盖不适，并会在暴雨之前加重。他说他的"关节炎"没有好转。他一直在服用非甾体抗炎药（NSAIDs），但没有得到缓解。他的家庭医生将他转诊给一位骨科医生进行进一步评估。

既往病史
D. S. 在高中和大学积极参加体育活动。他在大学期间踢足球时撕裂了前交叉韧带（anterior cruciate ligament，ACL），并从那时退出了大学校际体育竞赛。他的另一不适涉及右肩僵硬，他认为是高中打棒球时投球所致。目前使用NSAIDs治疗关节炎性疼痛，立普妥10mg治疗轻度高脂血症。

X线
双侧膝关节X线片显示中度退行性变化，左膝关节间隙变窄，右膝严重退行性变化和关节空间狭窄。

案例研究问题
多项选择。选择最佳答案，并在每个题号的左侧写上你选择的字母。

____ 1. The bi– in the word bilateral is a

    a. suffix

    b. root

    c. prefix

    d. combining form

____ 2. The –itis in the word arthritis is a

    a. root

    b. prefix

    c. derivation

    d. suffix

____ 3. Arthr/o is a(n)

    a. combining form

    b. acronym

    c. prefix

    d. suffix

____ 4. The AI in the abbreviation NSAID means (see Appendix 2)

    a. antacid

    b. antiinflammatory

    c. antiinfectious

    d. after incident

简答

5. Use Appendix 2 to find what the abbreviation ACL means.
___

6. Use Appendix 2 to find what the abbreviation c/o means.
___

7. Use Appendix 7 to find what the prefix hyper- means.
___

8. Use Appendix 2 to find what the abbreviation prn means.
___

9. Use Appendices 5, 6, and 7 to find what the word parts in hyperlipidemia mean.

   a. hyper- ___

   b. lip/o ___

   c. -emia ___

10. Use Appendix 3 to find what the word parts in orthopedic mean.

   a. orth/o ___

   b. ped/o ___

11. Use Appendix 7 to find what the prefix inter- means.
___

CHAPTER 2 后缀

预测试

多项选择。选择最佳答案，并在每个数字的左边写上您选择的字母。

____ 1. The suffix in the word hearing is
   a. hear
   b. ring
   c. ing
   d. ear

____ 2. The suffixes –ism, –ia, and –ist are found in
   a. verbs
   b. adjectives
   c. adverbs
   d. nouns

____ 3. The suffixes –ic, –ous, –al, and –oid are found in
   a. adjectives
   b. nouns
   c. verbs
   d. roots

____ 4. The suffix –form means
   a. excess
   b. origin
   c. resembling
   d. paired

____ 5. The plural of fungus is
   a. fungi
   b. fungal
   c. fungae
   d. funga

____ 6. The singular of ova（eggs）is
   a. ovi
   b. ovae
   c. ovum
   d. ovas

学习目标

学完本章后,应该能够:

1. ▶ 定义后缀。
2. ▶ 给出如何使用后缀将名词变成形容词和复数形式的示例。
3. ▶ 认识并应用医学术语中使用的通用名词、形容词和复数后缀。
4. ▶ 分析案例研究中使用的后缀。

Case Study: R. F.'s Encounter with a Cerebral Aneurysm
案例研究:R. F. 遇到脑动脉瘤

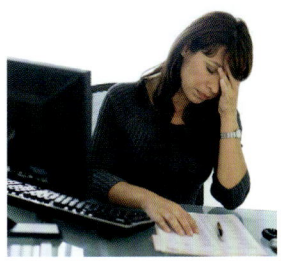

Chief Complaint
R. F., a 48-year-old financial analyst, has been complaining of atypical headaches for the past few weeks. With one of the headaches, she experienced vomiting that she could not attribute to the flu or something she had eaten. She does not have a history of migraines. R.F. had an appointment with a neurologist, who referred her to the neurosurgery clinic for evaluation of a possible cerebral hemorrhage.

Examination
Patient is a 48 y/o female c/o sudden and severe headaches over the past three to four weeks; one headache was accompanied with vomiting. Patient admits to recent photophobia and intermittent blurred vision. She has a history of venous thrombi (clots) following an emergency hip surgery for a fracture she suffered two years ago when she was in an automobile accident. Multiple vertebrae and her pelvis were also fractured. No other complications post-accident noted. Hypertensive with a BP of 154/86; neurologic and physical examination is otherwise normal. Diagnoses: hypertension and possible cerebral aneurysm.

Clinical Course
The neurologist ordered a CT scan that revealed a small saccular aneurysm measuring 4 mm near the cerebral arterial circle, the vascular pathway supplying the brain. R.F. was scheduled for a craniotomy and surgical insertion of a clip around the neck of the aneurysm to control bleeding and offer protection from rebleeding.

An aneurysm is a bulge in a weakened arterial wall that can rupture and cause damage. An aneurysm is illustrated later in this chapter when we learn more about R.F.'s medical care. There is more information on aneurysms and their potential effects in Chapters 9 and 17.

主诉
R. F. 是一名 48 岁的金融分析师,主诉过去几个星期非典型性头痛。在一次头痛中,她经历了呕吐,但不是由流行性感冒或饮食引起的。她没有偏头痛(migraines)的病史。R.F. 约见了神经科医生(neurologist),这位医生将她转到神经外科(neurosurgery)门诊评估脑出血(cerebral hemorrhage)。

检查
患者是 48 岁的女性,主诉在过去 3～4 周内发生突然和严重的头痛;一次头痛伴随呕吐。患者承认最近畏光(photophobia)和间歇性视力模糊。她在 2 年前的汽车事故中由于骨折进行了急诊髋关节手术后,有静脉血栓(venous thrombi)的病史,她的多个椎骨和骨盆也断裂了。事故后没有其他并发症。高血压(hypertensive),血压(blood pressure,BP)为 154/86,神经系统和体格检查正常。诊断:高血压和可能的脑动脉瘤(cerebral aneurysm)。

临床病程
神经科医生指示进行 CT 扫描,显示在脑动脉环(cerebral arterial circle)附近有 4mm 的小囊状动脉瘤,脑动脉环是供应大脑的血管通路。R.F. 计划进行开颅手术(craniotomy),并在颈部动脉瘤周围手术插入夹子以控制出血,并提供保护以防止再出血。

动脉瘤是弱化的动脉壁中的隆起,可能破裂并导致损伤。当我们更多地了解 R.F. 的医疗护理时,本章后面会用插图说明动脉瘤。有关动脉瘤及其潜在影响的更多信息,请参见第 9 章和第 17 章。

简介

后缀是修饰词根的单词结尾。一个后缀可能表示该单词是一个名词或形容词，经常还会决定如何定义该单词（框 2-1）。例如，使用词根 myel/o，意为"骨髓"，形容词结尾 -oid 构成单词 myeloid，意为"像或与骨髓相关"；名词结尾 -oma 构成单词 myeloma，意为"骨髓肿瘤"。加上另一个，代表起源或起因的词根 gen 和形容词结尾 -ous，构成单词 myelogenous，意为"发起于骨髓"。

本书给出的后缀是所有医学词汇的通用后缀，包括：

- 名词：人、地方或物
- 形容词：修饰名词的单词
- 复数：将单数名词变为复数的结尾

与疾病状态、医学治疗或具体身体系统相关的后缀将在其他章节给出。

名词后缀

下列通用后缀会将词根变为名词。表 2-1 给出了表示不同状态的后缀。请注意 -sis 可能与不同的组合元音一起出现，如 -osis、-iasis、-esis 或 -asis，前两个意味着不正常的状态。

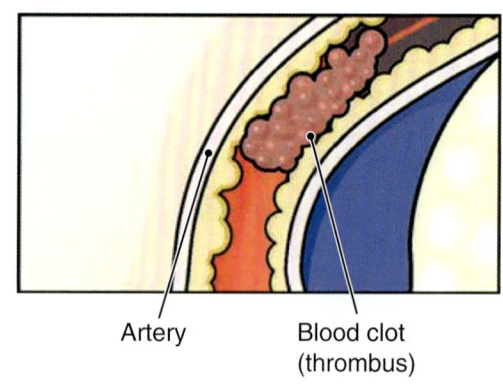

图 2-1 血栓形成（thrombosis）。本术语指的是血管内有血栓（thrombus）。单词 thrombosis 有名词后缀 –sis，意为"状态"

框 2-1

聚焦单词

有含义的后缀

有些后缀在加到不同的单词时会表示特定的含义。后缀 -thon 来自于希腊城市 Marathon，胜利的消息就是由一位长跑者从那里带来。该后缀被加在不同的单词上，以表示需要极大的忍耐力的竞赛。例如 bike-a-thon（自行车马拉松）、dance-a-thon（跳舞马拉松）、telethon（电视节目马拉松）等，甚至有大型慈善募捐活动被称为 thon-a-thon（马拉松的马拉松）。

形容词结尾 -ish 被用于显示某些特征，如 boyish（幼稚的）或 childish（孩子气的）。将 -ish 加到单词上表示一种不是很确切的估计，如 forty-ish（40 左右）或 blue-ish（偏蓝色的）。午餐约会的模糊时间可以被称为 noon-ish（中午其后）。

在医学中，后缀 -tech 被用于暗示高科技，如公司名称 Genentech。加上 -pure 被用于赋予信心，如 Multi-Pure water filter（多重净化水过滤器）。后缀 -mate 暗示有帮助，如 helpmate，在词典中被定义为有帮助的伙伴，更确切地就是妻子，或有时是丈夫。医疗设备 HeartMate 是一个用于帮助受损心脏的泵。

表 2-1 意为"状态"的后缀

后缀	示例	示例定义
-ia	dementia ［di'menʃə］	丧失（de-）智力功能（来自于拉丁语 mind），痴呆
-ism	racism ［'reisizm］	种族歧视
-sis	thrombosis ［θrɒm'bəʊsis］	血管中有血凝块（thrombus），血栓（图 2-1）
-y	atony ［'ætəni］	缺少（a-）肌张力，无力

练习 2-1

写出下列单词中意为"状态"的后缀,并读出每个单词。

1. phobia（unfounded fear; from G. phobos: fear）
   ['fəubiə]

2. psoriasis（skin disease）
   [sə'raiəsis]

3. egotism（exaggerated self-importance; from ego: self）
   ['egətizəm]

4. dystrophy（changes due to lack of nourishment; root: troph/o）
   ['distrəfi]

5. anesthesia（loss of sensation; root: esthesi/o, 图 2-2）
   [ˌænəs'θi:ziə]

6. parasitism（infection with parasites or behaving as a parasite）
   ['pærəsaitizəm]

7. stenosis（narrowing of a canal）
   [sti'nəusis]

8. tetany（sustained muscle contraction）
   ['tetəni]

9. diuresis（increased urination; root: ur/o）
   [ˌdaijuə'ri:sis]

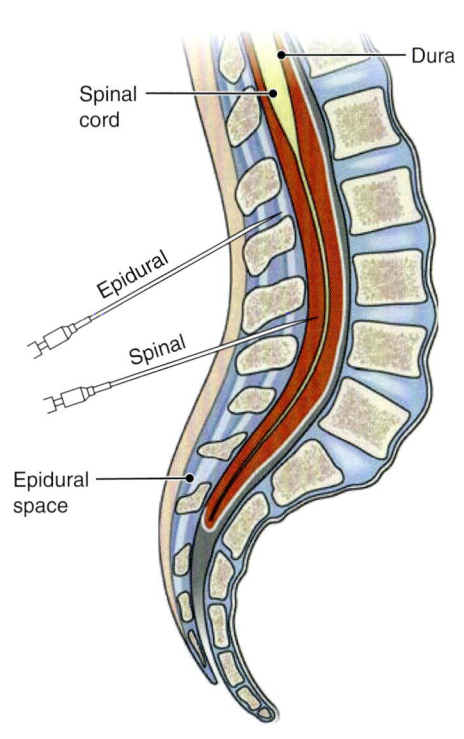

图 2-2 麻醉注射部位。单词 anesthesia 使用名词后缀 –ia,意思是"状态"。硬脑膜（dura）是脑脊膜（meninges）的一层,脑脊膜是覆盖脑和脊髓的膜。执行麻醉的人是麻醉师（anesthetist 或 anesthesiologist）

表 2-2 给出了将词根变为医学专科或专家的后缀。后缀 -logy 被用于医学以外的很多领域，它包含来自于希腊单词 logo 的词根 log/o，意为"单词"，一般意为一个领域的研究。例如 biology（生物学）、archeology（考古学）、terminology（名词学）、和 technology（制造学）。带有该结尾的单词也被用于确定一个机构部门或一个专科，如 cardiology（心内科）、dermatology（皮肤科）和 radiology（放射科）等。一些例子是生物学（biology）、考古学（archeology）、术语（terminology）和技术（technology），如框 2-2 所述。具有此结尾的术语也用于识别机构部门或专科，如在心脏科（cardiology）、皮肤科（dermatology）、放射科（radiology）等。两个结尾 -iatrics 和 -iatry 包含根 -iatr / o，基于一个希腊语意为愈合的单词，意为"医生"或"医疗"。

表 2-2　医学专科后缀

后缀	含义	示例	示例定义
-ian	研究领域的专家	physician　[fɪˈzɪʃən]	医生（来自于词根 physi/o，意为"自然"）
-iatrics	医学专科	pediatrics　[ˌpiːdiˈætrɪks]	儿科学，儿童疾病的研究与治疗（ped/o）（图 2-3）
-ics	医学专科	orthopedics　[ˌɔːθəˈpiːdɪks]	矫形学，骨骼和关节的研究和治疗（来源于词根 ped/o，意为"儿童"，和前缀 ortho-，意为"直接"）
-ist	研究领域的专家	podiatrist　[pəˈdaɪətrɪst]	足病医生（pod/o）
-logy	研究	physiology　[ˌfɪziˈɒlədʒi]	生理学，生物体功能的研究（来源于 physi/o，意为"自然"）

练习 2-2

写出下列单词中意为"……的研究""医学专科"或"一个研究领域专家"的后缀。

1. cardiologist（specialist in the study and treatment of the heart; root: cardi/o）
　[ˌkɑːdiˈɒlədʒɪst]　　　　　　　　　　　　　　　　　　　　＿＿＿＿＿＿

2. neurology（the study of the nervous system; root: neur/o）
　[njʊəˈrɒlədʒi]　　　　　　　　　　　　　　　　　　　　　＿＿＿＿＿＿

3. geriatrics（study and treatment of the aged; root: ger/e）（图 2-4）
　[ˌdʒeriˈætrɪks]　　　　　　　　　　　　　　　　　　　　　＿＿＿＿＿＿

4. dermatology（study and treatment of the skin, or derma）
　[ˌdɜːməˈtɒlədʒi]　　　　　　　　　　　　　　　　　　　　＿＿＿＿＿＿

5. optician（one who makes and fits corrective lenses for the eyes; root: opt/o）
　[ɒpˈtɪʃn]　　　　　　　　　　　　　　　　　　　　　　　　＿＿＿＿＿＿

6. anesthetist（one who administers anesthesia）（图 2-2）
　[əˈnesθɪtɪst]　　　　　　　　　　　　　　　　　　　　　　＿＿＿＿＿＿

写出下列领域专家的单词。

7. anatomy（study of body structure）
　[əˈnætəmi]　　　　　　　　　　　　　　　　　　　　　　　＿＿＿＿＿＿

8. pediatrics（care and treatment of children; root: ped/o）（图 2-3）
　[ˌpiːdiˈætrɪks]　　　　　　　　　　　　　　　　　　　　　＿＿＿＿＿＿

练习 2-2 续表

9. radiology (use of radiation in diagnosis and treatment)
   [ˌreɪdɪˈɒlədʒɪ] _____

10. psychology (study of the mind; root: psych/o)
    [saɪˈkɒlədʒɪ] _____

11. technology (practical application of science)
    [tekˈnɒlədʒɪ] _____

12. obstetrics (medical specialty concerning pregnancy and birth)
    [əbˈstetrɪks] _____

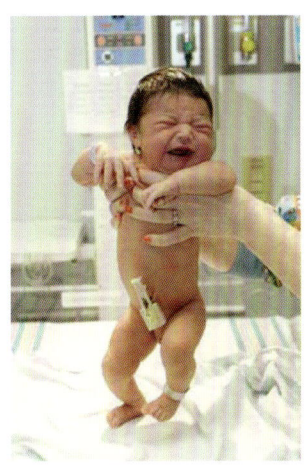

图 2-3 儿科（pediatrics）是儿童的护理和治疗。后缀 -ics 表示医学专科。在这张照片中，儿科医生（pediatrician）正在测试婴儿的反应。词根 ped/o 意为"儿童"

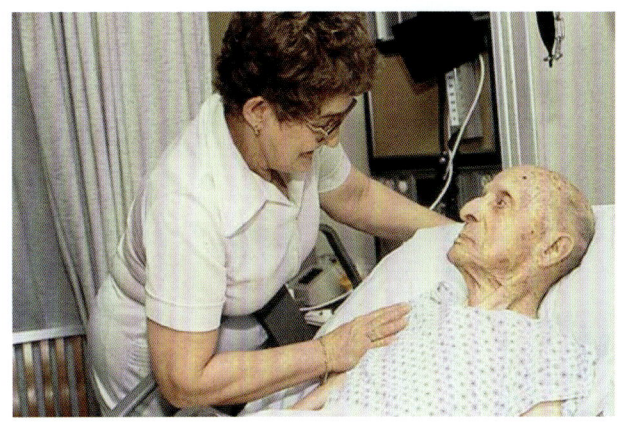

图 2-4 老年医学（geriatrics）是老年人的护理和治疗。该领域的专家是老年科医生（geriatrician）

框 2-2

健康职业
医学实验室技术

医学实验室技术领域包括广泛的临床科学。为医疗行业执行实验室测试的人可以遵循两个职业路径之一。临床实验室科学家（clinical laboratory scientist, CLS），也称为医学技术人员（medical technologist, MT），需要学士学位；临床实验室技术员（clinical laboratory technician），也称为医学实验室技术人员（medical laboratory technician），需要副学士学位。临床实验室技术员可能具有更有限的责任，并在比 CLS 更密切的监督下工作。两个培训计划都需要在毕业后在实验室实习。

根据美国临床病理学会（American Society of Clinical Pathology，ASCP），这些医疗保健专业人员从事各种工作，从简单的婚前血液检查到更复杂的疾病检测，包括 HIV 病毒/艾滋病、糖尿病和癌症。他们通过显微镜检查人体血液和组织标本寻找微生物，如细菌、寄生虫或癌细胞。他们可以匹配血液用于输血，并测试血液中的化学物质、药物和其他物质。医生依靠他们提供的信息来确定诊断并为他们的患者制订治疗计划。此外，这些实验室专业人员可以评估测试结果、开发和修改实验室程序，并建立和监测程序以确保测试的准确性。他们可能在实验室的几个领域工作，或专门在一个特定领域工作，如免疫学、微生物学或分子生物学。

在工作过程中，他们操作有价值的设备，包括计算机和精密仪器，如大功率显微镜和细胞计数器。因此，他们必须精通相关的仪器和电子技术。医学实验室科学职业需要完成由国家临床实验室科学认证机构（National Accrediting Agency of Clinical Laboratory Science，NAA-CLS）认可的 CLS 或医疗技术人员培训计划。一些州和一些雇主要求医疗实验室技术人员和临床实验室技术员持有许可证。许可证可能需要学士学位和通过考试。对于具体要求，请联系国家卫生部门或职业许可委员会。

形容词后缀

下面的形容词结尾意为"与……相关""相似"或"类似"（表 2-3）。没有什么规则规定给定的名词应该用哪个后缀。

请注意，以后缀 -sis 结尾的单词在加 -ic 变为形容词时，第一个 s 要变为 t，如 genetic，与 genesis（起源）相关；psychotic 与 psychosis（精神疾病）相关；或 diuretic 与 diuresis（多尿）相关。

表 2-3 意为"与……相关""相似"或"类似"的后缀

后缀	示例	示例定义
-ac	cardiac ['kɑ:diæk]	心脏的
-al	vocal ['vəʊk(ə)l]	声音的
-ar	nuclear ['nju:kliə]	原子核的
-ary	salivary ['sælivəri]	唾液的
-form	muciform ['mju:sifəm]	黏液状的
-ic	anatomic [ˌænə'tɒmik]	解剖学的（图 2-5）
-ical（ic + al）	electrical [i'lektrik(ə)l]	电的
-ile	virile ['virail]	男性的
-oid	lymphoid ['limfɒid]	淋巴的
-ory	circulatory ['sɜ:kjʊlət(ə)ri]	循环的
-ous	cutaneous [kju:'teiniəs]	皮肤的（来自于拉丁语 cutis：皮肤）

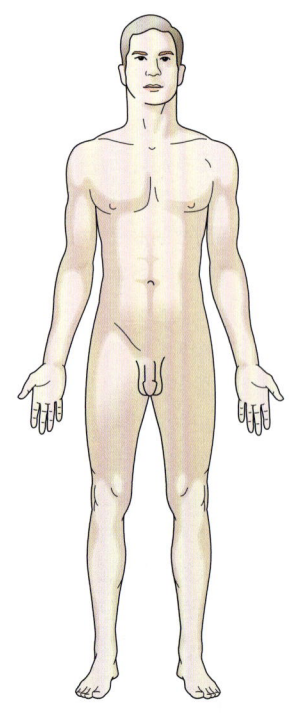

图 2-5 解剖位置。这种体位是解剖学研究中的标准。在该体位的人面朝前，手臂在两侧，掌心向前（anterior）。形容词后缀 –ic 意为"相关"

练习 2-3

识别下列单词中意为"相关""类似"或"相像"的后缀。

1. dietary（pertaining to the diet）
   ['daɪətəri]
2. neuronal（pertaining to a nerve cell, or neuron）（图 2-6）
   [n'jʊərənəl]
3. metric（pertaining to a meter or measurement; root metr/o means "measure"）
   ['metrɪk]
4. venous（pertaining to a vein; root: ven/o）
   ['viːnəs]
5. epileptiform（like or resembling epilepsy）
   [epɪ'leptɪfɔːm]
6. toxoid（like or resembling a toxin, or poison）
   ['tɒksɔɪd]
7. topical（pertaining to a surface）
   ['tɒpɪkl]
8. febrile（pertaining to fever）
   ['fiːbraɪl]
9. neurotic（pertaining to neurosis, a mental disorder）
   [njʊə'rɒtɪk]
10. surgical（pertaining to surgery）
    ['sɜːdʒɪkl]
11. muscular（pertaining to a muscle）
    ['mʌskjələ(r)]
12. urinary（pertaining to urine; root: ur/o）
    ['jʊərɪnəri]
13. respiratory（pertaining to respiration）
    [rə'spɪrətri]
14. pelvic（pertaining to the pelvis）（图 2-7）
    ['pelvɪk]
15. saccular（pouch-like, resembling a small sac）
    ['sækjʊlə]

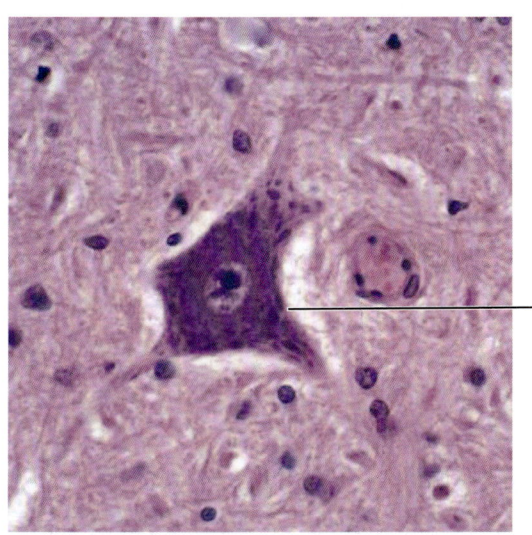

图 2-6 神经元（neuron）是神经细胞。neuron 的形容词形式是 neuronal

构成复数

基于单词的结尾，许多医学单词有特殊的复数形式。表 2-4 给出了一些通用规则和示例。表中第二列的复数结尾由第一列的单词结尾替换。请注意，单数结尾 -on 和 -um 都是变为 -a 成为复数。在将以 -a 结尾的复数名词改为单数时，必须记住具体单词的单数结尾。

表 2-4		复数结尾	
结尾	单数	示例	复数示例
a	ae	vertebra（脊骨）['vɜːtibrə]	vertebrae ['vəːtibriː]（图 2-8）
en	ina	lumen（内腔）['luːmen]	lumina ['ljuːminə]（图 2-9）
ex, ix, yx	ices	matrix（基质）['meitriks]	matrices ['meitrisiːz]
is	es	diagnosis（确定疾病或缺陷）[ˌdaiəɡˈnəʊsis]	diagnoses [ˌdaiəɡˈnəʊsiːz]
ma	mata	stigma（伤痕或伤疤）['stigmə]	stigmata ['stigmətə]
nx	nges	phalanx（指骨或趾骨）['fælæŋks]	phalanges [fæ'lændʒiːz]（图 2-10）
on	a	ganglion（神经节）['ɡæŋɡliən]	ganglia ['ɡæŋɡliə]
um	a	serum（稀薄的液体）['sirəm]	sera ['sirrə]
us	i	thrombus（血栓）['θrɒmbəs]（图 2-1）	thrombi ['θrɒmbi]

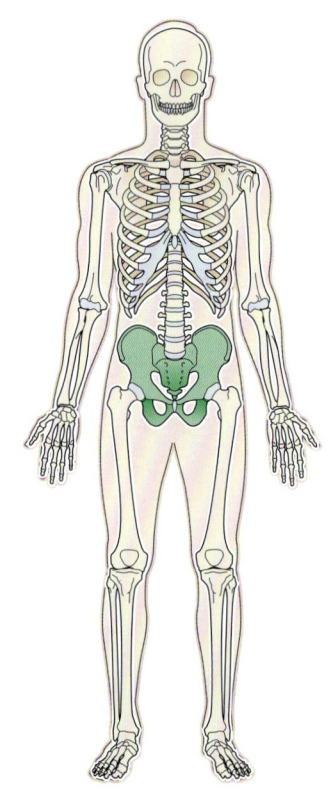

图 2-7 骨盆（pelvis）是骨髋关节带。pelvis 的形容词形式是 pelvic

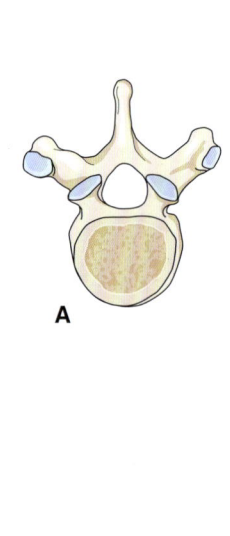

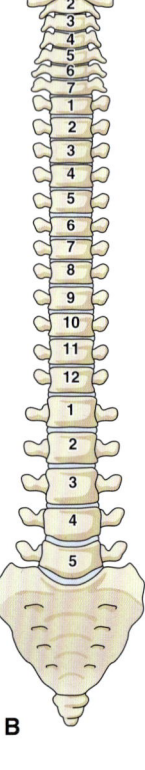

图 2-8 脊椎的骨骼。A. 脊柱的每块骨骼都是一根椎骨（vertebra）；B. 脊柱由 26 块椎骨构成，vertebra 的复数形式为 vertebrae

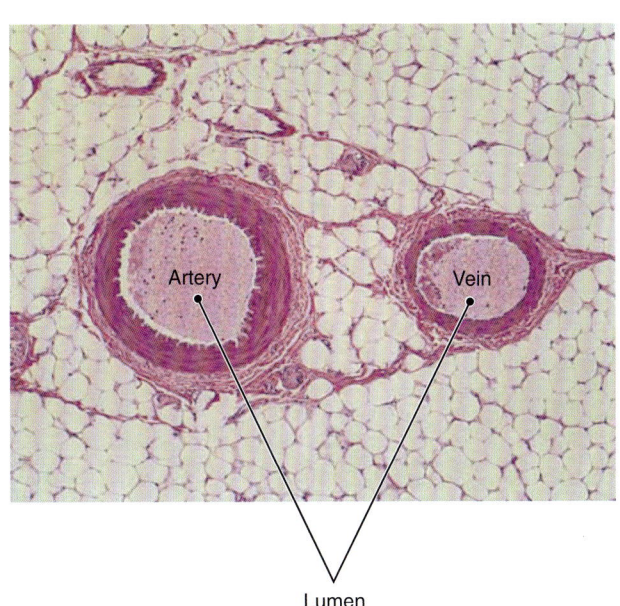

图 2-9 管腔是器官或血管的中心开口。图中示出了两根血管，一根动脉（Artery）和一个静脉（Vein）。Lumen 的复数形式是 lumina

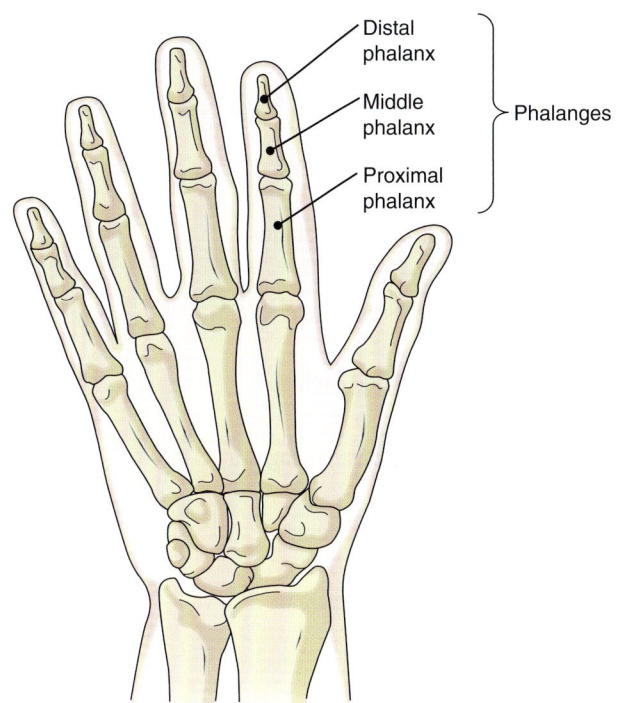

图 2-10 右手骨（前视图）。手指或脚趾的每块骨骼是指（趾）骨（phalanx）。每只手有 15 块指骨，phalanx 的复数形式是 phalanges

练习 2-4

写出下列单词的复数形式。每个单词的结尾有下划线。

1. patel<u>la</u>（kneecap）
   [pəˈtelə]

2. phenomen<u>on</u>（occurrence or perception）
   [fəˈnɒmɪnən]

3. oment<u>um</u>（abdominal membrane）
   [əʊˈmentəm]

4. progn<u>osis</u>（prediction of disease outcome）
   [prɒɡˈnəʊsɪs]

5. ap<u>ex</u>（tip or peak）
   [ˈeɪpeks]

6. ov<u>um</u>（female reproductive cell; egg）
   [ˈəʊvəm]

7. spermatoz<u>oon</u>（male reproductive cell; sperm cell）
   [ˌspɜːmətəˈzəʊən]

8. mun<u>inx</u>（membrane around the brain and spinal cord）
   [ˈmiːnɪŋks]

9. embol<u>us</u>（blockage in a vessel）
   [ˈembələs]

10. protoz<u>oa</u>（single-celled animals）
    [ˌprəʊtəˈzəʊə]

练习 2-4 续表

写出下列单词的复数形式。每个单词的结尾有下划线。

11. append<u>ices</u>（things added）
    [əˈpendisiːz]
12. adeno<u>mata</u>（tumors of glands）
    [ˌædiˈnəʊmətə]
13. fung<u>i</u>（simple, nongreen plants）
    [ˈfʌŋgiː]
14. pelv<u>es</u>（cup-shaped cavities）
    [ˈpelviːs]
15. foram<u>ina</u>（openings, passageways）
    [fəˈræmənə]
16. curric<u>ula</u>（series of courses）
    [kəˈrikjələ]
17. ind<u>ices</u>（directories, lists）
    [ˈindisiːz]
18. alveol<u>i</u>（small sacs）
    [ælˈviːəlai]

一些例外

构成复数的规则有一些例外，例如：sinus（空间）的复数是 sinuses，virus 的复数是 viruses，有时用 serums（稀薄的液体）替代 sera。后缀 -es 可以加在以 -ex 或 -ix 结尾的单词后形成复数，如 appendixes（附录）、apexes（尖端）和 indexes（索引）。

人们经常会用到一些不正确的复数形式，例如用了 stigmas 而不是 stigmata，用 referendums 取代了 referenda，stadiums 代替了 stadia。以 -oma 结尾的单词，意为"肿瘤"，变为复数要改成 -omata，但很多人只是简单地加一个 s 构成复数。例如，carcinoma（癌症）的复数应该是 carcinomata，但大家常用的是 carcinomas。

Case Study Revisited
案例研究再访

R.F.'s Postoperative Follow-Up

R.F. underwent a craniotomy in which a special clip was placed around the neck of the aneurysm. She was closely observed for postoperative neurologic deficits, including vascular spasm, a serious possible complication. She tolerated the procedure well with no complications.

R.F. 术后跟进

R.F. 进行了开颅手术，其中特殊的夹子放置在颈部的动脉瘤周围。她被密切观察术后是否有神经功能缺损，包括血管痉挛，这是一种严重可能的并发症。她很好地耐受了手术，没有并发症。

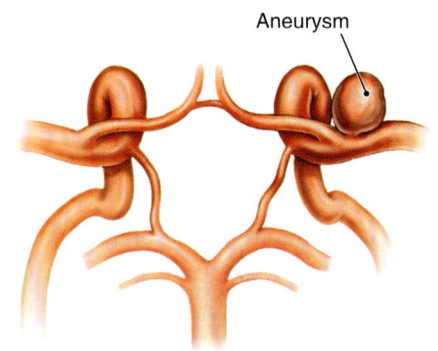

Aneurysm

Cerebral arterial circle

CHAPTER 2 复习

识别下列单词中意为"状态"的后缀。

1. alcoholism ['ælkəhɒlizəm] (alcohol dependence) _____
2. insomnia [in'sɒmniə] (inability to sleep; root: somn/o) _____
3. acidosis [ˌæsi'dəʊsis] (acid body condition) _____
4. dysentery ['disəntri] (intestinal disorder; root: enter/o) _____
5. psychosis [sai'kəʊsis] (disorder of the mind) _____
6. anemia [ə'ni:miə] (lack of blood or hemoglobin; root: hem/o) _____

给出下列单词中意为"专科"或"专家"的后缀。

7. psychiatry [sai'kaiətri] _____
8. orthopedics [ˌɔ:θə'pi:diks] _____
9. anesthesiologist [ˌænəsˌθi:zi'ɒlədʒist] _____
10. technician [tek'niʃn] _____
11. anatomist [ə'nætəmist] _____
12. obstetrician [ˌɒbstə'triʃn] _____

给出下列领域专家的名称。

13. dermatology [ˌdɜ:mə'tɒlədʒi] _____
14. pediatrics [ˌpi:di'ætriks] _____
15. physiology [ˌfizi'ɒlədʒi] _____
16. gynecology [ˌgaini'kɒlədʒi] _____

识别下列单词中意为"相关""类似"或"相像"的形容词后缀。

17. basic ['beisik] _____
18. oral ['ɔ:rəl] _____
19. anxious ['æŋkʃəs] _____
20. fibroid ['faibrɔid] _____
21. circular ['sɜ:kjələ(r)] _____
22. arterial [ɑ:'tiəriəl] _____
23. pelvic ['pelvik] _____
24. binary ['bainəri] _____
25. skeletal ['skelətl] _____
26. rheumatoid ['ru:mətɔid] _____
27. febrile ['fi:brail] _____
28. surgical ['sɜ:dʒikl] _____
29. vascular ['væskjələ(r)] _____
30. exploratory [ik'splɒrətri] _____

写出下列单词的复数形式，每个单词结尾都有下划线。

31. gingiva（gums）［dʒin'dʒaivə］_____
32. testis（male reproductive organ）［'testis］_____
33. criterion（standard）［krai'tiəriən］_____
34. lumen（central opening）［'lu:men］_____
35. locus（place）［'ləʊkəs］_____
36. ganglion（mass of nervous tissue）［'gæŋliən］_____
37. larynx（voice box）［'læriŋks］_____
38. vena（vein）［'vi:nə］_____
39. nucleus（center; core）［'nju:kliəs］_____

写出下列单词的单数形式，每个单词的结尾都有下划线。

40. thrombi（blood clots）［'θrɒmbai］_____
41. vertebrae（bones of the spine）［'vɜ:tibri:］_____
42. bacteria（type of microorganism）［bæk'tiəriə］_____
43. alveoli（air sacs）［æl'vi:əlai］_____
44. apices（high points, tips）［'episi:z］_____
45. foramina（openings）［fə'ræmənə］_____
46. diagnoses（identifications of disease）［ˌdaiəg'nəʊsi:z］_____
47. carcinomata（cancers）［kɑ:sinəʊ'mətə］_____

单词构建

利用给出的单词组成部分写出下列定义的单词，每个组成部分可多次使用。

| -ist   -ic   parasit   -ism   -y   log   -o |

48. pertaining to parasites_____
49. study of parasites_____
50. a condition of having parasites_____
51. One who studies parasites_____

单词分析

定义下列单词，并给出单词中每个组成部分的含义。如果需要，可以使用词典。

52. geriatrician［ˌdʒeriə'triʃn］_____
    a. ger/e_____
    b. iatr/o_____
    c. -ic_____
    d. -ian_____
53. anesthesia［ˌænəs'θi:ziə］_____
    a. an-_____
    b. esthesi/o_____
    c. -ia_____

54. photophobia [ˌfəʊtə'fəʊbɪə] _____
   a. phot/o _____
   b. phob（from Greek phobos）_____
   c. -ia _____

Additional Case Studies
补充案例研究

Case Study: C. R.'s Job-Related Breathing Problems
案例研究：C. R. 与工作相关的呼吸问题

Chief Complaint

C. R., a 54 y/o woman, has been having difficulty breathing (dyspnea) that was originally attributed to a left upper lobe (LUL) pneumonia. She was treated with an antibiotic, and after no improvement was noted in her breathing, C. R. had a follow-up chest x-ray that revealed a small LUL pneumothorax. She was referred to the respiratory clinic and saw Dr. Williams, a pulmonologist.

Past Medical History

C. R. has a history of smoking a pack a day for 30 years and stopped two years ago. She noticed an improvement in her breathing and tired less easily after she quit. About one month ago, she complained of general malaise, dyspnea, and a productive cough; she was expectorating pus-containing (purulent) sputum and was febrile. The chest radiograph and sputum cultures indicate that her symptoms had progressed into a bronchopneumonia with pulmonary edema complicated by a small pneumothorax in the LUL. A pea-size mass was identified in the left lobe. Also noted, C. R. is a hairstylist as well as a manicurist and recently went back to work in a beauty salon. She has complained that the fumes from the hair chemicals and nail products affect her breathing.

Clinical Course

Dr. Williams performed a bronchoscopic examination. During the examination, he took a biopsy of the mass, and the results were negative. Sputum cultures were also taken to determine the spectrum of action of an appropriate antibiotic. A respiratory therapist measured the patient's respiratory volumes and recorded any changes. The patient was told to drink plenty of liquids, get proper rest, and refrain from working for one week. She was told to wear a mask when she returned to work, avoid unventilated areas in the salon, and avoid the chemical fumes as much as possible. She is to return to the clinic in one month for follow-up.

主诉

C. R. 是一名54岁的女性，有呼吸困难（dyspnea），最初归因于左上肺叶（left upper lobe，LUL）肺炎（pneumonia）。她用抗生素治疗，在注意到呼吸没有改善之后，C. R. 做了胸部X线检查，显示左上肺叶气胸（pneumothorax）。她被转诊到呼吸科门诊（respiratory clinic），由Williams医生诊治，他是一名肺病专家（pulmonologist）。

既往病史

C. R. 有30年每天一包烟的吸烟史，2年前戒烟。在她戒烟后，她注意到呼吸改善，而且不太容易疲劳。大约1个月前，她主诉全身不适（general malaise）、呼吸困难和排痰性咳嗽；她咳脓（purulent）痰并发热。胸片和痰培养物表明她的症状已经发展为支气管肺炎（bronchopneumonia），伴有左上肺叶的小气胸并发肺水肿。在左叶中发现豌豆大小的肿块。另外，C. R. 是一名发型师兼美甲师，最近回到美容院工作。她抱怨美发化学品和指甲产品的气味影响了她的呼吸。

临床病程

Williams医生进行了支气管镜（bronchoscopic）检查。在检查期间，还对肿块进行了活检，结果是阴性。还采集了痰培养物以确定合适抗生素的抗菌谱。呼吸治疗师检测患者的呼吸量，并记录所有变化。告知患者要喝大量的液体，并要适当休息，并且1周内避免工作。她被告知返回工作时要戴口罩，避免室内不通风的区域，并尽可能避免化学烟雾。她将在1个月内返回诊所接受随访。

案例研究问题

多项选择，选择最佳答案，在题号的左侧写出选择的字母。

____ 1. The gh in the terms cough and radiograph is pronounced as

 a. g

 b. h

 c. f

 d. s

____ 2. The pn in the term bronchopneumonia is pronounced as

 a. p

 b. n

 c. f

 d. s

____ 3. Which of the following is a compound word?

 a. pulmonary

 b. pneumothorax

 c. respiratory

 d. antibiotic

____ 4. The suffix that means "condition of" in pneumonia is

 a. –nia

 b. –monia

 c. –ia

 d. –onia

____ 5. The plural of spectrum is

 a. spectra

 b. spectria

 c. spectrina

 d. spectrums

CHAPTER 3 前缀

预测试

多项选择。选择最佳答案，并在每个数字的左边写上您选择的字母。

____1. A word prefix appears
  a. in the middle of the word
  b. after a suffix
  c. at the end of the word
  d. at the beginning of the word

____2. The prefix in the words prefix and pretest means
  a. before
  b. final
  c. fixed
  d. superior

____3. The prefix in the word microscopic is
  a. mic
  b. scop
  c. micro
  d. pic

____4. The suffix in the word microscopic is
  a. –ic
  b. –scop
  c. –micro
  d. –ros

____5. The prefixes uni–, tri–, and poly– all refer to
  a. size
  b. number
  c. location
  d. shape

____6. The prefixes leuk/o–, cyan/o–, and erythr/o– all refer to
  a. dimensions
  b. area
  c. abnormalities
  d. color

____7. The opposite of hypoglycemia (low blood sugar) is
  a. hypoglucemia
  b. hyperglycemia
  c. hypocalcemia
  d. hypoglycemic

____8. The opposite of prenatal (before birth) is
  a. perinatal
  b. prenatural
  c. postnatal
  d. prepartum

学习目标

学完本章后, 应该能够:

1 ▶ 定义前缀, 并解释如何使用前缀。
2 ▶ 确认并定义医学术语中使用的一些前缀。
3 ▶ 在医学术语中使用前缀构成单词。
4 ▶ 分析案例研究中的前缀。

Case Study: T. S.'s Diving Accident and Spinal Cord Injury
案例研究: T. S. 的跳水事故和脊髓损伤

Chief Complaint
A 12-year-old male, T.S., was transported to the emergency room after diving into a shallow backyard cement pool. He c/o severe head and neck pain and has minimal movement of his arms. He is not able to move his legs.

Examination
A well-nourished 12-year-old male is awake and oriented, initially hypotensive and bradycardic, but vital signs are stabilizing. He reports being at a backyard pool party for his friend's birthday and remembers diving into the pool head first. The next thing he recalls is waking up on the deck of the pool with his friends standing all around him. He has a large erythematous and bruised area centered on the upper part of the forehead. T.S. has full head and neck movement with fair muscle strength. He has weak shoulder movement and is able to slightly flex his elbows and extend his wrists. His legs are areflexic and flaccid. He has no finger movement. Past medical history is noncontributory.

Clinical Course
T. S. is diagnosed with a burst or comminuted fracture of the C6 vertebra that may potentially result in quadriplegia. After surgical stabilization of the cervical fracture, T.S. was transferred to the spinal cord unit where his vital signs could be monitored closely along with frequent assessments for orthostatic hypotension and possible complications following spinal surgery. He will be moved to a rehabilitation center in about two weeks for physical and occupational therapy. His medical team consists of his primary physician (pediatrician), a neurosurgeon, a neurologist, and a physical medicine and rehabilitation (PM&R) specialist. T.S.'s condition will require a full complement of healthcare team members, including nurses, psychologists, physical and occupational therapists, pharmacists, and social workers.

A spinal cord injury can result in psychologic as well as permanent physical damage, as noted in T.S.'s follow-up study later in this chapter. There is more information on the spinal cord and behavioral disorders in Chapter 17.

主诉
T. S. 是一名 12 岁的男性,他在跳入浅浅的后院水泥池后被送到急诊室。他主诉严重的头部和颈部疼痛,并且手臂几乎不能运动,腿也不能移动。

检查
一名营养良好的 12 岁男性,意识清醒,且能够识别方向,最初有低血压(hypotensive)和心动过缓(bradycardic),但生命体征(vital sign)平稳。他主诉在一个后院泳池参加他的朋友的生日聚会,并记得头部首先潜入泳池。他回忆起的下一件事是在游泳池的地板上醒来时,他的朋友们站在周围。他的额头上部有一个大红斑(erythematous)和擦伤(bruised)。T.S. 的头和颈能够充分运动,肌肉力量正常。他的肩膀运动能力很弱,能够稍微弯曲肘部和伸出手腕。他的腿部柔软(flexic)和松弛(flaccid),手指不能运动。既往病史与当前病情无关。

临床病程
T. S. 被诊断为 C6 椎骨(vertebra)破裂或粉碎性骨折(comminuted fracture),可能导致四肢麻痹(quadriplegia)。术后颈部骨折稳定后,被转移到脊髓病房(spinal cord unit),在那里他的生命体征可以被密切监测,对于直立性(orthostatic)低血压和脊柱手术后可能的并发症也能得到快速评估。他将在大约 2 个星期内被转移到康复中心(rehabilitation center)进行物理和与职业相关的治疗。他的医疗团队由主管医生[儿科医生(pediatrician)]、一名神经外科医生(neurosurgeon)、一名神经科医生(neurologist)和一名物理医学和康复(physical medicine and rehabilitation, PM & R)专家组成。T.S. 的状况将需要一个完整的保健团队,包括护士、心理学家(psychologist)、物理和职业治疗师(physical and occupational therapist)、药剂师(pharmacist)和社会工作者。

如本章后面的 T.S. 的随访研究所指出,脊髓损伤可导致心理和永久性身体损伤。有关脊髓和行为障碍(behavioral disorder)的更多信息见第 17 章。

简介

前缀是加在单词或词根之前以修饰其含义的组成部分。例如：单词 lateral 意为"边、侧"，加上意为"一个"的前缀 uni- 构成单词 unilateral，含义为"影响或涉及一侧"；加上意为"相反或相对"的前缀 contra- 构成单词 contralateral，指的就是对侧，单词 equilateral 意为"有相等的边"。本书中的前缀后会跟一个短线 -，以表示它是构成单词的前缀。

表 3-1 至表 3-8 介绍了最常用的前缀。虽然列表很长，几乎所有你需要通过本书学习的前缀都在这里，另外一些前缀，包括与疾病有关的前缀，在后面的几章中给出。本章中许多前缀的含义您已经熟悉，如框 3-1 所示。你可能不知道练习中的所有单词，但最好猜一猜。表中的单词作为使用示例给出，几乎所有这些单词都会重新出现在其他章节中。如果您在工

框 3-1

聚焦单词
简化的前缀

近来，简化的前缀层出不穷。在日常生活中意为"电子"的前缀 e- 扩散很快，例如 e-mail（电子邮件）、e-commerce（电子商务）、e-zine（电子杂志）和 e-waste（电子垃圾等）。意为"极限"的 X- 则出现在 X-game（极限游戏）和 X-sport（极限运动）之中。

前缀 nan/o 意为"第十亿的"，却被常用于与非常小的粒子相关的名词中，例如 nanotechnology（纳米技术）。它还出现在其成分包含极细微粒（nanoparticles）的化妆品名称之中。Steri- 意为无菌或至少是清洁，被用于命名 Steri-Strip 绷带和其他保护性医疗产品和清洗材料。

在许多手术器械名称中，前缀 endo- 表示新的内窥镜设备，它们又细又长，更小的工作端用在微创面。例如 endoscissors（内镜切除器）、endosuture（内镜缝合）、endocautery（内镜烧灼）和 endosnare（内镜圈套）。

用于具体年龄人群的医疗产品也使用一些前缀。Geri- 与老年相关，例如 geriatrics（老年病学），还出现在 geri-chair（老年座椅）、geri-pads（老年衬垫）、geri-jacket（老年夹克）等。Pedi- 或 pedia- 意为"儿童"，出现在 pedi-cath（儿童导管）、pedi-dose（儿童剂量）和 pedi-set（儿童套装）等名词之中。

框 3-2

健康职业
注册护士

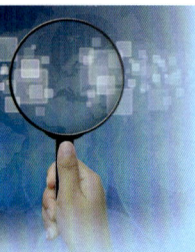

护理工作是所有医疗保健行业中最多样化的，拥有最多的从业者。约 60% 的护理工作在医院，其他地点包括办公室、诊所、救济院、家庭和私人公司。在这些环境中，护士可能专注于特殊的专业，如紧急或重症护理、手术、精神病学、儿科（pediatric）或老年（geriatric）护理。注册护士（registered nurse，RN）通常直接与患者接触，他们提供教育、健康和健康辅导，提供情感支持，维护患者记录和数据登记，帮助诊断测试，并提供随访和康复护理。在更广泛的范围内，他们会在工厂、监狱和学校工作。他们也在公共卫生、健康检查或免疫中心工作，管理献血工作或协调研究试验。

通向护理生涯的三种可能的教育途径是四年制本科学士学位（BSN）、来自社区或初级学院的 2~3 年副学士学位（ADN）或来自于医院护理培训项目的 2~3 年的文凭。虽然大多数护士毕业于被认可的 ADN 或 BSN 课程，但仍有数量有限的医院文凭课程，能够为学生的护理职业生涯做好准备。课程包括文学、科学、行为科学和护理。所有的教育项目都包括一个在医疗机构监督的临床培训。所有毕业生必须通过国家考试（NCLEX-RN），获得职业执照。

有些人以实习护士或护士助手的身份开始他们的职业生涯，然后返回学校获取注册护士学位。另一些人可能从副学士或培训文凭开始，然后在工作时参加学士学位课程，通常可从雇主那里获得学费报销。对于那些希望转变为护理职业的人，也有速成课程。

想要进一步提升自己职业和工作独立性的注册护士可以培训成为护士麻醉师、护士助产士、临床护士专家或护士执业人员（他们可以提供初级护理，在一些州能够开处方药物）。作为护理教育者和管理者的职业也需要高级培训。护理工作的前景非常好，特别是在医疗服务不足的地区、病例管理、护士信息学和家庭医疗保健等领域。护理职业的信息来源包括国家护理联盟（National League for Nursing）网站 www.nln.org、美国护理学院协会（American Association of Colleges of Nursing）网站 www.aacn.nche.edu 和美国护士协会（American Nurses Association）网站 http://nursingworld.org。

作时忘记前缀，则可以参考本章或附录 3 和附录 4 单词组成部分及其含义表。附录 7 仅给出了前缀。

所有医务人员都熟悉这些前缀。要了解特定的护理领域，参见框 3-2。

表 3-1　表示数字的前缀

前缀	含义	示例	示例定义
prim/i-	第一	primary ['praɪm(ə)rɪ]	主要的，第一的
mon/o-	一个	monocular [mə'nɒkjʊlə]	单眼的
uni-	一个	unite [juː'naɪt]	联合
hemi-	一半，一侧	hemisphere ['hemɪsfɪə]	半球（图 3-1）
semi-	一半，部分的	semipermeable [semɪ'pɜːmɪəbl]	半渗透的
bi-	两个，两次	binary ['baɪnərɪ]	由两部分构成，二元的
di-	两个，两次	diatomic [ˌdaɪə'tɒmɪk]	二原子的
dipl/o-	双，对	diplococci d [ˌdɪpləʊ'kɒksaɪ]	双球菌
tri-	三个	tricuspid [traɪ'kʌspɪd]	三尖瓣（图 3-2）
quadr/i-	四个	quadruplet ['kwɒdrʊplɪt]	四胞胎
tetra-	四个	tetralogy [tɪ'trælədʒɪ]	四联症
multi-	多个	multicellular [mʌltɪ'seljʊlə]	多细胞的（图 3-3）
poly-	多个，许多	polymorphous [ˌpɒlɪ'mɔːfəs]	多形的 (morph/o)

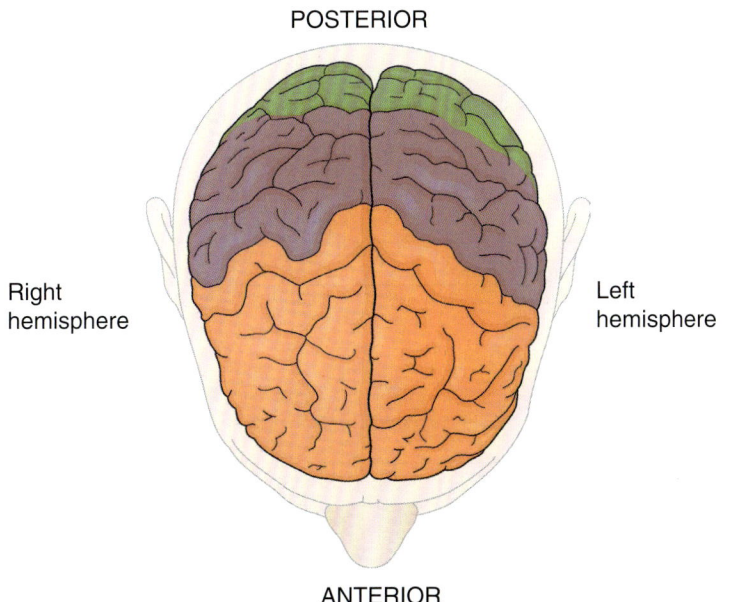

图 3-1　**脑半球。** 大脑的每一半都是一个半球（hemisphere），前缀 hemi- 意为一半或一侧

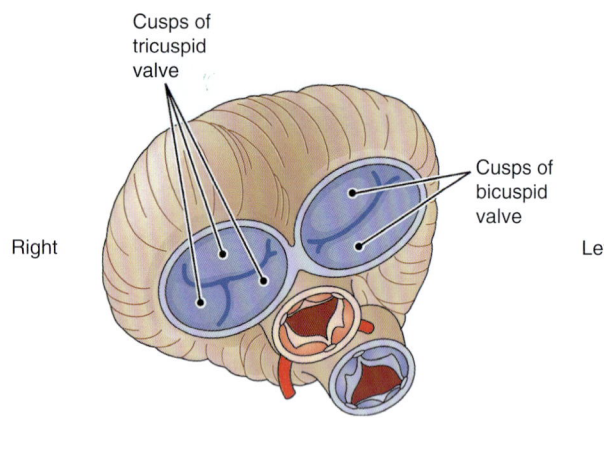

图 3-2 心脏瓣膜。心脏右侧的瓣膜三尖瓣（tricuspid），有三个尖（cusp）；心脏左侧的瓣二尖瓣（bicuspid），有两个尖。前缀 bi- 和 tri- 表示数字

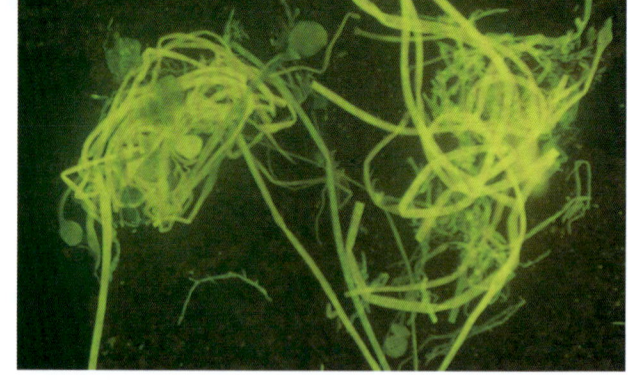

图 3-3 多细胞生物。这种真菌有一个以上的细胞，它是一个简单的多细胞（multicellular）生物

练习 3-1

填空，在做练习时，读出每个单词。

1. Place the following prefixes in order of increasing numbers: tri, uni-, tetra-, bi- _____
2. A binocular [bɪˈnɒkjələ(r)] microscope has _____ eyepieces.
3. A quadruped [ˈkwɒdruped] animal walks on _____ feet (ped/o).
4. The term unilateral [ˌjuːnɪˈlætrəl] refers to _____ side (later/o).
5. The term semilunar [ˈsemiˈluːnə] means shaped like a _____ moon.
6. A diploid [ˈdɪplɔɪd] organism has _____ sets of chromosomes (-ploid).
7. A tetrad [ˈtetræd] has _____ components.
8. A tripod [ˈtraɪpɒd] has _____ legs.
9. Monophonic [ˌmɒnəˈfɒnɪk] sound has _____ channel.

给出与下列前缀含义相似的一个前缀。

10. di- _____
11. poly- _____
12. hemi- _____
13. mon/o- _____

表 3-2　表示颜色的前缀

前缀	含义	示例	示例定义
cyan/o-	蓝色	cyanosis [ˌsaɪəˈnəʊsɪs]	紫绀（图 3-4）
erythr/o-	红色	erythrocyte [ɪˈrɪθrə(ʊ)saɪt]	血红细胞 (-cyte)
leuk/o-	白色、无色	leukemia [lʊˈkimɪə]	白血病
melan/o-	黑色、暗色	melanin [ˈmelənɪn]	黑色素
xanth/o-	黄色	xanthoma [zænˈθəʊmə]	黄色瘤 (-oma)

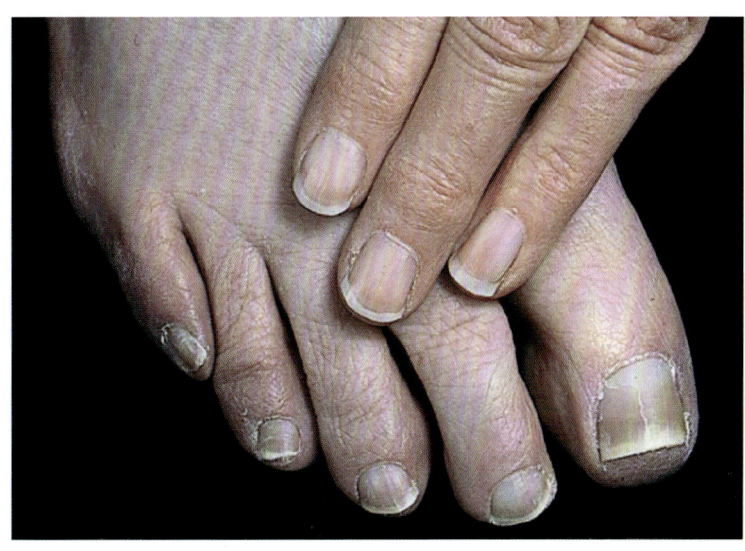

图 3-4　紫绀（cyanosis），蓝色变色。与指尖的正常颜色相比，在脚趾甲和脚趾中看到这种异常的颜色。前缀 cyan/o- 意为"蓝色"

练习 3-2

匹配以下术语，并在每个数字的左侧写入相应的字母。

____ 1. melanocyte [bɪˈnɒkjələ(r)]　　　　a. pertaining to bluish discoloration

____ 2. xanthoderma [zænθəˈdɜːmə]　　　b. redness of the skin

____ 3. cyanotic [ˌsaɪəˈnɒtɪk]　　　　　　c. yellow coloration of the skin

____ 4. erythema [ˌɛrɪˈθiːmə]　　　　　　d. cell that produces dark pigment

____ 5. leukocyte [ˈlʊkəˌsaɪt]　　　　　　e. white blood cell

表 3-3　否定性前缀

前缀	含义	示例	示例定义
a-、an-	不、没有、缺少、不在	anhydrous [æn'haidrəs]	脱水的 (hydr/o)
anti-	相反	antiseptic [ˌænti'septik]	抗菌的 (sepsis)
contra-	相反、相对、对立	contraindicated [ˌkɔntrə'indiˌkeitid]	禁忌，不建议
de-	向下、没有、去除、丧失	decalcify [ˌdi:'kælsifai]	除钙 (calc/i)
dis-	不在、去除、分离	dissect [di'sekt]	分离组织以进行解剖学研究
in-*、im-（用于 b、m、p 之前）	不	incontinent [in'kɔntinənt]	失禁
non-	不	noncontributory [ˌnɔnkən'tribjʊtəri]	不重要，对诊断没有贡献
un-	不	uncoordinated [ˌʌnkəʊ'ɔ:dineitid]	不在一起工作，不合作

* 在 inject（注射）和 inhale（吸气）中也意为 "进" 或 "进入"

练习 3-3

识别并定义下列单词中的前缀。

	Prefix	Meaning of Prefix
1. aseptic	a	not, without, lack of, absence
2. antidote		
3. amnesia		
4. disintegrate		
5. contraception		
6. inadequate		
7. depilatory		
8. nonconductor		

为下列单词加一个否定的前缀。

9. conscious	unconscious
10. significant	
11. infect	
12. usual	
13. specific	
14. congestant	
15. compatible	

表 3-4　表示方向的前缀

前缀	含义	示例	示例定义
ab-	远离	abduct [əbˈdʌkt]	使外展（图 3-5）
ad-	朝向、靠近	adduct [əˈdʌkt]	使内收（图 3-5）
dia-	穿过	diarrhea [ˌdaiəˈriə]	腹泻
per-	穿过	percutaneous [ˌpɜːkjʊˈteiniəs]	经由皮肤的
trans-	穿过	transected [trænˈsektid]	切穿或横切

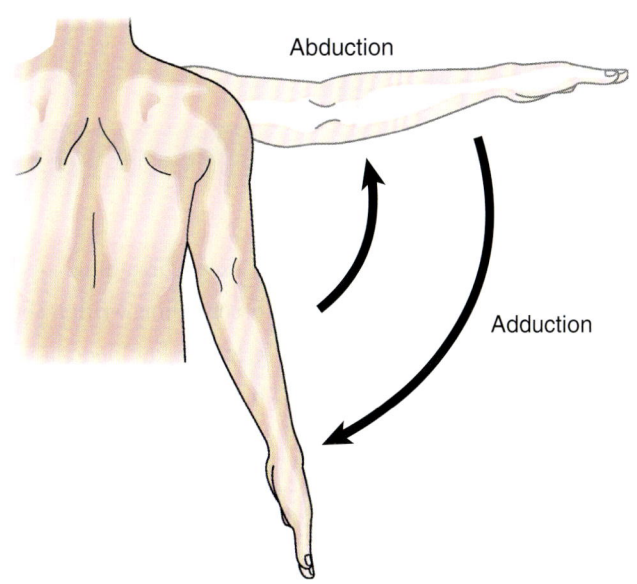

图 3-5　外展（abduction）和内收（adduction）。前缀 ab- 意为"远离"，手臂在外展中远离身体；前缀 ad- 意为"朝向"，手臂在内收中朝向身体移动

练习 3-4

识别并定义下列单词中的前缀。

	Prefix	Meaning of Prefix
1. dialysis	dia	through
2. percolate	_____	_____
3. adjacent	_____	_____
4. absent	_____	_____
5. diameter	_____	_____
6. transport	_____	_____

表 3-5　表示程度的前缀

前缀	含义	示例	示例定义
hyper-	之上、过量、不正常地高、升高	hyperthermia [ˌhaipə'θɜːmiə]	高体温
hypo-*	之下、低于、不正常地低、下降	hyposecretion [ˌhaipəusi'kriːʃn]	分泌不足
olig/o-	少、缺乏	oligospermia [ˌoligəu'spəːmiə]	少精子症
pan-	全部	pandemic [pæn'demik]	影响全人类的疾病
super-*	之上，过量	supernumerary [ˌsjuːpə'njuːmərəri]	过量

* 也表示位置，如 hypodermic（皮下的）和 superficial（表面的）

练习 3-5

匹配以下术语，并在每个数字的左侧写入相应的字母。

____ 1. hypotensive [ˌhaipəu'tensiv]
____ 2. oligodontia [ˌɒligəu'dɒnʃiə]
____ 3. panplegia [pæn'pliːdʒiə]
____ 4. superscript ['suːpəskript]
____ 5. hyperventilation [ˌhaipəˌventi'leiʃn]

a. excess breathing
b. something written above
c. having low blood pressure
d. total paralysis
e. less than the normal number of teeth

表 3-6　表示大小和比较的前缀

前缀	含义	示例	示例定义
equi-	相等，相同	equilibrium [ˌiːkwi'libriəm]	均衡
eu-	真实，好，舒服，正常	euthanasia [ˌjuːθə'neiziə]	安乐死 (thanat/o)
hetero-	其他，不同，不等的	heterogeneous [ˌhetərə(u)'dʒiːniəs]	由不同物质构成，不一致
homo-、homeo-	相同，不变	homograft ['həumədɡrɑːft]	同物种组织移植
iso-	相等，相同	isocellular [aisə'seljulə]	同族细胞的
macro-	大，不正常地大	macroscopic [ˌmækrə(u)'skɒpik]	肉眼可见的
mega-*、megalo-	大，不正常地大	megacolon [ˌmegə'kəulən]	结肠增大
micro-*	小，很小	microcyte ['maiˌkrəusait]	小红细胞 (-cyte)

表 3-6		表示大小和比较的前缀（续表）	
前缀	含义	示例	示例定义
neo-	新的	neonate ['niːə(ʊ)neit]	新生儿
normo-	正常	normovolemia [ˌnɔːməʊvəˈliːmiə]	正常血量
ortho-	直的，正确的，直立的	orthodontics [ˌɔːθəˈdɒntiks]	畸齿矫正学 (odont/o)
poikilo-	变化的，不规则的	poikilothermic [ˌpɔikiləʊˈθɜːmik]	有变化的体温 (therm/o)
pseudo-	假的	pseudoplegia [ˌsjuːdəʊˈpliɡiə]	假性麻痹 (-plegia)
re-	再次，反向	reflux [ˈriːflʌks]	反流

*Mega- 也意为一百万，如 megahertz（兆赫兹）。Micro- 也意为百万分之一，如 microsecond（微秒）

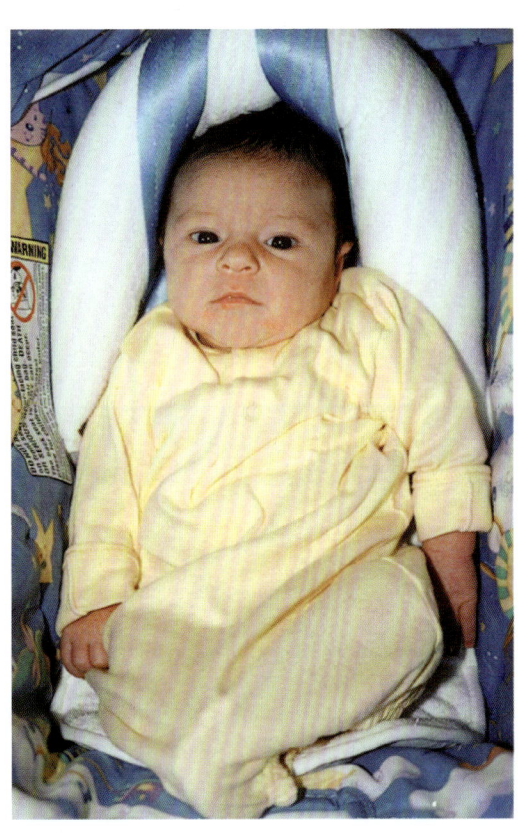

图 3-6　新生儿（neonate 或 newborn）。前缀 neo- 意为"新的"

练习 3-6

匹配以下术语，并在每个数字的左侧写入相应的字母。

___ 1. isograft ['aisəgrɔ:ft]
___ 2. orthotic [ɔ:'θɒtik]
___ 3. pseudoreaction [sju:dəur'iækʃn]
___ 4. poikiloderma [pɔikiləu'dʒ:mə]
___ 5. homothermic [həumə∪'θɜ:mik]

a. having a constant body temperature
b. irregular, mottled condition of the skin
c. false response
d. tissue transplanted between identical individuals
e. straightening or correcting deformity

识别并定义下列单词中的前缀。

	Prefix	Meaning of Prefix
6. homeostasis	homeo	same, unchanging
7. equivalent		
8. orthopedics		
9. rehabilitation		
10. euthyroidism		
11. neocortex		
12. megabladder		
13. isometric		
14. normothermic		

写出下列单词的反义词。

15. homogeneous (of uniform composition) [ˌhɒmə'dʒi:niəs] _____
16. macroscopic (large enough to see with the naked eye) [ˌmækrə'skɒpik] _____

表 3-7　表示时间和/或位置的前缀

前缀	含义	示例	示例定义
ante-	之前	antenatal [ænti'neit(ə)l]	出生前 (nat/i)
pre-	之前，在……前面	premature ['premətjʊə]	早产的、不成熟的
pro-	之前，在……前面	prodrome ['prəudrəum]	前驱症状
post-	之后，在……后面	postnasal [ˌpost'nezl]	鼻后 (nas/o)

练习 3-7

匹配以下术语，并在每个数字的左侧写入相应的字母。

____ 1. postmortem ['pəust'mɔ:tem]
____ 2. antedate [ˌænti'deit]
____ 3. progenitor [prəu'dʒenitə(r)]
____ 4. prepartum [pri'peərətm]
____ 5. projectile [prə'dʒektail]

a. to occur before another event
b. ancestor, one who comes before
c. before birth (parturition)
d. throwing or extending forward
e. occurring after death

识别并定义下列单词中的前缀。

	Prefix	Meaning of Prefix
6. prediction [pri'dikʃn]	pre	before，infront of
7. postmenopausal ['pəustmenəu'pɔ:zəl]		
8. procedure [prə'si:dʒə(r)]		
9. predisposing [ˌpri:di'spəuziŋ]		
10. antepartum [ˌænti'pa:təm]		

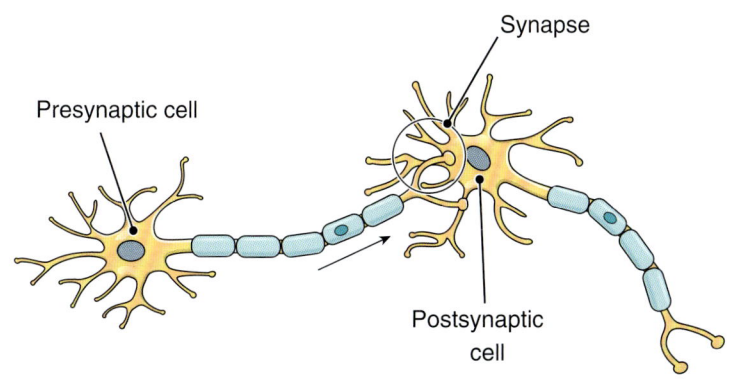

图 3-7　突触。神经细胞聚集在突触（synapse），如前缀 syn- 所示。突触前细胞（presynaptic）位于（前缀 pre-）突触之前；突触后（ostsynaptic）细胞位于（前缀 post-）突触之后

表 3-8		表示位置的前缀	
前缀	含义	示例	示例定义
dextr/o-	右	dextrogastria [ˌdekstrə'gæstriə]	胃 (gastr/o) 向右位移
sinistr/o-	左	sinistromanual [ˌsinistrə'mænjuəl]	左撇子
ec-、ecto-	外，外面	ectopic [ek'tɒpik]	异位的
ex/o-	远离，外面	excise ['eksaiz]	切断
end/o-	内，在……内	endoderm ['endə(ʊ)dɜ:m]	内胚层
mes/o-	中间	mesencephalon [ˌmesen'sef(ə)lɒn]	大脑的中央部位 (encephalon)，中脑
syn-、sym-（用在 b、m、p 之前）	在一起	synapse ['sainæps]	两个神经细胞的结合点
tel/e-、tel/o-	末端	telophase ['telə(ʊ)feiz]	末期 (mitosis)

练习 3-8

匹配以下术语，并在每个数字的左侧写入相应的字母。

____ 1. mesoderm ['mesədɜːm]
____ 2. symbiosis [ˌsimbai'əusis]
____ 3. sinistrocardia [sinistrəu'kɑːdiə]
____ 4. endoscope ['endəskəup]
____ 5. telephase ['teləfeiz]

a. displacement of the heart to the left
b. device for viewing the inside of a structure
c. two organisms living together
d. last stage of cell division (mitosis)
e. middle layer of a developing embryo

识别并定义下列单词中的前缀。

	Prefix	Meaning of Prefix
6. sympathetic [ˌsimpə'θetik]	sym	together
7. extract ['ekstrækt]		
8. ectoparasite [ˌektə'pærəsait]		
9. syndrome ['sindrəum]		
10. endotoxin [ˌendəu'tɒksin]		

写出下列单词的反义词。

11. exogenous (outside the organism)
    [ek'sɒdʒənəs]

12. dextromanual (right-handed)
    [dekst'rəumənjuəl]

13. ectoderm (outermost layer of the embryo)
    ['ektəuˌdɜːm]

Case Study Revisited
案例研究再访

T.S.'s Therapy

From the hospital, T.S. was transferred to a rehabilitation center for further evaluation and therapy. At this point in his recovery, he was unable to move his legs and had limited movement of his arms. He is participating in a plan of care with physical and occupational therapy and is working on performing basic activities of daily living. Within therapy, he is practicing wheelchair functional operations, transfers, and safe propulsions. The goal is to progress toward independence within his home lifestyle and regain status as an active member in his school and community. Despite the support and encouragement of his family and many friends, he remains depressed and anxious about his future.

T.S. 的治疗

T.S. 从医院被转移到康复中心进行进一步评估和治疗。这时，在康复方面，他不能移动腿，手臂的移动也有限。他正参与一项关于物理和职业治疗的护理计划，并正在执行基本的日常生活活动。在治疗中，他正在练习轮椅非功能性操作、转移和安全推进，目标是在自己的家庭生活中实现独立，并重新获得在学校和社区的积极活动成员的地位。尽管有家人和许多朋友的支持和鼓励，他仍然很沮丧，并对未来感到焦虑。

CHAPTER 3 复习

匹配以下术语，并在每个数字的左侧写入相应的字母。

___ 1. primitive   a. one-half or one side of the chest
___ 2. biceps   b. having two forms
___ 3. unify   c. combine into one part
___ 4. dimorphous   d. a muscle with two parts
___ 5. hemithorax   e. occurring first in time

___ 6. erythematous   a. cell with yellow color
___ 7. melanoma   b. having a bluish discoloration
___ 8. xanthocyte   c. darkly pigmented tumor
___ 9. cyanotic   d. red in color
___ 10. leukocyte   e. white blood cell

___ 11. telencephalon   a. total paralysis
___ 12. mesoderm   b. first stage of cell division
___ 13. panplegia   c. double vision
___ 14. prophase   d. middle layer of tissue
___ 15. diplopia   e. endbrain

匹配以下前缀及其含义。

___ 16. poikilo   a. good, true, easy
___ 17. eu   b. straight, correct
___ 18. ortho   c. false
___ 19. pseudo   d. few, scanty
___ 20. oligo   e. varied, irregular

填空

21. A monocle has _____ lens(es).
22. A triplet is one of _____ babies born together.
23. Sinistrad means toward the _____.
24. A disaccharide is a sugar composed of _____ subunits.
25. A contralateral structure is located on the side _____ to a given point.
26. A tetralogy is composed of _____ part(s).
27. The term in T.S.'s case study that describes his lack of reflexes is _____.

识别并定义下列单词中的前缀。

                                 Prefix   Meaning of Prefix

28. hyperactive   _____   _____

29. transfer _____ _____
30. distant _____ _____
31. posttraumatic _____ _____
32. regurgitate _____ _____
33. extend _____ _____
34. adhere _____ _____
35. unusual _____ _____
36. ectoderm _____ _____
37. detoxify _____ _____
38. semisolid _____ _____
39. premenstrual _____ _____
40. perforate _____ _____
41. dialysis (di-AL-ih-sis) _____ _____
42. antibody _____ _____
43. microsurgery _____ _____
44. disease _____ _____
45. endoparasite _____ _____
46. symbiotic (sim-bI-OT-ik) _____ _____
47. prognosis (prog-NO-sis) _____ _____
48. insignificant _____ _____

真假判断

检查以下语句。如果语句为真，则在第一个空白处写 T；如果语句为假，则在第一个空格中写 F，并通过替换第二个空格中带下划线的单词来更正语句。

	True or False	correct Answer
49. Immune cells are primed by their <u>first</u> exposure to a disease organism.	T	
50. A unicellular organism is composed of <u>10</u> cells.	F	one
51. To bisect is to cut into <u>two</u> parts.		
52. A tetrad has <u>five</u> parts.		
53. In Latin, the oculus dexter is the <u>left</u> eye.		
54. A triceps muscle has <u>six</u> parts.		
55. A polygraph measures <u>many</u> physiologic responses.		
56. In T.S.'s case study, quadriplegia refers to paralysis of <u>four</u> limbs.		
57. T.S.'s orthostatic hypotension would occur when he is <u>upright</u>.		

反义词

写出下列单词的反义词。

58. humidify _____
59. abduct _____
60. permeable _____

61. heterogeneous _____
62. exotoxin _____
63. microscopic _____
64. hyperventilation _____
65. postsynaptic _____
66. septic _____

同义词

写出下列单词的同义词。

67. supersensitivity _____
68. megalocyte (extremely large red blood cell) _____
69. antenatal _____
70. isolateral (having equal sides) _____

单词构建

利用给出的单词组成部分写出下列定义的单词，每个组成部分可以使用多次。

| mon/o   -al   dextr/o   end/o   macro   cardi   cyt   -ic   ecto   micro   -ia |

71. Pertaining to a very small cell _____
72. A condition in which the heart is outside its normal position _____
73. Pertaining to a cell with a single nucleus _____
74. Condition in which the heart is displaced to the right _____
75. Pertaining to the innermost layer of the heart _____
76. Pertaining to a very large cell _____
77. Condition in which the heart is extremely small _____

单词分析

定义下列单词，并给出每个单词组成部分的含义。如果需要，可以使用词典。

78. isometric [ˌaɪsəˈmɛtrɪk] _____
    a. iso- _____
    b. metr/o _____
    c. -ic _____
79. symbiosis [ˌsɪmbaɪˈəʊsɪs] _____
    a. sym- _____
    b. bio _____
    c. -sis _____
80. monoclonal [ˌmɒnəʊˈkləʊnəl] _____
    a. mon/o- _____
    b. clon(e) _____
    c. -al _____

Additional Case Studies
补充案例研究

Case Study 3-1: Displaced Fracture of the Femoral Neck
案例研究 3-1：股骨颈的骨折移位

While walking home from the train station, M.A., a 72 y/o woman with preexisting osteoporosis, tripped over a raised curb and fell. In the emergency department, she was assessed for severe pain, and swelling and bruising of her right thigh. A radiograph showed a fracture at the neck of the right femur (thigh bone) (Fig. 3-8). M.A. was prepared for surgery and given a preoperative injection of an analgesic to relieve her pain. During surgery, she was given spinal anesthesia and positioned on an operating room table, with her right hip elevated on a small pillow. Intravenous antibiotics were given before the incision was made. Her right hip was repaired with a bipolar hemiarthroplasty (joint reconstruction). Postoperative care included maintaining the right hip in abduction, fluid replacement, physical therapy, and attention to signs of tissue degeneration and possible dislocation.

当从火车站回家时，一名 72 岁的患有骨质疏松症（osteoporosis）的女性 M.A.，被一个凸起的路缘绊了一下并跌倒。在急诊科，她被评估为严重的疼痛、右大腿肿胀和瘀伤。X 线片显示右股骨（femur）颈骨折（fracture）（图 3-8）。医院准备给 M.A. 做手术，并给予术前注射镇痛药（analgesic）以缓解她的疼痛。在手术期间，她被给予脊髓麻醉（anesthesia），并且被置于手术台上，右臀部用一个小枕头垫高。在切开之前静脉内（intravenous）给予抗生素。她的右髋通过双极半关节成形术（hemiarthroplasty）被修复。术后护理包括在外展（abduction）运动中维护右髋、液体置换、物理治疗和注意组织变性和脱臼的可能（dislocation）。

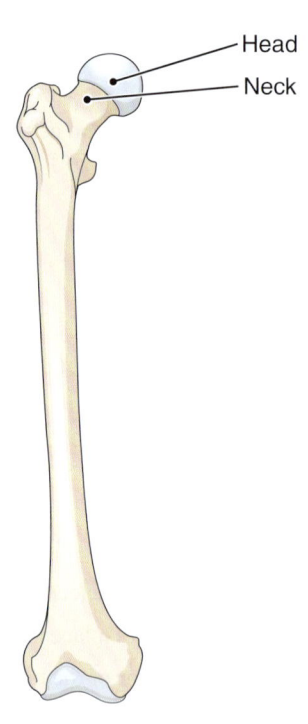

图 3-8　右股骨（femur）。案例研究 3-1 中的股骨颈（femoral neck）骨折

Case Study 3-2: Urinary Tract Infection
案例研究 3-2：泌尿系统感染

Chief Complaint

D. S. recently noticed some blood in her urine, and at the same time, she was experiencing some pain when she urinated. She thought she might have a fever and generally felt tired. She was not sleeping well since she frequently had to get up during the night to use the bathroom. She decided to make an appointment to see her primary care physician.

Past Medical History

A 33 y/o female nonsmoker, has two children, in a monogamous relationship, is a triathlete, and is in excellent health. Has a history of occasional urinary tract infections,

主诉

D. S. 最近注意到她的尿液中带血，同时，在排尿时伴随疼痛。她认为可能发热，并且经常觉得累。由于经常不得不在夜间去卫生间，导致睡眠不好。她决定预约初级保健医生。

既往病史

一名 33 岁的已婚女性，不吸烟，有两个孩子，是一个铁人三项运动员，并且健康状况极好。有偶尔的尿路感染，每年 1~2 次。现在出现排尿困难（dysuria）、

about one to two times a year. Presents now with dysuria (painful urination), hematuria (blood in the urine), and nocturia (nighttime urination).

Clinical Course

Urine analysis report showed cloudy urine with a large number of leukocytes and erythrocytes indicating a urinary tract infection. D.S. was given an antibiotic and told to increase her fluid intake. If symptoms persist beyond one week, D.S. is to return to the office.

血尿（hematuria）和夜尿（nocturia）。

临床病程

尿液分析报告显示，尿液混浊，有大量的白细胞和红细胞，提示有尿路感染。D.S. 被给予抗生素，并被告知增加液体摄入量。如果症状持续超过 1 周，D.S. 要再次就诊。

案例研究问题

识别并定义下列单词中的前缀。

	Prefix	Meaning of Prefix
1. preexisting		
2. analgesic, anesthesia		
3. dislocation		
4. replacement		
5. bipolar		
6. hemiarthroplasty		
7. degeneration		
8. antibiotic		
9. erythrocyte		
10. primary		

填空。

11. The suffixes in the words osteoporosis and anesthesia mean_____.

12. The suffixes in the words intravenous, femoral, and analgesic mean_____.

13. In a monogamous relationship, each person has_____partner.

14. A triathlete competes in an event with_____activities, such as swimming, bicycling, and running.

在案例研究中找出描述下列事物的单词。

15. The time period before surgery_____

16. The time period after surgery_____

17. A position away from the midline of the body_____

18. Another name for a white blood cell_____

CHAPTER 4

细胞、组织和器官

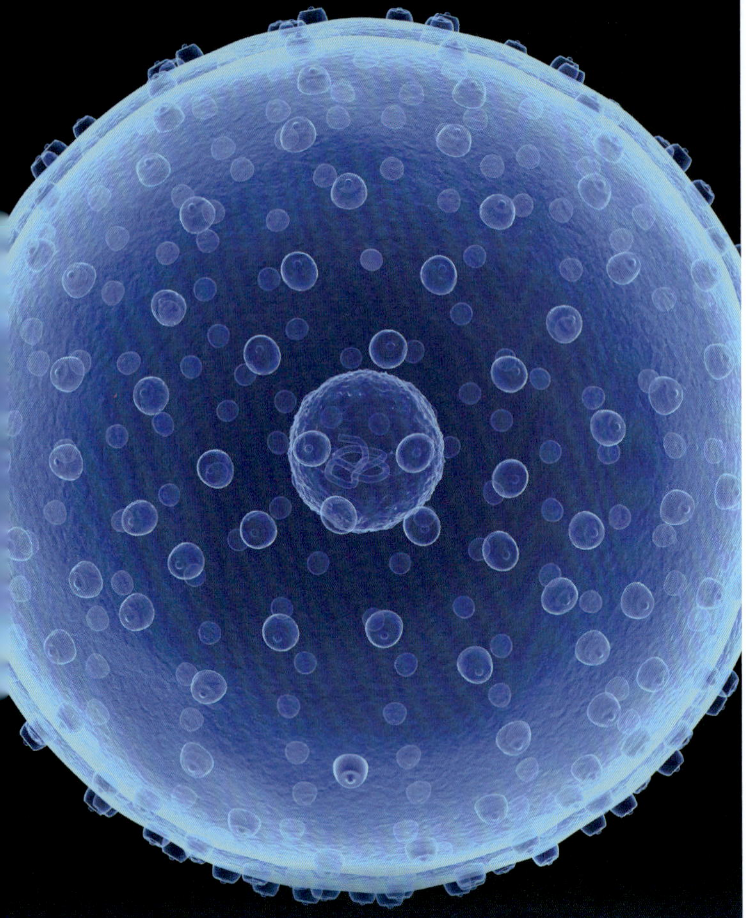

预测试

多项选择。选择最佳答案，并在每个数字的左边写上您选择的字母。

_____ 1. The root that means "cell" is
   a. spher
   b. aden
   c. cyt
   d. gen

_____ 2. The root that means "tissue" is
   a. hist
   b. fibr
   c. plas
   d. hem

_____ 3. The control center of the cell is the
   a. membrane
   b. lysosome
   c. ribosome
   d. nucleus

_____ 4. The process of body cell division is called
   a. separation
   b. segregation
   c. mitosis
   d. gestation

_____ 5. A compound that speeds the rate of a metabolic reaction is a(n)
   a. vitamin
   b. enzyme
   c. salt
   d. lipid

_____ 6. The substance that makes up the cell's genetic material is
   a. DNA
   b. mineral
   c. base
   d. neurons

_____ 7. Chemicals: cells: tissues:_____: systems: organism. What belongs in the blank?
   a. genes
   b. enzymes
   c. nuclei
   d. organs

_____ 8. The root morph/o means
   a. reproduction
   b. fat
   c. form
   d. balance

学习目标

学完本章后，应该能够：

1 ▶ 列出从最简单到最复杂的生物体水平。
2 ▶ 描述和定位细胞的主要组成部分。
3 ▶ 例举人体的四种基本组织类型，并描述其功能。
4 ▶ 定义与人体组织的结构和功能相关的基本术语。
5 ▶ 识别并使用与细胞、组织和器官相关的前缀、词根和后缀。
6 ▶ 分析案例研究中与细胞、组织和器官相关的医学单词。

Case Study: R. S.'s Self-Diagnosis
案例研究：R. S. 的自我诊断

Chief Complaint

R. S. is a second-year medical student who, until recently, has done well in school. Lately, he finds that he is always tired and unable to focus in class. He decides to self-diagnose and begins with a review of systems (ROS). He notes that he is not having any cardiovascular, lymphatic, or respiratory system symptoms, such as tissue swelling, coughing, or shortness of breath. He also has not noticed any changes in urinary system functions. He realizes that he has gained some weight recently and has also been a little constipated but has no other problems with his digestive system. He rules out anything concerning his musculoskeletal system because he has no muscle cramps, joint pain, or weakness. He thinks his skin is drier than usual. He worries that this is an integumentary system sign of hypothyroidism and becomes concerned about his endocrine system function. Unable to perform any imaging studies or laboratory tests on his own, he makes an appointment to see a campus health services physician.

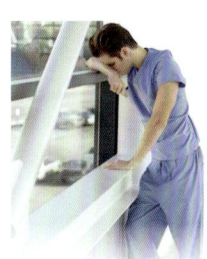

主诉

R. S. 是一名二年级的医学生，一直在学校做得很好。近来，他发现自己总是疲劳，无法在课堂上集中精力。他决定自我诊断，并从系统评价 (review of systems, ROS) 开始。他注意到，他没有任何心血管、淋巴或呼吸系统症状，如组织肿胀、咳嗽或呼吸急促，他也没有发现泌尿系统功能的任何变化。他意识到最近体重有所增加，也有轻微便秘，但没有其他消化系统问题。他排除了关于肌肉骨骼系统的所有问题，因为他没有肌肉痉挛、关节疼痛或虚弱。他认为他的皮肤比平时更干燥，怀疑这是甲状腺功能减退的表皮系统标志，并关注他的内分泌系统功能。因为无法自己进行任何成像研究或实验室检查，他预约了校园健康服务医生。

Examination

R. S. tells the doctor he feels he has a metabolic disorder. He thinks he might have an adenoma, a glandular tumor that is disrupting homeostasis, his normal metabolic state. The doctor takes a complete history and orders various blood tests to assist with the diagnosis. He completes a physical examination that reveals no abnormalities.

检查

R. S. 告诉医生他觉得患有代谢紊乱。他认为可能有一个腺瘤 (adenoma) 破坏体内平衡 (homeostasis)，也就是正常代谢状态。医生完整地记录了病史，并进行各种血液检查以协助诊断。他做了体格检查，没有显示异常。

Clinical Course

The blood glucose levels, complete blood count (CBC), and thyroid function tests are all normal. Nothing in the tests indicates anything physically wrong with the patient. There is no indication that any further cytologic or histologic tests are necessary. The doctor tells R.S. that he is sleep deprived from all his studying and that his weight gain can be explained by his poor food choices in the university cafeteria. In addition, the doctor advises R.S. to schedule some exercise into his daily routine. Lastly, he reminds R.S. that although he is studying to be a doctor, self-diagnosis at this point in his career could be inaccurate and could cause undue anxiety.

临床病程

血糖 (blood glucose) 水平、全血细胞计数 (complete blood count, CBC) 和甲状腺 (thyroid) 功能检查均正常。检查中没有任何迹象表明患者身体有问题，也没有迹象表明需要任何进一步的细胞学或组织学检查。医生告诉 R.S.，学习剥夺了睡眠，他的体重增加可以解释为大学食堂中仅有的食物选择。此外，医生建议 R.S. 在日常生活中安排一些锻炼。最后，他提醒 R.S.，虽然他正在学习成为一名医生，但在职业生涯的这一时期进行的自我诊断可能是不准确的，并可能导致不适当的焦虑。

人体组织

所有生物体的构成都是从简单到复杂（图4-1）。化学物质构成细胞，细胞是身体结构和功能单元。共同工作的一组细胞构成组织，组织构成具有特定功能的器官。器官成为不同系统的组成部分，所有系统共同组成这个生物体。本章讨论与细胞、组织和器官相关的术语。

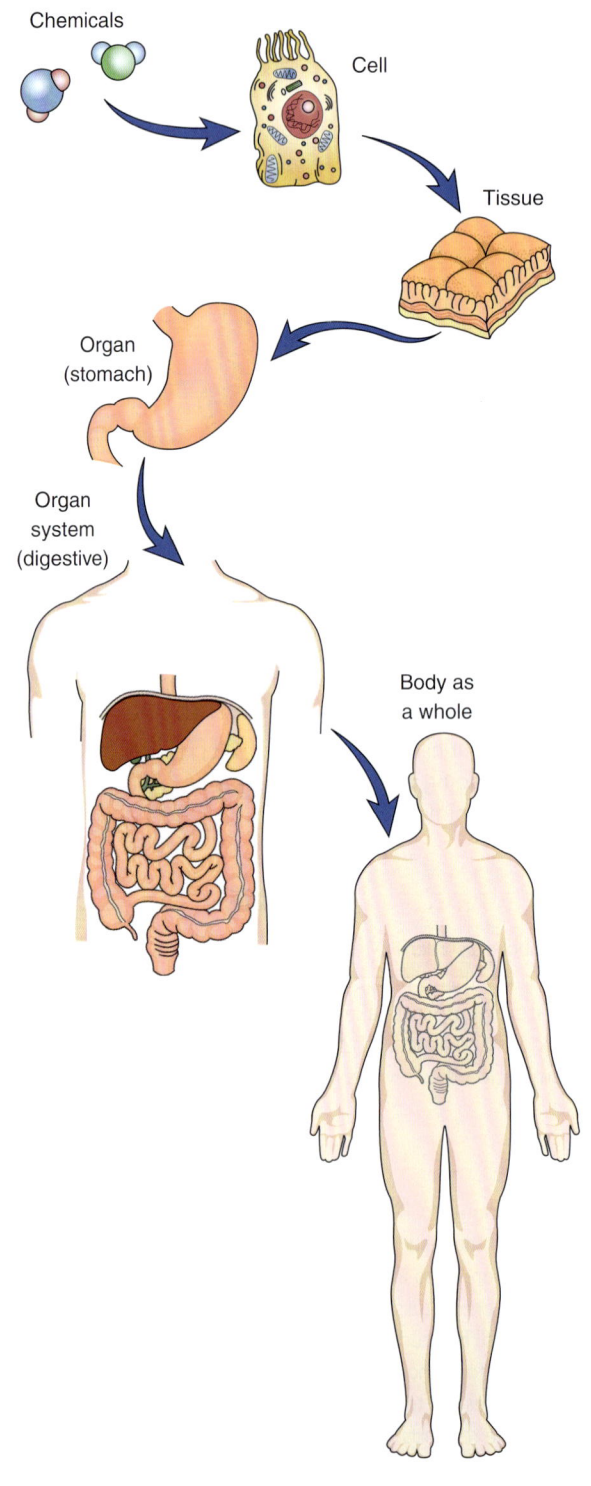

图4-1　组织级别（levels of organization）。人体的组织从简单的化学（chemicals）水平到最复杂的整个有机体水平。图中所示的器官是胃（stomach），是消化系统（digestive）的一部分

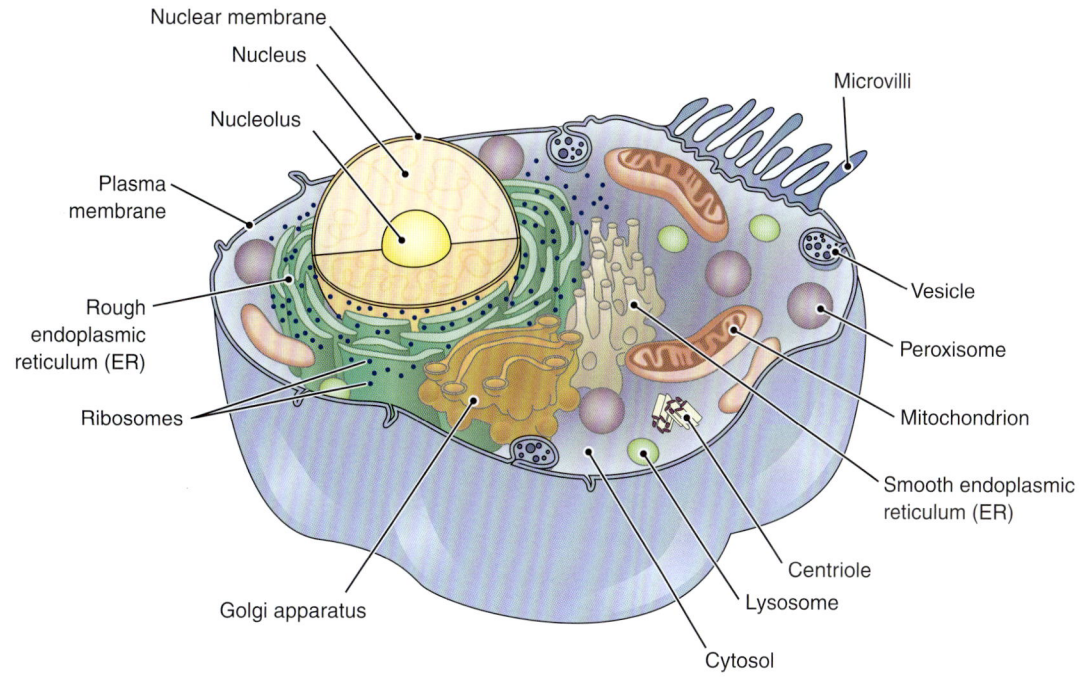

图 4-2 广义动物细胞（截面图）。图中显示的是主要的细胞器（organelle）

细胞

细胞是生物体的基本构成单位（图 4-2）。细胞完成所有活动并产生身体的所有组成部分，它们进行新陈代谢，而新陈代谢是身体所有物理和化学活动的总和，它们以三磷酸腺苷（adenosine triphosphate，ATP）的形式为新陈代谢提供能源，三磷酸腺苷被认为是细胞的能量化合物。构成器官的主要细胞有以下几类：

- **蛋白质**（protein），包括酶、某些激素和结构性物质。
- **碳水化合物**（carbohydrate），包括糖和淀粉，主要的碳水化合物是葡萄糖，它在血液中循环，为细胞提供能量。

框 4-1

供你参考
细胞结构

名称	说明	功能
plasma membrane ['plæzmə] 细胞膜	细胞外壳，主要由脂类和蛋白质构成	包含着细胞内的物质；规定哪些物质能够进入和离开细胞；参与许多活动，例如生长、繁殖和细胞之间的互动
microvilli [ˌmaɪkrəʊ'vɪlaɪ] 微绒毛	细胞膜微小的延伸	吸收物质进入细胞
nucleus ['njuːklɪəs] 细胞核	大的深色细胞器，位于细胞中心，由 DNA 和蛋白质构成	包含指导所有细胞活动的遗传单元——染色体
nucleolus [ˌnjuːkli'əʊləs] 细胞核仁	细胞膜中的小物体，由 RNA、DNA 和蛋白质构成	制造核糖体

续框 4-1

cytoplasm ['saɪtə(ʊ)plæz(ə)m] 细胞质	充满在细胞核膜与细胞膜之间的胶质悬浮液	许多细胞活动发生的场所，由细胞溶质和细胞器组成
cytosol ['saɪtə(ʊ)sɒl] 细胞溶质	细胞质的液体部分	包围细胞器
endoplasmic reticulum (ER) [ˌɛndoʊ'plæzmɪk rɪ'tɪkjʊləm] 内质网	细胞质之中的网膜。粗糙的内质网上附着有核糖体，平滑的没有	粗糙的内质网将蛋白质分类，并组合成复杂的化合物。平滑的内质网参与脂类合成
ribosomes ['raɪbə(ʊ)səʊmz] 核糖体	细胞质中自由的小物体，或附着于内质网，由 RNA 和蛋白质构成	产生蛋白质
mitochondria [ˌmaɪtəʊ'kɒndrɪə] 线粒体	大的细胞器，内有褶皱的膜	将营养中的能量转化为 ATP
Golgi apparatus ['ɡɔːldʒi] 高尔基体	层膜	制造包含蛋白质的化合物，将这些化合物分类，并将它们传送到细胞的其他部分或细胞之外
lysosomes ['laɪsəsəʊmz] 溶酶体	消化酶的小囊	在细胞内消化物质
peroxisomes [pə'rɒksɪsəʊmz] 过氧化物酶体	由膜包裹的细胞器，包含酶	破坏有害物质
vesicles ['vesɪk(ə)lz] 小泡	细胞质中带膜的小囊	储存物质，并将物质大量传入或传出细胞
centrioles ['sentrɪəʊlz] 中心粒	细胞核附近的杆状物体（通常是2个）	在细胞分裂期间帮助分离染色体
surface projections 表面突起	细胞延伸的结构	在细胞周围移动细胞或液体
cilia ['sɪlɪə(r)] 纤毛	细胞外短的、毛发样突起	在细胞周围移动液体
flagellum [flə'dʒeləm] 鞭毛	细胞外长的、鞭样突起	移动细胞

- **脂类**（lipid），包括脂肪。某些激素源自于脂类，脂肪组织被用于储存脂类。

在充满细胞的细胞质内是被称为细胞器（organelle）的亚单元，每个都有特定的功能（图4-2）。细胞的主要结构和名称如框4-1所示。疾病会影响特定的细胞部分，例如囊胞性纤维症和糖尿病会影响细

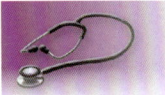

框 4-2

临床观点
细胞器与疾病

在细胞的处置与回收中起关键作用的两个细胞器可能也与疾病有关。溶酶体（lysosomes）包含能够分解碳水化合物、脂类、蛋白质以及核酸的酶，以安全地回收细胞结构。作为正常发育的一部分，溶酶体也会消化细胞自身。不再被需要的细胞会通过在其细胞质中释放溶酶体酶来"自我毁灭"。在家族性黑蒙性白痴（Tay-Sachs disease）患者身体中，神经细胞中的溶酶体缺乏能够分解特定脂类的酶。这些脂类在细胞中集结，引起功能不正常，导致大脑损伤、失明和死亡。

过氧化物酶体（peroxisomes）有点像溶酶体，但不包含不同类型的酶。它们分解进入细胞的有毒物质，例如毒品、酒精，以及正常新陈代谢的一些有害的副产品。如果溶酶体或过氧化物酶体错误地毁坏了细胞，就可能导致疾病。这可能发生在自身免疫（autoimmune）性疾病之中，患者身体发生一种对自己细胞的免疫反应，风湿性关节炎（rheumatoid arthritis）就是一个例子。

线粒体（mitochondria）有自己的DNA，因为在早期发育中它们可能是独立的生物体，DNA或细胞核DNA的突变（变化）控制线粒体活动，可能会干扰ATP的产生，并损害全身的器官。这些线粒体失调很难诊断，因为它们会引起不同的症状，会与癫痫（epilepsy）、脑瘫（cerebral palsy）和多发性硬化症（multiple sclerosis）混淆。

胞膜。其他一些失调源于线粒体（mitochondria）、内质网（endoplasmic reticulum，ER）、溶酶体（lysosomes）或过氧化物酶体（peroxisomes），如框4-2所示。

细胞核是细胞的控制区域，包含携带基因信息的染色体（chromosomes）（图4-3）。除生殖细胞外，每个人类细胞都包含46条染色体。染色体的线状结构由复杂的有机物质脱氧核糖核酸（deoxyribonucleic acid，DNA）构成，DNA组成单独的单元，被称为基因。基因控制蛋白质的合成，这些蛋白质大都是特别的酶，用于加速新陈代谢反应。为了促进蛋白质的产生，细胞使用了一种被称为核糖核酸（ribonucleic acid，RNA）的化合物，在化学上与DNA相关。基因或染色体的变化（突变）是遗传疾病的病源。

当细胞体发生有丝分裂时，染色体数量增加一倍，并被平均分配到两个子细胞。有丝分裂各阶段如图4-4所示，不分裂时，细胞处于分裂间隔期。发生癌变时，细胞不受控制地分裂，引起细胞增生和肿瘤。生殖细胞（卵和精子）会发生减数分裂（meiosis），染色体减半，为受精做准备。

细胞的研究被称为细胞学（cytology），基于词根 cyt/o，意为"细胞"。框4-3给出了细胞学领域的职业信息。

组织

细胞能组成四种执行特定功能的组织：

上皮（epithelial [ˌepɪ'θiːlɪəl]）组织如图4-5所示，

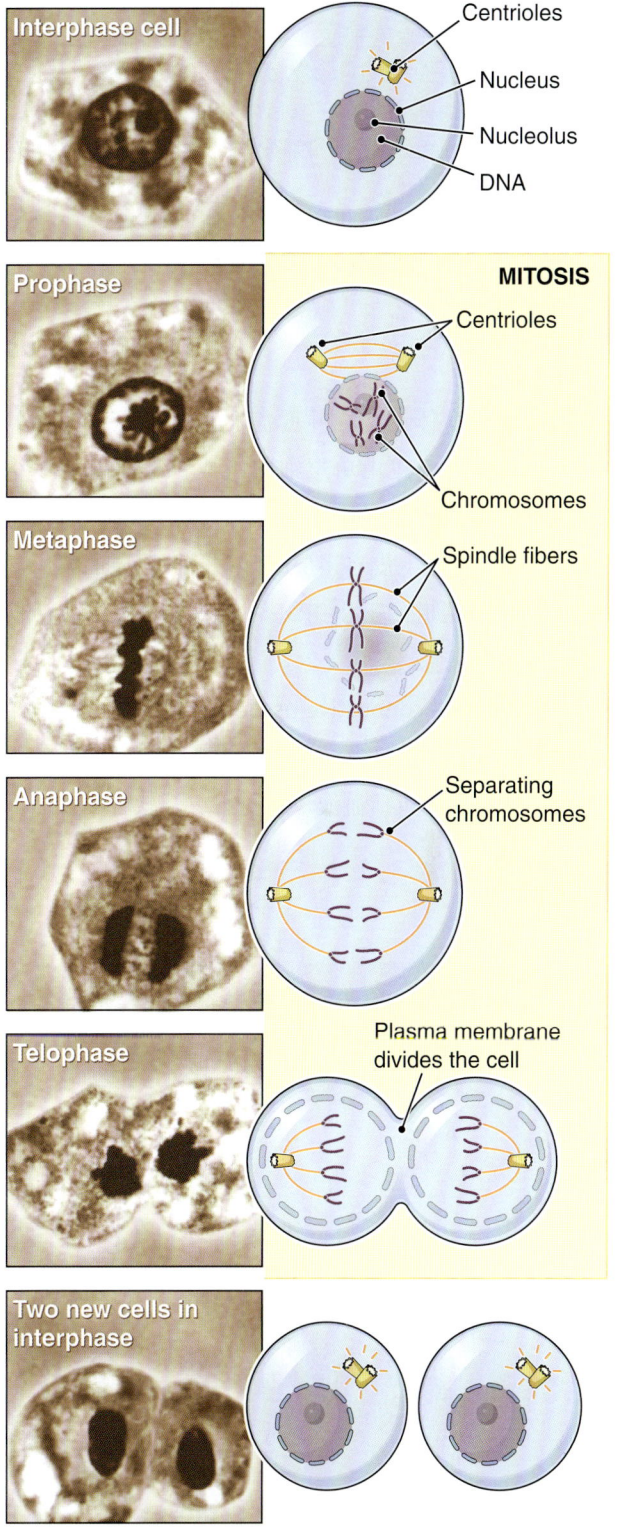

图4-4 **细胞分裂的阶段。** 当不进行有丝分裂（mitosis）时，细胞处于分裂间期。图中显示的细胞仅用于说明。它不是一个人类细胞，虽然有46条染色体

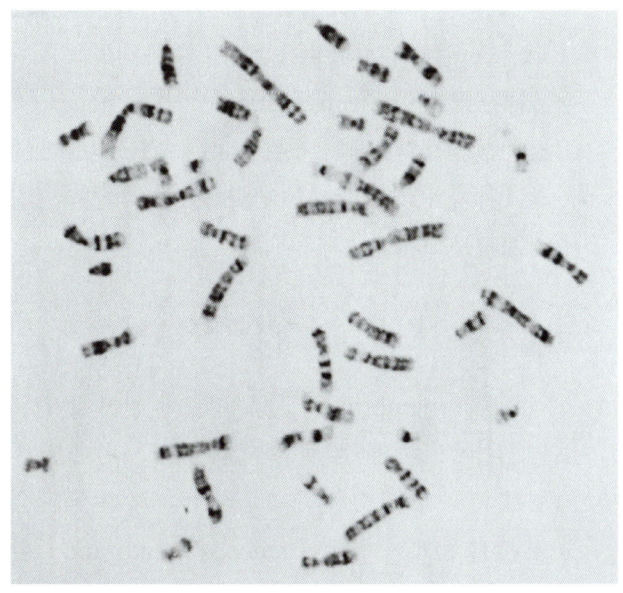

图4-3 **人类染色体。** 除殖细胞外每个人类细胞都包含46条染色体

> 框 4-3
>
> ### 健康职业
> #### 细胞技术人员
>
> 细胞技术是细胞的实验室研究。细胞技术人员（cytotechnologist）与病理学家（pathologist）合作，根据细胞变化诊断癌症、感染和其他疾病。这个职业最初开发用于研究宫颈涂片诊断宫颈癌，但后来扩展到包括来自许多其他身体部位，如腺体、淋巴结、器官和体腔的标本的分析。除了直接显微镜研究，细胞技术人员的工作现在还包括分子分析和免疫化学，通常涉及复杂的自动化和计算机化仪器。
>
> 对细胞技术职业有兴趣的人应该认真和独立，有高度的责任感，善于做出决定。这一领域需要学士学位，课程包括解剖学、化学、微生物学、组织学、数学或统计学，加上专业的实验室培训。成功完成课程后，毕业生有资格参加美国临床病理学会（American Society for Clinical Pathology, ASCP）注册局认证考试。对监督、管理或教学职位感兴趣的人需要高级学位和 3～5 年的专业经验，还应该获得细胞技术专家的 ASCP 认证。细胞技术认可的项目可在联合认证委员会（Commission on Accreditation on Allied Health Programs, CAAHEP）的网站上找到：http://www.caahep.org。美国细胞工程学会（American Society for Cytotechnology）开发了实践标准，监测监管问题，评估新技术，并为专业提供教育机会，他们的网站是 http://www.asct.com。

覆盖并保护身体结构，并覆盖器官、管道和腔体的内部。简单的上皮由单层细胞组成，功能是从一个系统吸收物质到另一个系统，如呼吸系统和消化系统的管道。复层上皮有多层细胞，保护深层的组织，如在口腔和阴道的上皮组织。腺体中的大多数活性细胞是上皮细胞。

结缔组织（connective tissue）支持并约束身体结构（图 4-6），它包含纤维和其他细胞之间的非生物物质。这类组织包括血液、脂肪组织、软骨和骨骼。

肌肉组织（muscle tissue）（词根：my/o）收缩产生运动（图 4-7）。肌肉组织分三类：

- 骨骼肌（skeletal muscle）移动骨骼，它有可见的交叉带或横纹状，参与肌肉的收缩。因为处于意识控制之下，也被称为随意肌（voluntary muscle）。
- 心肌（cardiac muscle）组成心脏，它不在意识控制之下，被称为非随意肌（involuntary muscle）。
- 平滑肌或内脏肌（smooth or visceral muscle）构成腹腔器官的壁，也是非随意肌肉。人体中的许多器官都有由平滑肌构成的壁，管道和血管也主要由平滑肌构成。

神经组织（nervous tissue）（词根：neur/o）组成大脑、脊髓和神经（图 4-8）。通过电脉冲的传导，神经组织协调并控制身体反应。神经组织中的细胞是神经元或神经细胞。

薄膜

薄膜（membrane）是简单的、非常薄的、柔韧的组织片。薄膜可以覆盖器官、形成腔体内层或将一个结构与另一个分开。某些薄膜会分泌特殊物质。黏膜（mucous membrane）会分泌一种润滑表面并保护其下组织的黏液，如覆盖在消化道和呼吸道内的黏膜。浆膜（serous membrane）会分泌稀薄的水状液体，构成身体腔

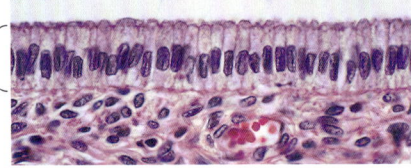
A

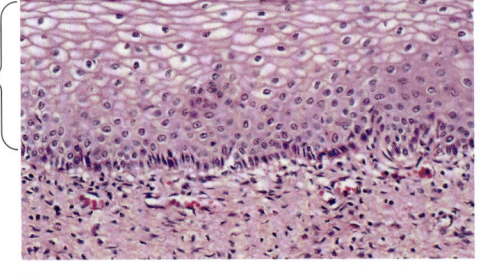
B

图 4-5　上皮组织。A. 简单上皮中的细胞在单层中，并且从一个系统到另一个系统吸收物质；B. 分层上皮中的细胞在多个层中，保护更深的组织

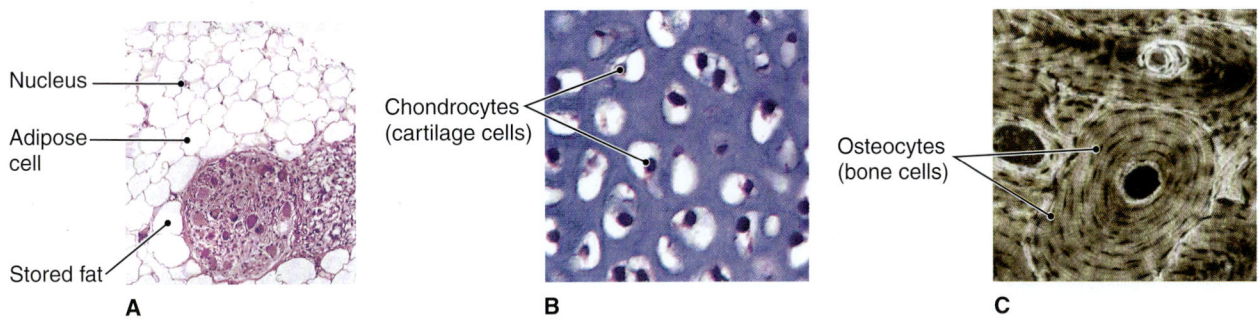

图4-6 结缔组织。(A)结缔组织的示例是储存脂肪组织(adipose tissue);(B)用于保护和加固的软骨(cartilage);(C)构成骨架的骨骼(bone)

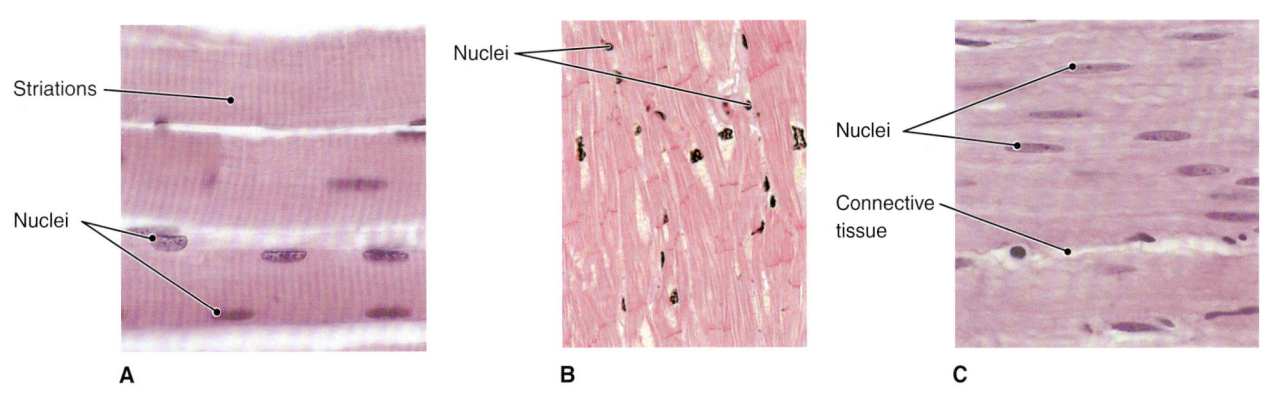

图4-7 肌肉组织。(A)骨骼肌移动骨骼,具有产生收缩的可见的条纹;(B)心肌构成心脏的壁;(C)平滑肌组成中空器官、管道和血管壁

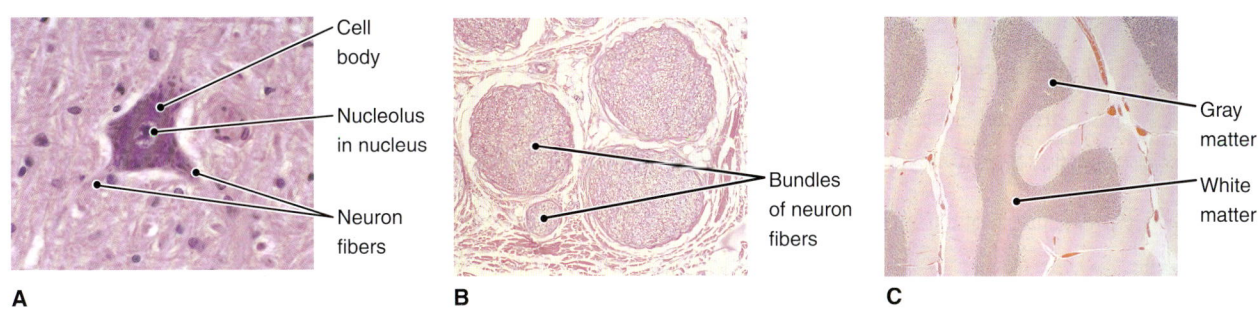

图4-8 神经组织。(A)神经系统的功能细胞是神经元;(B)神经元纤维结合形成神经;(C)神经组织也构成脊髓和大脑,分为灰质(gray matter)和白质(white matter)

体内膜并覆盖器官,包括心脏和肺周围的膜。纤维膜(fibrous membrane)覆盖并支撑器官,在骨骼、大脑和脊髓周围都有纤维膜。

组织的研究被称为组织学(histology),基于词根hist/o,意为"组织"。框4-4给出了组织学使用的一些名词。

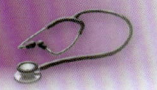

临床观点
组织的实验室研究

框 4-4

活组织检查（biopsy）就是将活的组织切下来并做检查，以确定诊断。这个名词也用于样本本身。Biopsy 源自于希腊单词 bio，意为"生命"，加上 opsis，意为"视力"。加在一起意为"活组织的形象"。

一些被用于细胞核组织的名词来源于拉丁语。体内（in vivo）意为"在活的身体中"，与体外（in vitro）正好相反，in vitro 的字面含义为"在镜中"，是指实验室中所做的实验和程序，与在活的生物体内所做的研究相对应。原位（in situ）意为"在其原始的位置"，用于指未扩散的肿瘤。

In toto 意为"整体"或"全部"，用于指被从体内完全切除的结构或器官。死后（postmortem）在字面上意为"死亡之后"，被用于指为确定死因所做的尸体解剖。

器官与器官系统

组织构成器官，器官具有特定的功能，并构成身体系统，图 4-9 给出了消化系统作为示例。根据功能的不同，身体系统如下：

循环（circulation）：
- 心血管系统（cardiovascular system），由心脏和血管组成。
- 淋巴系统（lymphatic system）、器官和管道帮助循环，并协助保护身体免受外来物种的侵害。

营养与体液平衡（nutrition and fluid balance）：
- 呼吸系统（respiratory system），获得新陈代谢所需的氧气，并排出新陈代谢的副产品二氧化碳。
- 消化系统（digestive system），摄入、分解并吸收营养，排出不能消化的废物。
- 泌尿系统（urinary system），排出可溶性废物，平衡体液的容量和成分。

产生后代（production of offspring）：
- 男性和女性生殖系统（the male and female reproductive systems）。

协调与控制（coordination and control）：
- 神经系统（nervous system），由大脑、脊髓和神经组成，包含传感系统。该系统接收和处理刺激，并指导身体的反应。
- 内分泌系统（endocrine system），由产生激素的各个腺体组成。

身体结构与运动（body structure and movement）：
- 骨骼系统（skeletal system），由骨骼和关节组成。
- 肌肉系统（muscular system），移动骨骼并建立器官、肌肉系统和骨骼共同保护生命器官。

身体覆盖（body covering）：
- 皮肤系统（the integumentary system），包括皮肤及其相关结构，例如头发、汗腺和油腺。该系统的功能是保护并协助调节体温。

人体是作为一个整体活动的，没有任何系统是独立的。这些系统共同维护身体的内在稳定性，这种稳定性被称为体内平衡。

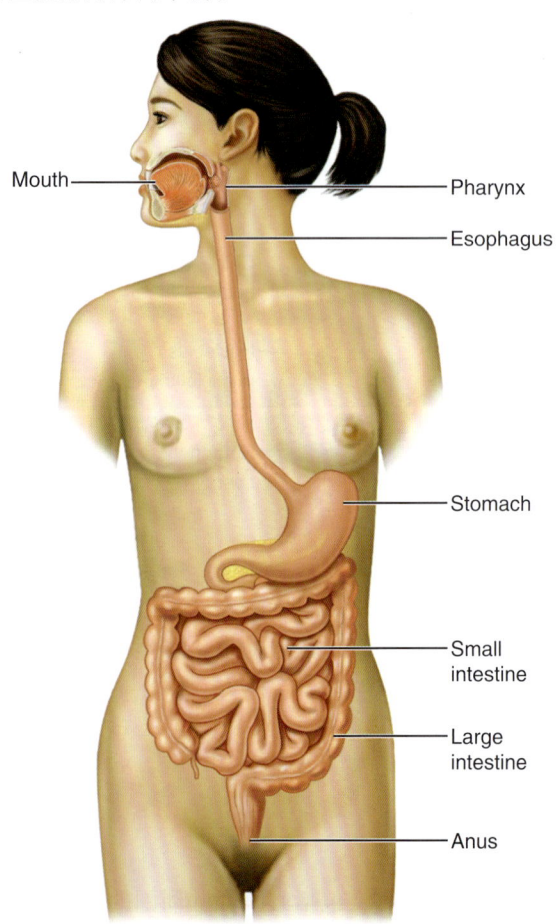

图 4-9 消化器官。其他器官和腺体有助于消化

Terminology 关键术语

ATP		三磷酸腺苷,细胞的能量化合物,储存细胞活动所需的能量;adenosine triphosphate [ə'denə(ʊ)si:n trai'fɑs,fet]
carbohydrate	[kɑ:bə'haidreit]	碳水化合物,一类有机化合物,包括糖和淀粉
cell	[sel]	细胞,生物体的基本结构和功能单元,是一种在显微镜下可见的单元,与其他细胞一起构成组织(词根 cyt/o)
chromosome	['krəʊməsəʊm]	染色体,细胞核中的线状物体,包含基因信息
cytology	[sai'tɒlədʒi]	细胞学,细胞的研究
cytoplasm	['saitə(ʊ)plæz(ə)m]	细胞质,充满细胞并支撑细胞器的液体
DNA		脱氧核糖核酸,细胞的基因化合物,构成基因;deoxyribonucleic [di:'ɔksi,raibəu'nju:kli:ik] acid
enzyme	['enzaim]	酶,加速新陈代谢反应的一种有机物质
gene	[dʒi:n]	基因,由 DNA 组成的遗传单元,与其他基因一起构成染色体
glucose	['glu:kəʊs]	葡萄糖,在血液中循环的一种单糖,新陈代谢的主要能量来源(词根 gluc/o,glyc/o)
histology	[hi'stɒlədʒi]	组织学,组织的研究
homeostasis	[ˌhəʊmiə(ʊ)'steisis]	体内平衡,一种稳定状态,内部稳定与恒定的状态
lipid	['lipid]	脂类,一类包括脂肪的有机化合物(词根 lip/o)
membrane	['membrein]	薄膜,一种简单、非常薄、柔韧的组织片,可以覆盖器官、构成腔体或分开身体结构
metabolism	[mi'tæbəliz(ə)m]	新陈代谢,生物体内发生的所有物理和化学反应的总和
mitosis	[mai'təʊsis]	细胞分裂
mucus	['mju:kəs]	黏液,由薄膜或腺体中的细胞分泌的一种黏稠的液体,润滑并保护组织(词根 muc/o,myx/o);形容词形式是 mucous
nucleus	['nju:kliəs]	细胞核,细胞的控制中心,基于其染色体包含的信息指导所有细胞活动
organ	['ɔ:g(ə)n]	器官,身体中具有特定功能的部分,是身体系统的组成部分
organelle	[ˌɔ:gə'nel]	细胞器,细胞质中的一种特殊结构
protein	['prəʊti:n]	蛋白质,一类有机化合物,包括结构性物质、酶和某些激素
RNA		核糖核酸,参与细胞内蛋白质生成的一种有机化合物;ribonucleic [ˌri:bəunju:'kli:ik] acid
tissue	['tisju:]	组织,一组为特定目的共同活动的细胞(词根 hist/o,histi/o)

与细胞、组织和器官相关的单词组成部分

见表 4-1 至表 4-3

表 4-1	细胞和组织的词根		
词根	含义	示例	示例定义
morph/o	形状	polymorphous [ˌpɒliˈmɔːfəs]	多形的
cyt/o, -cyte	细胞	cytologist [saiˈtɒlədʒist]	细胞学家
nucle/o	细胞核	nuclear [ˈnjuːkliə]	细胞核的
kary/o	细胞核	karyotype [ˈkæriə(ʊ)taip]	细胞染色体组型（图4-10）
hist/o, histi/o	组织	histocompatibility [ˌhistəʊkəmˌpætəˈbiləti]	组织兼容
fibr/o	纤维	fibrosis [faiˈbrəʊsis]	纤维变性
reticul/o	网	reticulum [riˈtikjʊləm]	网状物
aden/o	腺体	adenoma [ˌædiˈnəʊmə]	腺体肿瘤
papill/o	乳头	papilla [pəˈpilə]	乳头状突起
myx/o	黏液	myxadenitis [ˌmiksædiˈnaitis]	黏液腺炎
muc/o	黏液，黏膜	mucorrhea [məˈkəʊriə]	黏液外流
somat/o, -some	身体，小体	chromosome [ˈkrəʊməsəʊm]	染色体

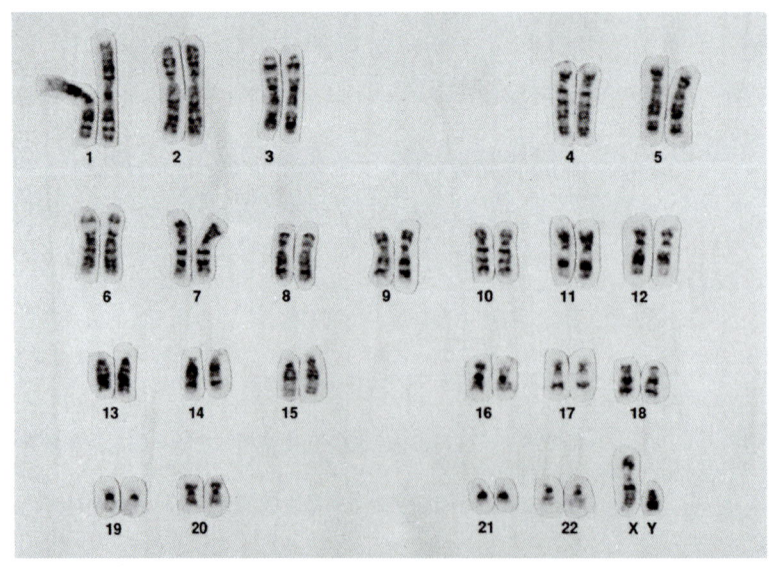

图 4-10　**人类染色体组型**。46条染色体按照大小排列成23对。XY性染色体，第23对在右下角，表明细胞来自男性；女性细胞为XX性染色体

练习 4-1

填空，并读出标有音标的单词。

1. Cytogenesis [ˌsaɪtəˈdʒenəsɪs] is the formation (genesis) of _____.
2. A fibril [ˈfaɪbrɪl] is a small _____.
3. A histologist [hɪˈstɒlədʒɪst] studies _____.
4. A dimorphic [daɪˈmɔːfɪk] organism has two _____.
5. Karyomegaly [ˌkærɪəˈmegəli] is enlargement (-megaly) of the _____.
6. Nucleoplasm [ˈnjuːklɪəˌplæzəm] is the substance that fills the _____.
7. Adenitis [ˌædəˈnaɪtɪs] is inflammation (-itis) of a (n) _____.
8. A papillary [pəˈpɪləri] structure resembles a (n) _____.
9. A myxoma [mɪksˈəʊmə] is a tumor of tissue that secretes _____.
10. A reticulocyte [rɪˈtɪkjʊləsaɪt] is a cell that contains a (n) _____.
11. The term mucosa [mjuːˈkəʊsə] is used to describe a membrane that secretes _____.
12. Somatotropin [ˌsəʊmətəʊˈtrəʊpɪn], also called growth hormone, has a general stimulating effect on the _____.

使用后缀 -logy 构建有下列含义的单词。

13. The study of form _____
14. The study of cells _____
15. The study of tissues _____

表 4-2 中的词根通常与一个简单的名词后缀（-in、-y 或 -ia）或形容词后缀（-ic）组合，被用于单词结尾。在本书中将这种日常作为词尾出现的组合视为后缀，例如 -trophy、-plasia、-tropin、-philic 和 -genic。

表 4-2 细胞活动的词根

词根	含义	示例	示例定义
blast/o, -blast	未成熟细胞、生产性细胞、胚胎细胞	histioblast [ˈhɪstɪəblɑːst]	成组织细胞
gen	起端、生成	karyogenesis [ˌkærɪə(ʊ)ˈdʒenɪsɪs]	细胞核生成
phag/o	吃、消化	autophagy [ɔːˈtɒfədʒi]	自噬
phil	吸引、吸收	basophilic [ˌbesəˈfɪlɪk]	嗜碱性的
plas	生成、成形、发育	hyperplasia [ˌhaɪpəˈpleɪzɪə]	增生
trop	对……有影响，影响	chronotropic [krɒnəˈtrɒpɪk]	变时性的
troph/o	喂食、成长、营养	atrophy [ˈætrəfi]	组织退化

练习 4-2

匹配以下各组中的术语，并在每个数字的左侧写入相应的字母。

____ 1. phagocyte ['fægəsait]
____ 2. histogenesis [ˌhisto'dʒɛnisis]
____ 3. leukoblast ['lju:kəblæst]
____ 4. genetics [dʒə'nɛtiks]
____ 5. hypertrophy [hai'pɜtrəfi]

a. overdevelopment of tissue
b. study of heredity
c. formation of tissue
d. cell that ingests waste
e. immature white blood cell

____ 6. neoplasia [ˌnio'pleʒir]
____ 7. gonadotropin [ˌgɔnədə'trɔpin]
____ 8. aplasia [ə'pleʒə]
____ 9. somatic [so'mætik]
____ 10. chromophilic [ˌkrəumɒu'filik]

a. attracting color
b. pertaining to the body
c. substance that acts on the sex glands
d. new formation of tissue
e. lack of development

识别并定义下列单词中的词根。

	Root	Meaning of Root
11. genesis ['dʒenəsis]	gen	origin, formation
12. esophagus [i'sɒfəgəs]		
13. normoblast ['nɔ:məblɑ:st]		
14. aplastic [ə'plæstik]		
15. dystrophy ['distrəfi]		

表 4-3　体内化学成分的后缀和词根

词根	含义	示例	示例定义
后缀			
-ase	酶	lipase ['lipeiz]	脂肪酶
-ose	糖	lactose ['læktəʊs]	乳糖
词根			
hydr/o	水、液体	hydration [hai'dreiʃən]	水合作用
gluc/o	葡萄糖	glucogenesis [ˌglu:kəʊ'dʒeni:sis]	葡萄糖生成
glyc/o	糖、葡萄糖	normoglycemia [ˌnɒməglai'si:miə]	血糖量正常
sacchar/o	糖	polysaccharide [ˌpɒli'sækəraid]	多糖
amyl/o	淀粉	amyloid ['æmilɒid]	淀粉状的
lip/o	脂类、脂肪	lipophilic [ˌlipə(ʊ)'filik]	亲脂的
adip/o	脂肪	adiposuria [ˌædi'pɒsju:riə]	脂肪尿
steat/o	脂肪的	steatorrhea [ˌstiətə'ri:ə]	脂肪痢
prote/o	蛋白质	protease ['prəʊtieiz]	蛋白酶

练习 4-3

填空。

1. A disaccharide [daiˈsækərid] is a compound that contains two _____.
2. The ending -ose indicates that fructose is a(n) _____.
3. Hydrophobia [ˈhaidrəˈfobiə] is an aversion (-phobia) to _____.
4. Amylase [ˈæmiˌles] is an enzyme that digests _____.
5. Liposuction [ˈliposʌkʃən] is the surgical removal of _____.
6. A glucocorticoid [ˌɡlʊkoˈkɔrtiˌkɔid] is a hormone that controls the metabolism of _____.
7. An adipocyte [ˈædipəʊˌsait] is a cell that stores _____.

识别并定义下列单词中的词根。

	Root	Meaning of Root
8. asteatosis [əstiəˈtəʊsis]	____	_____
9. lipoma [liˈpəʊmə]	____	_____
10. hyperglycemia [ˌhaipəɡlaiˈsiːmiə]	____	_____
11. glucolytic [gˈluːkəlaitik]	____	_____

Terminology 补充术语

amino acids [əˈmiːnəʊ]	氨基酸，能够生成蛋白质的含氮化合物
anabolism [əˈnæbəliz(ə)m]	合成代谢，一种制造身体物质的新陈代谢；新陈代谢的建立阶段
catabolism [kəˈtæbəliz(ə)m]	分解代谢，一种将物质分解成能量和简单化合物的新陈代谢
collagen [ˈkɒlədʒ(ə)n]	胶原蛋白，一种在结缔组织中发现的纤维蛋白
cortex [ˈkɔːteks]	皮质，器官的外层
glycogen [ˈɡlaikədʒ(ə)n]	糖原，肝糖一种储存在肝脏和肌肉中的复合糖化合物，当需要能量时被分解为葡萄糖
interstitial [ˌintəˈstiʃ(ə)l]	细胞间隙，组织内细胞之间的空隙
parenchyma [pəˈreŋkimə]	软组织，器官中的功能性组织
parietal [pəˈraiit(ə)l]	腔壁的，与腔体壁相关的，用于描述体腔内部的薄膜
soma [ˈsəʊmə]	躯体，身体
stem cell	干细胞，一种能够发育成任意不同类型细胞的未成熟细胞，一种前体细胞
visceral [ˈvis(ə)r(ə)l]	内脏的，与体内器官相关的，用于描述器官表面的薄膜

Case Study Revisited
案例研究再访

R. S.'s Return to Class Schedule

Following his appointment, R.S. decided to accept his doctor's advice. He started preparing at least two meals a day at home and often boxed a lunch to eat during the day on campus. The more nutritious meals provided him greater energy; he no longer felt sluggish. He visited the university gym to work out at least two to three times a week for 20 minutes and hoped to increase that time when his schedule permitted. He realized how important exercise is to feeling energized, upbeat, and more confident in his everyday activities. Finally, he recognized that a little knowledge is a dangerous thing and that it is not smart to try and diagnose oneself.

R.S. 返回课堂

约见医生后，R. S. 决定接受医生的建议。他每天在家准备至少两餐，并经常在校园吃自带的午饭。营养更丰富的饮食给他更多的能量，他不再感到倦怠。他经常去大学健身房，每周至少锻炼 2 ~ 3 次，每次 20 分钟，并希望在日程安排允许的时候增加锻炼时间。他意识到运动非常重要，在日常活动中感觉充满活力、乐观，且更有信心。最后，他认识到缺乏知识是一件危险的事情，试图自我诊断并不聪明。

CHAPTER 4 复习

标记练习

在相应的下划线上写出每个编号部分的名称。

Centriole
Cytosol
Golgi apparatus
Lysosome
Microvilli
Mitochondrion
Nuclear membrane
Nucleolus

Nucleus
Peroxisome
Plasma membrane
Ribosomes
Rough ER
Smooth ER
Vesicle

1. _____
2. _____
3. _____
4. _____
5. _____
6. _____
7. _____
8. _____
9. _____
10. _____
11. _____
12. _____
13. _____
14. _____
15. _____

匹配

匹配以下术语，并在每个数字的左侧写入相应的字母。

____ 1. ATP   a. small bodies that store fat

____ 2. DNA   b. material that holds the cellular organelles

____ 3. nucle oplasm   c. energy compound of the cells

____ 4. liposomes   d. genetic material

____ 5. cytoplasm   e. material that fills the nucleus

____ 6. blastocyte   a. immature cell

____ 7. ribosomes   b. organelles that produce ATP
____ 8. mitochondria   c. organelles that contain RNA
____ 9. mitosis   d. small cellular body containing digestive enzymes
____ 10. lysosome   e. cell division

____ 11. reticular   a. resembling a gland
____ 12. adenoid   b. fibrous tumor
____ 13. fibroma   c. cell with a very large nucleus
____ 14. megakaryocyte   d. pertaining to a network
____ 15. chromosome   e. structure that contains genes

____ 16. autotroph   a. resembling a nipple
____ 17. papilliform   b. having no specific form
____ 18. amorphous   c. wasting of tissue
____ 19. atrophy   d. pertaining to the body
____ 20. somatic   e. organism that can manufacture its own food

____ 21. fibroplasia   a. difficulty in eating
____ 22. hypoplasia   b. dissolving of fat
____ 23. dysphagia   c. underdevelopment of an organ or tissue
____ 24. cytogenesis   d. formation of fibrous tissue
____ 25. lipolysis   e. formation of cells

____ 26. adiposuria   a. presence of fat in the urine
____ 27. proteolytic   b. presence of glucose in the urine
____ 28. glucosuria   c. treatment using water
____ 29. polysaccharide   d. compound composed of many simple sugars
____ 30. hydrotherapy   e. destroying or dissolving protein

补充术语。

____ 31. amino acid   a. pertaining to the internal organs
____ 32. collagen   b. breakdown phase of metabolism
____ 33. visceral   c. fibrous protein in connective tissue
____ 34. cortex   d. outer region of an organ
____ 35. catabolism   e. building block of protein

填空。

36. The study of tissues is called _____.
37. The four basic tissue types are _____.
38. All the activities of a cell make up its _____.
39. The system that includes the kidneys and bladder is the _____.
40. The systems involved in circulation are the cardiovascular system and the _____.
41. The simple sugar that is the main energy source for metabolism is _____.
42. A thick cellular secretion that lubricates and protects tissues is called _____.

43. An organic compound that speeds the rate of metabolic reactions is a（n）_____.
44. A cytotoxic substance is poisonous or damaging to_____.
45. The term dehydration refers to a loss or deficiency of_____.
46. The study of form and structure is called _____.
47. A myxocyte is found in tissue that secretes _____.

真假判断

检查以下语句，如果语句为真，则在第一个空白处写 T；如果语句为假，则在第一个空格中写 F，并在第二个空格中通过替换带下划线的单词来更正语句。

	true or False	correct Answer
48. A megakaryocyte is a cell with a large <u>nucleus</u>.	_____	_____
49. Hydrophobia is an aversion to <u>fats</u>.	_____	_____
50. An adipocyte is a cell that stores <u>glucose</u>.	_____	_____
51. There are <u>46</u> chromosomes in each human cell, aside from the reproductive cells.	_____	_____
52. A whip-like extension of a cell is a <u>flagellum</u>.	_____	_____

单词构建

使用给出的单词组成部分写出下列定义的单词，每个组成部分可以使用多次。

```
-oid    amyl/o    muc/o    aden/o    -ase    lip/o    leuk/o    histi/o    blast
```

53. Like or resembling a gland _____
54. Immature white blood cell _____
55. Enzyme that digests fat _____
56. Resembling mucus _____
57. Cell that gives rise to tissue _____
58. Enzyme that digests starch _____
59. Resembling starch _____

单词分析

定义下列单词，并给出每个单词组成部分的含义，必要时可以使用词典。

60. homeostasis [ˌhomiəˈstesis]
        a. homeo_____   **b.** stat（from Greek states）_____   **c.** -sis_____
61. somatotropic [səmətətˈropik]
        a. somat/o_____   **b.** trop/o_____   **c.** -ic_____
62. autophagy [ɔˈtafədʒi]
        a. auto_____   **b.** phag/o_____   **c.** -y_____
63. asteatosis [əstirˈtousis]
        a. a-_____   **b.** steat/o_____   **c.** -sis_____

Additional Case Studies
补充案例研究

Case Study 4-1: Hematology Laboratory Studies
案例研究 4-1：血液学实验室研究

J. E. had a blood test as required for a preoperative anesthesia assessment in preparation for scheduled plastic surgery on her breasts. The report read as follows:

Complete blood count (CBC) and differential:

Red blood cell (RBC) count—4.5 million/mcL

Hemoglobin (Hgb)—12.6 g/dL

Hematocrit (Hct)—38 percent

White blood cell (WBC) count—8,500/mcL

Neutrophils—58 percent

Lymphocytes—34 percent

Monocytes—6 percent

Eosinophils—1.5 percent

Basophils—0.5 percent

Platelet count—200,000/mcL

Prothrombin time (PT)—11.5 seconds

Partial thromboplastin time (PTT)—65 seconds

Blood glucose—84 mg/dL

The surgeon reviewed these results and concluded that they were within normal limits (WNL).

J. E. 进行了术前麻醉评估所需的血液检查，以准备进行预约乳房整形手术。检查报告如下：

全血细胞计数（complete blood count，CBC）和差异：

红细胞（red blood cell，RBC）计数—4.5 million/mcl

血红蛋白（hemoglobin，Hgb）—12.6 g/dl

血细胞比容（hematocrit，Hct）—38 %

白细胞（white blood cell，WBC）计数—8,500/mcl

嗜中性粒细胞（neutrophils）—58 %

淋巴细胞（lymphocytes）—34 %

单核细胞（monocytes）—6 %

嗜酸性粒细胞（eosinophils）—1.5 %

嗜碱性粒细胞（basophils）—0.5 %

血小板（platelet）计数—200,000/mcl

凝血酶原时间（prothrombin time，PT）—11.5s

部分凝血活酶时间（partial thromboplastin time，PTT）—65s

血糖（blood glucose）—84 mg/dl

外科医生审查了这些结果，并得出结论，指标都在正常范围内。

Case Study 4-2: Needle Aspiration of Thyroid Tumor
案例研究 4-2：甲状腺肿瘤针吸术

Chief Complaint

D. S., a 65-year-old male, noticed a lump on the side of his neck and went to see his physician. He has a history of prostate cancer and had a prostatectomy four years ago. Bilateral lymph node dissection revealed no metastasis. His physician referred him to a surgeon for evaluation of a nodule on the thyroid gland.

Examination

Dr. Thompson, a general surgeon, examined D.S. and recommended a needle aspiration of the thyroid gland. The ultrasound-guided fine needle aspiration revealed atypical cells with abundant cytoplasm and prominent nuclei but no metastasis. However, the nuclei showed some morphologic changes. Histologic slides of the left thyroid showed clusters of epithelial cells associated with lymphocytes suggestive of

主诉

D. S. 是一名 65 岁的男性，他注意到脖子一侧的肿块，并去看他的医生。他有前列腺癌（prostate cancer）的病史，并在 4 年前进行了前列腺切除术（prostatectomy），双侧淋巴结解剖显示无转移。他的医生将他转诊给外科医生做甲状腺（thyroid gland）结节评估。

检查

普通外科医生 Dr. Thompson 检查了 D.S.，并推荐甲状腺针吸术（needle aspiration of the thyroid gland）。超声引导细针抽吸显示具有丰富细胞质和突出细胞核的非典型细胞，但没有转移。然而，细胞核显示一些形态变化。左侧甲状腺的组织学幻灯片显示有与淋巴

lymphocytic thyroiditis.

Clinical Course

D. S. underwent a total thyroidectomy and is healing well. A follow-up CT scan of the neck and chest showed no additional nodules or indications of metastatic disease.

细胞相关的上皮细胞簇，提示有淋巴细胞性甲状腺炎（lymphocytic thyroiditis）。

临床病程

D. S. 经历了全甲状腺切除术（thyroidectomy）并且愈合良好。颈部和胸部的后续 CT 扫描显示没有额外的结节或转移性疾病的迹象。

多项选择。选择最佳答案，并写上你选择的字母。

____ 1. J.E.'s blood test results were within normal limits. She could be described as being in a state of
   a. homeopathy
   b. neoplasia
   c. hematophilia
   d. homeostasis

____ 2. The suffix in glucose indicates that this compound is a（n）
   a. enzyme
   b. sugar
   c. protein
   d. fat

____ 3. The suffix in prostatectomy and thyroidectomy means
   a. removal or excision
   b. incision into
   c. inflammation
   d. resembling

____ 4. The singular form of nuclei is
   a. nucleolus
   b. nucleoli
   c. nucleum
   d. nucleus

识别并给出下列单词中前缀的含义。

	Prefix	Meaning of Prefix
5. atypical	____	____
6. prothrombin	____	____
7. bilateral	____	____
8. monocytes	____	____
9. dissection	____	____
10. metastasis	____	____

在案例研究中找出以下单词。

11. Three words that contain a root that means attract, absorb _____

12. Two words with a root that means formation, molding, development _____

13. A word with a root that means form _____

14. A word with a root that means tissue _____

15. Four words that contain a root that means cell _____

CHAPTER 5

身体结构

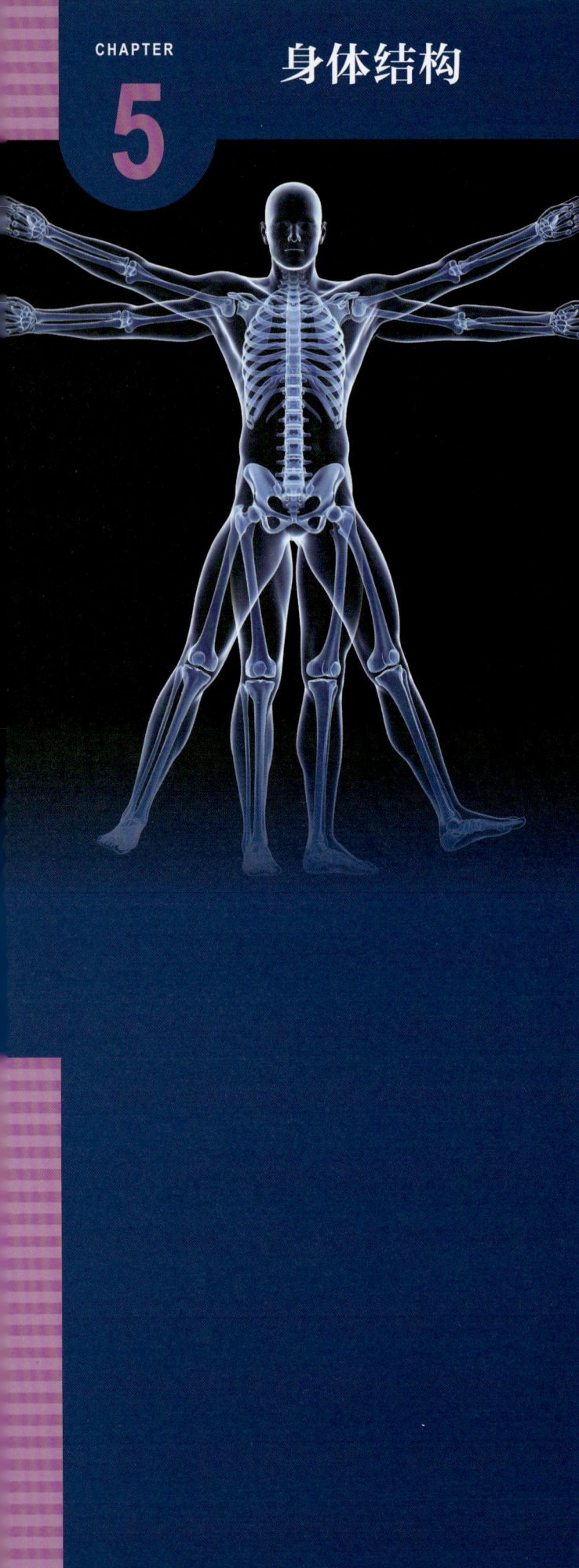

预测试

多项选择，选择最佳答案，并在每个数字的左边写上你选择的字母。

____ 1. In humans, dorsal is another term for
   a. lateral
   b. central
   c. anterior
   d. posterior

____ 2. A plane that divides the body into left and right parts is a
   a. coronal plane
   b. sagittal plane
   c. transverse plane
   d. frontal plane

____ 3. The scientific name for the chest cavity is
   a. cranial cavity
   b. dorsal cavity
   c. thoracic cavity
   d. pelvic cavity

____ 4. The brain and spinal cord are in which cavity?
   a. dorsal
   b. abdominal
   c. cervical
   d. ventral

____ 5. The root cephal/o refers to the
   a. spine
   b. head
   c. chest
   d. lungs

____ 6. The root brachi/o refers to the
   a. head
   b. spinal cord
   c. leg
   d. arm

____ 7. The prefix inter- means
   a. outside
   b. between
   c. around
   d. over

____ 8. The prefix supra- means
   a. above
   b. near
   c. behind
   d. below

学习目标

学完本章后，应该能够：

1 ▶ 定义解剖学中使用的主要方向性术语。
2 ▶ 描述人体的三个截面。
3 ▶ 定位背侧腔和腹侧腔的体腔。
4 ▶ 定位并为腹部的九个分区命名。
5 ▶ 定位并为腹部的四个象限命名。
6 ▶ 描述医学实践中使用的主要体位。
7 ▶ 定义描述人体结构的基本术语。
8 ▶ 认识并使用与人体部位相关的词根。
9 ▶ 认识并使用与体外和方向相关的前缀。
10 ▶ 识别案例研究中关于人体结构的医学单词和缩略语。

Case Study: B.K.'s Stomach Ache
案例研究：B. K. 的胃痛

Chief Complaint

It was summer vacation, and B. K. and his older brother were hosting a lemonade stand in front of their home. Late in the afternoon, B. K., a 4-year-old male, appeared agitated and complained to his mother that he had a stomach ache. His mother recalled that she had given him a peanut butter and jelly sandwich and an apple for lunch earlier in the day. He had had no problems eating his lunch. Later in the day, she saw her son curled up on the couch crying and holding his stomach, and she decided to take him to the after-hours clinic where the child's pediatrician was on staff.

Examination

Dr. Davies, B. K.'s pediatrician, had known the boy since he was a newborn. B. K.'s parents made certain that their son had physical examinations on a regular basis. His immunizations were current, and aside from a few earaches and colds, B. K. was a healthy young boy. Upon arrival in the clinic, the office medical assistant recorded that B.K.'s vital signs were within normal limits. Dr. Davies then saw the patient and had him lie supine on the examination table. He performed a cephalocaudal assessment. The only abnormality causing concern was the abdominal pain B. K. said he was experiencing. Dr. Davies asked B.K. to show him where it hurt the most. The boy first pointed to the left upper quadrant of his abdomen and then, somewhat confused, pointed to his right lower quadrant. The medical assistant returned and drew some blood for laboratory studies, which later showed normal results. Dr. Davies then ordered an abdominal x-ray.

Clinical Course

The x-ray revealed that B. K. had swallowed a nickel and a penny. The boy then confessed that he was trying to hide the money from his brother, so he had swallowed the coins. Dr. Davies explained to B. K. and his mother that he expected no serious complications and that the coins should be expelled in the next 24 hours or so.

In this chapter, we learn about body regions and orientations and become familiar with some of the terms healthcare professionals use to pinpoint exact locations on and within the body.

主诉

在暑假期间，B. K. 和他的哥哥在家门前开设了一个柠檬水站。下午晚些时候，4 岁的男孩 B. K. 似乎很激动，向母亲抱怨肚子疼。他的母亲回忆说，她早上给了他一个花生酱果冻三明治和一个苹果作为午餐，午饭后没有发生问题。当天晚些时候，她看到她的儿子蜷缩在沙发上捂着胃哭泣，她决定带他去那个下班后仍然营业的诊所看儿科医生。

检查

儿科医生 Davies 从 B. K. 一出生就知道。B. K. 的父母一直都安排他们的儿子做定期体格检查。他的免疫接种是最新的，除了几次耳痛和感冒，B. K. 是一个健康的男孩。一到达诊所，办公室医疗助理就记录了 B. K. 的生命体征，在正常范围内。然后 Davies 医生看了患者，让他仰卧（lie supine）在检查台上，进行了从头到脚的（cephalocaudal）评估。引起关注的唯一异常是 B. K. 说他正在经受腹部疼痛。Davies 医生要 B. K. 向他展示疼痛最严重的部位，男孩第一次指向他腹部的左上部，然后有点困惑，又指向他的右下部。医学助理抽取了血液进行实验室研究，结果显示正常。Davies 博士随后指示进行腹部 X 线检查。

临床病程

X 线显示 B. K. 吞下了一个五分和一个一分钱的硬币。男孩后来承认试图瞒着他的兄弟藏钱，所以他吞下了硬币。Davies 医生向 B. K. 和他的母亲说明他预测没有严重的并发症，并且硬币应该在接下来的 24 小时内被排出。

在本章中，我们要学习人体的部位和定位，并熟悉医疗保健专业人士用于确定身体内的确切位置的一些术语。

简介

所有医疗保健领域均需要身体方向和定位的知识。例如，医生、外科医生、护士、职业治疗师和物理治疗师必须完全熟悉用于描述身体位置和体位的术语。放射技术人员必须能够定位患者，并且能够指引行X线检查获得合适的图像用于诊断，如框5-1所示。

方向性术语

在描述身体中一个给定点的位置或方向时，总是假定主体处于解剖位置，也就是站立、面朝前、两臂处于身体两侧、掌心向前、双脚平行（图5-1），在这样的站位下，框5-2给出了用于确定相对位置的方向性术语。

框 5-1

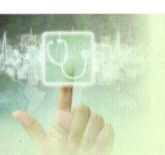

健康职业
放射技术人员

放射技术人员（radiologic technologist）通过对身体的X线片（radiograph）帮助诊断医学疾病。他们还使用CT扫描和其他成像技术对患者进行检查，以帮助医生诊断。根据机构的患者安全移动程序，他们必须使患者为放射学检查做好准备，将患者置于适当的位置；然后将设备调整到正确的角度和高度，并调整用于拍摄X线或其他诊断图像的设置。他们必须正确地定位图像，并在曝光后取出并处理图像。他们还要保存患者记录和维护设备。放射技术人员必须通过使用保护装置和发射最低可能的辐射量，为自身和患者尽可能降低辐射危害。他们佩戴徽章来监测辐射水平，并记录他们的暴露情况。

放射技术人员可以专门从事特定的成像技术，如骨密度测定（bone densitometry）、心血管介入放射成像（cardiovascular-interventional radiography）、计算机断层扫描（computed tomography）、乳腺X线照相术（mammography）、磁共振成像（magnetic resonance imaging）、核医学（nuclear medicine）和质量管理。其中一些将在后面的章节中描述。

大多数放射技术人员在医院工作，但也能在医生办公室、诊断成像中心（例如，做乳腺X线照相术）和门诊护理中心工作。放射技术人员最低必须具有副学士学位才有资格获得专业认证，监督或教学职位需要更高的学位。放射学技术教育联合审查委员会（Joint Review Committee on Education in Radiologic Technology）负责认可大多数教育项目。美国放射技术员注册处（American Registry of Radiologic Technologists，ARRT）在放射学以及其他成像技术（CT、核磁共振、核医学等）领域提供国家认证考试。在美国大多数州作为放射技术人员就业，都要求ARRT认证。目前，这个领域的工作机会良好。美国放射技术人员协会（American Society of Radiologic Technologists）在www.asrt.org网站上有关于这个职业的信息。

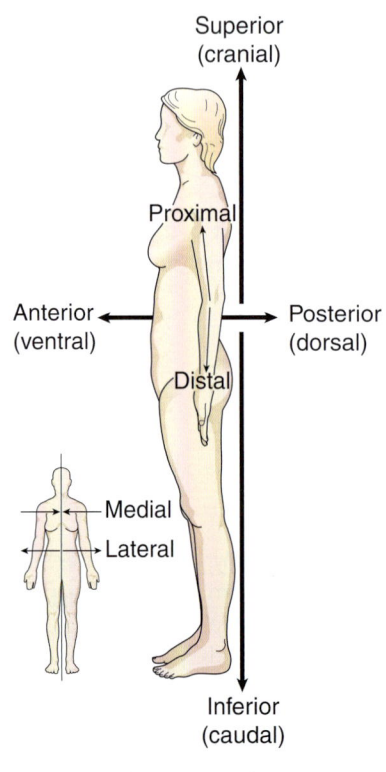

图 5-1　方向性术语

框 5-2

供你参考
解剖方位

名词	定义
anterior (ventral) 前面（腹部）	朝向或在身体前面（腹部）
posterior (dorsal) 后面（背部）	朝向或在身体后面（背部）
medial 中间	朝向身体中线
lateral 侧	朝向身体侧面
proximal 近轴的	靠近附着点或给定参考点
distal 远轴的	远离附着点或给定参考点
superior 在上的	在……之上，在较高的位置
inferior 在下的	在……之下，在较低的位置
cranial (cephalad) 颅侧的（向头侧）	朝向头部
caudal 尾侧	朝向脊椎的末端（拉丁语 cauda，意为"尾巴"）
superficial (external) 表面的（外部的）	靠近身体表面
deep (internal) 深处的（内部的）	靠近身体中心

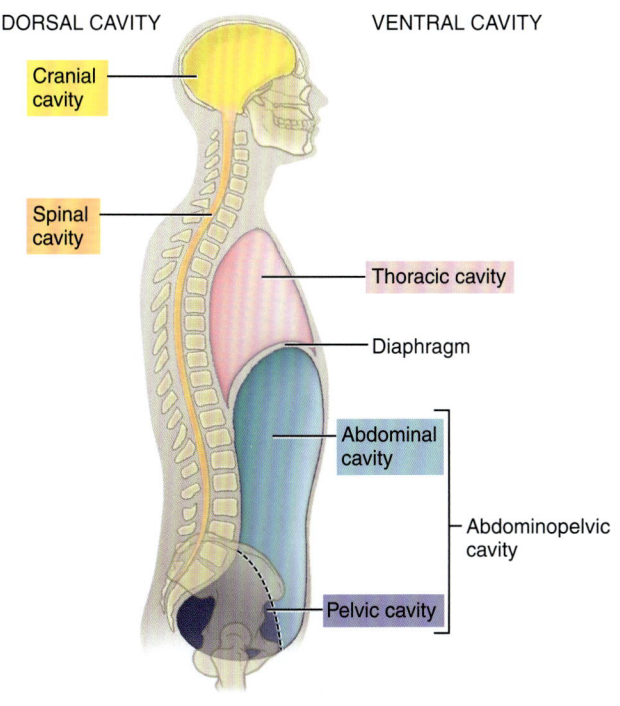

图 5-3　体腔侧视图。显示背侧腔和腹侧腔及其分区

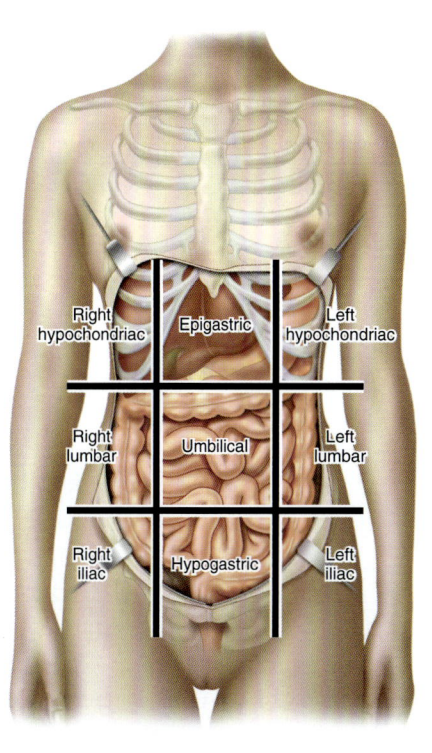

图 5-4　腹部的九个部位

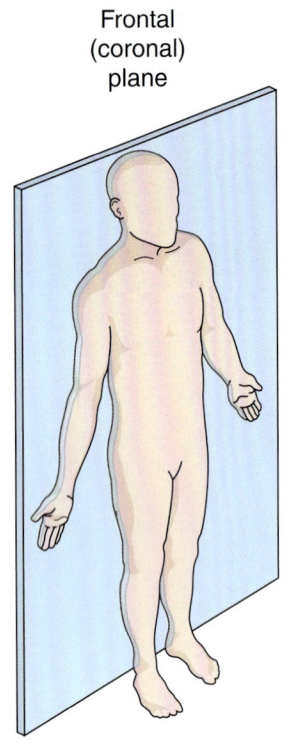
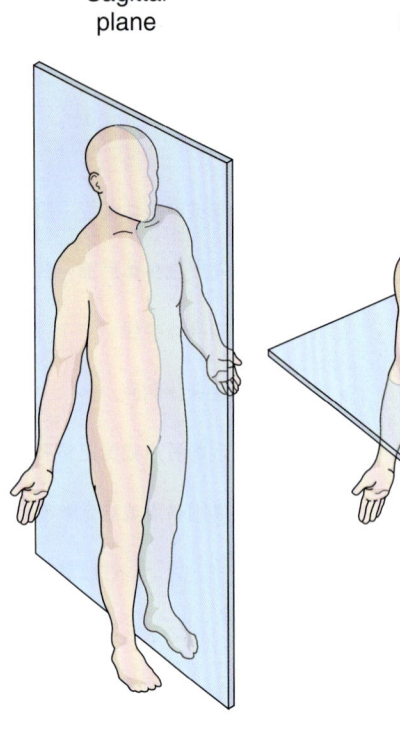
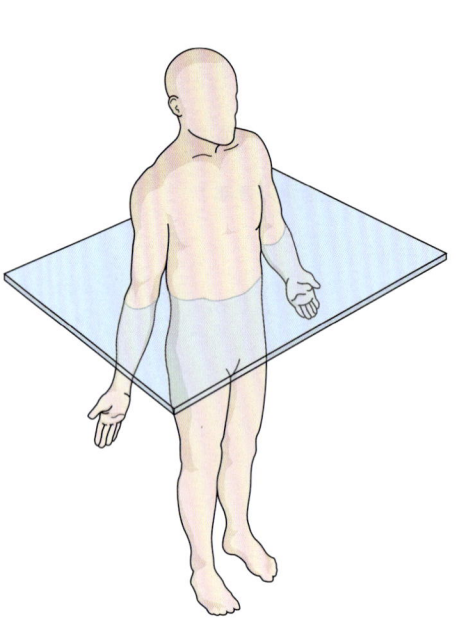

图 5-5　人体截面

图 5-2 示出了人体截面，即在不同方位切开身体的平面。正截面（frontal plane）也被称为冠截面（coronal plane），从上到下沿中线垂直方向将身体分为前部（anterior）和后部（posterior）。纵截面（sagittal plane）从前向后穿过身体，将身体分为左、右两个部分。如果纵截面穿过中线，就被称为中矢（midsagittal）截面或中（medial）截面。横截面水平穿过身体，将身体分为上（superior）、下（inferior）两个部分。

体腔

人体的内部器官处于背侧（dorsal）腔和腹侧（ventral）腔之中（图 5-3）。背侧腔包含颅腔（cranial cavity）中的大脑和髓腔（髓管）中的脊髓。腹侧腔的最上部是胸腔（the thoracic cavity），由横隔膜（diaphragm）将其与腹腔（abdominal cavity）分开，横隔膜是一块用于呼吸的肌肉。在腹腔和盆腔（pelvic cavity）没有解剖分割，共同构成腹盆腔（abdominopelvic cavity）。覆盖腹盆腔及其内部器官的薄膜是腹膜（peritoneum［ˌperɪtə'niːəm］）。

框 5-3

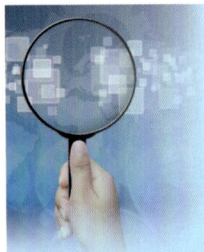

聚焦单词

把工作量减半

刚刚学医的学生会对需要学习的医学词汇量之大感到吃惊。由于人体基本上是两侧对称的，除了肝脏、脾脏、胃、胰腺和肠道等内部器官之外，人体右侧所有的任何东西在左侧几乎也都有，这在某种程度上减轻了学习负担。骨架可以象征性地沿着中心分开，在中线的两侧具有相同的结构。许多血管和神经都是成对的，这能够将工作量减半。

另外，在一个部位的许多血管和神经有相同的名称。桡动脉（radial artery）、桡静脉（radial vein）和桡神经（radial nerve）是平行的，都位于前臂的桡骨（radius）周围。血管通常会用它们所供血的器官命名，如肝脏的肝动脉（hepatic artery）和肝静脉（hepatic vein）、肺脏的肺动脉（pulmonary artery）和肺静脉（pulmonary vein）以及肾脏的肾动脉（renal artery）和肾静脉（renal vein）。

没有人能说学习医学词汇轻而易举，因为确实比较难。

腹部区域

为了区分方位，可以用想象中的线将腹部分为九个部位——三个中间区域和六个侧区域（图 5-4）。中间的三个部位是：

- 上腹部（epigastric [ˌepi'gæstrik]），位于胃之上。
- 脐部（umbilical [ʌm'bilik(ə)l]），因脐而得名。
- 下腹部（hypogastric [ˌhaipə'gæstrik]）位于胃之下。
- 左右两侧的部位有相同的名称（框 5-3），包括：
- 季肋部（hypochondriac [ˌhaipə(ʊ)'kɒndriæk]），由于位于肋骨，特别是肋骨的软骨（词根 chondr/o）附近而得名。
- 腰部（lumbar [ˈlʌmbə]），位于背部最窄的位置（腰椎）。
- 髂部（iliac [ˈiliæk]），因臀部最上端的骨骼——髂骨而得名。这些部位也被称为腹股沟

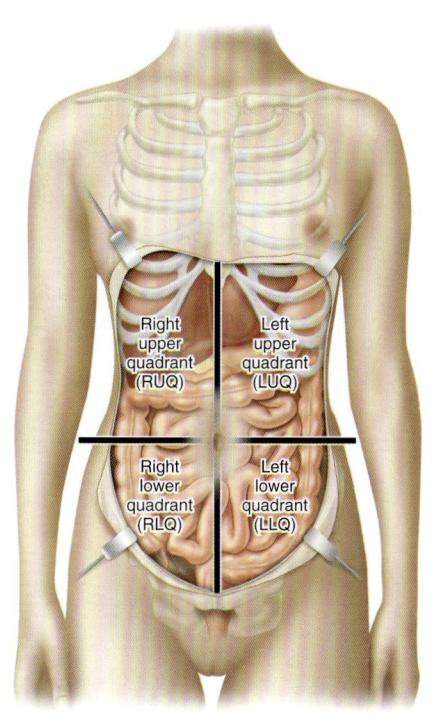

图 5-6　腹部的四个部分。图中显示了各部分中的一些器官

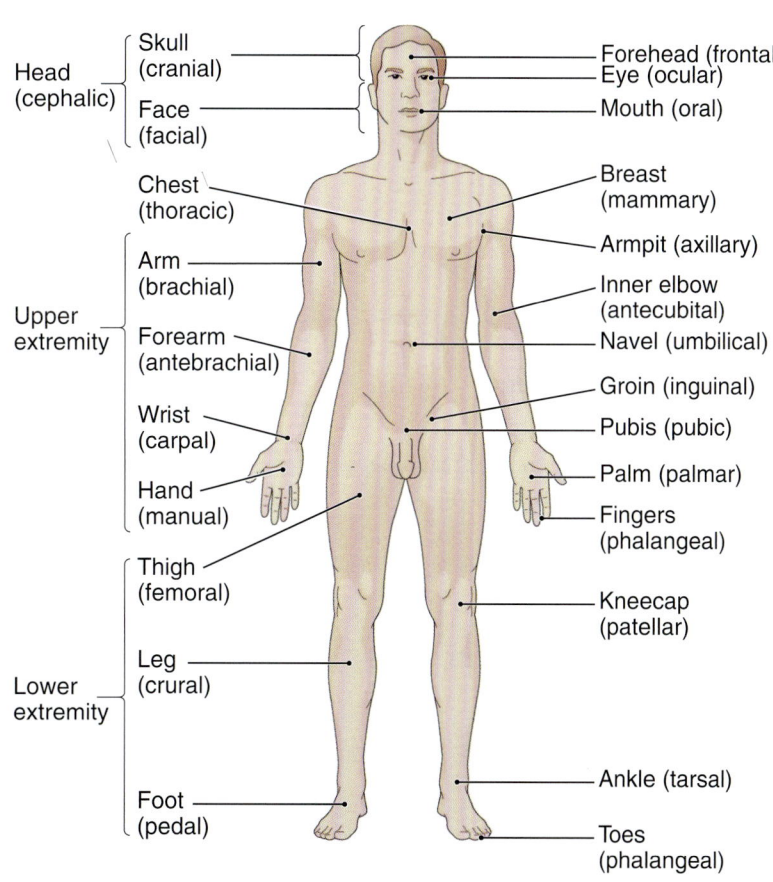

图 5-7　身体部位的常用术语，前视图。括号中是部位的解剖形容词

区（inguinal ['iŋgwin(ə)l]）。

为简单起见，腹部也可以用在肚脐处交叉的水平和垂直线不太精确地分为四个部分（图5-6），分别是右上部（RUQ）、左上部（LUQ）、右下部（RLQ）和左下部（LLQ）。

图5-7和图5-8给出了更多的关于身体部位的名词。

体位

除了解剖部位外，还有一些特殊目的，如检查、测试、手术或引流，而使人体处于的标准位置。最常见的体位及用途在框5-4中介绍。

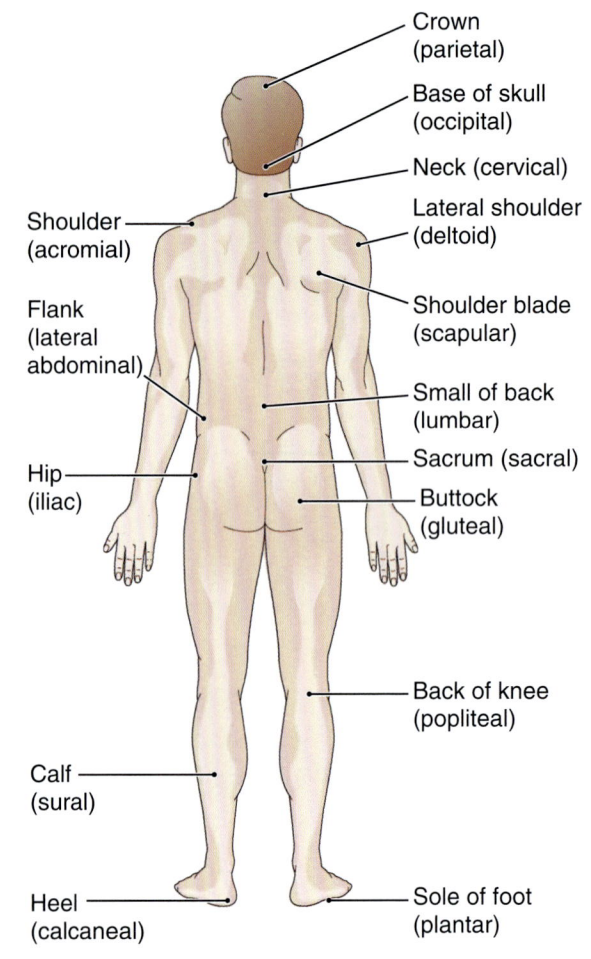

图5-8 身体部位的常用术语，后视图。括号中是部位的解剖形容词

供你参考
体位

框 5-4

体位	说明
anatomic position [ˌænə'tɒmɪk] 解剖体位	直立，脸朝前，两臂在两侧，掌心朝前，脚趾朝前；用于描述和研究身体
decubitus position [dɪ'kjuːbɪtəs] 卧位	躺下，根据接触床面的部位，可分为左侧卧位、右侧卧位、背卧位和俯卧位
dorsal recumbent position [rɪ'kʌmb(ə)nt] 屈膝背卧位	后背着床，腿弯曲并分开，双脚平放；用于妇产科检查
Fowler position 福勒体位	后背着床，床头抬起约50cm，膝盖抬高；用于放松呼吸和引流
jackknife position ['dʒæknaɪf] 折刀状卧位	后背着床，双肩抬高，双腿弯曲，大腿与腹部成直角；用于尿道插管

续框 5-4

体位	说明
knee–chest position 膝胸卧位	膝盖着床，头和胸上部在桌上，双臂交叉在头上；用于妇产科检查和肠道冲洗
lateral recumbent position 侧卧位	身体一侧着床，一腿弯曲，双臂位置可变
lithotomy position ［li'θɒtəmi］ 截石位	背部着床，双腿弯曲至腹部，大腿分开；用于妇科和泌尿外科手术
prone 俯卧位	躺下，脸朝下
Sims position 希姆斯体位	左侧着床，右腿向前伸并抬高，左臂贴后背，胸部向前置于床上；用于肾脏和子宫手术，结肠检查和灌肠
supine ［'s(j)u:pain］ 仰卧位	躺下，脸朝上
trendelenburg position ［tren'delənbɜ:g］ 头低脚高位	后背着床，通过将床倾斜 45°使头部位置降低；用于盆腔和腹部手术，休克治疗

Terminology 关键术语

abdominal cavity ［æb'dɒmɪn(ə)l］	腹腔，在横隔膜与盆腔以上的腹侧腔
abdominopelvic cavity ［æb͵dɒmɪnə'pelvɪk］	腹盆腔，在横隔膜与骨盆之间的腹侧腔，包括腹腔和盆腔
anatomic position ［͵ænə'tɒmɪk］	解剖体位，解剖学研究的标准体位，直立，脸朝前，两臂在两侧，掌心朝前，双脚平行
cranial cavity ［'kreɪnɪəl］	颅腔，包括大脑的背侧腔
diaphragm ［'daɪəfræm］	横隔膜，将胸腔与腹腔分开的肌肉
frontal (coronal) plane ［kə'rəʊn(ə)l］	正（冠）截面，将人体分为前（anterior）部与后（posterior）部的切面
pelvic cavity ［'pelvɪk］	盆腔，腹腔以下的腹侧腔
peritoneum ［͵perɪtə'niːəm］	腹膜，覆盖腹盆腔及其内部器官的大片薄膜
sagittal plane ［'sædʒɪt(ə)l］	纵截面，将人体分为左右两部分的切面
spinal cavity (canal) ［'spaɪn(ə)l］	髓腔，包含髓管的背侧腔
thoracic cavity ［θɔː'ræsɪk］	胸腔，横隔膜以上的腹侧腔
transverse (horizontal) plane ［trænz'vɜːs］	横（水平）截面，将人体分为上（superior）下（inferior）两部分的切面

与身体结构相关的单词组成部分

表 5-1 至表 5-3 提供了与身体结构相关的词根和前缀。

表 5-1　头部和躯干部位的词根

词根	含义	示例	示例定义
cephal/o	头部	megacephaly ［ˌmegəˈsefəli］	巨头畸形
cervic/o	颈部	cervicofacial ［ˌsɜːvikəʊˈfeiʃəl］	颈颜面的
thorac/o	胸部	thoracotomy ［θɔːrəˈkɒtəmi］	胸廓切开术
abdomin/o	腹部	intra-abdominal ［ˌintrəæbˈdɔminəl］	腹内的
celi/o	腹部	celiocentesis ［ˌseliəsənˈtesis］	腹腔穿刺术
lapar/o	腹壁	laparoscope ［ˈlæpərəʊskəʊp］	腹腔镜
lumb/o	腰部	thoracolumbar ［ˌθɔːrəkəʊˈlʌmbə］	胸腰部的
periton, peritone/o	腹膜	peritoneal ［ˌperitəʊˈniːəl］	腹膜的

练习 5-1

根据括号中给出的后缀，写出正确的形容词。

1. Pertaining to (-ic) the chest _____thoracic_____
2. Pertaining to (-ic) the head _____
3. Pertaining to (-al) the neck _____
4. Pertaining to (-al) the abdomen _____
5. Pertaining to (-ar) the lower back _____

填空。

6. Peritonitis ［ˌperitəˈnaitis］ is inflammation (-itis) of the _____.
7. The adjective celiac ［ˈsiːliˌæk］ pertains to the _____.
8. In B.K.'s opening case study, the doctor's cephalocaudal examination began at his _____.
9. In the opening study, B.K. was placed on his back in a _____ position for the doctor to examine his abdomen.
10. A laparotomy ［ˌlæpəˈrɒtəmi］ is an incision through the _____.

表 5-2　身体四肢的词根

词根	含义	示例	示例定义
acro	手足、末端	acrocyanosis ［ˌækrəusiə'nəusis］	手足发绀
brachi/o	臂	antebrachium ［ˌænti'breikiəm］	前臂
dactyl/o	手指、脚趾	polydactyly ［ˌpɒli'dæktili］	多指（趾）畸形
ped/o	足	pedometer ［pe'dɒmitə］	计步器
pod/o	足	podiatric ［pəu'daiətric］	足病学

练习 5-2

填空

1. Acrokinesia ［ˌækrəkai'ni:ziə］ is excess motion (-kinesia) of the _____.
2. Animals that brachiate ［b'reikieit］, such as monkeys, swing from place to place using their _____.
3. A dactylospasm ［dækti'lɒspæzəm］ is a spasm (cramp) of a(n) _____.
4. The term brachiocephalic ［breitʃi:əʊ'kefælik］ refers to the _____.
5. Sinistropedal ［sinist'rəʊpedl］ refers to the use of the left _____.

表 5-3　位置和方位的前缀

前缀	含义	示例	示例定义
circum-	周围	circumoral ［ˌsɜːkəm'ɔːrəl］	口周的
peri-	周围	periorbital ［ˌpəri'ɒbitl］	眶周的
intra-	内、在……之内	intravascular ［ˌintrə'væskjʊlə］	血管内的
epi-	上、在……之上	epithelial ［ˌepi'θi:liəl］	上皮的
extra-	在……之外	extrathoracic ［ˌekstrəɔː'ræsik］	胸外的
infra-*	在……之下	infrascapular ［ˌinfrə'skæpjulə］	肩胛下的
sub-*	在……之下	sublingual ［sʌb'liŋgw(ə)l］	舌下的
inter-	在……之间	intercostal ［ˌintə'kɒst(ə)l］	肋间的
juxta-	靠近、在……旁边	juxtaposition ［ˌdʒʌkstəpə'ziʃ(ə)n］	并列
para-	靠近、在……旁边	parasagittal ［ˌpærə'sædʒit(ə)l］	旁矢状面的
retro-	在……之后、向后	retrouterine ［ˌretrəʊ'ju:tərin］	子宫后的

续表 5-3	位置和方位的前缀		
前缀	含义	示例	示例定义
supra-	在……之上	suprapatellar [ˌsjuprəpəˈtelə]	髌上的

*也指程度

练习 5-3

同义词，写出与下列单词含义相同的单词。

1. perioral　　　　　　　　　　　　　circumoral
2. infrascapular　　　　　　　　　　　_____
3. perivascular　　　　　　　　　　　_____
4. subcostal　　　　　　　　　　　　_____
5. circumorbital　　　　　　　　　　_____

反义词，写出与下列单词含义相反的单词。

6. suprapatellar　　　　　　　　　　infrapatellar
7. extracellular　　　　　　　　　　_____
8. subscapular　　　　　　　　　　_____
9. intrathoracic　　　　　　　　　　_____

定义下列单词。

10. paranasal
    [pærəˈneizəl] _____
11. retroperitoneal
    [retrəuperitəˈni:əl] _____
12. supraabdominal
    [ˈsu:prə æbˈdɒminl] _____
13. intrauterine
    [ˌintrəˈju:tərain] _____

参考图 5-6 和图 5-7，定义下列术语。

14. periumbilical
    [piəriəmˈbilaikl] _____
15. intergluteal
    [intɜːrgluːˈti:l] _____
16. epitarsal
    [epiˈtɑːsl] _____
17. intraocular
    [ˌintrəˈɒkjulə] _____
18. parasacral
    [pæˈreiseikrəl] _____

Terminology 补充术语

digit	[ˈdɪdʒɪt]	手指或脚趾（形容词：digital）
epigastrium	[ˌepɪˈɡæstrɪəm]	上腹部
fundus	[ˈfʌndəs]	基底
hypochondrium	[ˌhaɪpəʊˈkɒndrɪəm]	季肋部
lumen	[ˈluːmen]	管腔
meatus	[mɪˈeɪtəs]	管道或开口
orifice	[ˈɒrɪfɪs]	体腔开口
os		口部、任何身体开口
septum	[ˈseptəm]	隔膜
sinus	[ˈsaɪnəs]	窦
sphincter	[ˈsfɪŋktə]	括约肌

Terminology 缩略语

LLQ	Left lower quadrant	左下四分之一
LUQ	Left upper quadrant	左上四分之一
RLQ	Right lower quadrant	右下四分之一
RUQ	Right upper quadrant	右上四分之一

Case Study Revisited 案例研究再访

Outcome of B. K.'s Case

Teased by his brother but reassured by the doctor, B.K. spent a quiet afternoon and evening and slept through the night. In the morning, he went into the bathroom and had a bowel movement. Examination of his stool showed that the coins had been expelled, and B.K. felt much better. Following this experience, B.K. deposited his earnings in his piggy bank.

B. K. 案例的结果

他的兄弟笑了，但医生放心了。B.K. 过了一个平静的下午和晚上，夜间睡得很好。早上，他走进卫生间排便，检查他的大便证实硬币已被排出，B.K. 感觉好多了。有了这一经历，B.K. 将他的收入存入他的存钱罐。

CHAPTER 5 复习

标记练习

方向性术语

写出每个编号对应的术语。

Anterior (ventral)　　Medial
Distal　　Posterior (dorsal)
Inferior (caudal)　　Proximal
Lateral　　Superior (cranial)

1. _____
2. _____
3. _____
4. _____
5. _____
6. _____
7. _____
8. _____

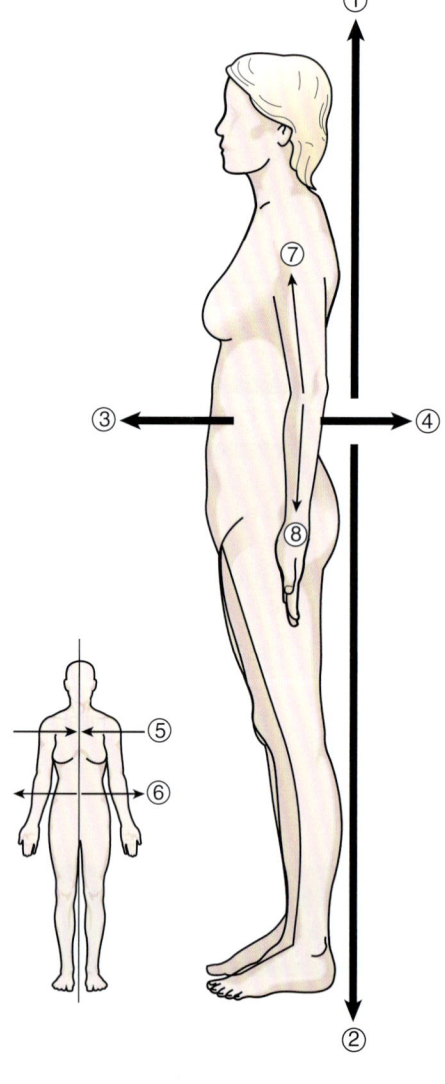

人体截面

写出每个编号对应的截面名称。

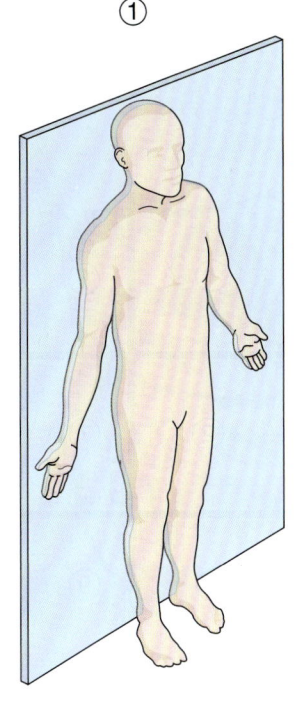
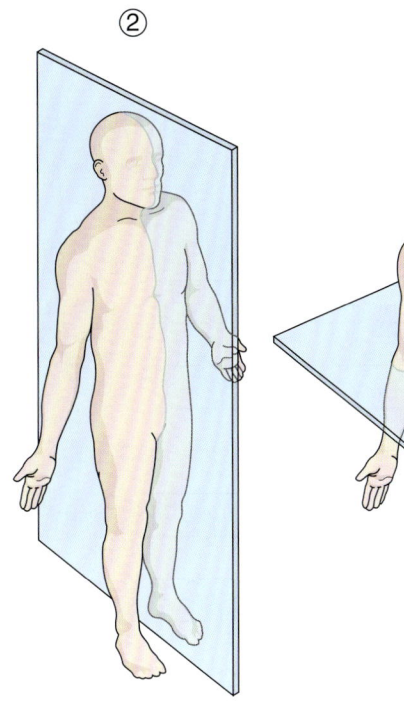
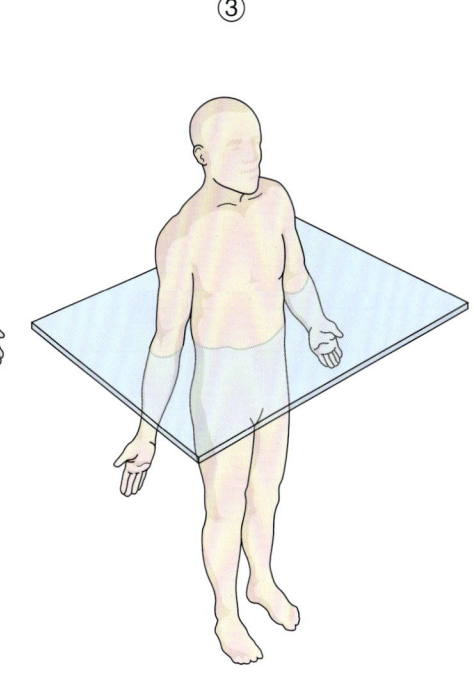

Frontal (coronal) plane   Transverse (horizontal) plane
Sagittal plane

1. _____
2. _____
3. _____

体腔，侧视图

写出每个编号对应的体腔名称。

Abdominal cavity   Pelvic cavity
Abdominopelvic cavity   Spinal cavity (canal)
Cranial cavity   Thoracic cavity
Dorsal cavity   Ventral cavity
Diaphragm

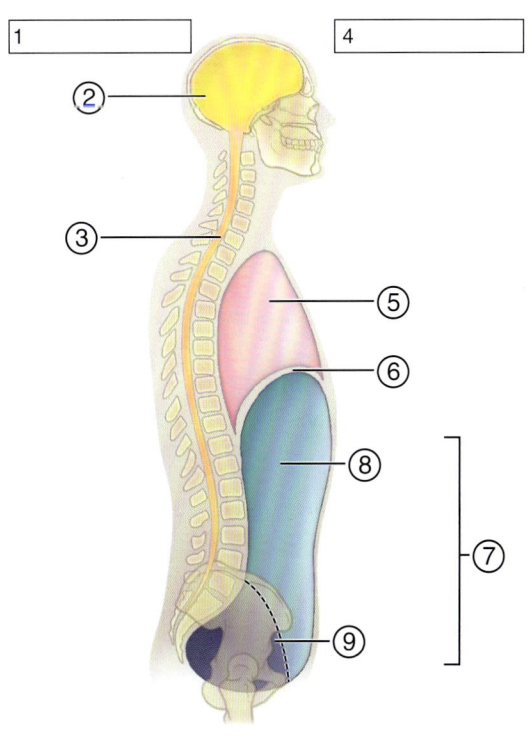

1. _____
2. _____
3. _____
4. _____
5. _____
6. _____
7. _____
8. _____
9. _____

腹部的九个部位

写出每个编号对应的部位名称。

Epigastric region   Right hypochondriac region
Hypogastric region   Right iliac (inguinal) region
Left hypochondriac region Right lumbar region
Left iliac (inguinal) region   Umbilical region
Left lumbar region

1. _____
2. _____
3. _____
4. _____
5. _____
6. _____
7. _____
8. _____
9. _____

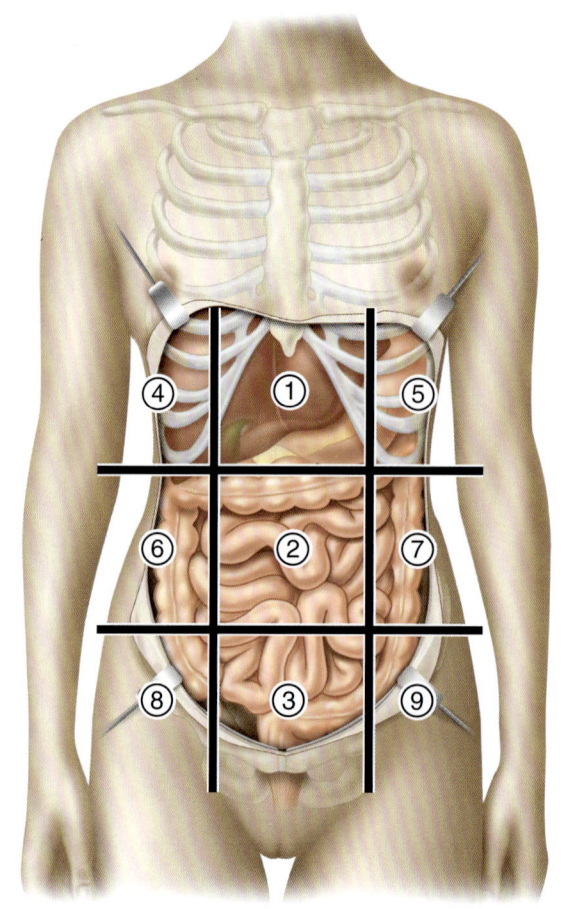

Abdominal regions

术语

匹配以下术语，并在每个数字的左侧写入相应的字母。

____ 1. thoracentesis   a. surgical puncture of the chest
____ 2. acrodermatitis   b. skin inflammation of the extremities
____ 3. laparoscopy   c. pertaining to the right foot
____ 4. dextropedal   d. examination through the abdominal wall
____ 5. caudal   e. toward the tail

____ 6. macropodia   a. circular cut
____ 7. subdermal   b. excessive size of the feet
____ 8. macrocephaly   c. beneath the skin
____ 9. celiotomy   d. abnormal largeness of the head
____ 10. circumcision   e. incision of the abdomen

补充术语

____ 11. fundus   a. passage or opening
____ 12. meatus   b. circular muscle that regulates an opening

____ 13. lumen   c. central opening of a tube
____ 14. sphincter   d. base of a hollow organ
____ 15. septum   e. dividing wall

真假判断

检查以下每个语句。 如果语句为真，则在第一个空白处写入 T；如果语句为假，则在第一个空格中写入 F，并在第二个空格中通过替换带下划线的单词来更正语句。

	true or False	correct Answer
16. The cranial and spinal cavities are the <u>ventral</u> body cavities.	F	dorsal
17. A <u>midsagittal plane</u> divides the body into equal right and left parts.		
18. The wrist is <u>proximal</u> to the elbow.		
19. A <u>transverse plane</u> divides the body into anterior and posterior parts.		
20. The abdominal cavity is <u>inferior</u> to the pelvic cavity.		
21. The hypogastric region is <u>inferior</u> to the umbilical region.		
22. When B.K. in the opening case study was lying in the supine position, he was lying <u>face down</u>.		
23. The right hypochondriac region is in the <u>RUQ</u>.		

形容词

命名以下形容词所指的人体部分。

24. celiac　　　　　_____
25. phalangeal　　　_____
26. popliteal　　　 _____
27. occipital　　　 _____
28. carpal　　　　　_____
29. cervical　　　　_____
30. lumbar　　　　　_____
31. brachial　　　　_____

定义

定义下列单词。

32. laparoscope　　　_____
33. suprapubic　　　 _____
34. infraumbilical　 _____
35. cervicofacial　　_____
36. sublingual　　　 _____
37. retroperitoneal　_____
38. bipedal　　　　　_____

同义词

写出下列单词的同义词。

39. posterior _____
40. circumocular _____
41. submammary _____
42. ventral _____

反义词

写出下列单词的反义词。

43. microcephaly _____
44. deep _____
45. proximal _____
46. subscapular _____
47. extracellular _____
48. superior _____

排除

在下面每组中，给与其他内容不相配的单词加下划线，并解释你选择的原因。

49. cervic/o — dactyl/o — brachi/o — acro — pod/o _____
50. umbilical region — hypochondriac region — epigastric region — cervical region — iliac region _____
51. jackknife — supine — transverse— decubitus — prone _____
52. thoracic cavity — spinal cavity — pelvic cavity — abdominal cavity — abdominopelvic cavity _____

单词构建

使用给出的单词组成部分写出下列定义的单词。

spasm   cephal   -o-   dactyl   extra-   -ic   infra-   syn-   thorac   a-   intra-   -y   poly

53. cramp of a finger or toe _____
54. below the chest _____
55. inside the chest _____
56. condition of having extra fingers or toes _____
57. fusion of the fingers or toes _____
58. pertaining to the head and chest _____
59. absence of a finger or toe _____
60. within the head _____
61. absence of a head _____

单词分析

定义下列单词，给出每个单词组成部分的含义。如果需要，可以使用词典。

62. mesocephalic ［ˌmezəʊsə'fælik］ _____

    a. mes/o _____

    b. cephal/o _____

    c. -ic _____

63. acrocyanosis [ækrəʊsaɪəˈnəʊsɪs] _____

    a. acro _____

    b. cyan/o _____

    c. –sis _____

64. antebrachial [æntebˈrəkjəl] _____

    a. ante- _____

    b. brachi/o _____

    c. -al _____

65. epigastric [ˌepiˈgæstrɪk] _____

    a. epi- _____

    b. gastr/o _____

    c. –ic _____

Additional Case Studies
补充案例研究

Case Study 5-1: Emergency Care
案例研究 5-1：紧急护理

During a triathlon, paramedics responded to a scene with multiple patients involved in a serious bicycle accident. B.R., a 20-year-old woman, lost control of her bike while descending a hill at approximately 40 mph. As she fell, two other cyclists collided with her, sending all three crashing to the ground.

At the scene, B. R. reported pain in her head, back, chest, and leg. She also had numbness and tingling in her legs and feet. Other injuries included a cut on her face and on her right arm and an obvious deformity to both her shoulder and knee. She had slight difficulty breathing.

The paramedic did a rapid cephalocaudal assessment and immobilized B.R.'s neck in a cervical collar. She was secured on a backboard and given oxygen. After her bleeding was controlled and her injured extremities were immobilized, she was transported to the nearest emergency department.

During transport, the paramedic in charge radioed ahead to provide a prehospital report to the charge nurse. His report included the following information: occipital and frontal head pain; laceration to right temple, superior and anterior to right ear; lumbar pain; bilateral thoracic pain on inspiration at midclavicular line on the right and midaxillary line on the left; dull aching pain of the posterior proximal right thigh; bilateral paresthesia (numbness and tingling) of distal lower legs circumferentially; varus (knockknee) adduction deformity of left knee; and posterior displacement deformity of left shoulder.

At the hospital, the emergency department physician ordered radiographs for B.R. Before the procedure, the radiology technologist positioned a lead gonadal shield centered on the midsagittal line above B.R.'s symphysis pubis to protect her ovaries from unnecessary irradiation by the primary beam. The technologist knew that gonadal shielding is important for female patients undergoing imaging of the lumbar spine, sacroiliac joints, acetabula, pelvis, and kidneys. Shields should not be used for any examination in which an acute abdominal condition is suspected.

在铁人三项赛期间，护理人员对一个涉及严重自行车事故的多患者现场做出反应。B.R.是一名20岁的女性，在以大约每小时40英里的速度沿着一个山坡下降时，她的自行车失去了控制。她摔倒时，另外两个骑自行车的人与她相撞，三人都撞倒在地。

在现场，B. R. 主诉头部、背部、胸部和腿部疼痛。她的腿和脚感到麻木和刺痛。其他伤处包括脸与右臂上的伤口，肩膀与膝盖有明显的畸形，呼吸微弱。

护理人员进行了快速全面评估，并将B.R.的颈部固定在颈圈中。她被固定在背板上并给予氧气。在她的出血得到控制并且受伤的四肢被固定后，她被运送到最近的急诊部。

在运输期间，负责护理的医务人员提前向监护护士提供了入院前报告。他的报告包括以下信息：枕骨和额头疼痛，撕裂从太阳穴延伸到右耳的前上部，腰痛，吸气时右锁骨中线到左腋中线双侧胸痛，右腿近端钝性疼痛，双侧下肢远端感觉异常（麻木和刺痛），左膝内翻（knockknee）内收畸形，左肩后位移畸形。

在医院，急诊科医生在手术前为 B.R. 安排了放射线检查，放射科医生在 B.R. 的耻骨联合上方的中线上放置了一个铅制性腺屏障以保护她的卵巢免受原射线束不必要的照射。放射科医生知道，性腺屏蔽对于经历腰椎、骶髂关节、髋臼、骨盆和肾脏成像的女性患者是重要的。屏障不应用于怀疑有急性腹部疾病的任何检查。

Case Study 5-2: Medical Assistant in Training
案例研究 5-2：培训中的医疗助理

P. K. is a student in a local medical assistant training program. She was beginning her clinical rotations and was scheduled in a busy outpatient clinic. During the first week, she was assigned to follow a clinical medical assistant (CMA) who was prepping patients for examination by the physician. One of the goals for the week was to learn about body positioning for the various examinations.

P. K. 是一名在地方医疗助理培训计划中学习的学生。她开始了临床轮换，并被安排在一个繁忙的门诊诊所。在第一周，她被分配跟随一名临床医疗助理（CMA），该助理正在使患者做好准备接受医生检查。本周的目标之一是学习各种检查的身体体位。

The first day, P. K. assisted the CMA with a patient who came in for a gynecologic examination. After the physician completed the history, he asked P. K. and the medical assistant to help the patient into a lithotomy position.

The next morning, an elderly patient who came in with suspected pneumonia was escorted to an examination room. She was lying on her back on the examination table waiting for the physician. P. K. placed the patient into a Fowler position to aid the patient's breathing.

Later that afternoon, P.K. heard the CMA call for assistance with a patient whose blood pressure was lower than normal. P.K. walked in, and the patient had already been placed into a Trendelenburg position.

The next day, a patient came in to have some stitches or sutures removed. The patient previously had a cyst removed from his lumbar region. P.K. assisted the patient into a prone position in preparation for the nurse clinician to remove the sutures.

By the end of the week, P. K. felt comfortable with positioning patients for the various physical examinations.

第1天，P. K. 和 CMA 协助一名患者进行妇科检查。医生记录病历后，P. K. 和医疗助手要求并帮助患者处于截石体位。

第2天早上，一名疑似患有肺炎的老年患者被护送到检查室。她躺在检查桌上等待医生，P.K. 将患者置于半坐卧位以帮助患者呼吸。

那天下午晚些时候，P. K. 听到 CMA 呼叫为血压低于正常的患者提供帮助。P. K. 走进来时，患者已经被置于头低足高体位。

第3天，来了一名拆线患者。该患者曾经切除了腰部囊肿，P.K. 帮助他置于俯卧位以准备护士和临床医生拆除缝合线。

截止到周末，P.K. 了解了患者各种身体检查的体位。

案例研究问题

多项选择。根据案例研究 5-1，选择最佳答案，并在每个题号左侧写上你选择的字母。

____ 1. The term for the timespan between injury and admission to the emergency department is

  a. preoperative

  b. prehospital

  c. pretrauma

  d. intrainjury

____ 2. A cephalocaudal assessment goes from

  a. front to back

  b. head to toe

  c. side to side

  d. skin to bone

____ 3. The victim's injured extremities were immobilized before transport. Immobilized means

  a. abducted as far as possible

  b. internally rotated and flexed

  c. adducted so that the limbs are crossed

  d. held in place to prevent movement

____ 4. A cervical collar was placed on the victim to stabilize and immobilize the

  a. uterus

  b. shoulders

  c. neck

  d. pelvis

____ 5. The singular form of acetabula is

  a. acetabulum

  b. acetabia

  c. acetab

  d. acetabulae

对于与案例研究相关的每个问题，在一个或两个图上画出或遮盖适当的区域。

6. Draw dots over the areas of the victim's occipital and frontal head pain.

7. Draw a dash (—) over the area of the right temporal laceration—superior and anterior to the right ear.

8. Crosshatch the area of lumbar pain.

9. Place an X over the area of thoracic pain at the anterior left midaxillary line.

10. Draw a star at the area of the pain on the right proximal posterior thigh.

11. Shade the area of the bilateral paresthesia of the distal lower legs, circumferentially.

12. Draw an arrow to show the direction of the varus adduction of the left knee.

13. Draw an arrow to show the direction of the posterior displacement of the left shoulder.

14. Draw a fig leaf to show the gonadal shield on the midsagittal line above the symphysis pubis.

15. Draw a circle around the area of the sacroiliac joints.

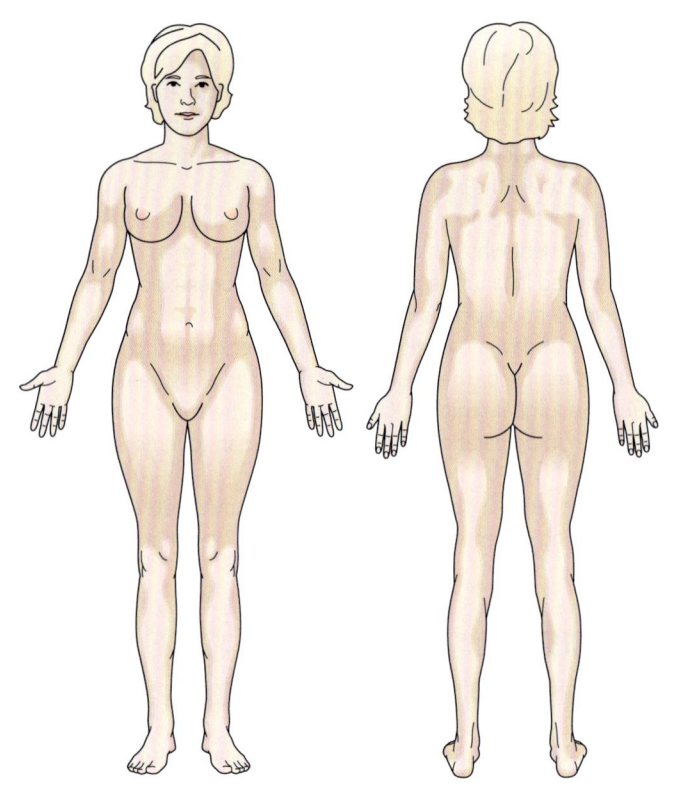

多项选择。选择最佳答案，并在每个数字的左边写上你选择的字母。

_____ **16.** The patient was placed in a Fowler position to

    a. aid breathing

    b. perform urologic surgery

    c. examine the colon

    d. palpate the vertebrae

_____ **17.** The lumbar region refers to the

    a. lower abdomen

    b. chest

    c. lateral abdomen

    d. small of the back

描述下列体位置。

18. lithotomy_____

19. Trendelenburg_____

20. lateral recumbent_____

PART 2 疾病与治疗

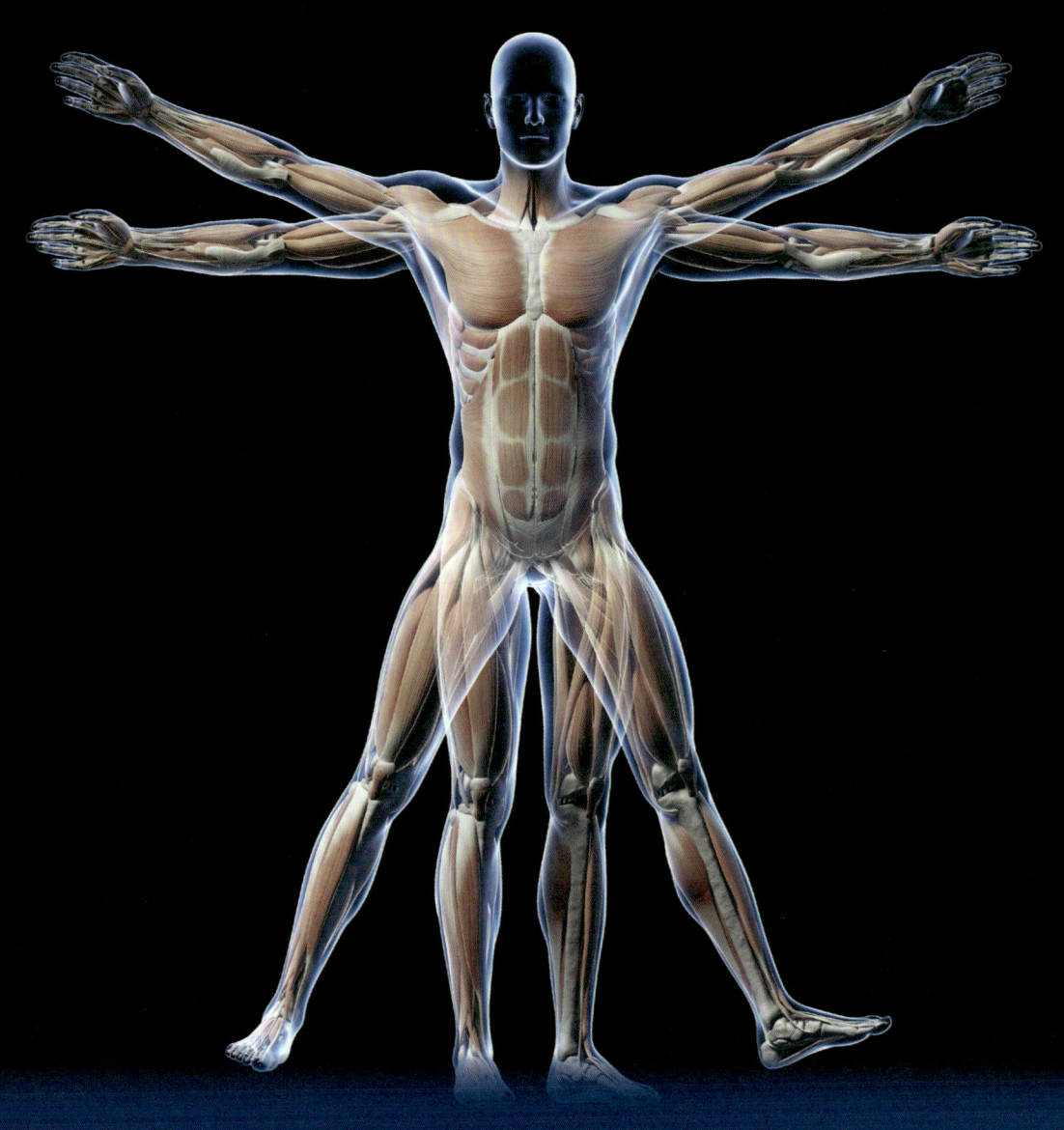

Chapter 6 ▶ Disease
第 6 章　疾病

Chapter 7 ▶ Diagnosis and Treatment; Surgery
第 7 章　诊断、治疗与手术

Chapter 8 ▶ Drugs
第 8 章　药物

CHAPTER 6

疾病

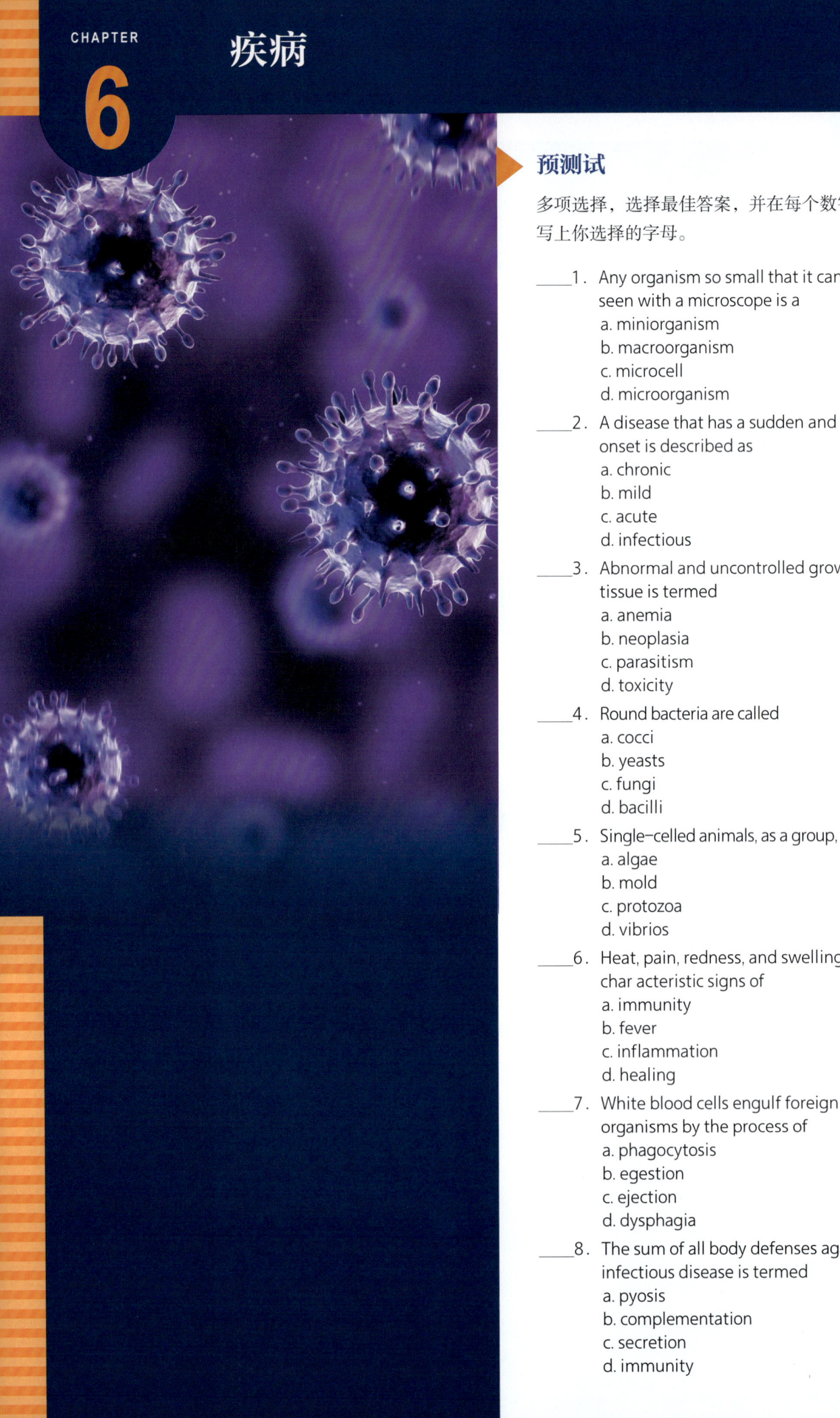

预测试

多项选择，选择最佳答案，并在每个数字的左边写上你选择的字母。

____1. Any organism so small that it can only be seen with a microscope is a
 a. miniorganism
 b. macroorganism
 c. microcell
 d. microorganism

____2. A disease that has a sudden and severe onset is described as
 a. chronic
 b. mild
 c. acute
 d. infectious

____3. Abnormal and uncontrolled growth of tissue is termed
 a. anemia
 b. neoplasia
 c. parasitism
 d. toxicity

____4. Round bacteria are called
 a. cocci
 b. yeasts
 c. fungi
 d. bacilli

____5. Single-celled animals, as a group, are called
 a. algae
 b. mold
 c. protozoa
 d. vibrios

____6. Heat, pain, redness, and swelling are the char acteristic signs of
 a. immunity
 b. fever
 c. inflammation
 d. healing

____7. White blood cells engulf foreign organisms by the process of
 a. phagocytosis
 b. egestion
 c. ejection
 d. dysphagia

____8. The sum of all body defenses against infectious disease is termed
 a. pyosis
 b. complementation
 c. secretion
 d. immunity

学习目标

学完本章后,应该能够:

1 ▶ 列出主要的疾病类型。
2 ▶ 对比常见的微生物感染类型,并列出每种微生物引起的疾病。
3 ▶ 描述常见的疾病反应。
4 ▶ 定义并给出肿瘤的示例。
5 ▶ 定义与疾病相关的主要术语。
6 ▶ 识别并使用与疾病相关的单词组成部分。
7 ▶ 分析案例研究中出现的疾病术语。

Case Study: Infected on an African Safari
案例研究:在非洲野生动物园被感染

Chief Complaint

J. N., a 56-year-old female, was on a month-long safari vacation with her husband in South Africa. During the last week of the trip, she began to experience a low-grade fever, abdominal cramping, and foul-smelling diarrhea. She returned home and promptly saw her internist.

Examination

The internist took a history, and J.N. recounted the events leading up to the acute onset of abdominal spasms and other intestinal symptoms. She explained that she and her husband went on an African safari and visited some pretty remote areas. Sanitation was a concern of hers, and she was careful to consume only bottled beverages. J.N. did admit though that she tried some of the native cuisine in the high mountain villages. The internist ordered the following laboratory tests: complete blood count (CBC), liver enzymes, and a stool specimen. The stool specimen was checked for protozoa, helminths such as hookworm, and other parasites that may have been endemic to the region in which J.N. and her husband had traveled. The CBC showed an elevated white blood count (WBC), and the stool specimen was positive for the protozoan Giardia lamblia. No indications of hepatitis or any other signs of pathology were noted.

Clinical Course

J. N.'s internist explained the results of the tests and said that she most likely contracted the illness from contaminated water in the mountain villages she visited. He prescribed the drug Tindamax, also known as tinidazole, and told her to take the medicine on an empty stomach. He cautioned her about transmitting the infection. Lastly, he reinforced strict personal hygiene and instructed her to wash her hands meticulously after having a bowel movement. She was to notify the office if symptoms persisted.

In this chapter, we learn about different categories of diseases, including infectious diseases, such as the protozoal disease J.N. contracted. We also discuss how the body responds to disease and learn about word parts contained in disease terminology. Diseases often require medical intervention, such as drug treatment, as in J. N.'s case. Medical treatment in general is the subject of Chapter 7, and drugs are specifically discussed in Chapter 8.

主诉

J. N. 是一名56岁的女性,与她丈夫在南非的野生动物园度假1个月。在旅行的最后1周,她经历了低热、腹部绞痛(abdominal cramping)和恶臭的腹泻(diarrhea)。她返回家中,并迅速去见她的内科医生。

检查

内科医生记录了病历,J.N.描述了导致腹部痉挛(abdominal spasm)和其他肠道症状(intestinal symptom)的急性发作(acute onset)事件。她解释说,她和她丈夫去了一个非洲野生动物园,并访问了一些相当偏僻的地区。她很关注卫生(sanitation),很小心地只喝瓶装饮料。J.N. 承认她品尝了一些在高山村庄的当地美食。内科医生指示做以下实验室检查:全血细胞计数(CBC)、肝酶(liver enzyme)和粪便标本(stool specimen)。粪便样本检查原生动物(protozoa)、蠕虫(helminth),例如钩虫(hookworm)以及其他寄生虫(parasite),这些寄生虫在 J.N. 和她丈夫旅行的区域可能是当地流行的(endemic)。全血细胞计数显示白细胞计数(WBC)升高,并且粪便标本对于原生动物贾第鞭毛虫(Giardia lamblia)阳性。没有肝炎或任何其他病理迹象。

临床病程

J. N. 的内科医生解释了检查的结果,并说她最有可能是在所访问的山区村庄受到污染水源的感染。他开了处方药替硝唑,也称为磺甲硝咪唑,并告诉她在空腹时服药。他告诫她感染会传播。最后,他再次强调了严格的个人卫生,并指示她在排便后仔细洗手。如果症状持续,她要通知医生。

在本章中,我们要学习不同类型的疾病,包括传染性疾病,例如 J.N. 感染的原生动物疾病。我们还将讨论身体如何对疾病做出反应,并了解疾病术语中包含的单词组成部分。疾病通常需要医疗干预,例如药物治疗,就像 J.N. 的情况。一般的医学治疗见第7章,药物治疗在第8章中具体讨论。

疾病类型

疾病是人体正常功能的任何失调。疾病可以被分为不同的类型，但在分类上通常会有一些重叠。

- 感染性（infectious）疾病：由特定的有害微生物和其他寄生在另一种生命体中的寄生物（parasites）所引起。任何致病介质都被称为病原体（parasites）。
- 退行性（degenerative）疾病：因可能造成损害（创伤）和坏死（组织死亡）的损耗、老化或外伤（受伤）所导致。常见病例包括关节炎（arthritis）、心血管问题和气肿（emphysema）这样特定的呼吸系统疾病。先天畸形（congenital malformations）、脱垂（prolapse）或疝气（hernia）等结构性畸形也可能是退行性变化所导致的。
- 肿瘤（neoplasia）：组织异常且不受控制地生长。
- 免疫失调（immune disorder）：这类疾病包括免疫系统失效、过敏和自身免疫病，自身免疫病患者体内会制造针对自身组织的抗体。
- 新陈代谢紊乱（metabolic disorder）：由缺少细胞功能所需的酶或其他因素所导致。许多遗传性疾病属于这一类别。因营养摄入不足或身体不能吸收并利用营养引起的营养不良也会扰乱新陈代谢。（代谢性疾病在第12章中进行更详细地讨论，遗传性疾病在第15章中讨论）。
- 激素失调（hormonal disorder）：因激素产量过低或过高，或激素不能正常发挥功能所导致。糖尿病（diabetes mellitus）就是一个例子。（第16章有更多关于激素失调的细节。）
- 精神和情感障碍（mental and emotional disorder）：影响智力和适应个体所在环境的疾病。（第17章进一步讨论行为障碍。）

框6-1介绍了一些疾病的命名方式。

导致疾病的是其病因（etiology [ˌiːtiˈɒlədʒi]），许多疾病都有多个相互作用的病因。急性疾病是突发且严重的，持续时间短。慢性疾病持续时间长，进展缓慢。紧急医疗技术员是一个处理急性疾病的直接影响健康的专业（框6-2）。

感染性疾病

感染性疾病（infectious disease）是由病毒（virus）、细菌（bacterium）、真菌（fungus）（霉菌和酵母菌）、原生动物（protozoa）（单细胞动物）和虫子（worm）（蠕虫）引起的（框6-3）。感染性生物会通过不同的途径或感染门户进入人体，包括损伤的皮肤、呼吸道、消化道以及泌尿和生殖道。被感染人体的排泄物可能包含这些感染性微生物，通过空气、食物、水或直接接触扩散感染。微生物通常通过它们释放的毒素导致疾病，有害微生物或其毒素在人体内的存在被称为败血症（sepsis）。

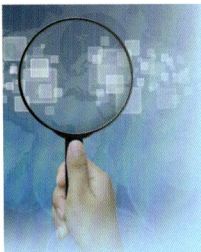

框 6-1

聚焦单词
疾病的命名

疾病命名方式有很多。有些是因其最初被发现的地方命名，例如莱姆病（Lyme disease）由康涅狄格州的莱姆镇（Lyme）而得名，西尼罗河病（West Nile disease）和里夫特裂谷热（Rift Valley fever）是因非洲的地名而得名，汉坦病毒发热（hantavirus fever）则因韩国一条河的名称而得名。还有一些是由第一个描述该疾病的人名而命名，例如库利贫血（Cooley anemia），炎症性肠道疾病克罗恩病（Crohn disease）和淋巴系统的霍奇金病（Hodgkin disease）。

许多疾病是基于它们所引起的症状命名的。结核病（tuberculosis）会在肺和其他组织中造成，被称为结节（tubercles）的小损伤。皮肤炭疽（skin anthrax）产生的损伤会变黑，其名称来源于无烟煤（anthracite coal）相同的词根。镰状细胞性贫血（sickle cell anemia）患者的红细胞在释放氧气之后会扭曲成新月状，失去了光滑的原形，挤在一起阻断小血管，使组织不能获得氧气。

黑死病（bubonic plague）会引起疼痛，使淋巴结变大，被称为腹股沟淋巴结炎（buboes）。红斑狼疮（lupus erythematosus）是一种系统性自免疫疾病，名称来源于拉丁语单词lupus（意为：狼），因为患者脸上形成的红疹使他们像狼。黄热病（yellow fever）、猩红热（scarlet fever）和风疹（rubella）的名称都与这些疾病症状的颜色相关。

健康职业
急救医疗技术员

急救医疗技术人员（emergency medical technician，EMT）是第一个到达汽车事故、心脏病发作或其他紧急情况现场的健康专业人员。急救医疗技术人员必须快速评估和应对医疗危机，记录病历、进行身体格检查、安抚患者，并在必要时将患者运送到最近的医疗机构。

为了执行救生职责，急救医疗技术人员需要全面的培训，包括彻底了解解剖学和生理学。急救医疗技术人员必须知道如何使用专用设备，例如用于固定损伤的背板、用于监测心脏活动的心电图仪，以及用于治疗心脏骤停的除颤仪。他们还必须精通静脉输液，给予氧气和某些抢救药物。在医疗机构，急救医疗技术人员在报告病史、体格检查以及为稳定患者所采取的措施中与医生和护士密切合作。大多数急救医疗技术人员在大学或技术学校接受培训，并且必须在他们受雇的地方获得认证。

随着美国人口老龄化和集中在城市中心，事故和其他紧急情况的发生率预计会上升，因此，对急救医疗技术人员的需求仍然很高。有关这个职业的更多信息，请参照国家紧急医疗技术员协会（National Association of Emergency Medical Technicians）http://www.naemt.org。

框 6-2

供你参考
常见感染性微生物

框 6-3

生物类别	说明	引发疾病示例
bacterium [bæk'tɪərɪəm]	细菌，遍布世界的微小的生物，某些细菌能够导致疾病，单数形式为 bacterium [bæk'tɪərɪəm]	
cocci ['kɒksaɪ]	球菌，可能成团（staphylococci，葡萄球菌）、成链（streptococci，链球菌）或其他形式，单数形式为 coccus ['kɒkəs]	肺炎（pneumonia）、风湿热（rheumatic fever）、食物中毒、败血症（septicemia）、尿路感染、淋病（gonorrhea）
bacilli [bə'sɪlaɪ]	杆菌，单数形式为 bacillus [bə'sɪləs]	伤寒（typhoid）、痢疾（dysentery）、沙门氏菌病（salmonellosis）、结核病、肉毒中毒（botulism）、破伤风（tetanus）
vibrios ['vɪbrɪəʊ]	弧菌	霍乱（cholera）、肠胃炎（gastroenteritis）
spirochetes ['spaɪərəʊkiːt]	螺旋菌	莱姆病、梅毒（syphilis）、文森氏口炎（Vincent disease）
chlamydia [klə'mɪdɪə]	衣原体，生长在活细胞中的极其微小的细菌，有着复杂的生命周期，与病毒不同，对抗生素敏感	结膜炎（conjunctivitis）、沙眼（trachoma）、盆腔炎和其他性传播疾病
rickettsia [rɪ'ketsɪə]	立克次体，生长在活细胞中的极小的细菌，对抗生素敏感	斑疹伤寒（typhus）、洛基山斑疹热（Rocky Mountain spotted fever）
virus ['vaɪərəs]	病毒，只能在活细胞中生存并繁殖的亚微观传染性病原体	感冒、疱疹（herpes）、肝炎（hepatitis）、麻疹（measles）、水痘（varicella）、流行性感冒、艾滋病
fungus ['fʌŋɡəs]	真菌，简单的非绿色植物，其中一些是寄生的，包括酵母菌和霉菌，单数形式是 fungus ['fʌŋɡəs]	念珠菌病（candidiasis）、皮肤感染、溪谷热（valley fever）
protozoa [ˌprəʊtə'zəʊə]	原生物，单细胞动物，单数形式为：protozoon [ˌprəʊtə(ʊ)'zəʊən]	痢疾、滴虫感染、疟疾（malaria）
helminths ['helmɪnθ]	寄生虫	旋毛虫病（trichinosis）、蛔虫、蛲虫、钩虫造成的感染

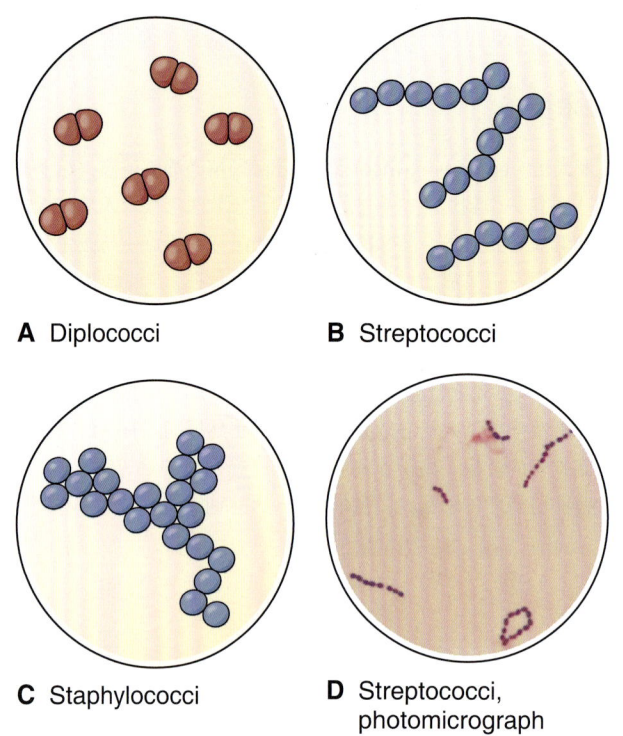

图 6-1 圆的细菌,革兰氏染色球菌(cocci)。A. 成对的细胞,双球菌(diplococci);B. 成链的细胞,链球菌(streptococci);C. 细胞群,葡萄球菌(staphylococci);D. 在显微镜下在显微镜下观察链球菌(streptococci)。革兰氏阳性细胞为紫色;革兰氏阴性细胞为红色

细菌

根据形状,细菌可分为:

- 圆的,球菌,如图 6-1 所示。
- 杆状的,杆菌,如图 6-2 所示。
- 弯曲的,包括弧菌和螺旋菌,如图 6-3 所示。

细菌可根据其形状命名,也可以根据它们组合的方式命名,还可以根据它们在实验室染色时所呈现的颜色命名。最常见的实验室染色是革兰氏染色,用革兰氏阳性的有机染色紫和革兰氏阴性的有机染色红。

衣原体(chlamydia)和立克次体(rickettsia)比一般的细菌小,只能在活的宿主细胞中生长(框 6-3)。

疾病反应

炎症

对感染和其他一些疾病的常见反应是炎症(inflammation)。当细胞受损时,它们会释放化学

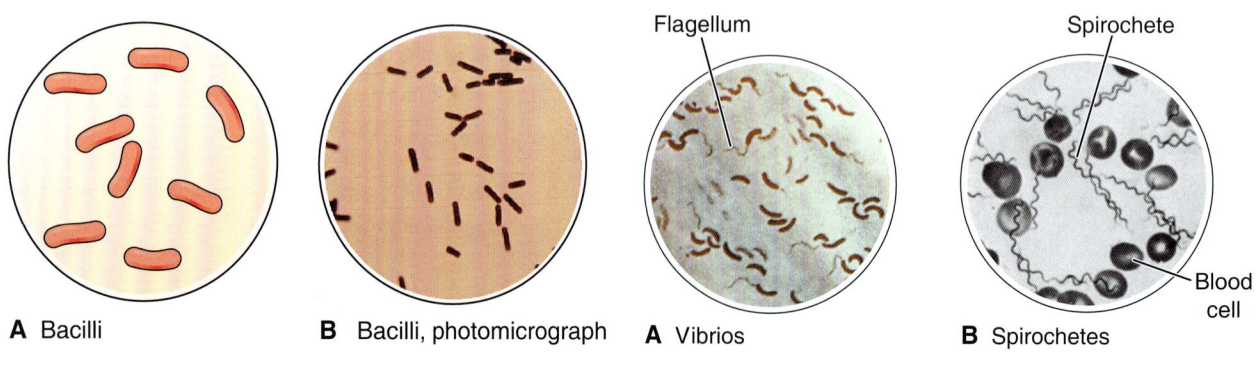

图 6-2 杆菌(bacilli),杆状细菌。A. 杆菌的绘图;B. 杆菌的显微照片

图 6-3 弯曲的细菌。A. 弧菌(vibrio)是短弯的杆状;B. 螺旋体(spirochete)是螺旋形的

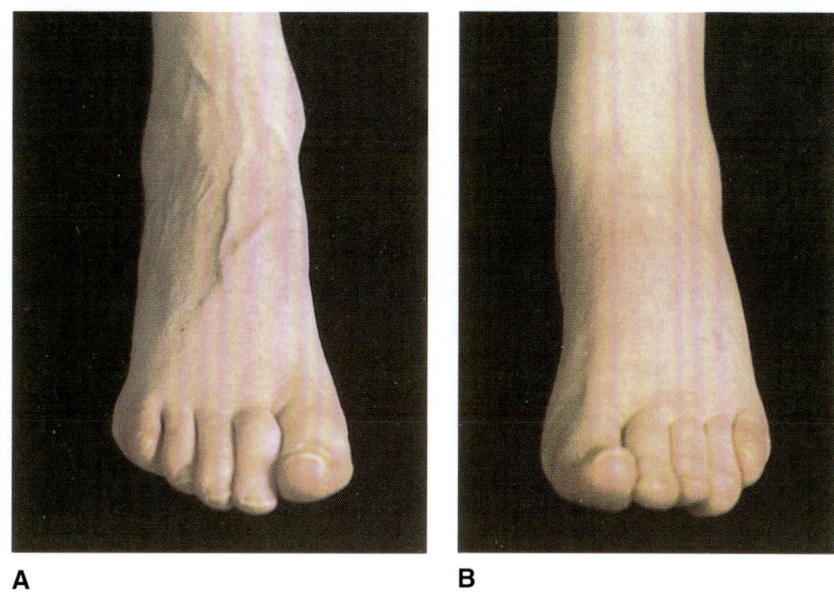

图 6-4 水肿。A. 正常脚显示静脉、肌腱和骨骼；B. 水肿（edema）模糊了表面特征

物质，允许血液的细胞和液体进入组织。这一血液流动造成炎症的四个症状：

- 发热（heat）
- 疼痛（pain）
- 发红（redness）
- 肿胀（swelling）

后缀 -itis 表示炎症，例如：appendicitis（阑尾炎）和 tonsillitis（扁桃体炎）。

炎症是水肿（edema）发生的可能原因之一，水肿是组织中液体的隆起或积累（图 6-4）。水肿的其他原因包括液体堵塞、心脏衰竭和体内液体成分失去平衡。

吞噬作用

人体用吞噬作用（phagocytosis [ˌfægə(ʊ)saiˈtəʊsis]）来摆脱入侵微生物、受损的细胞和其他有害碎片。特定的白细胞能够吞噬这些东西，并将其彻底摧毁（图 6-5）。巨噬细胞在血液、组织和淋巴系

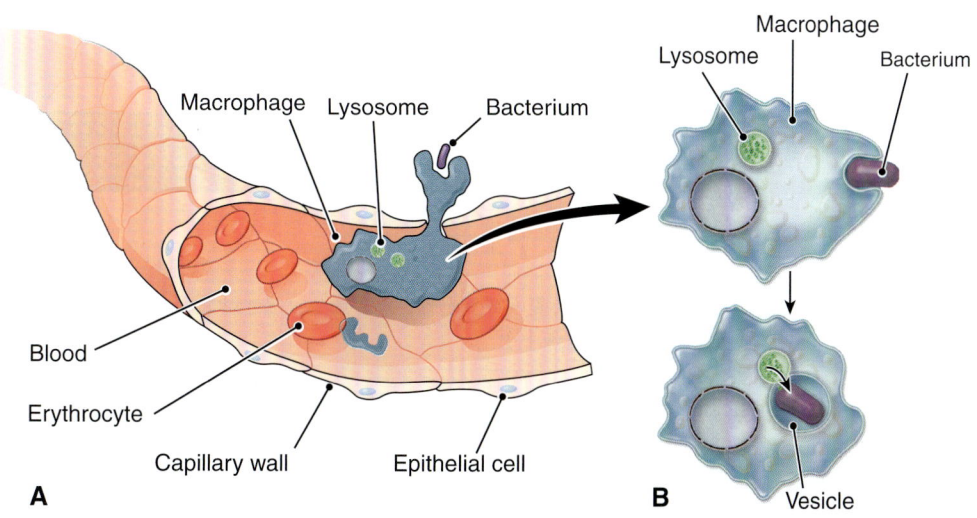

图 6-5 吞噬作用。A. 一个吞噬白细胞挤压通过毛细管壁吞噬细菌；B. 细菌被包封在囊泡中，并被溶酶体酶破坏

统中循环。吞噬作用的残余物包括体液和白细胞，它们的混合物被称为脓（pus）。

免疫

免疫（immunity）是指对所有感染性疾病的抵抗。炎症和吞噬作用是内生或内在保护性机制的示例，它们基于个人的基因构成，并不需要预先暴露于致病微生物。属于这类免疫的抵抗还有机械性壁垒，例如完整的皮肤和黏膜，以及人体分泌物，例如胃酸和唾液和眼泪中的酶。

在我们暴露于致病微生物期间发展起来的免疫，被称为获得性免疫（acquired immunity）或适应性免疫（adaptive immunity），这类免疫对自然暴露于的或服用疫苗获得的特定致病微生物有效（参见第10章）。负责适应性免疫的系统由血液中的细胞、淋巴系统和其他组织构成。这些细胞识别外来的入侵者，通过直接攻击消灭它们，并通过产生循环抗体（antibody）使入侵者不能移动，协助摧毁它们。免疫系统还持续监视人体的异常和失效的细胞，例如癌症细胞。免疫系统可能会反应过激而产生过敏，还可能左右自身的组织，导致自身免疫病。

肿瘤形成

上面提到，肿瘤（neoplasm）是异常且不受控制的组织增长。良性（benign）肿瘤不扩散，也就是说不向其他组织转移，尽管在其生长处可能造成损害。侵害性肿瘤可能向其他组织转移，被认为恶性

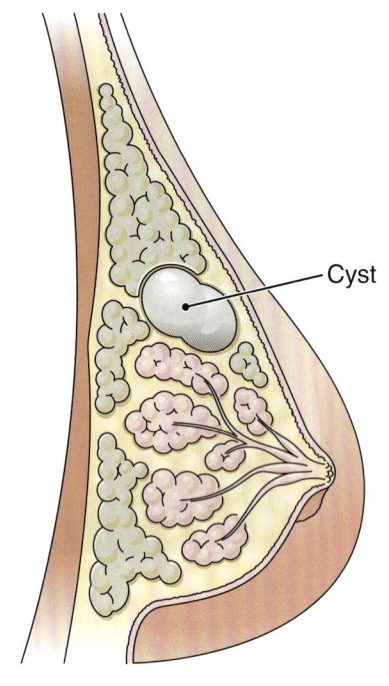

图6-6　乳腺囊肿（cyst）

（malignant）的，通常被称为癌症（cancer）。涉及上皮的恶性肿瘤是癌。如果肿瘤发生在腺上皮，就是恶性腺瘤（adenocarcinoma，词根 aden/o 意为"腺体"），色素上皮细胞癌（melanocytes）就是黑色素瘤。涉及结缔组织或肌肉的肿瘤被称为肉瘤（sarcoma）。血液、淋巴系统和神经系统的癌症要根据其涉及的细胞类型和其他临床特征来分类。

囊肿（cyst）是充满液体或半固体物质的液囊（sac）或水泡（pouch），常被误认为是异常的，但不是癌变（图6-6）。囊肿通常发生在乳房、皮肤的脂肪腺和卵巢。囊肿的成因包括感染或导管阻塞。

Terminology 关键术语

acute [ə'kju:t]	急性的，突然、严重，病期短
benign [bi'nain]	良性的，不会复发或变恶性，利于康复；描述肿瘤不向其他组织扩散（metastasize [mə'tæstəsaiz]）
carcinoma [ˌkɑ:si'nəʊmə]	癌，由上皮细胞组成的恶性肿瘤（源自于希腊词根 carcino，意为"蟹"，形容词形式为：carcinomatous）
chronic ['krɒnik]	慢性的，发展缓慢
cyst [sist]	囊肿，异常充满的液囊或水泡（图6-6，词根 cyst/o）

Terminology 关键术语

edema [ɪˈdiːmə]	水肿，组织中液体的积累，肿胀；形容词为：edematous [ɪˈdiːmətəs]（图 6-4）
etiology [ˌiːtiˈɒlədʒi]	病因，致病源
Gram stain	革兰氏染色，实验室染色程序，将细菌分为两类，革兰氏阳性，紫色；革兰氏阴性，红色（图 6-1）
hernia [ˈhɜːniə]	疝，器官通过异常开口突出（图 6-7）
inflammation [ɪnfləˈmeɪʃ(ə)n]	炎症，对组织受伤的局部反应，特征是发热、疼痛、发红和肿胀
lesion [ˈliːʒ(ə)n]	病变，明显的受损组织、受伤处或伤口
malignant [məˈlɪɡnənt]	恶性的，错误生长、有害、可能致死，描述可能向其他组织扩散的入侵性肿瘤
metastasis [mɪˈtæstəsɪs]	转移，从身体的一部分扩散到另一部分，癌症的特征；动词形式为 metastasize [məˈtæstəsaɪz]，形容词为 metastatic [ˌmetəˈstætɪk]
microorganism [ˌmaɪkrəʊˈɔːɡ(ə)nɪz(ə)m]	微生物，不使用显微镜就无法看到的生物
necrosis [neˈkrəʊsɪs]	坏死，（词根 necr/o，意为"死亡"）；形容词形式为：necrotic [neˈkrɒtɪk]
neoplasm [ˈniːə(ʊ)plæz(ə)m]	肿瘤，异常的、不受控制的组织生长，可能是良性的，也可能是恶性的。前缀 neo- 意为"新的"，词根 plasm 意为"形成"。词根 onc/o 和后缀 -oma 都指肿瘤
parasite [ˈpærəsaɪt]	寄生虫，生长在另一个生物（宿主）之上或之中的生物，会给宿主带来危害
pathogen [ˈpæθədʒ(ə)n]	病原体，能够致病的生物（词根 path/o 意为"疾病"）
phagocytosis [ˌfæɡə(ʊ)saɪˈtəʊsɪs]	吞噬作用，摄取例如入侵的细菌或细胞碎片等生物和废物（词根 phag/o 意为"吃"），巨噬细胞（phagocyte）然后摧毁它们（图 6-5）
prolapse [ˈprəʊlæps]	脱垂，器官下降或向下位移
pus [pʌs]	脓，炎症的产物，包含液体和白细胞（词根 py/o）
sarcoma [sɑːˈkəʊmə]	肉瘤，结缔组织中发生的恶性肿瘤（源自于希腊词根 sarco 意为"肉"），形容词为 sarcomatous
sepsis [ˈsepsɪs]	腐败作用，败血症，在血液或其他组织中存在有害微生物或其毒素，形容词为 septic
toxin [ˈtɒksɪn]	毒素，形容词为 toxic（词根 tox/o，toxic/o）
trauma [ˈtrɔːmə]	创伤，身体或心理的伤口或伤害

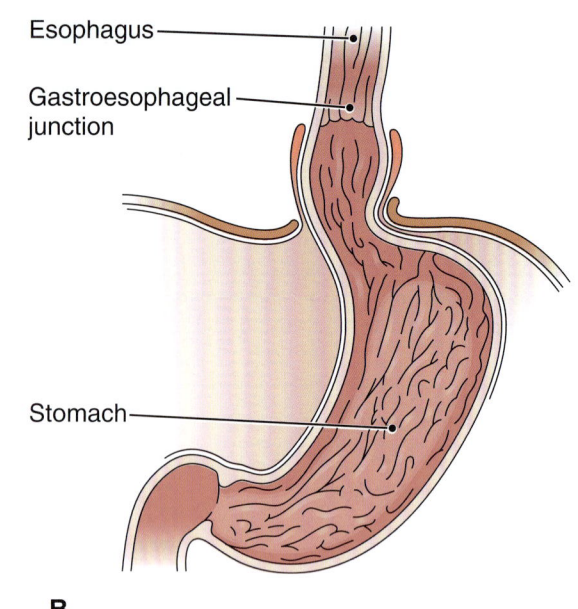

图 6-7 疝（hernia）。A. 正常胃 B. 食管裂孔疝；胃通过隔膜突出到胸腔中，提高了食道和胃之间的连接的水平

与疾病相关的单词组成部分

（表 6-1 至 6-5）

表 6-1	与疾病相关的词根		
词根	含义	示例	示例定义
alg/o, algi/o, algesi/o	疼痛	algesia ［æl'dʒisiə］	疼痛的状态
carcin/o	癌症，癌	carcinoid ［'kɑːsinɒid］	与癌类似
cyst/o	充满的液囊或水泡、囊肿、囊状物	cystic ［'sistik］	囊肿的或有囊肿
lith	结石、石头	lithiasis ［li'θaiəsis］	结石病
onc/o	肿瘤	oncogenic ［ˌɔŋkəu'dʒenik］	致瘤的
path/o	疾病	athogen ［'pæθədʒ(ə)n］	病原体
py/o	脓	pyocyst ［pai'əusist］	脓囊肿
pyr/o, pyret/o	发热，火	pyrexia ［pai'reksiə］	发热
scler/o	硬的	sclerosis ［skliə'rəusis］	组织硬化
tox/o, toxic/o	毒	endotoxin ［'endəuˌtɒksin］	内毒素

练习 6-1

识别并定义下列单词中的词根。

	Root	Meaning of Root
1. toxicology [ˌtɒksiˈkɒlədʒi]	_____	_____
2. pyorrhea [ˌpaiəˈriə]	_____	_____
3. lithotomy [liˈθɒtəmi]	_____	_____
4. pathologist [pəˈθɒlədʒist]	_____	_____

填空。

5. Arteriosclerosis [ɑːtiəriəusklə'rəusis] is a(n)_____ of the arteries.
6. A urolith [ˈjuərəliθ] is a(n)_____ in the urinary tract (ur/o).
7. A cystotome [sisˈtəutəum] is an instrument for incising the_____.
8. The term pathogenic [ˈpæθəˈdʒenik] means producing_____.
9. A carcinogen [kɑːˈsinədʒən] is a substance that causes_____.
10. An exotoxin [ˌeksəu'tɒksin] is a(n)_____secreted by bacterial cells.
11. Pyoderma [paiəu'dɜːmə] is a skin disease associated with_____.
12. An algesimeter [ˈældʒesimiːtər] is used to measure sensitivity to_____.
13. An oncogene [ˈɒŋkədʒiːn] is a gene that causes a(n)_____.
14. A pyrogenic [pairəu'dʒenik] agent induces_____.

表 6-2　与疾病相关的前缀

前缀	含义	示例	示例定义
brady-	缓慢	bradypnea [bræˈdipniə]	呼吸过慢
dys-	异常、疼痛、困难	dysplasia [disˈpleiziə]	发育不良
mal-	坏的、差的	malabsorption [ˌmæləbˈsɔpʃən]	吸收不良
pachy-	厚的	pachycephaly [ˌpækəˈsefəli]	颅骨肥厚
tachy-	快的	tachycardia [ˌtækiˈkɑːdiə]	心动过速
xero-	干的	xeroderma [ˌziərə(ʊ)ˈdɜːmə]	干皮病

练习 6-2

匹配以下术语，并在每个数字的左侧写入相应的字母。

____ 1. tachycardia ［ˌtæki'kɑ:diə］ a. abnormal thickness of the fingers
____ 2. pachydactyly ［pæ'kidəktili］ b. abnormal nourishment of tissue
____ 3. bradypnea ［b'reidipniə］ c. difficulty in swallowing
____ 4. dystrophy ［'distrəfi］ d. slow breathing
____ 5. dysphagia ［dis'feidʒiə］ e. rapid heart rate

识别并定义下列单词中的前缀。

	Prefix	Meaning of Prefix
6. xerosis ［ziə'rəusis］	____	____
7. dysentery ［'disəntri］	____	____
8. maladjustment ［ˌmælə'dʒʌstmənt］	____	____

表 6-3　与疾病相关的后缀

后缀	含义	示例	示例定义
-algia	疼痛	neuralgia ［ˌnjʊə'rældʒə］	神经痛（neur/o）
-cele	疝、局部扩张	gastrocele ［'gætrəsel］	胃膨出（gastr/o）
-clasis, -clasia	破裂	karyoclasis ［ˌkəriəʊ'klæsis］	核破裂（kary/o）
-itis	炎症	cystitis ［si'staitis］	膀胱炎（cyst/o）
-megaly	扩大	hepatomegaly ［ˌhipætə'mɛgəli］	肝大（hepat/o）
-odynia	疼痛	urodynia ［jurəʊ'dainiə］	尿痛（ur/o）
-oma*	肿瘤	lipoma ［li'pəʊmə］	脂肪瘤
-pathy	疾病的	nephropathy ［nə'frɒpəθi］	肾病（nephr/o）
-rhage†, -rhagia†	喷出、过量流动	hemorrhage ［'heməridʒ］	大出血
-rhea†	流动、排泄	pyorrhea ［ˌpaiə'ri:ə］	脓漏
-rhexis†	断裂	amniorrhexis ［ˌæmniɒ'reksis］	羊膜破裂
-schisis	裂缝、分裂	retinoschisis ［ˌritinəʊ'ʃaisis］	视网膜劈裂症

* 复数：-omas，-omata
† 在词根上加此后缀时要双写字母 r

练习 6-3

匹配以下术语，并在每个数字的左侧写入相应的字母。

____ 1. adipocele ['ædipəʊseli:]　　　　　a. hernia containing fat
____ 2. blastoma [blɑːs'təmə]　　　　　 b. fissure of the chest
____ 3. thoracoschisis [θɔːrə'kɒskisis]　c. breaking of a bone
____ 4. melanoma [ˌmelə'nəʊmə]　　　 d. tumor of immature cells
____ 5. osteoclasis [ˌɒsti'ɒkləsis]　　　 e. tumor of pigmented cells

____ 6. gastrodynia ['gæstrəʊdiniə]　　 a. local dilatation containing fluid
____ 7. menorrhagia [ˌmenə'reidʒiə]　　b. pain in the stomach
____ 8. hydrocele ['haidrəsiːl]　　　　　c. pain in the head
____ 9. cephalgia [sep'hældʒə]　　　　 d. profuse menstrual flow
____ 10. hepatorrhexis [hepətəʊ'reksis]　e. rupture of the liver

词根 my/o 意为"肌肉"，请定义下列术语。

11. myalgia [mai'ældʒə] _____
12. myopathy [mai'ɒpəθi] _____
13. myorrhexis [maiə'reksis] _____
14. myodynia [ma'iɒdiniə] _____
15. myoma [mai'əʊmə] _____

一些与疾病有关的单词在组合单词中被用作后缀（表6-4）。后缀是出现在单词尾部的一个组成部分，可能是一个简单的后缀（例如 -y、-ia、-ic），也可能是一个词根加后缀的组合，例如 -megaly、-rhagia、-pathy 等。

表 6-4　被用作后缀的单词

单词	含义	示例	示例定义
dilation*, dilatation*	扩大、放宽	vasodilation [ˌvæzəʊdai'leiʃən]	血管舒张（vas/o）
ectasia, ectasis	扩大、扩张、膨胀	gastrectasia [gæs'trekteiʒə]	胃胀（gastr/o）
edema	液体积累、肿胀	cephaledema [ˌsefəli'diːmə]	脑水肿
lysis	分开、放松、分解、破坏	dialysis [ˌdai'æləsis]	透析
malacia	软化	craniomalacia ['kreiniəʊmə'leisiə]	颅骨软化（crani/o）
necrosis	组织死亡	osteonecrosis [ˌɒstiəʊne'krəʊsis]	骨坏死（oste/o）

续表 6-4　被用作后缀的单词

单词	含义	示例	示例定义
ptosis	下降、向下位移、脱垂	blepharoptosis ［ˌblefərə'təusis］	眼睑下垂（blephar/o，图 6-8）
sclerosis	硬化	phlebosclerosis ［ˌflebəuskli'rəusis］	静脉硬化（phleb/o）
spasm	突然收缩、痉挛	arteriospasm ［ɑ:'tiəriəu'spæz(ə)m］	动脉痉挛
stasis	萎缩、阻塞	menostasis ［ˌmenə'stæsis］	绝经（men/o）
stenosis	变窄、压缩	bronchostenosis ［ˌbrɒŋkəusti'nəusis］	支气管狭窄
toxin	有毒的	nephrotoxin ［ˌnefrəu'tɒksin］	肾毒素

*也可能意味着治疗

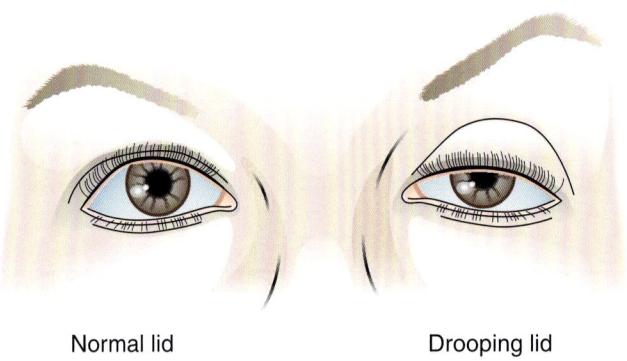

Normal lid　　　Drooping lid

图 6-8　眼睑下垂（blepharoptosis）。下垂（ptosis）意为向下位移

练习 6-4

匹配以下术语，并在每个数字的左侧写入相应的字母。

____ 1. myolysis ［ma'iɒlisis］　　　　　a. destruction of blood cells
____ 2. osteomalacia ［ˌɒstiəumə'leiʃə］　b. death of heart tissue
____ 3. cardionecrosis ［kɑ:daiənek'rəusis］　c. stoppage of blood flow
____ 4. hemolysis ［hi'mɒlisis］　　　　d. softening of a bone
____ 5. hemostasis ［ˌhi:mə'steisis］　　e. dissolving of muscle

词根 splen/o 意为"脾"，请定义下列术语。

6. splenomalacia ［spli:nɒ'mæleiʃə］ _____
7. splenoptosis ［spli:nɒp'təusis］ _____
8. splenotoxin ［ˌspli:nə'tɒksin］ _____

表 6-5	与感染性疾病有关的前缀和词根		
单词组成部分	含义	示例	示例定义
前缀			
staphy/o	葡萄样的、团	staphylococcus [ˌstæfilə(ʊ)'kɒkəs]	葡萄球菌
strept/o	扭曲的链	streptobacillus [ˌstreptəʊbə'siləs]	链杆菌
词根			
bacill/i, bacill/o	杆菌	bacilluria [bə'siljʊəriə]	杆菌尿
bacteri/o	细菌	bacteriostatic [bækˌtiriəs'tætik]	抑制细菌的
myc/o	真菌、霉菌	mycotic [mai'kɔtik]	真菌病
vir/o	病毒	viremia [vai'ri:miə]	病毒血症

练习 6-5

填空。

1. A bactericidal [bækˌtirə'saidl] agent kills _____.
2. A mycosis [mai'kosis] is any disease caused by a(n) _____.
3. The term bacillary ['bæslˌɛri] means pertaining to _____.
4. The prefix strepto- means _____.
5. The prefix staphylo- means _____.

使用后缀 -logy 写出下列含义的单词

6. Study of fungi _____
7. Study of viruses _____
8. Study of bacteria _____

Terminology 补充术语

acid-fast stain	抗酸性染色法，主要用于鉴定结核生物
communicable [kə'mju:nikəb(ə)l]	会传染的
endemic [en'demik]	地方病（源自于 en-，意为"在……之内"和希腊单词 demo，意为"民族"）
epidemic [epi'demik]	流行病，在给定地区同时影响很多人，在给定时间内在大部分人群中暴发
exacerbation [ekˌsæsə'beiʃən]	恶化，疾病或其症状的急性发作

Terminology 补充术语（续表）

iatrogenic [ai,ætrə(ʊ)'dʒenik]	医源性的（源自于希腊词根 iatro-，意为"医生"）
idiopathic [ˌidiə(ʊ)'pæθik]	先天的、原发的（词根 idio 意为"源于自身"）
in situ [in'saitju:]	在原地，局部、非侵害性的；用于说明肿瘤不扩散
normal flora ['flɔrə]	正常菌群，这些生物一般是无害的，通常还是有益的，但在特殊情况下可能会引发疾病，如受伤或免疫系统失效
nosocomial [ˌnosə'komiəl]	院内感染（词根 nos/o 意为"疾病"，comial 指医院）。这种感染可能是一个严重问题，特别是如果它们对抗生素有抵抗性。例如，目前没有针对耐甲氧西林的金黄葡萄球菌（methicillin-resistant Staphylococcus aureus，MRSA）和耐万古霉素的金黄葡萄球菌（vancomycin-resistant S. aureus，VRSA）的染色法，这两种细菌在医院环境中会引起危险的感染
opportunistic [ˌɒpətju:'nistik]	机会性的，描述患者由于身体条件较差或处于变化时期发生的感染
pandemic [pæn'demik]	普遍流行的疾病，描述一种疾病在整个地区或全世界流行
remission [ri'miʃ(ə)n]	缓解
septicemia [ˌsepti'si:miə]	败血症
systemic [si'stemik]	全身的

疾病的表现形式

abscess ['æbsis]	脓肿
adhesion [əd'hi:ʒ(ə)n]	粘连
anaplasia [ˌænə'pleʒə]	间变
ascites [ə'saiti:z]	腹水
cellulitis [ˌseljʊ'laitis]	蜂窝织炎
effusion [i'fju:ʒ(ə)n]	渗出
exudate ['egzjʊdeit]	渗出物
fissure ['fiʃə]	裂缝
fistula ['fistjʊlə]	瘘管
gangrene ['gæŋgri:n]	坏疽
hyperplasia [ˌhaipə'pleiziə]	增生
hypertrophy [hai'pɜ:trəfi]	肥大
induration [ˌindjʊ'reiʃən]	硬化
metaplasia [ˌmetə'pleiziə]	组织变形（前缀 meta- 意为"改变"）

Terminology 补充术语（续表）

polyp [ˈpɒlip]		息肉
purulent [ˈpjʊərʊl(ə)nt]		化脓性的
suppuration [ˌsʌpjəˈreʃən]		化脓

Terminology 缩略语

AF	Acid fast	抗酸
CA, Ca	Cancer	癌症
CIS	Carcinoma in situ	原位癌
FUO	Fever of unknown origin	不明原因的发热
Gm^+	Gram-positive	革兰氏阳性
Gm^-	Gram-negative	革兰氏阴性
MRSA	Methicillin-resistant Staphylococcus aureus	耐甲氧西林的金黄色葡萄球菌
Staph	Staphylococcus	葡萄球菌
Strep	Streptococcus	链球菌
VRSA	Vancomycin-resistant Staphylococcus aureus	耐万古霉素的金黄色葡萄球菌

Case Study Revisited 案例研究再访

J. N.'s Follow-Up

J. N. took the full course of drug therapy, and her symptoms subsided. She brought in a stool specimen to her follow-up office visit. Test results were negative for the offending pathogen.

J. N. 的随访

J. N. 完成了药物治疗的过程，她的症状消退了。她随访时带来了一个粪便标本，测试结果显示入侵病原体为阴性。

CHAPTER 6 复习

匹配

匹配以下术语，并在每个数字的左侧写入相应的字母。

____ 1. cardiomegaly	a. pertaining to profuse flow of blood
____ 2. neuroma	b. fear of cancer
____ 3. carcinophobia	c. tumor of a nerve
____ 4. encephalitis	d. enlargement of the heart
____ 5. hemorrhagic	e. inflammation of the brain

____ 6. sclerotic	a. stone formation
____ 7. oncolysis	b. dry
____ 8. analgesia	c. destruction of a tumor
____ 9. xerotic	d. absence of pain
____ 10. lithiasis	e. hardened

____ 11. dysphagia	a. swelling of the fingers or toes
____ 12. apyrexia	b. thickness of the skin
____ 13. pyorrhea	c. discharge of pus
____ 14. dactyledema	d. difficulty in swallowing
____ 15. pachyderma	e. absence of fever

____ 16. blepharoptosis	a. local wound or injury
____ 17. hemostasis	b. stoppage of blood flow
____ 18. toxoid	c. dropping of the eyelid
____ 19. lesion	d. like a poison
____ 20. ectasia	e. dilatation

____ 21. spasm	a. resembling cancer
____ 22. carcinoid	b. hardening of a vein
____ 23. venosclerosis	c. any disease of a gland
____ 24. cardiorrhexis	d. sudden contraction or cramp
____ 25. adenopathy	e. rupture of the heart

补充术语

____ 26. nosocomial	a. abnormal passageway
____ 27. iatrogenic	b. escape of fluid into a cavity
____ 28. fistula	c. tumor attached by a thin stalk
____ 29. polyp	d. acquired in a hospital
____ 30. effusion	e. caused by effects of treatments

____ 31. idiopathic   a. localized collection of pus
____ 32. purulent   b. having no known cause
____ 33. ascites   c. worsening
____ 34. abscess   d. fluid in the abdominal cavity
____ 35. exacerbation   e. forming or containing pus

填空

36. Heat, pain, redness, and swelling are the four major signs of _____.
37. Any abnormal and uncontrolled growth of tissue, whether benign or malignant, is called a(n) _____.
38. The spreading of cancer to other parts of the body is the process of _____.
39. Protrusion of an organ through an abnormal opening is a(n) _____.
40. Toxicology is the study of _____.
41. Death of tissue is called _____.
42. An oncoprotein is a protein associated with a(n) _____.
43. Referring to J.N.'s opening case study, the suffix and its meaning in the word diarrhea is _____.
44. The plural of protozoon is _____.
45. The common name for a helminth is a(n) _____.

定义

使用后缀 -genesis 写出下列含义的单词。

46. Formation of cancer _____
47. Origin of any disease _____
48. Formation of pus _____
49. Formation of a tumor _____

词根 bronch/o 与肺中的支气管相关，在该词根上添加一个后缀，形成下列含义的单词。

50. Excessive flow or discharge from a bronchus _____
51. Inflammation of a bronchus _____
52. Narrowing of a bronchus _____
53. Sudden contraction of a bronchus _____

使用意为"骨骼"的词根 oste/o 构成下列含义的单词。

54. Pain in a bone _____
55. Death of bone tissue _____
56. Tumor of a bone _____
57. Breaking of a bone _____
58. Softening of a bone _____

真假判断

检查以下语句。如果语句为真，则在第一个空白处写入 T；如果语句为假，则在第一个空格中写入 F，并在第二个空格中通过替换带下划线的单词来更正语句。

	true or false	correct answer
59. A mycosis is an infection with <u>a protozoon</u>.	_____	_____
60. Round bacteria in chains are <u>streptococci</u>.	_____	_____
61. A sudden disease of short duration is <u>chronic</u>.	_____	_____
62. A tumor that does not metastasize is termed <u>benign</u>.	_____	_____
63. A slower than normal heart rate is <u>tachycardia</u>.	_____	_____
64. A tumor of connective tissue is classified as a <u>sarcoma</u>.	_____	_____

排除

在下列每一组中，为与其余单词不相配的单词加下划线，并说明你选择的理由。

65. cocci — helminths — chlamydia — bacilli — vibrios

66. neoplasm — tumor — carcinoma — pathogen — oncology

67. septicemic — endemic — metastatic — opportunistic — epidemic

单词构建

使用给出的单词组成部分构建下列定义的单词。

| tox | pyr | gen | o | py | -oma | -y | path | nephr | -logy | -ic |

68. poisonous for the kidney _____
69. producing pus _____
70. tumor of the kidney _____
71. study of disease _____
72. producing fever _____
73. study of the kidney _____
74. producing disease _____
75. any disease of the kidney _____
76. producing kidney tissue _____

单词分析

定义下列单词，并给出每个单词组成部分的含义。如果需要，可以使用词典。

77. phagocytosis [ˌfæɡəsaiˈtosis]

    a. phag/o _____

    b. cyt/o _____

    c. -sis _____

78. hypoplasia [ˌhaipəˈpleʒə]
   a. hypo-_____
   b. plas _____
   c. –ia _____
79. antipyretic [ˌæntipaiˈrɛtik]
   a. anti-_____
   b. pyret/o_____
   c. -ic _____
80. arteriosclerosis [ɑrˌtirioskləˈrosis]
   a. arterio/o_____
   b. scler/o_____
   c. -sis _____
81. dysbiosis [disˈbaiəsis] Imbalance in the normal flora of microorganisms
   a. dys-_____
   b. bio _____
   c. –sis _____

Additional Case Studies
补充案例研究

Case Study 6-1: HIV Infection and Tuberculosis
案例研究 6-1： HIV 感染与结核病

T. H., a 48-year-old man, was an admitted intravenous (IV) drug user and occasionally abused alcohol. Over four weeks, he had experienced fever, night sweats, malaise, a cough, and a 10-lb weight loss. He was also concerned about several discolored lesions that had erupted weeks before on his arms and legs.

T. H. made an appointment with a physician assistant (PA) at the neighborhood clinic. On examination, the PA noted bilateral anterior cervical and axillary lymphadenopathy and pyrexia. T.H.'s temperature was 102.2° F. The PA sent T.H. to the hospital for further studies.

T. H.'s chest radiograph (x-ray image) showed paratracheal adenopathy and bilateral interstitial infiltrates, suspicious of tuberculosis (TB). His blood study results were positive for human immunodeficiency virus (HIV) and showed a low lymphocyte count. Sputum and bronchoscopic lavage (washing) fluid were positive for an acid-fast bacillus (AFB); a PPD (purified protein derivative) skin test result was also positive. Based on these findings, T.H. was diagnosed with HIV, TB, and Kaposi sarcoma related to past IV drug abuse.

T. H. 是一名 48 岁的男性，他是一个静脉（IV）药物允许使用者，偶尔滥用酒精。在 4 个多星期中，他经历了发热、盗汗、不适、咳嗽和 10 磅体重减轻。他还担心数周前在他的胳膊和腿上出现的几个变色的病变。

T. H. 预约了邻近诊所的医生助理（physician assistant）。检查时，医生助理注意到 T.H. 双侧前路颈椎和腋窝淋巴结肿大和发热。T.H. 的体温为 102.2°F。助理将 T.H. 转到医院进行进一步检查。

T. H. 的胸部 X 线片（radiograph）显示气管旁腺病（paratracheal adenopathy）和双侧间质性浸润（interstitial infiltrates），怀疑是结核病（tuberculosis，TB）。他的血液分析结果显示人类免疫缺陷病毒（human immunodeficiency virus，HIV）阳性，并显示淋巴细胞计数较低。痰和支气管灌洗液（bronchoscopic lavage）对于抗酸杆菌（acid-fast bacillus，AFB）阳性；纯化蛋白衍生物（purified protein derivative，PPD）皮肤试验结果也是阳性。基于这些发现，T. H. 被诊断为与过去静脉药物滥用相关的 HIV 感染、结核病和卡波西肉瘤。

Case Study 6-2: Endocarditis
案例研究 6-2： 心内膜炎

D. A., a 37 y/o man, sought treatment after experiencing several days of high fever and generalized weakness on return from his vacation. D. A.'s family doctor suspected cardiac involvement because of D. A.'s history of rheumatic fever. The doctor was concerned because D. A.'s brother had died of acute malignant hyperpyrexia during surgery at the age of 12. D. A. was referred to a cardiologist, who scheduled an electrocardiogram (ECG) and a transesophageal echocardiogram (TEE).

D. A. was admitted to the hospital with subacute bacterial endocarditis (SBE) and placed on high-dose IV antibiotics and bed rest. He had also developed a heart murmur, which was diagnosed as idiopathic hypertrophic subaortic stenosis (IHSS).

D. A. 是一名 37 岁的男性，度假返回后经历了几天的高热和全身乏力，寻求治疗。因为 D. A. 有风湿热（rheumatic fever）病史，家庭医生怀疑 D. A. 的心脏受到了影响。医生很担心，因为 D. A. 的兄弟在 12 岁的手术期间死于急性恶性高热。D. A. 被转诊给心脏病科医生（cardiologist），心脏病科医生为他安排了心电图（electrocardiogram，ECG）和经食管超声心动图（transesophageal echocardiogram，TEE）检查。

D. A. 因亚急性细菌性心内膜炎（subacute bacterial endocarditis，SBE）入院，并给予高剂量静脉抗生素和卧床休息。他还出现了一种心脏杂音（heart murmur），被诊断为特发性肥厚性主动脉瓣下狭窄（idiopathic hypertrophic subaortic stenosis，IHSS）。

案例研究问题

多项选择，选择最佳答案，写在每个题号的左侧。

____ 1. The term axillary refers to the
  a. armpit
  b. groin
  c. wrist
  d. bladder

____ 2. In referring to tissues, the term interstitial means
  a. around cells
  b. under cells
  c. between cells
  d. within cells

____ 3. The cervical region is the region of the
  a. head
  b. leg
  c. heart
  d. neck

____ 4. The term pyrexia refers to a
  a. fever
  b. stone
  c. tumor
  d. poison

____ 5. Paraesophageal and paratracheal refer to a position _____ the esophagus and trachea.
  a. under
  b. near
  c. superior to
  d. in between

____ 6. The endocardium is the tissue lining the heart's chambers. Endocarditis refers to a(n) _____ of this lining.
  a. narrowing
  b. inflammation
  c. overgrowth
  d. thinning

____ 7. D.A.'s heart murmur was caused by a stenosis, or _____ of the heart's aortic valve.
  a. narrowing
  b. inflammation
  c. overgrowth
  d. cancer

____ 8. The term for a condition or disease of unknown etiology is
  a. hypertrophic
  b. chronic
  c. acute
  d. idiopathic

填空。

9. Adenopathy is any disease of a(n) _____.
10. Tuberculosis is caused by a bacterium that is rod-shaped, thus described as a(n) _____.
11. A malignant neoplasm arising from muscle or connective tissue is a(n) _____.
12. A potentially fatal disease condition characterized by a very high fever is called _____.

给出下列缩略语的含义。

13. HIV _____
14. PPD _____
15. ECG _____
16. AFB _____

CHAPTER 7 诊断、治疗与手术

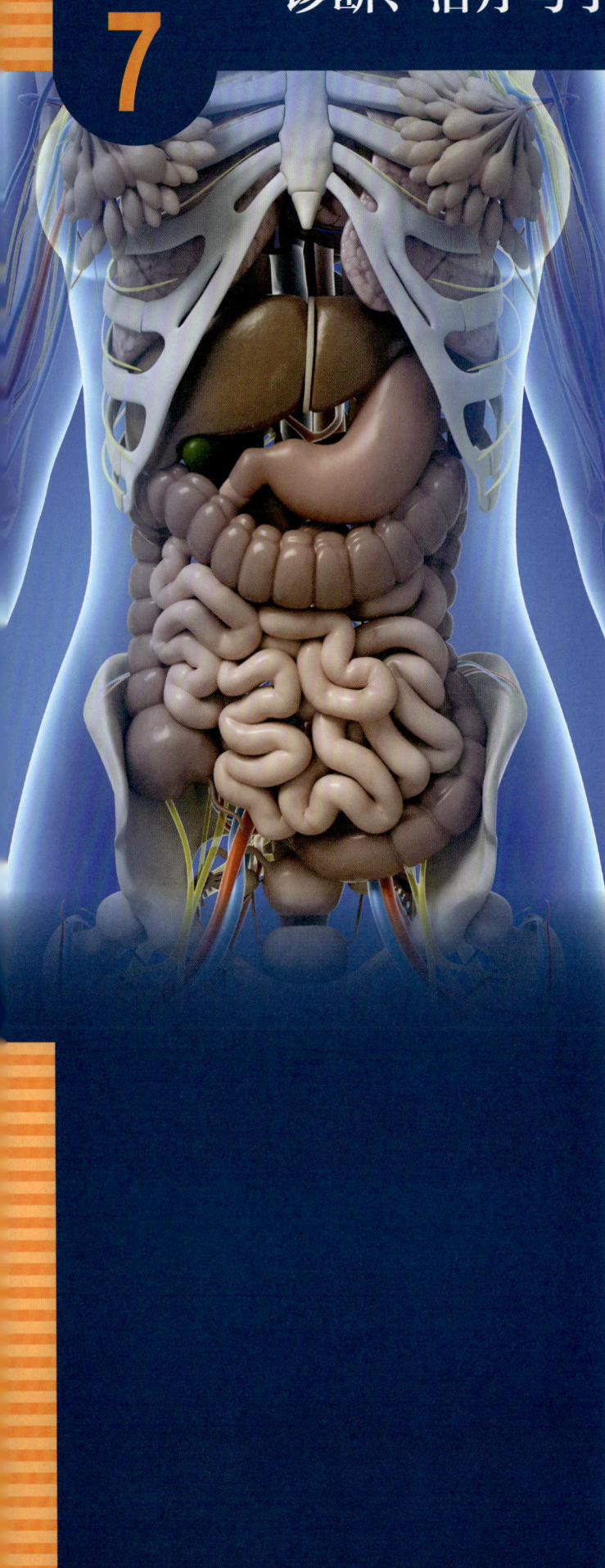

预测试

多项选择，选择最佳答案，并在每个数字的左边写上你选择的字母。

____ 1. Determination of a disease's nature and cause is called
   a. admission
   b. diagnosis
   c. titration
   d. prognosis

____ 2. Measurements of the basic functions needed to maintain life, such as breathing and pulse, together are called
   a. respiration
   b. health signs
   c. vital signs
   d. etiology

____ 3. A simple device for listening to sounds within the body is a
   a. cystoscope
   b. stethoscope
   c. barometer
   d. speculum

____ 4. Removal of tissue for microscopic study is a(n)
   a. biopsy
   b. aeration
   c. endoscopy
   d. CT scan

____ 5. Appendicitis is
   a. therapy of the appendix
   b. imaging of the appendix
   c. measurement of the appendix
   d. inflammation of the appendix

____ 6. A tracheotomy is
   a. surgical incision of the trachea
   b. placement of a tracheal tube
   c. removal of a tracheal tube
   d. removal of the trachea

学习目标

学完本章后，应该能够：

1. ▶ 列出病历的主要组成部分。
2. ▶ 描述患者检查使用的主要方法。
3. ▶ 指出并描述九种成像技术。
4. ▶ 指出可能的治疗方式的名称。
5. ▶ 描述替代性和补充性医疗的理论，以及在这些领域中的一些治疗方法。
6. ▶ 描述癌症的分期和分级系统。
7. ▶ 定义与医学检查、诊断和治疗相关的术语。
8. ▶ 识别并使用与诊断和手术相关的词根和后缀。
9. ▶ 解释诊断和治疗中使用的符号和缩略语。
10. ▶ 分析案例研究中与诊断和治疗相关的医学术语。

Case Study: M. L.'s Rollerblading Mishap
案例研究：M. L. 的滑旱冰事故

Chief Complaint

M. L., an active 59-year-old woman, was rollerblading early one morning. When attempting to avoid some loose gravel, she fell, injuring her right wrist and knee. She immediately experienced pain in her wrist and knee and noticed that her knee was swelling. She was able to use her cell phone and call her husband who came and took her to a nearby emergency room.

Examination

The physician assistant (PA) in the emergency room obtained the following history (Hx) of the incident:

M. L. was rollerblading on a path early that morning and skated into some loose gravel, causing her to fall forward. She attempted to break the fall with her arms and ended up landing with her right hand and knee bearing the impact of the fall. She was able to take off the rollerblades and, favoring her right leg, make her way over to a nearby bench, where she used her cell phone to contact her husband for help. M.L. was not wearing a helmet or any protective pads on her knees, elbows, or wrists.

The PA inspected the wrist, which was deformed and edematous. She palpated the wrist area and documented that M. L. complained of pain, weakness, and slight tingling in the fingers. There was limited range of motion (ROM) of the fingers. Next, the PA examined the knee that was now quite swollen. M.L. could not bear much weight on the right leg and complained of considerable pain. The PA explained the prognosis to M.L. and her husband and then proceeded to order some diagnostic tests.

Clinical Course

M. L. was taken to the radiology department, where an x-ray of the right wrist revealed a fracture. An MRI was ordered for the knee and showed no fractures or ligament tears. The PA explained to the patient that she might need to have an arthrocentesis, a tap to remove fluid in the knee joint, which would relieve some of the pain. She also explained that an endoscopic examination of the joint, an arthroscopy, might be required, but that the orthopedic surgeon who had already been consulted would determine whether or not this procedure was necessary.

主诉

M. L. 是一名 59 岁的女性，性格活泼，一天早晨她在溜旱冰，在试图避免一些松散的石砾时，她跌倒了，右手腕和膝盖受了伤。她立即感到手腕和膝盖疼痛，并发现膝盖肿胀。她能够使用手机打电话给丈夫带她去附近的急诊室。

检查

急诊室的医生助理（physician assistant，PA）获得了下列的病历（Hx）：

那天清晨 M. L. 在一条小路上滑旱冰，滑进一些松散的沙砾，使她向前摔倒。她试图用手臂避免摔倒，结果她的右手和膝盖着地，承受了摔倒的冲击。她能脱下旱冰鞋，靠她的右腿支撑走到附近的长凳上，在那里她用手机联系她的丈夫寻求帮助。M.L. 没有戴头盔，也没有在她的膝盖、肘部或手腕上佩戴任何保护垫。

医生助理检查了变形并肿胀的手腕。她对 M. L. 的手腕区域做了触诊（palpation），并记录了 M. L. 主诉疼痛、无力和手指轻微刺痛。手指的运动范围（range of motion，ROM）受到限制。接下来，医生助理检查了当时相当肿胀的膝盖。M. L. 的右腿上不能承受很大的重量，并主诉非常疼痛。助理向 M.L. 和她丈夫解释了预后（prognosis），然后着手安排一些诊断性检查。

临床病程

M. L. 被带到放射科，右手腕的 X 线片显示骨折。膝盖核磁共振（MRI）显示没有骨折或韧带撕裂。医生助理向患者说明她可能需要做关节穿刺术（arthrocentesis），用穿刺来消除膝关节中的积液，以缓解疼痛。她还解释说，可能需要对关节进行内窥镜（endoscope）检查，即关节镜检查（arthroscopy），已经咨询过的骨科医生将决定该检查是否必要。

简介

医疗起始于对疾病的评估，评估的基础是从患者和一系列测试和检查中所获得的信息。基于评估结果，推荐一个治疗方法，可能包括手术。

诊断

医疗诊断是对疾病性质和起因的确定，起始于患者的病历。病历包括带有症状描述（疾病的证据）的当前病史、既往病史和家庭及社会历史。

身体检查包括所有系统的审查以及任何疾病迹象的观察，随后是病历记录。在体格检查中，医生会利用以下技能：

- 检查（inspection）：视觉审查。
- 触诊（palpation）：有手或手指接触身体（图7-1）。
- 叩诊（percussion）：轻敲身体，根据所产生的声音评估组织是否健康（图7-2）。
- 听诊（auscultation）：用听诊器聆听身体内的声音（图7-3）。

医生会记录患者的生命体征（vital signs，VS），并与正常范围进行比较。生命体征反应了维持生命的基本必要功能，包括：

- 体温（temperature，T）。
- 脉率（pulse rate），单位是次/min（bpm）。

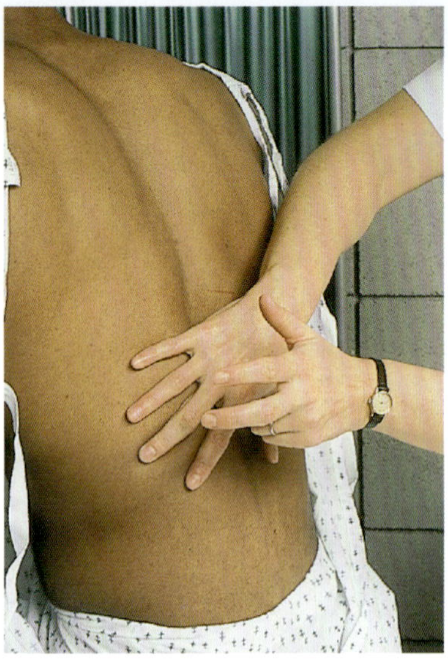

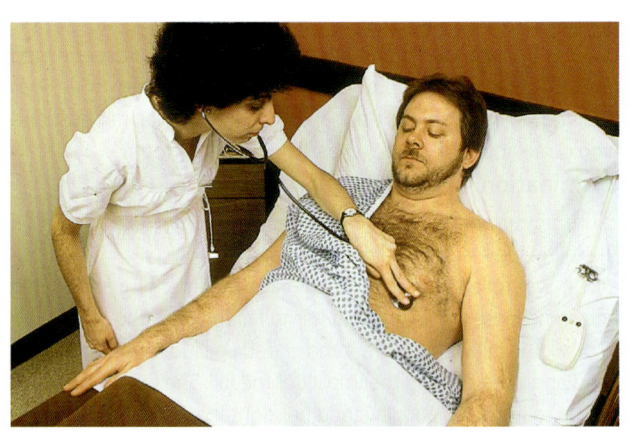

图7-2 叩诊。医生敲击身体以评估组织

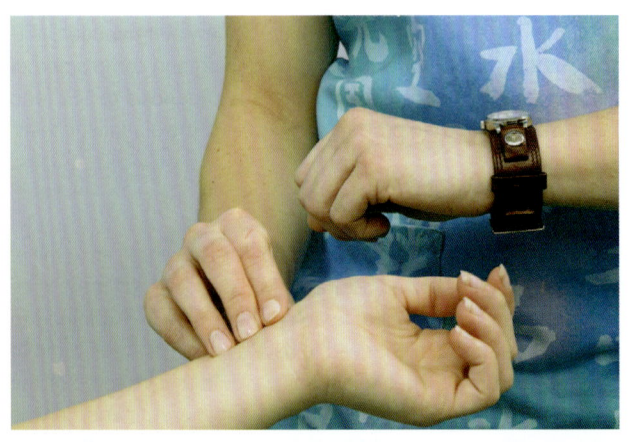

图7-3 听诊。医生使用听诊器听诊

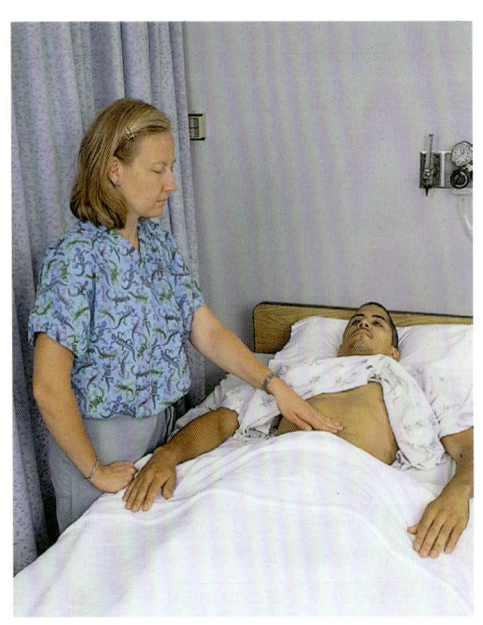

图7-1 触诊。医生用手或手指触摸体表

图7-4 脉率。医生触诊动脉以测量每分钟脉率

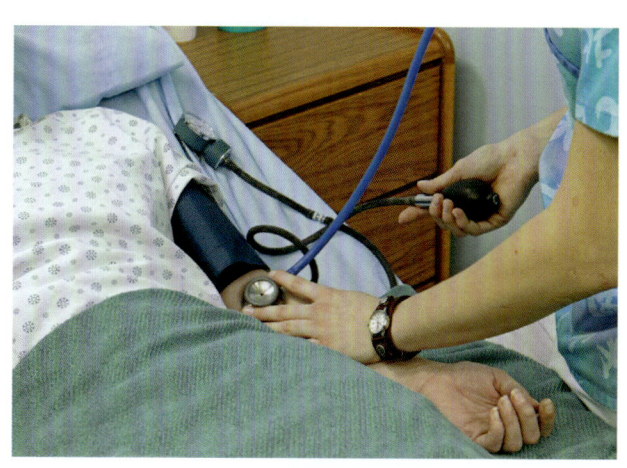

图 7-5　血压。医生使用血压计袖带（血压计）和听诊器来测量收缩压和舒张压

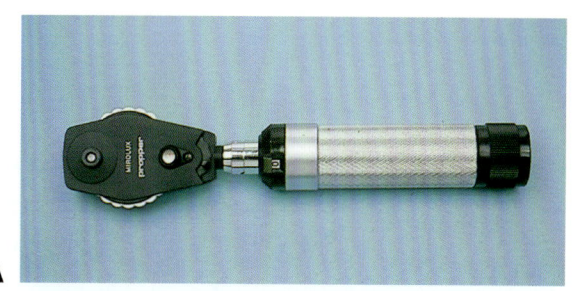
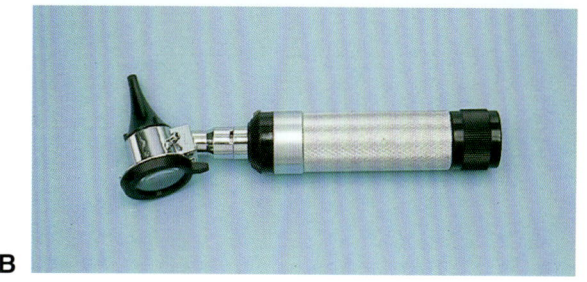

图 7-6　检查工具。A. 眼底镜做眼睛检查；B. 耳镜做耳朵检查

脉率通常与心率（heart rate，HR）相对应，就是每分钟心跳的次数（图 7-4）。

- 呼吸频率（R），单位是次 /min。
- 血压（BP），单位是毫米汞柱（mmHg），分别记录心脏在收缩（收缩压, systolic pressure）和舒张（舒张压, diastolic pressure）时的血液压力（图 7-5）。检查者通常会使用听诊器和血压计袖带，或血压计（sphygmomanometer［ˌsfɪgməʊməˈnɒmɪtə］）来测量血压。新型血压计能够直接测量血压，并显示数字结果。

在体格检查中使用的其他工具包括检查眼睛的眼底镜（ophthalmoscope）（图 7-6A）、检查耳朵的耳镜（otoscope）（图 7-6B）和检测反射的小锤。

皮肤、头发和指甲反应个人健康状态提供易于观察的指征。例如颜色、纹理、厚度和损伤（局部受伤）等皮肤特征在身体检查过程中都会被记录下来。

实验室测试结果会进一步帮助诊断。这些测试包括血压、尿液和其他体液的测试，以及感染性生物的鉴定。还有一些测试包括大脑和心脏电活动的研究、通过内窥镜（endoscope）检查体腔（图 7-7）和成像技术。活组织检查是从人体中取出组织，做显微镜检查。活组织检查样本可以通过以下方式获得：

- 针头抽取（吸出）体液，例如从胸腔或囊肿中抽取。

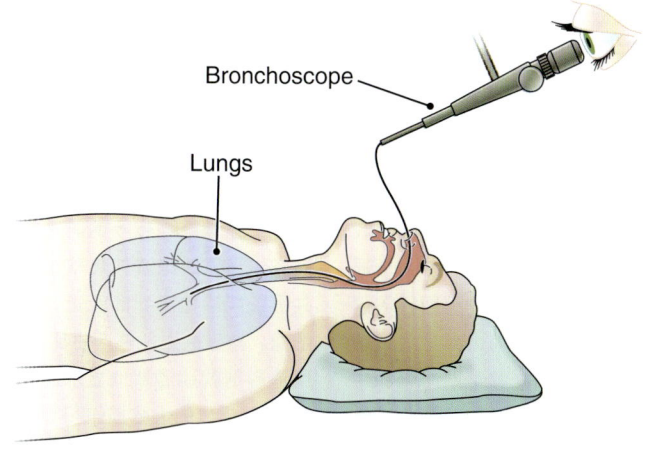

图 7-7　内窥镜。支气管镜（bronchoscope）是一种用于检查呼吸支气管的内窥镜

> 框 7-1
>
>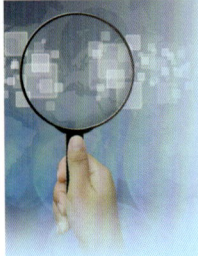
>
> **聚焦单词**
> **医学词汇的演变**
>
> 医学科学从来不是停滞不前的，其词汇也是这样。谁也不能说他或她已经学会了所有的医学词汇，因为随着新的诊断、治疗和技术的发明和发展，新的词汇不断增加。
>
> 50年以前，基因疗法、基因工程、体外受孕、克隆和干细胞研究还不为大众所知。正电子发射层析扫描（PET scans）、核磁共振（MRI）、DNA指纹、放射免疫检定法（radioimmunoassay）、鉴定骨质疏松的骨密度扫描，以及其他诊断技术也还都没有应用。一些新型药品，如降低胆固醇的他汀类药物（statins）、抗病毒制剂、治疗溃疡的抗组胺药（histamine antagonists）、治疗高血压的血管紧张素转换酶抑制剂（ACE inhibitors）和乳腺癌预防措施还都没有发明。与特定形式的癌症和特定遗传异常相关的基因也尚未分离。
>
> 每一项新的进步都会带来新词汇的使用，每一个要及时了解最新医学词汇的人都要活到老、学到老。

- 一个小穿孔，例如取一片皮肤。
- 内窥镜，例如经呼吸道或消化道。
- 手术取出，例如肿瘤或结节。

当出现新的测试时，医学词汇表中就会出现新的词汇（框7-1）。

成像技术

成像技术利用各种形式的能量产生可视的身体图像。最基本的成像方法是放射线照相术（radiography）（图7-8），利用X线在胶片上产生一个图像，或产生一个能够在显示器上观察的数字图像。对高密度组织，例如骨骼成像而

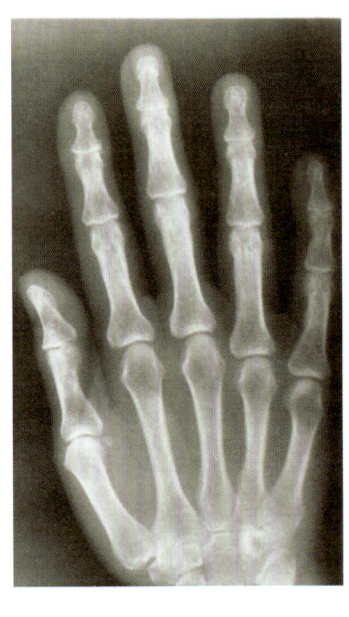

图7-8 X线成像。作用于感光胶片上的X线产生了正常右手的图像（X线片）

> 框 7-2
>
>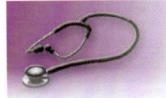
>
> **临床观点**
> **医学成像**
>
> 使医学发生革命性变化的三种成像技术是放射线照相术、计算机断层扫描（computed tomography，CT）与核磁共振。有了它们，今天的医生能够"看到"人体内部，而不需要做任何切口。
>
> 最老的技术是放射线照相术，一台机器发出X线，穿过人体到达胶片，其成像结果被称为X线片（radiograph）。较暗的区域表明射线穿过人体使胶片曝光，较亮的区域说明射线没有穿过人体。致密的组织（骨骼、牙齿）会吸收大部分X线，阻止其在胶片上曝光。因此，X线片常用于显示骨折和龋齿，也用于像肿瘤这样异常致密的组织。放射线照相术不能提供软组织的清晰图像，因为大部分射线都超过了组织在胶片上曝光，不过造影剂能够帮助血管和中空器官这样的结构显示得更加清晰，例如，硫酸钡（能够吸收X线）被摄入后能够附着在消化道上。
>
> 在CT扫描期间，一台围绕患者的机器发射X线波束穿过人体到达检测器。检测器记录射线波束的无数图像，一台计算机将这些图像组成横切面图像，或称为"切片"图像。与通常的放射线照相术不同的是，CT能够生成例如大脑、肝脏和肺脏等软结构的清晰图像，它常被用于显示大脑的损伤和肿瘤，造影剂有时甚至用于血管。
>
> 核磁共振利用强磁场和无线电波。行核磁共振的患者躺在一个充满高强磁场的舱室，患者软组织中的分子与磁场对齐。当无线电波加热软组织时，对齐的分子发射出核磁共振仪能够检测到的能量，再由计算机将这些信号转变为图像。核磁共振能够产生比CT更为清晰的软组织图像，不用造影剂就能清晰地显示血管的细节。核磁共振能够显示CT可能错过的大脑损伤和肿瘤。

言，放射线照相术是优选的方法。一些软组织结果也能显现，但需要使用例如钡合剂的造影剂以加强可视性。用于产生诊断成像的其他形式的能量包括声波、放射性同位素、无线电波和磁场。框 7-2 介绍了最常用的成像方法，框 7-3 是对这些应用中的成像技术的总结。

治疗

如果诊断已经确定，治疗［也被称为疗法（therapy）］就该开始了。治疗可能包括劝导、药物治疗、手术、理疗、物理疗法、职业疗法、心理治疗或以上方式的不同组合。缓解性疗法是提供缓解的治疗，但不旨在治愈。例如对终期患者，可以使用减轻疼痛和提供舒适的治疗方法，但不能指望改变疾病的结果。在诊断和整个治疗期间，会评估患者以建立预后（prognosis），也就是疾病结果的预测。

手术

手术是通过人工操作治疗疾病或伤害的一种方法。手术可以在现有的人体开口上进行，但在切割过程中，通常会涉及用锋利的设备切开或刺穿组织。框 7-4 介绍了常用是手术设备（图 7-11）。手术通常需要某种形式的麻醉或以减轻或消除疼痛。在手术之后，切口必须缝合以适当地愈合。传统上，外科医

框 7-3 供你参考
成像技术

成像方法	说明
cineradiography ［sinə'reidjugrəfi］ 放射性电影照相术	在荧光屏上产生连续的动画图像
computed tomography（CT）［tə'mɒgrəfi］ 计算机断层扫描	大量的 X 线以不同的角度穿过人体，利用计算机生成图像；能够获得人体横截面的三维图像；能够比简单的放射线照相术揭示更多的软组织细节（图 7-9A）
fluoroscopy ［flʊ(:)ə'rɒskəpi］ 荧光透视	利用 X 线检查深层组织机构；观察 X 线穿过人体后在荧光屏上产生的阴影
magnetic resonance imaging (MRI) 核磁共振	通过利用磁场和无线电波产生图像；通过分子性质的不同，揭示软组织的特性；消除了 X 线和造影剂的使用（图 7-9B）
positron emission tomography (PET) 正电子发射计算机断层扫描	通过服用一种由发射正电子的同位素标记的自然物质，如葡萄糖，来产生人体的截面图像；随后发射的射线由计算机翻译显示所服用物质在体内的分布；PET 被用于跟踪血液在器官中的流动，并监测器官内不同条件下的新陈代谢活动
radiography ［ˌreidi'ɒgrəfi］ 放射线照相术	利用 X 线通过人体生成内部结构的可视性记录，可以是感光胶片上，也可以是数字的。技术发展后，也被称为 roentgenography ［ˌrʌntdʒə'nɒgrəfi］光线照相术
scintigraphy ［sin'tigrəfi］ 闪烁成像	在内服一种放射性物质（radionuclide ［ˌreidiəʊ'njuːklaid］，放射线同位素）后组织中放射性物质的分布图像；图像是通过闪烁照相机获得的；其记录被称为闪烁扫描图（scintiscan），常用于确定需要检查的部分或用于测试的同位素，如骨骼扫描和镓同位素扫描
single-photon emission computed tomography (SPECT) 单光子发射计算机断层成像	能够查看跨截面放射性同位素分布的闪烁扫描术
ultrasonography ［ˌʌltrəsə'nɒgrəfi］ 超声波扫描术	从高频声波通过不同组织产生的回波产生可视化图像；也被称为声呐扫描术 sonography ［sə'nɒgrəfi］或回波扫描术 echography ［ɛ'kɒgrəfi］（图 7-10）

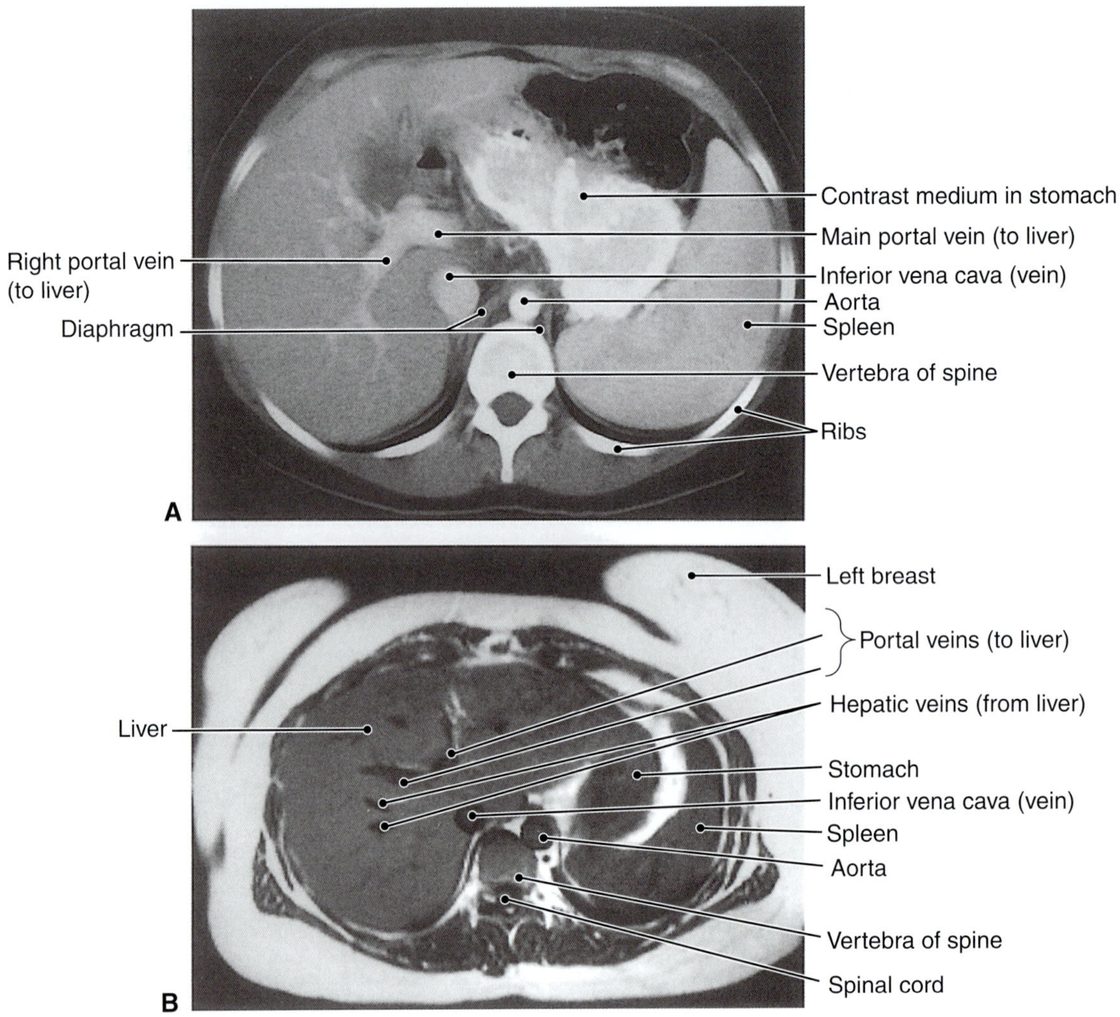

图 7-9 成像技术。图中示出了穿过肝和脾的横截面。A. 计算机断层扫描（CT）；B. 磁共振成像（MRI）

生会用缝线缝合伤口，但现在也会使用胶带、钢丝钉和皮肤胶。

现在许多类型的手术都使用激光。有些过程需要用有害的制剂来消灭一些组织，例如在烧灼过程中需要用加热或化学物品。对特定的手术，外科医生越来越多地使用计算机辅助的自动设备。在这类手术中，

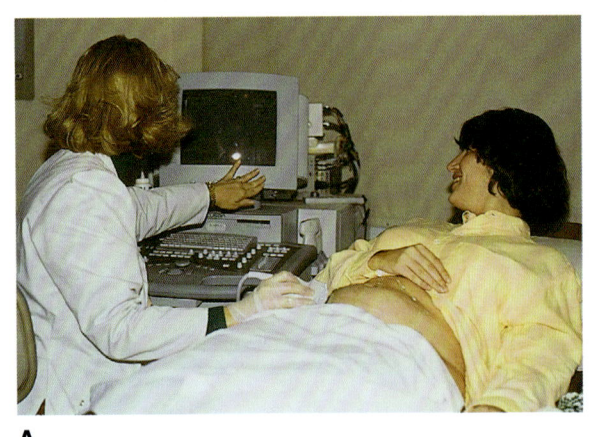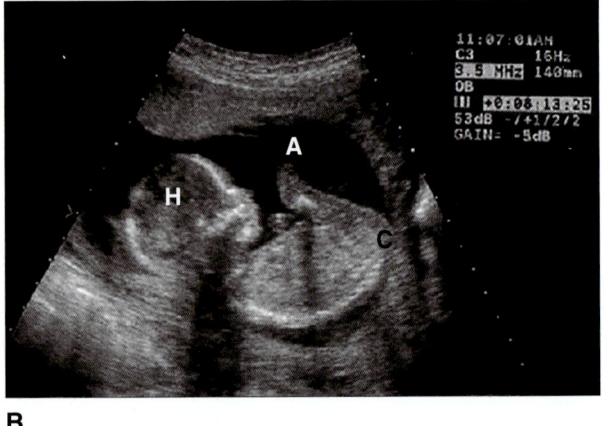

图 7-10 超声波检查。A. 医生正在使用超声波监测怀孕；B. 10~11 周怀孕子宫的超声波扫描图显示羊膜腔充满羊水（A），在纵截面中看到胎儿显示出头部（H）和尾骨（C）

> **供你参考**
> 手术器械

框 7-4

器械	说明
bougie ['buːʒi] 探条	细长、灵活的设备,用于探查和扩展管道
cannula ['kænjʊlə] 套管	包含一个套管针的导管,在去掉套管针后允许液体或空气流出
clamp [klæmp] 钳子	用于挤压组织的设备
curet (curette) [kju'ret] 刮匙	勺形设备,用于从腔壁或其他表面去除物质
elevator ['eliveitə] 起子	用于提起组织或骨骼的设备
forceps ['fɔːseps] 镊子	用于抓住或抽出的设备
gigli saw 钢丝锯	灵活的线锯
hemostat ['hiːməstæt] 止血钳	用于阻止血管血流的小钳子
rasp [rɑːsp] 锉刀	外科锉刀
retractor [ri'træktə] 牵引器	通过分开伤口并阻拦器官或组织以保持外露的设备
rongeur [rəun'ʒəː] 骨钳	圆凿钳
scalpel ['skælp(ə)l] 手术刀	有锋利刀刃的外科刀具
scissors ['sizəz] 剪刀	有两个相对刀片的切割设备
sound [saʊnd] 探针	用于探查腔体或管道的设备
trocar ['trəʊkɑː] 套管针	包含一个套管的尖锐设备,用于腔体穿孔

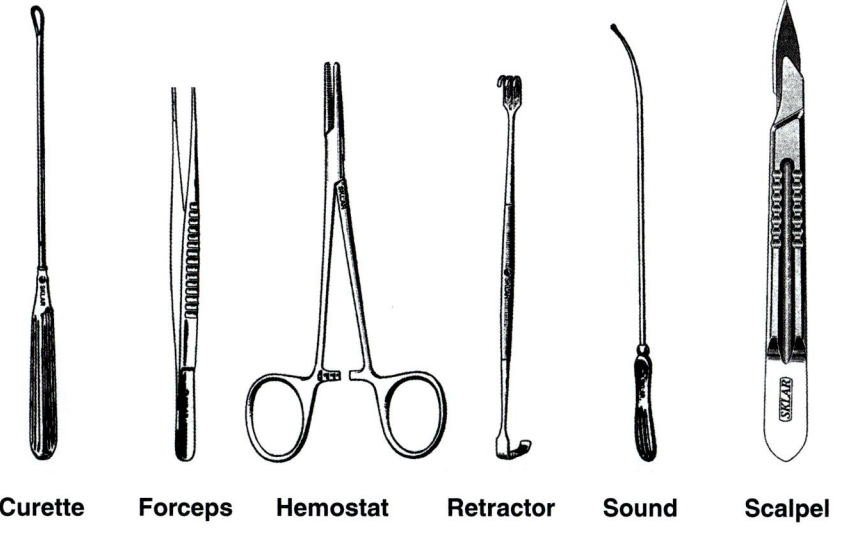

Curette   Forceps   Hemostat   Retractor   Sound   Scalpel

图 7-11 手术器械

外科医生使用远程操控或计算机控制的全自动设备，比标准的手术侵入少、引起的出血也比较少。这种方法主要用于泌尿生殖外科手术某些关节置换术、特定的心脏异常矫正术和胆囊切除术。

手术的主要目的包括：

- 治疗：切除（excision）患病或异常的组织，例如肿瘤或发炎的阑尾。手术也被用于修复伤口和损伤，例如烧伤后的植皮或骨折后的复位。手术还被用于矫正循环系统的问题和将组织结构放回它们正常的位置，例如在外科固定手术中抬升一个脱垂的器官，如膀胱。
- 诊断：为进行活组织检查切下部分组织进行实验室研究。因为有了先进的非侵入性诊断和成像技术，用于检查症状起因的探查性手术现在很少做了。
- 恢复：手术可以补偿损失的功能，如在结肠造口术（colostomy）中一段肠道被改道，在气管造口术（tracheostomy）处入一根导管以保持呼吸，插入食管或移植器官。外科医生可能执行整形或重建手术，以安装假肢、恢复适当的外观或起到美容的作用。
- 缓解：缓解性手术能够缓解疼痛或不适，如通过切断对一个器官的神经分布或通过缩小肿瘤的大小以降低压力。

框 7-5 给出了手术技术职业中的一些信息。

手术可能在急诊或紧急危险的状况下进行，如严重外伤或严重阻塞。其他手术，例如眼睛白内障摘除术，可以计划安排在方便时进行。选择性或非必需的手术即使推迟或不做，也不会引起严重后果。

随着时间的推移，手术超出了传统的医院手术室，已经扩展到医院的其他区域和私人手术设施之中，在那里患者可以在当天被作为门诊患者进行治疗。手术之前要给予术前护理，包括体格检查、获得患者对手术的知情同意和入院前检查。术后护理包括麻醉后苏醒、跟进评估和家庭护理指导。

替代性和补充性医疗

在过去的一个世纪，发达国家的主要致死原因从感染性疾病逐渐转移到心血管和呼吸系统的慢性疾病以及癌症。除了年龄的增长，生活习惯和环境对此产生了很大的影响。因此，许多人开始考虑用其他哲学和文化的替代和补充的医疗方法来完善传统的西医，包括整骨疗法（osteopathy）、自然疗法（naturopathy）、顺势疗法（homeopathy）和整脊疗法（chiropractic），针灸（acupuncture）、生物反馈（biofeedback）、按摩（massage）和冥想（meditation）技术也被采用，还有草药（herbal remedies）以及饮食、维生素和矿物质的营养指导。补充性和替代性疗法着眼于保持健康，而不是治疗疾病并为身体提供自我治疗的机会。因为人除了物理需求外，还具有情感、社会和精神需求，这些思想与整体健康护理的理念结合在一起，改善了对于个人的医疗，并鼓励人们参与自身的健康维护。

美国政府在国立卫生研究院（National Institutes of Health，NIH）内建立了国家补充和替代医疗中心（National Center for Complementary and Alternative Medicine，NCCAM），专门研究这些疗法。

框 7-5

健康职业
手术技术员

手术技术员（surgical technologist），也称为手术室技术员，在外科医生和护士的监督下准备和协助外科手术。他们准备手术室、手术器械和设备。他们帮助手术团队擦洗并穿上手术服，戴手套和面具。他们还为患者做术前准备，帮助把患者置于手术台上，并用无菌床单覆盖。在手术期间，手术技术员向外科医生递送器械和其他材料，维持手术用品供应和操作特殊设备。最后，他们还帮助计数材料以确保在手术结束时所有材料已经从患者体内移除，并协助缝合。他们还负责为实验室检查取出的样本。这项工作需要耐力，反应需灵活和快速。

手术技术员职业需要接受手术技术项目和认证的培训。培训的准备应包括基础科学、数学和计算机应用课程。手术技术员协会（Association of Surgical Technologists）在 www.ast.org 有关于这个职业的更多信息。

癌症

用于诊断癌症的方法包括身体检查、活组织检查、成像技术和与特定类型的恶性肿瘤（malignancies）相关的异常，或"标记物（markers）"的实验室检查。有些癌症标记物是副产品，例如酶、激素和细胞蛋白，它们本身异常或生成量异常。研究者也将特定的基因变异（genetic mutation）与特定形式的癌症相联系。

肿瘤医生（oncologists）或癌症专家使用分级法（grading）和分期法（staging）来区分癌症，选择与评估治疗方法，并预测疾病转归。分级法是基于在显微镜观察肿瘤细胞时发现的细胞（组织）变化，根据细胞异常的增加分为1~4级。

分期法是一个确立肿瘤扩散的临床严重程度的方法，既考虑在肿瘤原发位置的扩散，也考虑在身体其他部分的扩散（转移）。常用的是 TNM 系统，T 代表原发肿瘤（primary tumor），N 代表局部淋巴结（regional lymph nodes），M 代表远处转移（distant metastases），这些变量的评估对每种类型的肿瘤都有所不同。基于 TNM 结果，将严重程度分为 1~4 期。血液、淋巴系统和神经系统的癌症使用不同的标准进行评估。

治疗癌症最广泛使用的方法是手术、放疗（radiation therapy）和化疗（chemotherapy，使用化学物品进行治疗）。比较新的免疫疗法（immunotherapy）利用一些物质刺激人体的整体免疫系统，或使用针对特定肿瘤的疫苗。激素疗法（hormone therapy）对特定的癌症也可能有效。一旦不再有疾病存在的活跃迹象，癌症就称为处于缓解期（remission）。

Terminology 关键术语

anesthesia	[ˌænisˈθiːziə]	麻醉，通过使用药物使人丧失感知疼痛的能力
auscultation	[ˌɔːsk(ə)lˈteiʃ(ə)n]	听诊，倾听体内的声音，通常是胸部和腹部内的（图7-3）
biopsy	[ˈbaiɒpsi]	活组织检查，切下一小块组织做显微镜检查
cautery	[ˈkɔːt(ə)ri]	烧灼，通过有害化学品、加热或电流等破坏组织；烧灼术
chemotherapy	[ˌkemə(ʊ)ˈθerəpi]	化疗，利用化学品治疗疾病，通常用于指使用化学药品治疗癌症
diagnosis	[ˌdaiəgˈnəʊsis]	诊断，确定疾病起因和性质的过程
endoscope	[ˈendəskəʊp]	内窥镜，通过一个人体开口或小切口检查器官或腔体内部的仪器，大多数使用光纤进行观察（图7-7）
excision	[ikˈsiʒ(ə)n]	切除（后缀 -ectomy）
fixation	[fikˈseiʃ(ə)n]	固定（后缀 -pexy）
grading	[ˈgreidiŋ]	分级法，基于显微镜检查细胞评估肿瘤的方法
immunotherapy	[ˌimjʊnəʊˈθerəpi]	免疫疗法，涉及特定或非特定地刺激或压制免疫系统的治疗方法
incision	[inˈsiʒ(ə)n]	切口，切开（后缀 -tomy）
inspection	[inˈspekʃn]	观察
laser	[ˈleizə]	激光
ophthalmoscope	[ɒfˈθælməskəʊp]	眼底镜，检查眼睛内部的仪器（图7-6A）
otoscope	[ˈəʊtəskəʊp]	耳镜，检查耳朵的仪器（图7-6B）

Terminology	关键术语（续表）
palliative [ˈpæliətiv]	缓解，但不能治愈
palpation [pælˈpeiʃn]	触诊，通过将手或手指接触人体表面来检查皮肤肌理、体温、运动和坚实性等特性（图 7-1）
percussion [pəˈkʌʃ(ə)n]	叩诊，轻轻但快速地敲击人体,通过获得的声音评估敲击处下面组织的状况（图 7-2）
prognosis [prɒɡˈnəʊsis]	预后，疾病进程和结果的预测
radiography [ˌreidiˈɒɡrəfi]	放射线照相术
remission [riˈmiʃ(ə)n]	缓解期，疾病症状减轻；疾病症状发生减少或没有迹象显示疾病存在的阶段
sign [sain]	病证、迹象，可以被观察或检测到的疾病的客观迹象，例如发热、皮疹、高血压和血压或尿液异常
sphygmomanometer [ˌsfiɡməʊməˈnɒmitə]	血压计或血压计袖带，当心脏收缩（收缩压）和心脏舒张（舒张压）时，以毫米汞柱（mmHg）读取血压，并且报告为收缩/舒张压（图 7-5）
staging [ˈsteidʒiŋ]	分期法，诊断、治疗和预测恶性肿瘤的分类过程
stethoscope [ˈsteθəskəʊp]	听诊器（图 7-3）
surgery [ˈsɜːdʒ(ə)ri]	手术，通过手动操作治疗疾病或损伤的方法
suture [ˈsuːtʃə]	缝合，缝合线（后缀 -rhaphy）
symptom [ˈsim(p)təm]	症状，疾病的任何证据；有时局限于个人体验到的疾病的主观迹象，例如疼痛、头晕和虚弱
therapy [ˈθerəpi]	疗法、治疗
vital signs	生命体征
Alternative and Complementary Medicine	替代性和补充性医疗
acupuncture [ˈækjʊˌpʌŋ(k)tʃə]	针灸，古老的中国疗法，将针插入人体特定的穴位，以解除疼痛、引起麻醉或改善治疗；类似的效果可以通过点穴技术，用手指用力按压人体表面特点的位置来获得
biofeedback [baiəʊˈfiːdbæk]	生物反馈，一种学习控制非自主生理反应的方法，利用电子设备检测身体变化，并将这一信息反馈给个人
chiropractic [ˌkairə(ʊ)ˈpræktik]	脊椎按摩疗法，一种在诊断和治疗疾病中强调神经系统状态的学科；通常通过推拿脊椎以校正错位，大多数患者为治疗肌肉骨骼疼痛或头痛（源自于希腊语"cheir"，意为"手"）
holistic health care [həʊˈlistik]	整体医疗，将人作为一个具有肉体、情感、社会和精神需求的整体进行治疗的方法。强调综合护理、介入个人自身的护理，以及良好健康的维护而不是疾病的治疗

Terminology 关键术语（续表）

homeopathy [ˌhəʊmiˈɒpəθi]	顺势疗法，一种治疗疾病的理念，服用高度稀释的药品同时改善健康生活习惯和环境（源自于 home/o，意为"相同"和 path/o，意为"疾病"）
massage [məˈsɑːdʒ]	按摩，推拿身体或身体的一些部位以镇静、解除紧张，增进循环并刺激肌肉
meditation [ˌmediˈteɪʃ(ə)n]	冥想，通过聚焦自身，同时控制呼吸，或许还要重复一个字词或短语来清理思想的过程
naturopathy [ˌneɪtʃəˈrɒpəθi]	物理疗法，通过开发健康生活方式帮助人们自我治愈的治疗理念；物理疗法可能也会使用一些常规医疗方法（源自于 path/o，意为"疾病"）
osteopathy [ˌɒstiˈɒpəθi]	整骨疗法，基于人体在正常结构、有利的环境和适当的营养条件下能够克服疾病的治疗理论系统；整骨疗法诊断和治疗中应用标准的医学疗法，但强调有缺陷的身体结构的确认与矫正（源自于 oste/o，意为"骨骼"和 path/o，意为"疾病"）

与诊断和治疗相关的单词组成部分

见表 7-1 至表 7-3。

表 7-1　物理作用力相关的词根

词根	含义	示例	示例定义
aer/o	空气、气体	aerobic [eəˈrəʊbik]	有氧的
bar/o	压力	barometer [bəˈrɒmitə]	气压计
chrom/o, chromat/o	颜色、染色	chromatic [krəˈmætik]	有色的
chron/o	时间	chronologic [ˌkrɒnəˈlɒdʒik]	按时间顺序的
cry/o	冷	cryoprobe [ˈkraɪəʊˌprəʊb]	冷冻器
electr/o	电	electrolysis [ˌilekˈtrɒlisis]	电解
erg/o	工作	synergistic [ˌsinəˈdʒistik]	协作
phon/o	声音、语音	phonograph [ˈfəʊnəgrɑːf]	声音描记像
phot/o	光	photoreaction [ˌfəʊtəriˈækʃən]	光反应
radi/o	放射、X 线	radiology [ˌreɪdiˈɒlədʒi]	放射学
son/o	声音	sonogram [ˈsəʊnəgræm]	超声波扫描图
therm/o	热、温度	hypothermia [ˌhaɪpə(ʊ)ˈθɜːmiə]	低体温

练习 7-1

匹配下列术语，在每个题号的左侧写上适当的字母。

___ 1. hyperthermia ［ˌhaɪpəˈθɜːmɪə］　　a. abnormally high body temperature
___ 2. hyperbaric ［ˌhaɪpəˈbærɪk］　　　b. any pigmented cell
___ 3. synchrony ［ˈsɪŋkrəni］　　　　　c. pertaining to increased pressure
___ 4. radioactive ［ˌreɪdɪəʊˈæktɪv］　　d. occurrence at the same time
___ 5. chromocyte ［ˈkrəʊməsaɪt］　　　e. giving off radiation

识别并定义下列单词中的词根。

	Root	Meaning of Root
6. sonographer ［ˈsɒnəɡrɑːfə］	___	___
7. chronic ［ˈkrɒnɪk］	___	___
8. homeothermic ［həʊmɪəʊˈθɜːmɪk］	___	___
9. exergonic ［ˌeksəˈɡɒnɪk］	___	___
10. anaerobic ［ˌæneəˈrəʊbɪk］	___	___
11. achromatic ［ˌækrəʊˈmætɪk］	___	___

填空。

12. The term electroconvulsive ［ɪˌlektrəʊkənˈvʌlsɪv］ means causing convulsions by means of_____.
13. A photograph ［ˈfəʊtəɡrɑːf］ is an image produced by means of_____.
14. Cryotherapy ［ˌkraɪəʊˈθerəpi］ is treatment using _____.
15. Barotrauma ［ˈbærətrɔːmə］ is injury caused by _____.
16. Phonetics ［fəˈnetɪks］ is the study of_____.

表 7-2　与诊断相关的后缀

后缀	含义	示例	示例定义
-graph	记录数据的设备	polygraph ［ˈpɒlɪɡrɑːf］	多种波动扫描器、测谎仪
-graphy	记录数据的动作 *	echography ［eˈkɒɡrəfi］	回波描记术
-gram†	数据的记录	electrocardiogram ［ɪˌlektrəʊˈkɑːdɪəɡræm］	心电图
-meter	测量设备	calorimeter ［ˌkæləˈrɪmɪtə］	热量计
-metry	……的测量	audiometry ［ˌɒdɪˈɒmətri］	听力测量（audi/o），词根 metr/o 意为"测量"
-scope	用于观察或检查的设备	bronchoscope ［ˈbrɒŋkəskəʊp］	支气管镜
-scopy	……的检查	celioscopy ［ˌsiːiˈɒskəpi］	体腔（celi/o）镜检查

续表 7-2	与诊断相关的后缀

* 这个后缀不仅常用于表示数据的记录，还表示对数据的评估与解读
† 只使用 X 线产生的图像被称为 radiograph。当利用特殊技术使用 X 线为一个器官或区域产生图像时，后缀 -gram 与代表该区域的词根一起组合，例如 urogram（尿路造影照片）、angiogram（血管造影片）和 mammogram（乳房 X 线片）

练习 7-2

匹配下列术语，在每个题号的左侧写上适当的字母。

____ 1. microscope ['maɪkrəskəʊp] 　　a. examination of the abdomen
____ 2. ergometry [ɜː'ɡɒmɪtri] 　　b. a record of sound
____ 3. thermometer [θə'mɒmɪtə(r)] 　　c. measurement of work done
____ 4. laparoscopy [ˌlæpə'rɒskəpi] 　　d. instrument for measuring temperature
____ 5. sonogram ['sɒnəɡræm] 　　e. instrument for examining very small objects

____ 6. endoscope ['endəskəʊp] 　　a. a record of sound
____ 7. electroencephalograph [ɪˌlektrəʊen'sefələˌɡræf] 　　b. instrument for measuring time
____ 8. audiometer [ˌɔːdi'ɒmɪtə] 　　c. instrument for viewing the inside of a cavity or organ
____ 9. phonogram ['fəʊnəɡræm] 　　d. instrument used to measure hearing
____ 10. chronometer [krə'nɒmɪtə(r)] 　　e. instrument used to record the brain's electrical activity

表 7-3	与手术相关的后缀		
后缀	含义	示例	示例定义
-centesis	刺、敲	thoracentesis [θɔːrəsen'tiːsɪs]	胸腔穿刺术（thorac/o）
-desis	结合、融合	pleurodesis [plʊə'rəʊdiːsɪs]	胸膜固定术
-ectomy	切除、手术切除	hepatectomy [ˌhepə'tektəmi]	肝切除术（hepat/o）
-pexy	手术固定	hysteropexy [hɪstə'rɒpeksi]	子宫固定术（hyster/o）
-plasty	整形修复、整形手术	rhinoplasty ['raɪnəˌplæsti]	鼻成形术（rhin/o）
-rhaphy	手术修复、缝合	herniorrhaphy [hɜːni'ɔːrəfi]	疝修补术（herni/o）
-stomy	手术制造开口	tracheostomy [ˌtreɪki'ɒstəmi]	气管造口术（trache/o）
-tome	切割设备	microtome ['maɪkrətəʊm]	切片机
-tomy	切开、切割	laparotomy [ˌlæpə'rɒtəmi]	剖腹术（lapar/o）
-tripsy	压轧	neurotripsy ['njʊərəʊtrɪpsi]	神经压轧术（neur/o）

练习 7-3

匹配下列术语，在每个题号的左侧写上适当的字母。

____ 1. nephropexy ['nefrə,peksi]　　　　　　a. crushing of a stone

____ 2. rhinoplasty ['rainə,plæsti]　　　　　　b. surgical fixation of the kidney

____ 3. lithotripsy ['laiθəutripsi]　　　　　　c. puncture of the abdomen

____ 4. adenectomy [,ædə'nektəmi]　　　　　d. excision of a gland

____ 5. celiocentesis [si:liəusen'ti:sis]　　　　e. plastic surgery of the nose

词根 cyst/o 意为"膀胱"，使用该词根写出下列含义的单词。

6. Incision into the bladder_____

7. Surgical fixation of the bladder_____

8. Plastic repair of the bladder_____

9. Surgical repair of the bladder_____

10. Creation of an opening into the bladder_____

词根 arthr/o 意为"关节"，使用该词根写出下列含义的单词。

11. Plastic repair of a joint_____

12. Instrument for incising a joint_____

13. Incision of a joint_____

14. Puncture of a joint_____

15. Fusion of a joint_____

使用给出的词根写出下列定义的单词

16. Incision into the trachea (trache/o)_____

17. Surgical repair of the stomach (gastr/o)_____

18. Creation of an opening into the colon (col/o)_____

Terminology　补充术语

症状

clubbing ['klʌbiŋ]	杵状指，手指或脚趾因为指甲的软组织增生而膨胀，在很多疾病中可见，尤其是肺和心脏的疾病（图 7-12）
colic ['kɒlik]	绞痛，伴有平滑肌痉挛
cyanosis [,saiə'nəusis]	发绀，因为缺氧导致的皮肤青紫色
diaphoresis [,daiəfə'ri:sis]	发汗
malaise [mə'leiz]	不适或不安的感觉，通常显示有感染或其他疾病（mal-，意为"坏的"）
nocturnal [nɒk't3:nl]	夜间的（词根 noct/i 和 nyct/o，意为"夜晚"）

Terminology 关键术语

pallor	[ˈpælə(r)]	苍白，失色
prodrome	[ˈprəʊdrəʊm]	前驱症状
sequela	[siˈkwiːlə]	后遗症（复数：sequelae）
syncope	[ˈsiŋkəpi]	昏厥，由于大脑缺血导致的暂时性意识丧失

诊断

alpha-fetoprotein (AFP)	[ˈælfəfetˈɒprəʊtiːn]	甲胎蛋白
bruit brew		杂音，听诊器中听到的异常声音
facies	[ˈfeiʃiiz]	面容
febrile	[ˈfiːbrail]	发热的
nuclear medicine		核医学，利用放射性物质进行诊断、治疗和研究的医学分支
radiology	[ˌreidiˈɒlədʒi]	放射学
radionuclide	[ˈreidiəʊˈnjuːklaid]	放射性同位素
speculum	[ˈspekjələm]	窥镜用于检查管道的仪器（图 7-13）
syndrome	[ˈsindrəʊm]	综合征，一组显示疾病特性的迹象和症状

治疗

catheter	[ˈkæθitə(r)]	导管，用于将液体导入或导出人体（图 7-14）
clysis	[kˈlisis]	灌肠，也指灌肠使用的溶液
irrigation	[ˌiriˈgeiʃn]	用液体冲洗管道、腔体或区域（图 7-14）
lavage	[ˈlævidʒ]	灌洗
normal saline (NS)		生理盐水
paracentesis	[ˌpærəsenˈtiːsis]	穿刺术
prophylaxis	[ˌprɒfiˈlæksis]	预防疾病

手术

drain	[drein]	引流，使液体离开伤口或腔体的设备
ligature	[ˈligətʃə(r)]	绷带，捆绑的过程
stapling	[ˈsteipliŋ]	在手术中使用钢丝钉接合组织
surgeon	[ˈsɜːdʒən]	外科医生

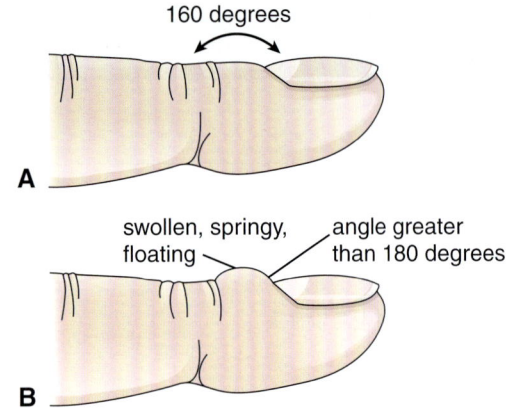

图 7-12 杵状指。A. 正常；B. 杵状指，由于指甲周围的软组织生长，手指的末端扩大

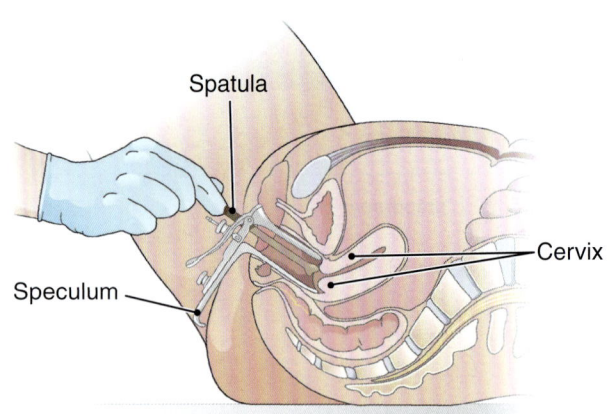

图 7-13 阴道窥镜。该设备用于检查阴道和子宫颈，并获得用于测试的宫颈样本

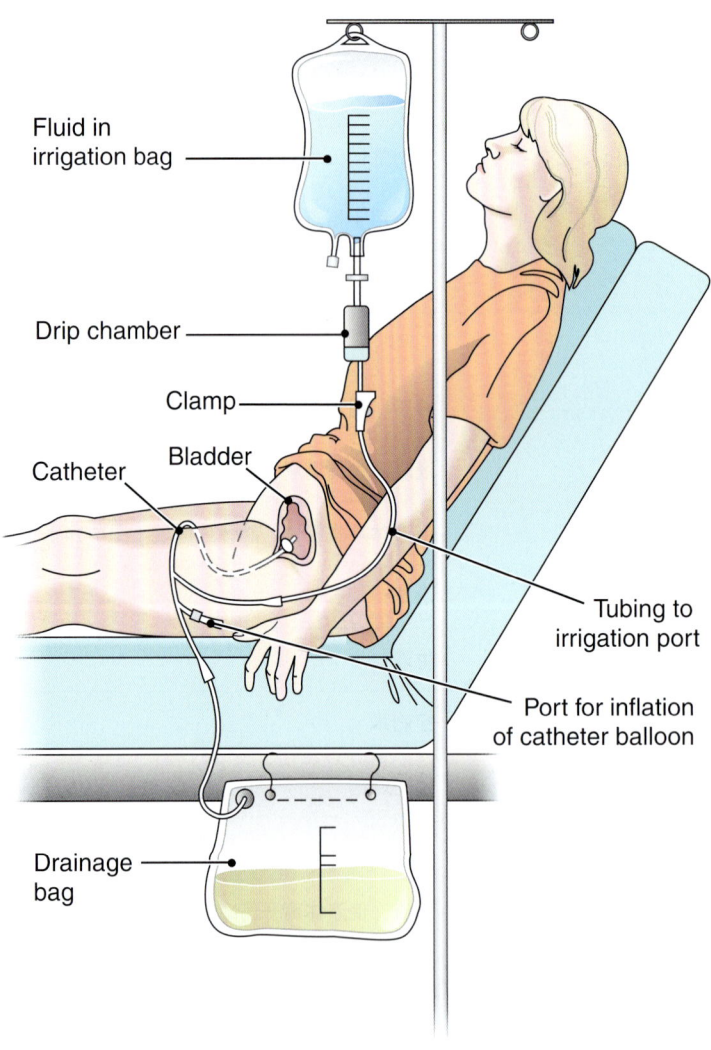

图 7-14 使用导管连续膀胱灌洗

Symbols 符号

1°	primary	原发	°	degree	度
2°	secondary (to)	继发	∧	above	以上
Δ	change	变化	∨	below	以下
L	left	左	=	equal to	等于
®	right	右	≠	not equal to	不等于
↑	increase(d)	上升	±	doubtful, slight	怀疑，轻微
↓	decrease(d)	下降	~	approximately	大约
♂	male	男性	×	times	倍数
♀	female	女性	#	number, pound	数字，磅数

Terminology 缩略语

病历和体格检查

ADL	Activities of daily living	日常生活活动
BP	Blood pressure	血压
bpm	Beats per minute	滴/分钟
C	Celsius	摄氏度
CC	Chief complaint	主诉
c/o, co	Complains (complaining) of	主诉
EOMI	Extraocular muscles intact	眼外肌完整
ETOH	Alcohol (ethyl alcohol)	酒精（乙醇）
F	Fahrenheit	华氏度
HEENT	Head, eyes, ears, nose, and throat	头、眼、耳、鼻、喉
HIPAA	Health Insurance Portability and Accountability Act	健康保险携带和责任法案
h/o	History of	……的病历
H & P	History and physical	病历和身体检查
HPI	History of present illness	当前病史
HR	Heart rate	心率

Terminology 缩略语（续表）

Hx	History	病史，病历
I & O	Intake and output	测量与记录，摄取与排泄
IPPA	Inspection, palpation, percussion, auscultation	检查、触诊、叩诊和听诊
IVDA	Intravenous drug abuse	静脉注射毒品
NAD	No apparent distress	无明显病痛、未查出疾病
NKDA	No known drug allergies	无已知药物过敏
P	Pulse	心跳
PE	Physical examination	体格检查
PE(R) RLA	Pupils equal (regular) react to light and accommodation	瞳孔（正常）对光的反应和调节
PMH	Past medical history	既往病史
pt	Patient	患者
R	Respiration	呼吸
R/O	Rule out	排除
R/O	Rule out	排除
T	Temperature	温度、体温
TPR	Temperature, pulse, respiration	体温、心跳、呼吸
VS	Vital signs	生命体征
WD	Well developed	发育良好
WNL	Within normal limits	在正常范围内
w/o	Without	没有
YO, y/o	Years old, year-old	年龄

诊断与治疗

ABC	Aspiration biopsy cytology	抽吸活检细胞学
AFP	Alpha-fetoprotein	甲胎蛋白
BS	Bowel sounds, breath sounds	肠鸣音、呼吸音
bx	Biopsy	活组织检查
CAM	Complementary and alternative medicine	补充性和替代性医疗
Ci	Curie (unit of radioactivity)	居里（放射性的单位）

Terminology 缩略语（续表）

C & S	Culture and (drug) sensitivity (of bacteria)	（细菌的）培养和（药物）敏感
CT	Computed tomography	计算机断层扫描
D/C, dc	Discontinue	中断
Dx	Diagnosis	诊断
EBL	Estimated blood loss	估计失血量
ICU	Intensive care unit	重症监护病房
I & D	Incision and drainage	切开和引流
MET	Metastasis	转移
MRI	Magnetic resonance imaging	核磁共振
NCCAM	National Center for Complementary and Alternative Medicine	国家补充与替代药物中心
NS, N/S	Normal saline	生理盐水
PCA	Patient-controlled analgesia	患者自控镇痛
PET	Positron emission tomography	正电子发射断层扫描术
PICC	Peripherally inserted central catheter	外周中心静脉置管
postop	Postoperative	手术后
preop	Preoperative	手术前
PSS	Physiologic saline solution	生理盐水溶液
RATx	Radiation therapy	放射疗法
Rx	Drug, prescription, therapy	药品，处方，疗法
TNM	(Primary) tumor, (regional lymph) nodes, (distant) metastases	（原发）肿瘤、（区域淋巴）节、（远距离）扩散
UV	Ultraviolet	紫外线

X 线片观察

AP	Anteroposterior	正前位
LL	Left lateral	左侧位
PA	Posteroanterior	后前位
RL	Right lateral	右侧位

Terminology 缩略语（续表）

Orders 医嘱

AMA	Against medical advice	违反医嘱
AMB	Ambulatory	救护车
BRP	Bathroom privileges	卫浴权限
CBR	Complete bed rest	完全卧床休息
DNR	Do not resuscitate	不能复苏
KVO	Keep vein open	保持静脉通畅
NPO	Nothing by mouth	禁食
OOB	Out of bed	不卧床
QNS	Quantity not sufficient	数量不足
QS	Quantity sufficient	数量足够
STAT	Immediately	立即
TKO	To keep open	保持开放

Case Study Revisited 案例研究再访

M. L.'s Injury Follow-Up

M. L. was seen by the orthopedic surgeon, who reduced her wrist fracture and applied a short arm cast. She was scheduled for an arthrocentesis to remove fluid from the right knee. Following the procedure, M. L. was discharged and sent home with instructions to rest and to keep the right wrist and leg elevated. She was directed to take an antiinflammatory medication (NSAID) for the inflammation and pain. It was recommended that in the future M. L. wear protective padding when she rollerblades.

M. L. 受伤随访

骨科医生看了 M. L.，为她固定了腕部的骨折并使用了短手臂石膏。她被安排进行关节穿刺术以从右膝盖清除液体。按照程序，M. L. 出院并被送回家，被告知要休息并使右手腕和腿抬高。M. L. 被指示服用抗炎药（NSAID）治疗炎症和疼痛，并建议她在未来溜旱冰鞋时穿戴保护垫。

CHAPTER 7 复习

匹配

匹配下列术语，在每个题号的左侧写上适当的字母。

____ 1. electrolyte   **a.** substance that conducts electric current
____ 2. staging   **b.** evidence of disease
____ 3. symptom   **c.** classification of malignant tumors
____ 4. syndrome   **d.** a group of symptoms that characterizes a disease
____ 5. suture   **e.** to unite parts by stitching them together

____ 6. cautery   **a.** a removal of tissue for microscopic study
____ 7. scintiscan   **b.** pain caused by cold
____ 8. cryalgesia   **c.** destruction of tissue with a damaging agent
____ 9. vasotripsy   **d.** image obtained with a radionuclide
____ 10. biopsy   **e.** crushing of a vessel

____ 11. ergometer   **a.** instrument used to cut bone
____ 12. osteotome   **b.** organism that produces color
____ 13. acupuncture   **c.** instrument to measure work output
____ 14. biofeedback   **d.** method for controlling involuntary responses
____ 15. chromogen   **e.** treatment by insertion of thin needles

补充术语。

____ 16. sequelae   **a.** partial excision
____ 17. prophylaxis   **b.** prevention of disease
____ 18. clubbing   **c.** symptom indicating an approaching disease
____ 19. prodrome   **d.** lasting effects of disease
____ 20. resection   **e.** enlargement of the ends of the fingers and toes

____ 21. catheter   **a.** thin tube
____ 22. colic   **b.** feeling of discomfort
____ 23. diaphoresis   **c.** acute abdominal pain
____ 24. malaise   **d.** washing out of a cavity
____ 25. lavage   **e.** profuse sweating

词根

识别并定义下列单词的词根。

	Root	Meaning of Root
26. chromocyte	_____	_____

27. anaerobic _____ _____
28. radiodense _____ _____
29. thermalgia _____ _____
30. chronology _____ _____
31. allergy _____ _____
32. ultrasonic _____ _____

填空

33. The PA in M.L.'s case evaluated her wrist by touching it. The term for this examination technique is_____.
34. Following her examination, the PA predicted the outcome of M.L.'s injuries; that is, she gave a(n)_____.
35. Referring to M.L.'s opening case study, the adjective form of diagnosis is_____.
36. In the same case study, the adjective form of edema is_____.
37. Another word for treatment is_____.
38. Photochromic eyeglass lenses change color in response to_____.
39. Plastic repair of the stomach is called_____.
40. Fusion of a joint is_____.
41. Surgical creation of an opening in the colon is a(n)_____.

使用意为"肝"的词根 hepat/o 写出下列单词。

42. Incision of the liver_____
43. Excision of liver tissue_____
44. Surgical fixation of the liver_____
45. Surgical repair of the liver_____

真假判断

检查一下语句，如果语句为真，在第一个空格内写上 T；如果语句为假，在第一个空格内写上 F，并通过在第二个空格上替代带下划线的单词更正语句。

	True or False	Correct Answer
46. Nephrectomy is surgical removal of a <u>gland</u>.	_____	_____
47. A baroreceptor is sensitive to <u>temperature</u>.	_____	_____
48. An otoscope is used to examine the <u>eye</u>.	_____	_____
49. An image produced by x-rays is a <u>radiogram</u>.	_____	_____
50. An echogram is produced by <u>ultrasound</u>.	_____	_____
51. Arthroscopy is endoscopic examination of a <u>joint</u>.	_____	_____

排除

在下列每组中，为与其他不相配的单词加下划线，并解释选择的理由。

52. percussion — inspection — palpation — remission — auscultation

53. ophthalmoscope — sphygmomanometer — stethoscope — syncope — endoscope

54. curette — forceps — speculum — scalpel — hemostat

55. TNM — MRI — PET — CT — SPECT

缩略语

写出本章开头 M.L. 的案例研究中下列缩略语的含义。

56. PA

57. MRI

58. Hx

59. ROM

60. NSAID

单词构建

使用给出的单词组成部分写出下列定义的单词。

lith/o -rhaphy neur/o -tripsy -tome r -pexy -scopy cyst/o

61. Crushing of a nerve

62. Surgical repair of the bladder

63. Surgical fixation of the bladder

64. Surgical repair of a nerve

65. Crushing of a stone

66. Bladder stone

67. Endoscopic examination of the bladder

68. Instrument used to incise a nerve

69. Instrument used to incise the bladder

单词分析

定义下列单词，并给出每个单词组成部分的含义。如果需要，可以使用词典。

70. isochromatophilic [ˌaisəkrəʊmætɒˈfilik]

    a. iso-

    b. chromat/o

    c. phil

    d. -ic

71. synchronous [ˈsiŋkrənəs]

    a. syn-

    b. chron/o

    c. -ous

72. asymmetric [ˌeisiˈmetrik]

    a. a-

    b. sym-

    c. metr/o _____

    d. -ic _____

73. chromogenesis ［ˌkrəʊməˈdʒenisis］ _____

    a. chrom/o _____

    b. gen/e _____

    c. –sis _____

Additional Case Studies
补充案例研究

Case Study 7-1: Comprehensive History and Physical
案例研究 7-1：综合病历与身体检查

C. F., a 46 YO married Asian woman, works as an office manager for an insurance company. This morning, she had a follow-up visit with her oncologist and was sent to the hospital for immediate admission for possible recurrence or sequelae of her ovarian cancer. She is alert, articulate, and a reliable reporter.

CC: C. F. presents with mild, low, aching pelvic pain and low abdominal fullness. She states, "I feel like I have cramps and am bloated. Sometimes I'm so tired I cannot do my work without a short nap."

HPI: C. F. has been in remission for 14 months from aggressively treated ovarian carcinoma. She presents with mild abdominal distention and tenderness on deep palpation of the lower pelvis. C. F. claims a feeling of fullness in the lower abdomen, loss of appetite, and inability to sleep through the night. She is afraid that her cancer was not cured. Sometimes her heart races and she cannot catch her breath, but with two children in college, she cannot afford to miss work.

MEDS: Therapeutic vitamin × 1/day. Valium 5 mg every six hours (q6h) as needed (prn) for anxiety. Benadryl 25 mg at bedtime (hs) prn for insomnia. Echinacea tea 3 cups/day to prevent colds or flu. Ginkgo biloba tea 3 cups/day for energy.

ALLERGIES: NKDA, no food allergies

PMH: C. F. was diagnosed with ovarian CA four years ago and treated with surgery, radiation, and chemotherapy. A total abdominal hysterectomy (removal of the uterus) with bilateral removal of the oviducts and ovaries was performed. At the time of surgery, the pelvic lymph nodes tested negative for disease. Chemotherapy and radiation therapy occurred after surgical recovery. C. F. has been well and capable of full ADL until four weeks ago. Childhood history is unremarkable, with normal childhood diseases, including measles, mumps, and chicken pox. C.F. was born and raised in this country. She has no other adult diseases, surgery, or injuries.

CURRENT HEALTH Hx: Denies tobacco, ETOH, or recreational drugs or substances. She exercises three to five times per week with aerobic exercise class and treadmill. She is a vegetarian and drinks one to five cups of green tea per day. Immunizations are up to date, unsure of last tetanus booster. Recent negative mammogram and negative TB test (PPD).

FAMILY Hx: Both parents alive and well. Maternal aunt died of "stomach tumor" at age 37.

TPR & BP & PAIN: 37C-96 – 22, 126/72, in no acute distress.

C. F. 是一名 46 岁的已婚亚洲妇女，担任保险公司的办公室经理。今天早上，因为其卵巢癌可能复发或发现后遗症，C. F. 与她的肿瘤科医生做了随访，并被立即送到医院。她是一名聪明、思维清晰和可靠的记者。

主诉：C. F. 说她有轻度的骨盆疼痛，并感觉下腹部胀满。她说："我觉得有些痉挛和肿胀。有时候我太累了，不打个盹儿就无法工作。"

当前病史：C. F. 已从积极治疗的卵巢癌病情中缓解了 14 个月。她在对下盆骨的深度触诊中表现轻微的腹部膨胀和压痛。C. F. 声称在下腹部有肿胀感觉，食欲不振，并且在夜间无法入睡。她害怕她的癌症没有治愈。她有时心跳加速，喘不上气，但是有两个孩子上大学，她不能失去工作。

药物治疗：维生素治疗每日 1 次。根据焦虑情况的需要（prn），每 6 小时（q6h）服用 5mg 安定。根据失眠情况需要，在睡前（hs）服用 25mg 苯那君。紫锥菊茶 3 杯/d，以防止感冒或流行性感冒。银杏叶茶每天 3 杯，以获得能量。

过敏史：无已知药物过敏，无食物过敏史

既往病史：C. F. 4 年前被诊断为卵巢癌，并接受手术、放射治疗（放疗）和化学治疗（化疗），进行了全面的腹部子宫切除术（去除子宫），双侧切除输卵管和卵巢。在手术时，盆腔淋巴结检查结果为阴性。化疗和放疗在手术恢复后进行。直到 4 周前，C. F. 康复状况很好，日常生活能够完全自理。童年病史无特别之处，有常见儿童疾病，包括麻疹、腮腺炎和水痘。C. F. 在这个国家出生和长大，没有其他成年疾病、手术或伤害。

当前健康史：拒绝烟草、酒精或娱乐性药物或物质。她每周锻炼 3~5 次，上有氧运动课和跑步机。她是一个素食者，每天喝 1~5 杯绿茶。免疫接种是最新的，不能确定最后的破伤风加强免疫。最近的乳房 X 线检查为阴性，结核试验（PPD）为阴性。

家族病史：父母健在，姨母在 37 岁死于胃癌。

体温、心率、呼吸 & 血压 & 疼痛：37℃，96，72，

HEENT: WNL. Mesocephalic; fundi benign; PERRLA; uncorrected 20/20 vision; mouth clear; good dental health; neck supple w/o rigidity, thyromegaly, or cervical lymphadenopathy; trachea midline. No carotid bruits.

LUNGS: All lobes clear to auscultation and percussion. HEART: Rate 96 bpm, regular; no murmurs, gallops, or rubs.

BREASTS: Symmetrical, w/o masses or discharge.

ABDOMEN: Skin intact with healed suprapubic midline surgical incision and a symmetrical area of discoloration and dermal thickness from radiation therapy. Bowel sounds active and normal. Suprapubic tenderness on palpation. No hepatosplenomegaly. Absence of inguinal lymph nodes on palpation. Kidneys palpable. Rectal examination WNL. Hemoccult test (stool test for blood) result negative.

GU: Unremarkable. Surgical menopause.

MUSCULOSKELETAL: WNL. No weakness, limitation of mobility, joint pain, stiffness, or edema.

NEUROLOGIC: All reflexes intact. No syncope, paralysis, numbness.

DIAGNOSTIC IMPRESSION: Possible recurrence of ovarian CA, ascites.

TREATMENT PLAN: Send blood for CA-125 (genetic marker for ovarian cancer). Schedule abdominal paracentesis and second-look diagnostic laparoscopy with biopsy and tissue staging. D/C all herbal supplements.

126/72，无急性疼痛

头、眼、耳、鼻、喉：正常。中型头；眼底良性；瞳孔等大；未校正视力 20/20；口腔清洁；牙齿健康；颈部柔软没有僵硬的甲状腺肿或颈淋巴结肿大，气管居中。无颈动脉杂音。

肺：所有肺叶对听诊和叩诊均清晰。心脏：心跳 96 次 /min，正常；无杂音、无跳音、无摩擦音。

乳房：对称，没有肿块或分泌物。

腹部：皮肤完好，耻骨上中线手术切口愈合良好，放射治疗造成的变色和真皮增厚区域对称。肠鸣音活跃和正常。触诊上耻骨触痛，无肝脾肿大，触诊发现腹股沟淋巴结缺失，肾脏可触及。直肠检查正常。隐血检查（粪便潜血检查）结果阴性。

生殖泌尿系统：无明显问题。手术绝经。

肌肉骨骼系统：正常，无虚弱、运动受限、关节疼痛、僵硬或水肿。

神经系统：所有反射完好，无昏厥、麻痹、麻木。

诊断印象：卵巢癌可能复发，腹水。

治疗计划：做血液 CA-125（卵巢癌基因标记）测试。安排腹腔穿刺术和二次腹腔镜诊断检查，做活检和组织分期。停用所有草药补充剂。

Case Study 7-2: Diagnostic Laparoscopy
案例研究 7-2：腹腔镜诊断

For a laparoscopy, C. F. was given general anesthesia and her trachea was intubated. She was placed in lithotomy position with arms abducted. Her abdomen was insufflated with carbon dioxide (CO_2) through a thin needle placed below the umbilicus. Three trocar punctures were made to insert the telescope with camera and the cutting and grasping instruments. Biopsies were taken of several pelvic lymph nodes and sent to the pathology laboratory. There were many adhesions from prior surgery, which were lysed to mobilize her organs and enhance visualization. A loop of small bowel, which had adhered to the anterior abdominal wall, had been punctured when the trocar was introduced. The surgeon repaired the defect with an endoscopic stapler and irrigated the abdomen with 3 L of NS mixed with antibiotic solution.

为了做腹腔镜检查 C. F. 被全身麻醉，并做气管插管。她被置于截石体位，上臂外展。她的腹部通过放置在脐部下面的细针吹入二氧化碳（CO_2）。进行了三个套管针穿刺以插入带有照相机和切割及抓握器械的内窥镜。对几个盆腔淋巴结做了活检，并送到病理实验室。先前的手术造成的许多粘连已经被细胞溶解，使其器官能够移动并增强了可视性。当引入套管针时，已经粘附到前腹壁的小肠环已经被穿刺。外科医生用内窥镜吻合器修复缺损并用 3L 的生理盐水混合抗生素溶液冲洗腹部。

案例研究问题

写出来自于补充案例研究的单词，以完成下列语句。

1. Secondary conditions, complications, or lasting effects of C. F.'s cancer would be called _____.
2. Examination by listening to body sounds with a stethoscope is called_____.
3. The size and shape of C. F.'s head was described as_____.
4. A collection of abdominal fluid (ascites) is drained by a cavity puncture and drainage procedure called a(n) _____.
5. Removal of tissue for microscopic examination is_____.
6. A surgical procedure in which an endoscope is inserted through the abdominal wall to visualize the abdominal cavity and determine the cause of a disorder is a(n)_____.
7. For her examination, C. F. was placed in a supine position with knees bent. This position is used for gynecologic and urologic surgery and is called the _____.

多项选择，选择正确的答案，写在每个题号的左侧。

____ 8. C. F.'s cancer was in a state of apparent cure with no active signs of disease. This state is called
   a. tumor staging
   b. syndrome
   c. remission d. sequelae

____ 9. The abbreviation NKDA refers to allergies to
   a. dust
   b. wheat
   c. eggs
   d. drugs

____ 10. C. F. claimed that her heart races and she cannot catch her breath. The terms for these conditions are, respectively,
   a. tachypnea and dyspnea
   b. tachycardia and dyspnea
   c. dyspnea and tachycardia
   d. tachycardia and bradypnea

____ 11. Syncope is
   a. fainting
   b. nosebleed
   c. palpitations
   d. anxiety

____ 12. Hepatosplenomegaly means
   a. removal of the liver and spleen
   b. prolapse of the heart and spleen
   c. hemorrhage of the liver and spleen
   d. enlargement of the liver and spleen

____ 13. C. F.'s abdominal cavity and organs were bound with fibrous tissue bands, which had to be lysed during surgery. These attachments are called
   a. sequelae
   b. adhesions
   c. ascites
   d. fibroids

____ 14. The accidental puncture of the intestine was not an expected outcome of surgery. It was an incident that occurred despite attempts to protect C.F. from harm. The term for this type of disorder is (see Chapter 6)
   a. iatrogenic
   b. nosocomial
   c. idiopathic
   d. etiologic

给出下列缩略语的含义。

15. HPI _____
16. CA _____
17. TPR _____
18. ADL _____
19. bpm _____
20. WNL _____
21. D/C _____
22. NS _____

CHAPTER 8

药物

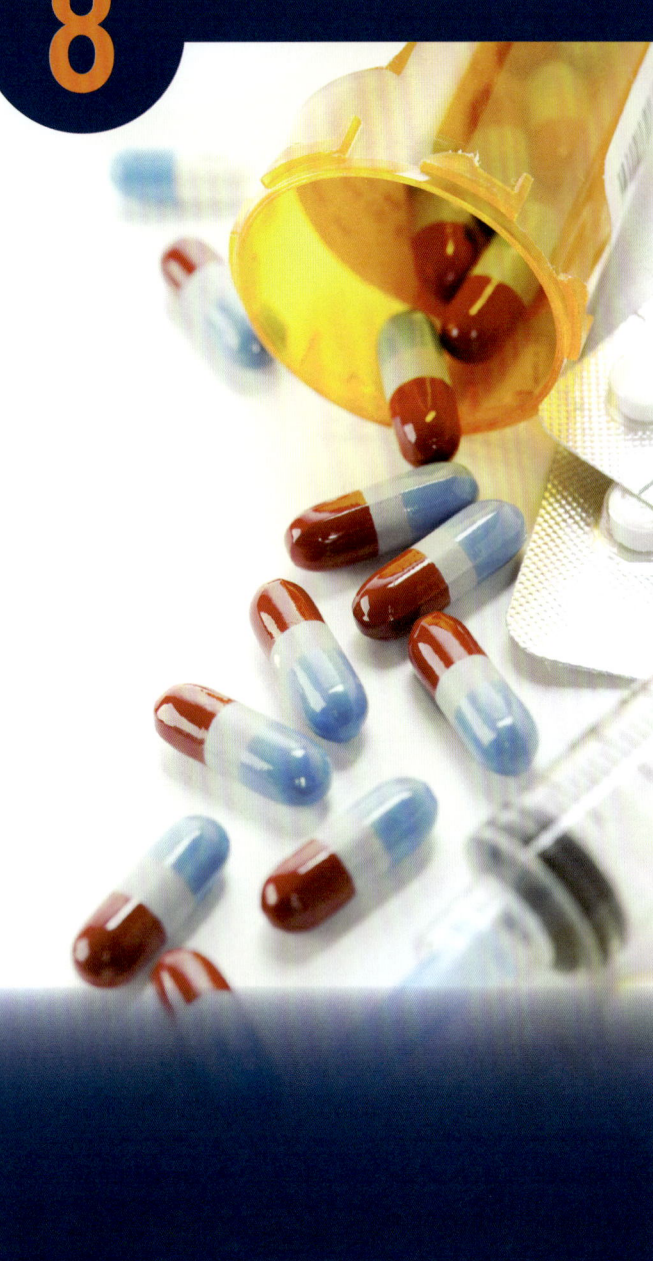

预测试

多项选择，选择正确的答案，在每个题号的左侧写出你选择的字母。

_____ 1. The federal agency that approves drugs for sale is the
   a. Occupational Safety and Health Adminis tration
   b. U.S. Department of Agriculture
   c. Department of Health and Human Services
   d. Food and Drug Administration

_____ 2. A reason for not using a specific drug is a
   a. prescription
   b. contraindication
   c. counter-purpose
   d. prognosis

_____ 3. A manufacturer's registered name for a drug is its
   a. chemical name
   b. generic name
   c. brand name
   d. over-the-counter name

_____ 4. The word root for drug or medicine is
   a. pharm
   b. scop
   c. log
   d. lapar

_____ 5. An analgesic is a drug used for
   a. fractures
   b. water retention
   c. pain
   d. coma

_____ 6. An antihypertensive drug affects
   a. blood pressure
   b. diet
   c. growth
   d. ovulation

_____ 7. The solvent in an aqueous solution is
   a. acid
   b. water
   c. salt
   d. base

_____ 8. The abbreviation tid means
   a. as needed
   b. once a day
   c. at bedtime
   d. three times a day

学习目标

学完本章后，应该能够：

1. ▶ 介绍处方药物与非处方药物的区别。
2. ▶ 列出药物的三种可能的不良反应。
3. ▶ 解释药物发生作用的两种方式。
4. ▶ 解释药物通用名称与商品名称的区别。
5. ▶ 列出三类药物参考信息。
6. ▶ 描述与草药相关的五个安全性问题。
7. ▶ 定义与药物及其作用相关的基本术语。
8. ▶ 识别并使用与药物相关的单词组成部分。
9. ▶ 定义与药物及其作用相关的缩略语。
10. ▶ 认识主要的药物种类及作用原理。
11. ▶ 列出常用的草药名称以及作用原理。
12. ▶ 列出常用的给药途径。
13. ▶ 列出药物制备的标准液体和固体剂型。
14. ▶ 分析几个案例研究中与药物相关的术语。

Case Study: P. L.'s Cardiac Disease and Crisis
案例研究：P. L. 的心脏病和危机

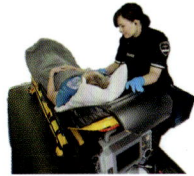

Chief Complaint

P. L. was having chest pain and had taken two nitroglycerin tablets without relief. Her family called an ambulance, and she was brought to the emergency room with chest pain that radiated down her arm, dyspnea, and syncope.

Examination

While P. L. was being admitted to the emergency room, her family provided a history to the triage nurse. They related that P.L. had a four-year history of heart disease. Her routine medications included Lanoxin to slow and strengthen her heartbeat, Inderal to support her heart rhythm, Lipitor to decrease her cholesterol, Catapres to lower her hypertension, nitroglycerin prn for chest pain, HydroDIURIL to eliminate fluid and decrease the heart's workload, Diabinese for her diabetes, and Coumadin to prevent blood clots. She also took Tagamet for her stomach ulcer and several OTC preparations, including an herbal sleeping formulation that she mixed in tea and Metamucil mixed in orange juice every morning for her bowels. Her family indicated that P. L. also took a number of other herbal and OTC medications, but they were unable to recall their names.

While P. L. was having a 12-lead ECG, her blood pressure dropped, and her heart rate deteriorated into a full cardiac arrest.

Clinical Course

Immediate resuscitation was instituted with cardiopulmonary resuscitation (CPR), defibrillation, and a bolus of IV epinephrine. Between shocks, she was given a bolus of lidocaine and a bolus of diltiazem plus repeated doses of epinephrine every five minutes. P. L. did not respond to resuscitation, and she was pronounced dead 55 minutes after arrival to the emergency room.

主诉

P. L. 有胸痛，服用 2 片硝酸甘油片没有得到缓解。她的家人叫救护车将她带到急诊室，她的胸部疼痛放射到手臂，伴随呼吸困难和晕厥。

检查

当 P. L. 被送进急诊室时，她的家人向分诊护士提供了病史。他们说到 P. L. 有 4 年的心脏病病史。她的常规药物包括：减缓并加强心功能的地高辛、支持心律的维拉帕米、降低胆固醇的立普妥、降低高血压的可乐定、因胸痛需要的硝酸甘油、消除液体和减轻心脏负荷需要的氢氯噻嗪、治疗糖尿病的氯磺丙脲和预防血栓的香豆素。她还服用西咪替丁和几种非处方制剂治疗胃溃疡，包括她在茶中混合的草药睡眠制剂，以及每天早上用橙汁混合的欧车前亲水胶以便于排便。她的家人表示 P. L. 还服用了一些其他草药和非处方药物，但他们不能记得名字。当 P. L. 做 12 导联的心电图时，她的血压下降，心率恶化为完全的心脏骤停。

临床病程

用心肺复苏术（CPR）、除颤和静脉注射肾上腺素立即进行复苏。在休克期间，每隔 5 分钟给予利多卡因和大剂量地尔硫卓加上重复剂量的肾上腺素。P. L. 对复苏没有反应，在到达急诊室 55 分钟后她被宣布死亡。

药物的基本概况

药物（drug）是改变人体功能的物质。传统上，药物源自于自然的植物、动物和矿物资源。现在，大多数药物是药品公司合成生产的，一些激素和酶是由基于工程产生的。许多药物是非处方（over-the-counter，OTC）药，不用持有医生开具的处方就可以购买；其他药物则需要医生的处方（prescription，Rx）才能购买。联邦食品和药物管理局（Food and Drug Administration，FDA）对在美国出售的药物的安全性和有效性负责，所有药物在销售之前必须获得批准。

药物的不良反应

药物或其他治疗形式的非预期作用就是副作用（side effect）。大多数药物在使用前必须评估其不良反应。另外，基于特定个人的身体状态、目前的用药情况、敏感性或家庭病史，可能存在某些禁忌证（contraindication）或原因不能使用某种特定的药物。患者处于治疗期间，必须警惕不良反应，例如消化不良、血液变化或过敏迹象等。变态反应（anaphylaxis）是药物可能引起的即时的严重过敏反应，可能会导致威胁生命的呼吸窘迫（respiratory distress）和循环衰竭（circulatory collapse）。

由于给定组合中药物可能会相互影响，医生在开具处方时必须了解患者正在使用的任何药物。在某些情况下，药物组合可能导致协同（synergy）或增强（potentiation），意味着不同的药物一起使用会有比单独使用更强的效果。在另外一些情况下，一种药物可能成为另一种药物的对抗剂（antagonist），干扰其效果。

药物也可能与特定的食物或交际中使用是物质产生不良反应，例如酒精和烟草。作用于中枢神经系统的药物可能会导致心理或身体依赖，患者会对药物产生长期或强迫性需求，而无视其不良反应。重复使用一种药物，可能会产生药物耐受性（drug tolerance），持续服用会降低效果，必须提高剂量以产生最初的效果。停药后会导致药物戒断（withdrawal）症状，特定症状与特定的药物相关。

药物名称

药物有各自的通用名称（generic name）或商品名称（brand name，框8-1给出了药物命名的信息）。通用名称通常是简单版本的药物化学名称，商品名称是生产商的注册商标名称。品牌名称受到专利保护，只有持有该专利的公司才能在其品牌名称下生产并销售该药物，直至专利到期。本章后面的框8-3是许多通用名称和商品名称的示例。请注意，同一药物可能由不同的公司以不同的商品名称上市销售。

药物信息

在美国，药物信息的标准是《美国药典》（United States Pharmacopeia，USP）。该药典由国家药理

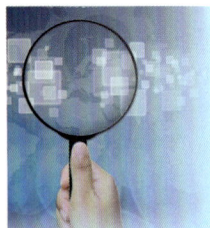

框 8-1

聚焦单词
药物因何而得名？

药物名称的来源有多种方式。有些药物因其起源而命名，例如肾上腺素（adrenaline）就根据其发源处肾上腺（adrenal gland）而得名，即使其通用名称 epinephrine，也提示我们它来自于肾（nephr/o）之上（epi-）的腺体。催产素（pitocin）是用于引产的药物，因其发源于脑垂体（pituitary gland）而命名，与激素的化学名称 oxytocin 组合而成。肉毒杆菌毒素（botox）目前被用于皮下注射以消除皱纹，它是一种能够引起肉毒杆菌中毒的微生物的毒素。阿司匹林（aspirin）是一种抗炎药，紫杉醇（taxol）是一种抗肿瘤药，洋地黄（digitalis）用于治疗心脏衰竭，阿托品（atropine）是一种平滑肌松弛剂，它们都是因其来源的植物而得名。阿司匹林由绣线菊（spiraea）的花朵而命名，阿司匹林是从这种花中提取的。紫杉醇来自于一种常绿的紫衫（taxus）属植物，洋地黄类来自于（digitalis）紫色毛地黄，阿托品来自于植物颠茄（atropa belladonna）。

一些名称表明了药物自身或其作用。优泌林是一种由基因工程产生的胰岛素，其名称 humulin 说明它是一种人工胰岛素，而不是源自于动物的激素。复方苯乙哌啶（lomotil）降低肠蠕动（motility），被用于治疗腹泻。颠茄的名称 Belladonna 来自于意大利语，意为"窈窕淑女"，因为该药物扩散眼睛的瞳孔，使女士们看起来更漂亮。

学家和其他科学家委员会出版，包含在美国销售的药物的配方，药物效力、质量和纯度的测试标准和药物的制备和配制标准。美国医院药剂师协会（American Society of Health System Pharmacists，ASHP）每年出版扩展的药物信息《医生桌上参考（Physicians' Desk Reference）》，包含药物生产商的信息。还有很多在线的药物信息可供使用。关于制药的职业信息请参见框8-2。

草药

人类使用植物治疗疾病有数百年的历史了，这种做法被称为草药（herbal medicine）或植物药（phytomedicine）。在发达国家，许多人将草药作为常规医药的替代或补充。尽管植物是很多常规药物的来源，制药公司通常会提纯、测量并调整或合成这些植物中的有效成分（active ingredient），而不是简单地呈现它们的自然状态。

使用草药的增多带来了一些问题，包括对其纯度（purity）、安全性（safety）、浓度（concentration）和有效性（efficacy）的质疑。另一个问题是药物的相互作用。医疗保健机构在记录患者的用药史时应该询问关于草药的使用，在接受治疗期间，患者应当报告其使用的所有草药。FDA并不测试和监管草药，也没有报告不良反应的要求。不过，草药生产商可以做出健康声明限制。政府建立了膳食补偿剂办公室（Office of Dietary Supplements，ODS），支持并协调该领域的研究。

框 8-2

健康职业
药剂师和药房技术员

药物是旨在治疗疾病和提高生活质量的化学品。药剂师（pharmacist）和药房技术员（pharmacy technician）的作用是确保患者获得正确的药物治疗方法和教育，以达到他们预期的健康状况。

作为医疗团队的主要成员，药剂师需要具有深厚的临床背景，并深入理解化学、解剖学和生理学。一些药剂师在社区或零售环境中工作，其他的在医院工作。不同的职位有不同的职责。所有药剂师都分发处方药物，监测患者对药物的反应，并指导患者适当地使用药物。通过订购和监测实验室结果以及根据需要调整药物剂量，医院药剂师陪同医生进行治疗和管理药物治疗方案。药剂师与其他卫生专业人员分享其专业知识，并可参与药物及其作用的临床研究。

药房技术人员协助药剂师履行职责。他们的培训也需要有完整的基础科学背景。各个州的规章制度不同，但药房技术人员可以执行许多与分配药物相关的任务，例如准备以及用适当的标签和使用说明包装药物。

因为对医疗保健的需求的增长，药剂师和药房技术员的工作前景很好。事实上，药剂师预计是美国增长最快的职业之一。有关药学职业的更多信息，请联系美国药学院学院协会（American Association of Colleges of Pharmacy），网址为www.aacp.org。

Terminology 关键术语

anaphylaxis	[ˌænəfiˈlæksis]	变态反应，极度的过敏反应，可能导致呼吸窘迫、循环衰竭和死亡
antagonist	[ænˈtæɡənist]	拮抗剂，干扰或对抗药物作用的物质
contraindication	[ˌkɒntrəˌindiˈkeiʃn]	禁忌证，使得一种药物的使用不合要求或可能造成危险的因素
drug	[drʌɡ]	药物，改变身体功能的物质
efficacy	[ˈefikəsi]	功效，产生特定结果的能力
generic name	[dʒəˈnerik]	通用名，药物的非专有名称，通常是简化的化学名称

Terminology 关键术语（续表）

phytomedicine [ˌfəʊtəʊ'medɪs(ə)n]		植物药，草药的另一个名称（词根 phyt/o 意为"植物"）
potentiation [pətenʃɪ'eɪʃən]		增强，两种药物共同作用产生的效力提高
prescription (Rx) [prɪˈskrɪpʃn]		处方，书面并署名的药物订单，附带服用说明
side effect		不良反应，与预期作用不相关或扩大了的药物治疗或其他治疗结果，通常用于治疗的不良作用
substance dependence		物质依赖，长期使用一种药物可能导致的一种状态，使人对该药物产生长期或强迫性需求，而无视其不良反应；依赖可以是心理的，也可以是身体上的
synergy [ˈsɪnədʒɪ]		协同，两种或多种药物共同作用产生的效果，比任何一种药物单独的作用更大；形容词 synergistic [ˌsɪnəˈdʒɪstɪk]
tolerance		耐药性，长期使用一种药物导致的有效性下降的状况，要获得最初的反应必须增加剂量
withdrawal		戒断，突然停止或减少原来常规使用的药物导致的状况

与药物相关的单词组成部分

表 8-1 列出了与药物相关的单词组成部分

表 8-1 与药物相关的单词组成部分

	含义	示例	示例定义
后缀			
-lytic (-lysis 的形容词形式)	溶解，减少、松弛	thrombolytic [θrɒmbəʊ'lɪtɪk]	溶栓
-mimetic	拟态的，模拟的	sympathomimetic [ˌsɪmpəθəʊmaɪ'metɪk]	拟交感神经
-tropic	作用于	psychotropic [ˌsaɪkə'trəʊpɪk]	作用于神经的（psych/o）
前缀			
anti-	对抗	antiemetic [æntɪmetɪk]	止吐药（emesis）
contra-	对抗，相反，对立	contraceptive [ˌkɒntrə'septɪv]	避孕
counter-	对抗、对立	countertransport [kaʊntətræns'pɔːt]	逆向转运
词根			
alg/o, algi/o, algesi/o	疼痛	algesia [ælˈdʒiːsɪə]	痛觉
chem/o	化学	chemotherapy [ˌkiːməʊ'θerəpɪ]	化疗
hypn/o	睡眠	hypnosis [hɪp'nəʊsɪs]	催眠

续表 8-1　与药物相关的单词组成部分

词根	含义	示例	示例定义
narc/o	麻痹	narcotic [nɑːˈkɒtik]	麻醉剂
pharm, pharmac/o	药物、医药	pharmacy [ˈfɑːməsi]	药房
pyr/o, pyret/o	发热	antipyretic [ˌæntipaiˈretik]	退热剂
tox/o, toxic/o	毒药，毒素	toxicity [tɒkˈsisəti]	毒性
vas/o	血管	vasodilation [ˌveizəʊdaiˈleiʃn]	血管舒张

练习 8-1

识别并定义下列单词的后缀。

	suffix	Meaning of suffix
1. hemolytic [hiːˈmɒlitik]	_____	_____
2. hydrotropic [ˌhaidrəˈtrɒpik]	_____	_____
3. parasympathomimetic [ˌpærəsimpəθəʊmiˈmetik]	_____	_____

使用表 8-1 中列出的前缀，写出下列单词的反义词。

4. bacterial_____
5. lateral_____
6. septic_____
7. act_____
8. emetic_____
9. pyretic_____

识别并定义下列单词的词根。

	Root	Meaning of Root
10. narcosis [nɑːˈkəʊsis]	_____	_____
11. chemistry [ˈkemistri]	_____	_____
12. analgesia [ˌænəlˈdʒiːziə]	_____	_____
13. toxicology [ˌtɒksiˈkɒlədʒi]	_____	_____
14. hypnotic [hipˈnɒtik]	_____	_____

定义下列单词。

15. vasodilation [ˌveizəʊdaiˈleiʃn] _____
16. pharmacology [ˌfɑːməˈkɒlədʒi] _____
17. mucolytic [ˌmjʊkəˈlitik] _____
18. gonadotropic [ˌɡɒnədəˈtrɒpik] _____

Terminology 缩略语

Drug and drug formulations 药物和药物配方

APAP	Acetaminophen	对乙酰氨基酚
ASA	Acetylsalicylic acid (aspirin)	乙酰水杨酸（阿司匹林）
ASHP	American Society of Health System Pharmacists	美国医院药剂师协会
cap	Capsule	胶囊
elix	Elixir	酏剂
FDA	Food and Drug Administration	食品和药物管理局
INH	Isoniazid (antituberculosis drug)	异烟肼（抗结核药）
MED(s)	Medicine(s), medication(s)	医药，药物
NSAID(s)	Nonsteroidal antiinflammatory drug(s)	非甾体抗炎药
ODS	Office of Dietary Supplements	美国膳食补充剂办公室
OTC	Over-the-counter	非处方
PDR	Physicians' Desk Reference	医生桌上参考
Rx	Prescription	处方
supp	Suppository	栓剂
susp	Suspension	混悬剂
tab	Tablet	片剂
tinct	Tincture	酊剂
ung	Ointment	膏剂
USP	United States Pharmacopeia	《美国药典》

Dosages and Directions 剂量和说明

a	Before (Latin, ante)	之前（拉丁语 ante）
aa	Of each (Greek, ana)	每个（希腊语 ana）
ac	Before meals (Latin, ante cibum)	餐前（拉丁语 ante cibum）
ad lib	As desired (Latin, ad libitum)	如预期（拉丁语 ad libtium）
aq	Water (Latin, aqua)	水（拉丁语 aqua）
bid, b.i.d.	Twice a day (Latin, bis in die)	每日 2 次（拉丁语 bis in die）
c̄	With (Latin, cum)	带有（拉丁语 cum）

Terminology 缩略语（续表）

DAW	Dispense as written	按医嘱配药
D/C, dc	Discontinue	不连续
DS	Double strength	2 倍浓度
hs	At bedtime (Latin, hora somni)	卧床时（拉丁语 hora somni）
ID	Intradermal(ly)	皮内注射
IM	Intramuscular(ly)	肌内注射
IU	International unit	国际单位
IV	Intravenous(ly)	静脉注射
LA	Long-acting	长效
mcg	Microgram	微克
mg	Milligram	毫克
ml	Milliliter	毫升
p	After, post	之后
pc	After meals (Latin, post cibum)	餐后（拉丁语 post cibum）
po, PO	By mouth (Latin, per os)	口服（拉丁语 per os）
pp	Postprandial (after a meal)	餐后
prn	As needed (Latin, pro re nata)	根据需要（拉丁语 pro re nata）
qam	Every morning (Latin, quaque ante meridiem)	每天早晨（拉丁语 quaque ante meridiem）
Qh	Every hour (Latin, quaque hora)	每小时（拉丁语 quaque hora）
q	h Every hours	每 小时
qid, q.i.d.	Four times a day (Latin, quater in die)	每日 4 次（拉丁语 quater in die）
s̄	Without (Latin, sine)	没有（拉丁语 sine）
SA	Sustained action	持续作用
SC, SQ, subcut	Subcutaneous(ly)	皮下
SL	sublingual(ly)	舌下
SR	Sustained release	缓释
s̄s̄	Half (Latin, semis)	一半（拉丁语 semis）
tid, t.i.d.	Three times per day (Latin, ter in die)	每日 3 次（拉丁语 ter in die）

Terminology 缩略语（续表）

U	Unit(s)	单位
x	Times	次数

药物参考信息

上面给出了药物的概要介绍和药物及药物使用的相关词汇。后面的信息框给出了一些药物参考信息。框 8-3 给出了主要的药物类别、通用名称和商品名称，框 8-4 列出了一些常用的草药及其使用方法，框 8-5 至框 8-7 是给药途径、药物制剂和注射用药的信息（图 8-1 至图 8-6）。

供你参考 — 常用药及其作用 （框 8-3）

药物类别	作用及应用	通用名称	商品名称
adrenergics ［'ədrənədʒiks］（sympathomimetics ［ˌsɪmpəθəʊmɪ'metɪk］）肾上腺素的	模拟交感神经系统的作用，对压力做出反应；用于治疗支气管痉挛、过敏反应和低血压	epinephrine 肾上腺素 phenylephrine 苯肾上腺素 pseudoephedrine 伪麻黄碱 dopamine 多巴胺	Bronkaid Neo-Synephrine Sudafed Intropin
analgesics ［ˌænəl'dʒi:ziks］镇痛药	减轻疼痛		
narcotics ［nɑ:'kɒtiks］麻醉剂	降低中枢神经系统的痛感；长期使用可能导致身体依赖	codeine 可待因 morphine 吗啡 meperidine 哌替啶 oxycodone 氧可酮 hydrocodone 氢可酮	 Demerol OxyContin, Percocet Vicodin, Lortab
nonnarcotics ［nɒn nɑ:'kɒtiks］非麻醉剂	从外围发生作用抑制前列腺素（局部激素）；也可以作为抗炎药和退热剂。环氧化酶-2 抑制剂限制引起炎症的酶，而不影响保护胃壁的酶	aspirin (ASA) 阿司匹林 acetaminophen (APAP) 醋氨酚 ibuprofen 布洛芬 celecoxib (Cox-2 inhibitor) 塞来昔布	 Tylenol Motrin, Advil Celebrex
anesthetics ［ænɪs'θɪtiks］麻醉剂	降低或消除感觉（esthesi/o）	局部：lidocaine 利多卡因 　　　bupivacaine 布比卡因 通用：nitrous oxide 氧化亚氮 　　　midazolam 咪达唑仑 　　　thiopental 硫喷妥钠	Xylocaine Marcaine Versed Pentothal
anticoagulants ［ˌænti:kə'væɡjʊlənts］抗凝剂	阻止凝结和形成血块	heparin 肝素 warfarin 华法令阻凝剂 apixaban 艾吡沙班	 Coumadin Eliquis

> **供你参考**
> 常用药及其作用

药物类别	作用及应用	通用名称	商品名称
anticonvulsants [ˌæntikən'vʌls(ə)ntz] 抗痉挛剂	压制或降低发作的次数和/或强度	phenobarbital 苯巴比妥 phenytoin 苯妥英 carbamazepine 卡马西平 valproic acid 丙戊酸	Dilantin Tegretol Depakene
antidiabetics ['ænti,daiə'betiks] 抗糖尿病药	预防或减轻糖尿病	Insulin 胰岛素 glyburide 格列本脲 acarbose 阿卡波糖 glipizide 格列吡嗪 metformin 二甲双胍	Humulin (注射) Diabeta Tradjenta Glucotrol Glucophage
antiemetics [æntimetiks] 止吐药	缓解恶心的症状，防止呕吐（emesis）	ondansetron 奥坦西隆 dimenhydrinate 茶苯海明 prochlorperazine 丙氯拉嗪 scopolamine 东莨菪碱 promethazine 异丙嗪	Zofran Dramamine Compazine TRANSDERM-SCOP Phenergan
antihistamines [ænti:his'tæminz] 抗组胺药	防止组织胺引发的反应：过敏和感染反应	diphenhydramine 苯海拉明 fexofenadine 非索非那定 loratadine 氯雷他定 cetirizine 西替利嗪	Benadryl Allegra Claritin Zyrtec
antihypertensives ['ænti:haipə'tensivz] 抗高血压药	通过降低心输出量、扩张血管或改善肾排泄降低血压。血管紧张素转换酶抑制剂阻止引起血压升高的物质的生成	amlodipine 氨氯地平 atenolol 阿替洛尔 clonidine 可乐宁 prazosin 哌唑嗪 minoxidil 米诺地尔 captopril 卡托普利 enalapril 依那普利 lisinopril 赖诺普利 losartan 氯沙坦 valsartan 缬沙坦	Norvasc Tenormin Catapres Minipress Loniten Capoten Vasotec Zestril, Prinivil Cozaar Diova
antiinflammatory drugs [æntiinf'læmətri] 抗炎药	抗感染和水肿		
corticosteroids [ˌkɔ:tikəʊs'tiɔid] 激素类	来自于肾上腺皮层的激素，由于过敏、呼吸和血液疾病，受伤以及恶性肿瘤；压制免疫系统功能	dexamethasone 地塞米松 cortisone 可的松 prednisone 泼尼松 hydrocortisone 氢化可的松 fluticasone 氟替卡松	Decadron Cortone Deltasone Hydrocortone, Cortef, Solu-cortef Flonase
nonsteroidal ['nɒnstərɔidl] anti-inflammatory drugs (NSAIDs) 非甾体抗炎药	通过介入前列腺素的合成降低感染和疼痛；也是退热剂	aspirin 阿司匹林 ibuprofen 布洛芬 indomethacin 吲哚美辛 naproxen 萘普生 celecoxib 塞来昔布	Motrin, Advil Indocin Naprosyn, Aleve Celebrex

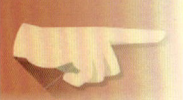

供你参考
常用药及其作用

续框 8-3

药物类别	作用及应用	通用名称	商品名称
antiinfective agents 抗感染药物	杀死或阻止感染性微生物的生长		
antibacterials［ˌænti:bæk'tiəriəlz］抗菌药 antibiotics［ˌæntibai'ɒtiks］抗生素	有效抵抗细菌	amoxicillin 阿莫西林 penicillin V 苯氧甲基青霉素 erythromycin 红霉素 vancomycin 万古霉素 gentamicin 庆大霉素 cephalexin 头孢氨苄 tetracycline 四环素 ciprofloxacin (for ulcer-causing Helicobacter pylori) 环丙沙星（治疗幽门螺旋杆菌引起的溃疡） isoniazid (INH) (tuberculosis) 异烟肼（抗结核）	Polymox Pen-Vee K Erythrocin Vancocin Garamycin Keflex Achromycin Cipro
antifungals［ˌænti'fʌŋgəls］抗真菌药	有效抵抗真菌	amphotericin B 两性霉素 B miconazole 咪康唑 nystatin 制霉菌素	Fungizone Monistat Nilstat
antiparasitics［ænti:pærə'sitik］抗寄生虫药	有效抵抗寄生虫：原生动物，蠕虫	iodoquinol (amebae) 双碘喹啉（针对阿米巴虫） quinacrine 阿的平	Yodoxin Atabrine
antivirals［ˌænti'vairəls］抗病毒药	有效抵抗病毒	acyclovir 阿昔洛韦 zanamivir (influenza) 扎那米韦（治疗流行性感冒） zidovudine (HIV) 齐多夫定（治疗艾滋病） indinavir (HIV protease inhibitor) 印地那韦（HIV 蛋白酶抑制剂）	Zovirax Relenza Retrovir Crixivan
antineoplastics［'ænti ˌni:əʊ'plæstiks］抗肿瘤药	摧毁癌细胞；它们对所有细胞都有毒性，但对活跃增长并分裂的细胞效果更强；激素与激素抑制剂也被用于减缓肿瘤的生长	cyclophosphamide 环磷酰胺 doxorubicin 阿霉素 methotrexate 甲氨蝶呤 vincristine 长春新碱 tamoxifen (estrogen inhibitor) 它莫西芬（雌激素抑制剂）	Cytoxan Adriamycin Oncovin Nolvadex
cardiac drugs 心脏病药 antiarrhythmics［ænʃiə'riðmiks］抗心律不齐药	作用于心脏 校正或防止心律异常	quinidine 奎尼丁 lidocaine 利多卡因 digoxin 地高辛	Quinidex Xylocaine Lanoxin
beta-adrenergic blockers［'bi:tə'ədrənədʒik］β- 肾上腺素能受体阻滞剂	抑制交感神经系统；降低心率并强迫心脏收缩	propranolol 普萘洛尔 metoprolol 美托洛尔 atenolol 阿替洛尔	Inderal Toprol-XL Tenormin

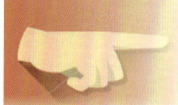

供你参考
常用药及其作用

药物类别	作用及应用	通用名称	商品名称
calcium-channel blockers ['kælsiəm] 钙通道阻滞剂	扩张冠状动脉，降低心率，减小收缩	diltiazem 地尔硫卓 nifedipine 硝苯地平 verapamil 维拉帕米	Cardizem Procardia Veralan, Calan
hypolipidemics [hi'pɒlipaidemiks] 降血脂药	降低高血清水平患者单靠饮食不能控制的胆固醇；他汀类药物	ovastatin 洛伐他汀 pravastatin 普伐他汀 atorvastatin 阿托伐他汀 lsimvastatin 辛伐他汀	Mevacor Pravachol Lipitor Zocor
nitrates ['naitreitz] 硝酸盐 antianginal agents [æn'ti:ənginl] 抗心绞痛药	通过降低血压和减少静脉回流扩张冠状动脉，并降低心脏负荷	nitroglycerin 硝酸甘油 isosorbide 异山梨醇	Nitrostat Isordil
CNS stimulants 中枢神经兴奋剂	刺激中枢神经系统	methylphenidate 哌醋甲酯 amphetamine 安非他明（长期使用可能导致药物依赖）	Ritalin Adderall, Dexedrine
diuretics [dai'juəretiks] 利尿剂	改善水、钠和其他电解质通过肾的排泄；用于减轻水肿和降低血压	furosemide 呋塞米 ethacrynic acid 依他尼酸 mannitol 甘露醇 hydrochlorothiazide (HCTZ) 氢氯噻嗪 triamterene + HCTZ 氨苯喋啶 + 氢氯噻嗪	Lasix Edecrin Osmitrol HydroDIURIL Dyazide
gastrointestinal drugs [ˌgæstrəʊin'testinl] 胃肠道药物	作用于消化道		
antidiarrheals [æntidə'ri:lz] 止泻药	通过减少肠蠕动或吸收刺激物并舒缓肠内壁治疗或阻止腹泻	Diphenoxylate+ atropine 苯乙哌啶 + 阿托品 loperamide 洛派丁胺 attapulgite 硅镁土	Lomotil Imodium Kaopectate
histamine H₂ antagonists ['histəmi:n] 组胺 H₂ 受体拮抗剂	通过干扰 H₂ 受体组胺的作用减少胃酸的分泌；用于治疗溃疡和其他胃肠道疾病	famotidine 法莫替丁 ranitidine 雷尼替丁	Pepcid Zantac
laxatives ['læksətivz] 通便剂	改善大肠的排泄，包括 　兴奋剂 　高渗剂（保水） 　大便软化剂 　成形剂	bisacodyl 比沙可啶 lactulose 乳果糖 docusate 多库酯钠 psyllium 洋车前子	Dulcolax Constilac, Chronulac Colace, Surfak Metamucil
proton pump inhibitors 质子泵抑制剂	通过阻滞氢离子（质子）传输进入胃降低胃的酸性	esomeprazole 埃索美拉唑 lansoprazole 兰索拉唑 omeprazole 奥美拉唑	Nexium Prevacid Prilosec

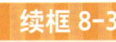

供你参考

常用药及其作用
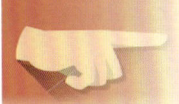

药物类别	作用及应用	通用名称	商品名称
muscle relaxants 肌肉松弛药	压抑神经系统对骨骼肌肉的刺激；用于控制肌肉痉挛和疼痛	baclofen 巴氯芬 carisoprodol 卡立普多 methocarbamol 美索巴莫	Lioresal Soma Robaxin
psychotropics [saikət'rɒpiks] 精神药物	影响大脑，改变精神活动、精神状态或行为		
antianxiety agents [ænti:əŋ'zaiəti] 抗焦虑药	降低或驱散焦虑；镇静剂	lorazepam 劳拉西泮 chlordiazepoxide 甲氨二氮䓬 diazepam 地西泮 hydroxyzine 羟嗪 alprazolam 阿普唑仑 buspirone 丁螺环酮	Ativan Librium Valium Atarax Xanax BuSpar
antidepressants [ænti:dip'resænts] 抗抑郁药	通过提高大脑神经递质（神经系统中活跃的化学物质）的水平减轻压抑	amitriptyline 阿米替林 imipramine 丙咪嗪 fluoxetine 氟西汀 paroxetine 帕罗西汀 sertraline 舍曲林	Elavil Tofranil Prozac Paxil Zoloft
antipsychotics [æntipsai'ʃɒtiks] 抗精神病药	作用于神经系统减轻神经病的症状	chlorpromazine 氯丙嗪 haloperidol 氟哌啶醇 risperidone 利培酮 olanzapine 奥氮平	Thorazine Haldol Risperdal Zyprexa
respiratory drugs 呼吸系统药物	作用于呼吸系统		
antitussives [ˌænti'tʌsivz] 止咳药	抑制咳嗽	dextromethorphan 右美沙芬	Benylin DM
asthma maintenance drugs 哮喘维持药物 bronchodilators [b'rɒntʃədaileitəz] 支气管扩张剂	用于预防哮喘发作和哮喘的长期治疗；通过放松支气管平滑肌防止或消除支气管痉挛；用于治疗哮喘发作和支气管炎	fluticasone 氟替卡松 montelukast 孟鲁斯特 albuterol 沙丁胺醇 epinephrine 肾上腺素 metaproterenol 间羟异丙肾上腺	Flovent Singulair Proventil Alupent Spiriva
expectorants [eks'pektərənts] 祛痰药	引发富有成效的咳嗽以排除呼吸系统的分泌物	guaifenesin 愈创甘油醚	Robitussin
mucolytics [mjʊkəʊ'litik] 化痰药	稀释痰液以方便排出	acetylcysteine 乙酰半胱氨酸	Mucomyst
sedatives/hypnotics ['sedətivz] / [hip'nɒtiks] 镇静剂/安眠药	引发放松和睡眠；较低（镇静）剂量改善放松状态，导致睡眠；较高（安眠）剂量引发睡眠；也用作抗焦虑药	phenobarbital 苯巴比妥 zolpidem 唑吡坦	Ambien

续框 8-3

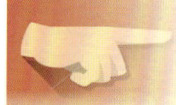

供你参考

草药的治疗应用

框 8-4

名称	被使用的部分	治疗应用
aloe ［ˈæləʊ］芦荟	叶	治疗烫伤和减轻皮肤刺激
black cohosh ［ˈkəʊhɒʃ］黑升麻	根	减少更年期潮热
chamomile ［ˈkæməmail］甘菊	花	抗炎药，防治胃肠道痉挛，镇静剂
echinacea ［ˌekəˈneiʃiə］紫锥菊	全部	降低感冒的严重性并缩短生病时间，可以刺激免疫系统，常用于伤口愈合
evening primrose oil ［ˈprimrəʊz］月见草油	种子	对心血管系统健康很重要的脂肪酸的来源，治疗经前综合征、类风湿性关节炎和皮肤病
Flax 亚麻	种子	是维持血液中适当的脂类（如胆固醇）很重要的脂肪酸的来源
ginger ［ˈdʒindʒə(r)］姜	根	减轻恶心和晕车，治疗感冒和喉咙痛
ginkgo ［ˈɡiŋkgəʊ］银杏	叶	改善大脑内血液循环和功能，改善记忆，用于治疗痴呆，抗焦虑药，保护神经系统
ginseng ［ˈdʒinseŋ］人参	根	缓解压力，降低血液胆固醇和血糖
green tea 绿茶	叶	抗氧化剂，抵抗胃肠道和皮肤癌症，口腔抗菌剂，减少龋齿
kava ［ˈkɑːvə］卡瓦胡椒	根	抗焦虑药，镇静剂
milk thistle ［ˈθisl］奶蓟草	种子	保护肝脏，抗毒，抗氧化剂
saw palmetto ［pælˈmetəu］锯棕榈	浆果	用于治疗良性前列腺增生症
slippery elm 榆树	树皮	作为含片治疗喉咙发炎，治疗胃肠道发炎和不适，保护发炎的皮肤
soy 大豆	豆	丰富的营养来源；在更年期综合征、骨质疏松和心血管疾病和预防癌症中有保护雌激素作用
St. John wort 圣约翰草	花	治疗焦虑和抑郁，具有抗菌和抗病毒性质（请注意，它能够与多种药物产生相互作用）
tea tree oil 茶树油	叶	抗菌，抑郁治疗伤口、皮肤感染和烫伤
valerian ［vəˈliəriən］缬草	根	镇静剂，辅助睡眠

框 8-5

供你参考
给药途径

途径	说明
通过吸收	
absorption ［əbˈsɔːpʃn］ 吸收	药物通过消化道或跨隔膜传输进入循环
inhalation ［ˌinhəˈleiʃn］ 吸入	通过呼吸系统用药，例如吸入气溶胶或喷雾器喷雾（图 8-1）
instillation ［ˌinstiˈleiʃən］ 滴注	液体滴入或注入体腔或身体表面，例如滴入耳朵或眼睛结膜（图 8-2）
oral ［ˈɔːrəl］ 口服	经口给药，peros（po）
rectal ［ˈrektəl］ 直肠给药	通过直肠栓剂或灌肠给药
sublingual (SL) ［sʌbˈliŋgwəl］ 舌下	舌下给药
topical ［ˈtɒpikl］ 外用	用于皮肤表面
transdermal ［ˈtrænzdɜːməl］ 经皮肤给药	通过皮肤吸收，例如从置于皮肤上的贴剂吸收
通过注射	
injection ［inˈdʒekʃn］ 注射	通过针头和注射器给药（图 8-3），被称为非肠道给药途径
epidural ［ˌepiˈdjʊərəl］ 脊膜外	注射到脊膜（包围脊髓的薄膜）与脊髓之间空间
hypodermoclysis ［haipəʊdɜːˈmɒklisis］ 皮下输液	通过皮下注入溶液给药；作为静脉输液的替代用于液体输送
intradermal (ID) ［ˌintrəˈdɜːməl］ 皮内注射	注射进入皮肤
intramuscular (IM) ［ˌintrəˈmʌskjələ(r)］ 肌内注射	注射进入肌肉
intravenous (IV) ［ˌintrəˈviːnəs］ 静脉注射	注射进入静脉
spinal (intrathecal) ［ˌintrəˈθiːkl］ 鞘内注射	穿过脊膜进入脊髓液
subcutaneous (SC) ［ˌsʌbkjuˈteiniəs］ 皮下注射	穿过皮肤注射

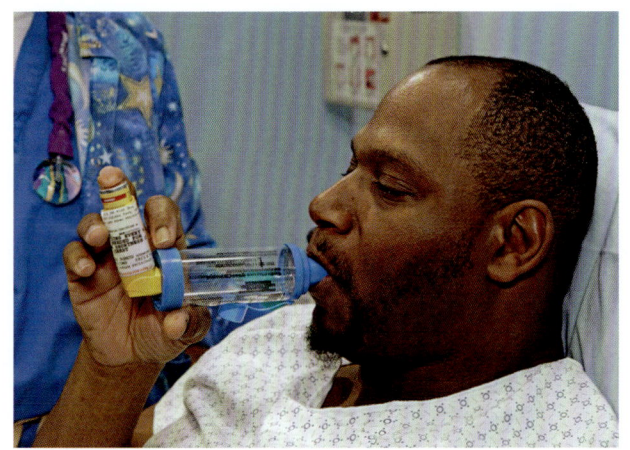

图 8-1 吸入药物。患者使用定量雾化吸入器给药

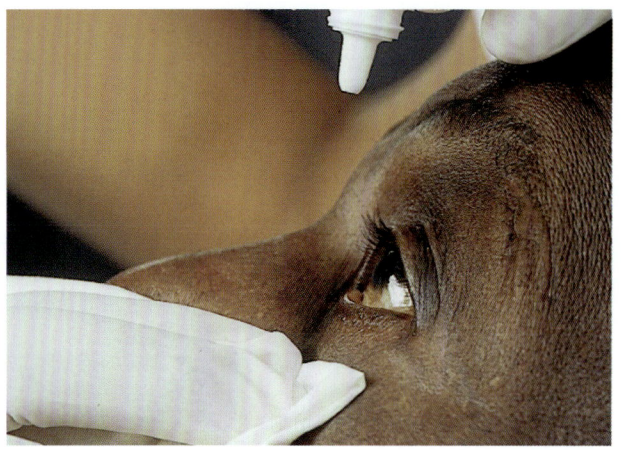

图 8-2 滴注药物。医生拉下下眼睑将眼药水滴入下结膜囊

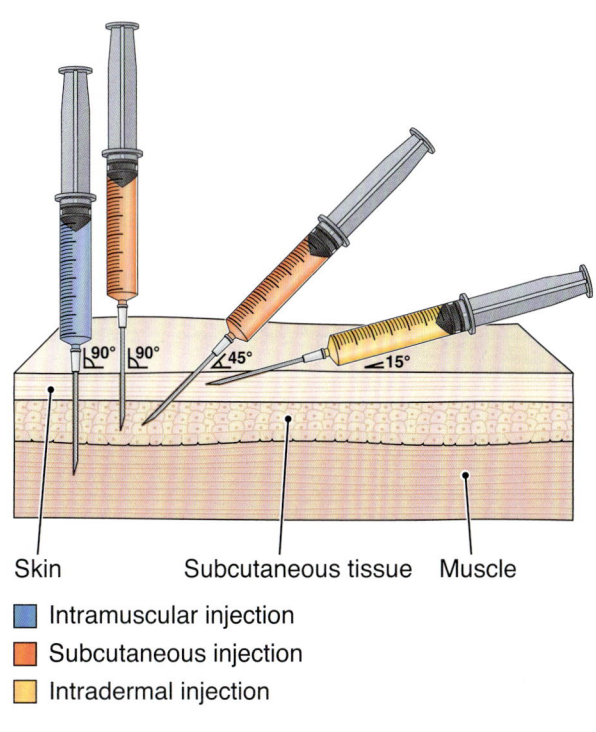

Skin　　Subcutaneous tissue　　Muscle

- Intramuscular injection
- Subcutaneous injection
- Intradermal injection

图 8-3 注射。比较肌内、皮下和皮内注射的插入角度

框 8-6

供你参考
药物配制

形式	说明
液体	
aerosol ['eərəsɒl] 气溶胶	能够被吸入的雾化溶液
aqueous solution ['eikwiəs] 水溶液	药物溶解在水中
elixir (elix) [i'liksə(r)] 酏剂	清澈的、有着令人愉快香味的甜的水醇性液体，用于口服

供你参考
续框 8-6
给药途径

形式	说明
emulsion ［iˈmʌlʃn］乳剂	混合物,其中一种液体分散于而不是溶解于另一种液体
lotion ［ˈləʊʃn］洗剂	为外用准备的溶液
suspension (susp) ［səˈspenʃn］悬浮液	细微的药物颗粒分散在液体中,使用前必须摇匀
tincture (tinct) ［ˈtɪŋktʃə(r)］酊剂	药物的酒精溶液
半固体	
cream 乳膏	外用的半固体乳剂
ointment (ung) ［ˈɔɪntmənt］软膏	药物溶于一种基质,使其能够保持与皮肤的接触
固体	
capsule (cap) 胶囊	药物包在明胶容器中,以便在胃中吸收
lozenge ［ˈlɒzɪndʒ］锭剂	在口中溶解的味道宜人的药片,例如咳嗽糖
suppository (supp) ［səˈpɒzətri］栓剂	药物与基质混合成型,插入身体开口时易于融化
tablet (tab) ［ˈtæblət］片剂	包含纯药物或与非活性成分混合并压制成型的固体剂型,也被称为药丸(pill)

供你参考
框 8-7
与注射用药相关的术语

词汇	含义
ampule ［ˈæmpuːl］安瓿	一个封闭的玻璃或塑料容器,用于容纳无菌静脉注射溶液(图 8-4)
bolus ［ˈbəʊləs］药丸	用于快速静脉注射的诊断或治疗药物的浓缩剂量
catheter ［ˈkæθɪtə(r)］导管	插入体腔、器官或血管的薄壁管(图 8-5)
syringe ［sɪˈrɪndʒ］注射器	注射液体用的设备(图 8-4)
vial ［ˈvaɪəl］小瓶	小的玻璃或塑料容器(图 8-4A)

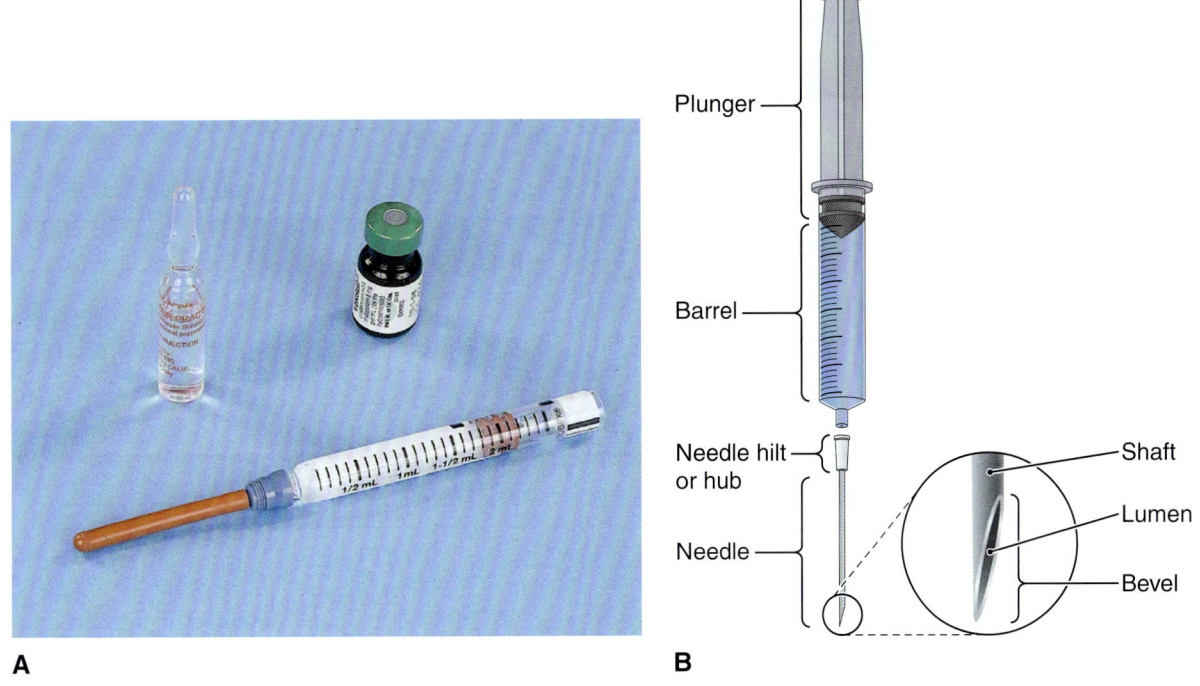

图 8-4 可注射药物材料。A. 可注射药物容器，示出了安瓿（左上）、小瓶（右上）和注射器（下图）；B. 针和注射器的部件

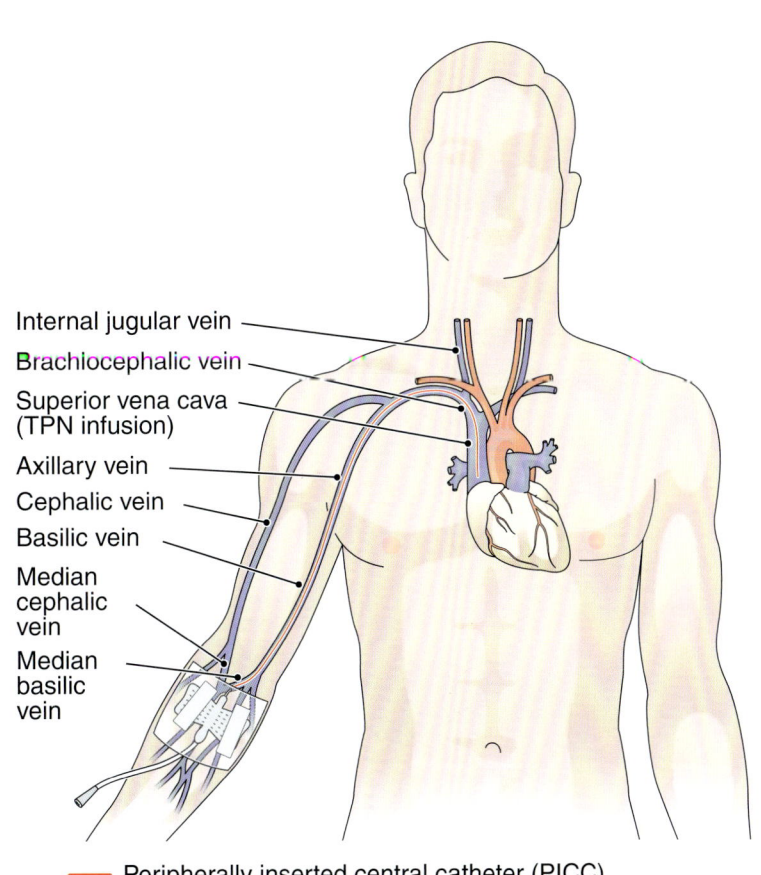

图 8-5 插管。图中示出了外周中心静脉置管（PICC）的安置

Case Study Revisited
案例研究再访

Following Up on P. L.'s Death

As the emergency room physician was documenting the course of events in P. L.'s death, he reviewed the patient's history and details provided by the family. He wondered if the patient routinely consumed any other OTC and herbal medications and thought about what potentiating effects the various drug combinations may have had. On the death certificate, her primary cause of death was listed as cardiac arrest. Multiple secondary diagnoses were listed, including polypharmacy.

P. L. 死亡随访

在急诊室医生记录 P. L. 死亡事件的过程中，他回顾了患者的病史和家属提供的细节。他想知道患者是否经常服用其他非处方药和草药，并考虑各种药物组合可能具有的增强作用。在死亡证明上，她的主要死因被列为心脏骤停。列出了多个次级诊断，包括复方用药。

CHAPTER 8 复习

匹配

匹配下列术语，在每个题号的左侧写上适当的字母。

____ 1. hyperpyrexia   a. abnormally high body temperature
____ 2. diuretic   b. combined drug action to greater effect
____ 3. potentiation   c. agent that prevents vomiting
____ 4. antiemetic   d. flowing in an opposite direction
____ 5. countercurrent   e. promoting excretion of water

____ 6. chronotropic   a. sympathomimetic
____ 7. vasomotor   b. affecting timing
____ 8. adrenergic   c. extreme allergic reaction
____ 9. anaphylaxis   d. effectiveness
____ 10. efficacy   e. pertaining to vessel movement

____ 11. ASA   a. aspirin
____ 12. bid   b. without
____ 13. aq   c. as needed
____ 14. $\bar{s}$ d. twice a day
____ 15. prn   e. water

____ 16. valerian   a. sedative
____ 17. aloe   b. source of fatty acids
____ 18. ginger root   c. antimicrobial
____ 19. tea tree oil   d. used to treat burns, irritation
____ 20. flax seed   e. relieves nausea

多项选择

选择正确的答案，在每个题号的左侧写上你选择的字母。

____ 21. NSAIDs are used to treat
    a. inflammation
    b. convulsions
    c. nausea
    d. hypertension

____ 22. A hypolipidemic drug
    a. lowers cholesterol
    b. increases urination
    c. diminishes sensation
    d. reduces inflammation

____ 23. Proton pump inhibitors
    a. are used to treat asthma
    b. relax muscle spasms
    c. reduce stomach acidity
    d. are used to administer drugs

____ 24. An ampule is a
    a. concentrated amount given rapidly
    b. mist to be inhaled
    c. tablet to dissolve in the mouth
    d. small sealed contain

___ 25. A drug that is administered topically is
   a. swallowed
   b. injected
   c. applied to the skin
   d. placed under the tongue

___ 26. Another term for hypodermic is
   a. intrathecal
   b. spinal
   c. epidural
   d. subcutaneous

___ 27. Another term for brand name is
   a. indicated name
   b. generic name
   c. trade name
   d. chemical name

___ 28. Drug administration by injection is described as
   a. instilled
   b. parenteral
   c. encapsulated
   d. nebulized

___ 29. P. L.'s nitroglycerine in the opening case study is ordered as prn SL. This means
   a. as needed, under the tongue
   b. at bedtime, under the tongue
   c. as needed, on the skin
   d. before meals, on the skin

___ 30. P. L. took several OTC preparations. OTC means
   a. on-the-cutaneous
   b. off-the-cuff
   c. over-the-counter
   d. requires a prescription

___ 31. During P. L.'s resuscitation, epinephrine was given in an IV bolus. This means it was administered
   a. intrathecally in a rapid concentrated dose
   b. parenterally as a topical solution
   c. intravenously in a continuous drip
   d. intravenously in a rapid concentrated dose

___ 32. P. L.'s herbal sleeping formulation was mixed into tea and taken at bedtime. The dissolved mixture is called a (n) ____ and is taken at ____.
   a. elixir, QAM
   b. emulsion, bid
   c. suspension, hs
   d. aqueous solution, hs

___ 33. P. L. had a secondary diagnosis of polypharmacy. This means that she
   a. used more than one drug store
   b. had polyps
   c. used more prescription than OTC drugs
   d. used many different drugs

填空

34. The study of drugs and their actions is called_____.
35. A toxicologist is one who studies_____.
36. A transdermal route of administration is through the_____.
37. Phytomedicine is the practice of treating with_____.
38. When a drug has lost its effect at a constant dose, the patient has developed_____.
39. An analgesic is used to treat_____.
40. An intravenous injection is given into a(n)_____.
41. An antipyretic drug counteracts_____.
42. With reference to drug interactions, another term for synergy is_____.

排除

在下列每组中，为与其他不相配的单词加下划线，并解释你选择的理由。

43. anesthetic — analgesic — narcotic — adrenergic — sedative

44. solution — elixir — tincture — emulsion — tablet

45. antineoplastics — nitrates — antiarrhythmics — calcium-channel blockers — beta-blockers

46. antitussive — histamine H_2 antagonist — expectorant — mucolytic — bronchodilator

定义

定义下列单词。

47. hemolytic

48. psychotropic

49. bronchoconstriction

反义词

写出下列单词的反义词。

50. emetic

51. vasodilation

52. balance

53. bacterial

54. indicated

55. neoplastic

缩略语

定义下列缩略语。

56. FDA

57. DAW

58. Rx

59. USP

60. D/C

单词构建

使用给出的单词组成部分写出下列定义的单词。

| narc/o | -lytic | thromb/o | muc/o | toxic/o | -sis | anxi/o | hypn/o |

61. an induced sleep-like state

62. reducing anxiety

63. condition caused by poisoning

64. dissolving a blood clot

65. condition of having a blood clot

66. a state of stupor

67. dissolving mucus

单词分析

定义下列单词，并给出每个单词组成部分的含义。如果需要，可以使用词典。

68. anaphylaxis ［ˌænəfiˈlæksis］ _____
    a. ana- _____
    b. phylaxis _____
69. pharmacokinetic ［ˌfɑːməkəukiˈnetik］ _____
    a. pharmac/o _____
    b. kinet/o _____
    c. -ic _____
70. adrenergic ［ˌædrəˈnɜːdʒik］ _____
    a. adren/o _____
    b. erg/o _____
    c. -ic _____
71. hypodermoclysis ［haipəudɜːˈmɒklisis］ _____
    a. hypo- _____
    b. derm/o _____
    c. clysis _____

Additional Case Studies
补充案例研究

Case Study 8-1: Inflammatory Bowel Disease
案例研究 8-1：炎症性肠病

A. E., a 19-year-old college student, was diagnosed at the age of 13 with Crohn disease, a chronic inflammatory disease that can affect the entire gastrointestinal tract from mouth to anus. A.E.'s disease is limited to his large bowel. During a nine-month period of disease exacerbation characterized by severe cramping and bloody stools, he took oral corticosteroids (prednisone) to reduce the inflammatory response. He experienced many of the drug's side effects, but has been in remission for four years. Currently, A. E.'s condition is managed on drugs that reduce inflammation by suppressing the immune response. He takes Pentasa (mesalamine) 250 mg 4 caps po bid. Pentasa is of the 5-ASA (acetylsalicylic acid or aspirin) group of antiinflammatory agents, which work topically on the inner surface of the bowel. It has an enteric coating, which dissolves in the bowel environment. He also takes 6-mercaptopurine (Purinethol) 75 mg PO daily and a therapeutic vitamin with breakfast. A.E. may take acetaminophen for pain but must avoid NSAIDs, which will irritate the intestinal mucosa (inner lining) and cause a flare-up of the disease.

A. E. 是一名 19 岁的大学生，在 13 岁时被诊断为克罗恩病，这是一种会影响从口到肛门的整个胃肠道的慢性炎性疾病。A.E. 的病只限于他的大肠。在以严重绞痛和血便为特征的 9 个月的疾病恶化期间，他口服皮质类固醇（泼尼松）以减少炎症反应。他经历了许多药物的不良反应，但已经缓解了 4 年。目前，A. E. 的病症用通过抑制免疫反应来减轻炎症的药物来控制。他口服 4 片 250mg 的 Pentasa（美沙拉嗪），每日 2 次。Pentasa 是 5-ASA（乙酰水杨酸或阿司匹林）抗炎剂，它们在肠的内表面上局部起作用，具有肠溶衣，溶解在肠道环境中。他还每天口服 75mg 的 6- 巯基嘌呤（Purinethol），早餐补充维生素治疗。为镇痛 A.E. 可以服用对乙酰氨基酚，但必须避免非甾体抗炎药，因为这类药物会刺激肠黏膜（内壁）并引起疾病的爆发。

Case Study 8-2: Asthma
案例研究 8-2：哮喘

E. N., a 20 YO woman with asthma, visited the preadmission testing unit one week before her cosmetic surgery to meet with the nurse and anesthesiologist. Her current meds included several bronchodilators, which she takes by mouth and by inhalation, and a tranquilizer that she takes when needed for nervousness. She sometimes receives inhalation treatments with Mucomyst, a mucolytic agent. On E.N.'s preoperative note, the nurse wrote:

Theo-Dur 1 cap 200 mg tid

Flovent inhaler 1 spray (50 mcg each nostril b.i.d.)

Ativan (lorazepam) 1 mg po bid

Albuterol metered-dose inhaler 2 puffs (180 mcg) prn

q4 – 6h for bronchospasm and before exercise

E. N. stated that she has difficulty with her asthma when she is anxious and when she exercises. She also admitted to occasional use of marijuana and ecstasy, a hallucinogen and mood-altering illegal recreational drug. The anesthesiologist wrote an order for lorazepam 4 mg IV one hour preop. The plastic surgeon recommended

E.N. 是一名 20 岁的哮喘女性，在她的整容手术前 1 周来到了入院前检查病房，与护士和麻醉师会面。她目前使用的药物包括几种支气管扩张剂，她通过口服和吸入给药，在神经紧张时还需要服用镇静剂。她有时接受黏液溶解剂 Mucomyst 的吸入治疗。在 E.N. 的术前说明中，护士写道：

茶碱缓释片 200mg，1 片，每日 3 次

氟替卡松吸入器 1 喷雾（50μg，每个鼻孔每日 2 次）

劳拉西泮 1mg 口服，每日 2 次

沙丁胺醇定量吸入器盆 2 次（180μg），必要时

支气管痉挛或锻炼前每 4~6 小时

E. N. 说她在焦虑和运动时会有哮喘。她还承认偶尔使用大麻和摇头丸，摇头丸是一种迷幻剂和改变情绪的非法娱乐药物。麻醉师开了处方，手术前劳拉西泮 4mg 静脉滴注 1 小时。整形外科医生为她的手术和恢复建议使用一些补充剂。他开了一种高效维生素处方，早餐和

several supplements to complement her surgery and her recovery. He ordered a high-potency vitamin, 1 tab with breakfast and dinner, to support tissue health and healing. He also prescribed bromelain, an enzyme from pineapple, to decrease inflammation, one 500 mg cap po qid three days before surgery and postoperatively for two weeks. Arnica montana was prescribed to decrease discomfort, swelling, and bruising; three tabs sublingual tid the evening after surgery and for the following 10 days.

晚餐各 1 片，以支持组织健康和康复。 他还开了菠萝蛋白酶以减少炎症，手术前 3 天和术后 2 个星期 500mg 口服，每日 4 次。山金车被用于减少不适、肿胀和淤伤，手术后和以后的 10 天舌下含服 3 片，每日 3 次。

案例研究问题

多项选择，选择正确的答案，在每个题号左侧写上你选择的字母。

____ 1. A. E. takes several drugs to prevent or act against his inflammatory response. These agents are described as

　　a. contrainflammatory

　　b. counterinflammatory

　　c. antiinflammatory

　　d. proinflammatory

____ 2. A. E. presented with several untoward results or risks from the corticosteroid therapy. These sequelae are called

　　a. contraindications

　　b. side effects

　　c. antagonistic effects

　　d. exacerbations

____ 3. A. E. takes four 250-mg capsules of Pentasa po bid. How many capsules does he take in one day?

　　a. 2,000

　　b. 1,000

　　c. 4

　　d. 8

____ 4. A. E. must avoid NSAIDs because in cases of inflammatory bowel disease, these drugs are

　　a. contraindicated

　　b. indicated

　　c. prescriptive

　　d. synergistic

____ 5. E. N. used a mucolytic drug when needed. This drug's action is to

　　a. increase mucus secretion

　　b. decrease spasms

　　c. calm anxiety

　　d. eliminate mucus

____ 6. E.N.'s Flovent inhaler is indicated as 1 spray of 50 mcg in each nostril bid. How many micrograms (mcg) does she get in one day?

　　a. 100 mcg

　　b. 200 mcg

　　c. 250 mcg

　　d. 500 mcg

____ 7. The Ativan that E.N. takes for nervousness is a(n) _____ drug.

　　a. anxiolytic

　　b. antiemetic

　　c. analgesic

　　d. bronchodilator

____ 8. The anesthesiologist ordered lorazepam (Ativan) to be given IV preop to decrease anxiety and to smooth E.N.'s anesthesia induction. The complementary way that lorazepam and anesthesia work together is called

　　a. antagonistic

　　b. complementary medicine

　　c. synergy

　　d. tolerance

____ **9.** Bromelain and Arnica montana are supplements that can be described as all of the following except

   a. phytopharmaceutical

   b. alternative

   c. chronotropic

   d. complementary

____ **10.** Arnica montana was prescribed three tabs SL tid. How many tablets would E.N. take in one day?

   a. 6

   b. 33

   c. 12

   d. 9

____ **11.** Flovent is administered as an inhalant. The form in which the drug is prepared is called a(n)

   a. aerosol

   b. elixir

   c. unguent

   d. emulsion

定义下列缩略语。

12. po_____

13. mg_____

14. NSAIDs_____

15. mcg_____

16. IV_____

PART 3 人体系统

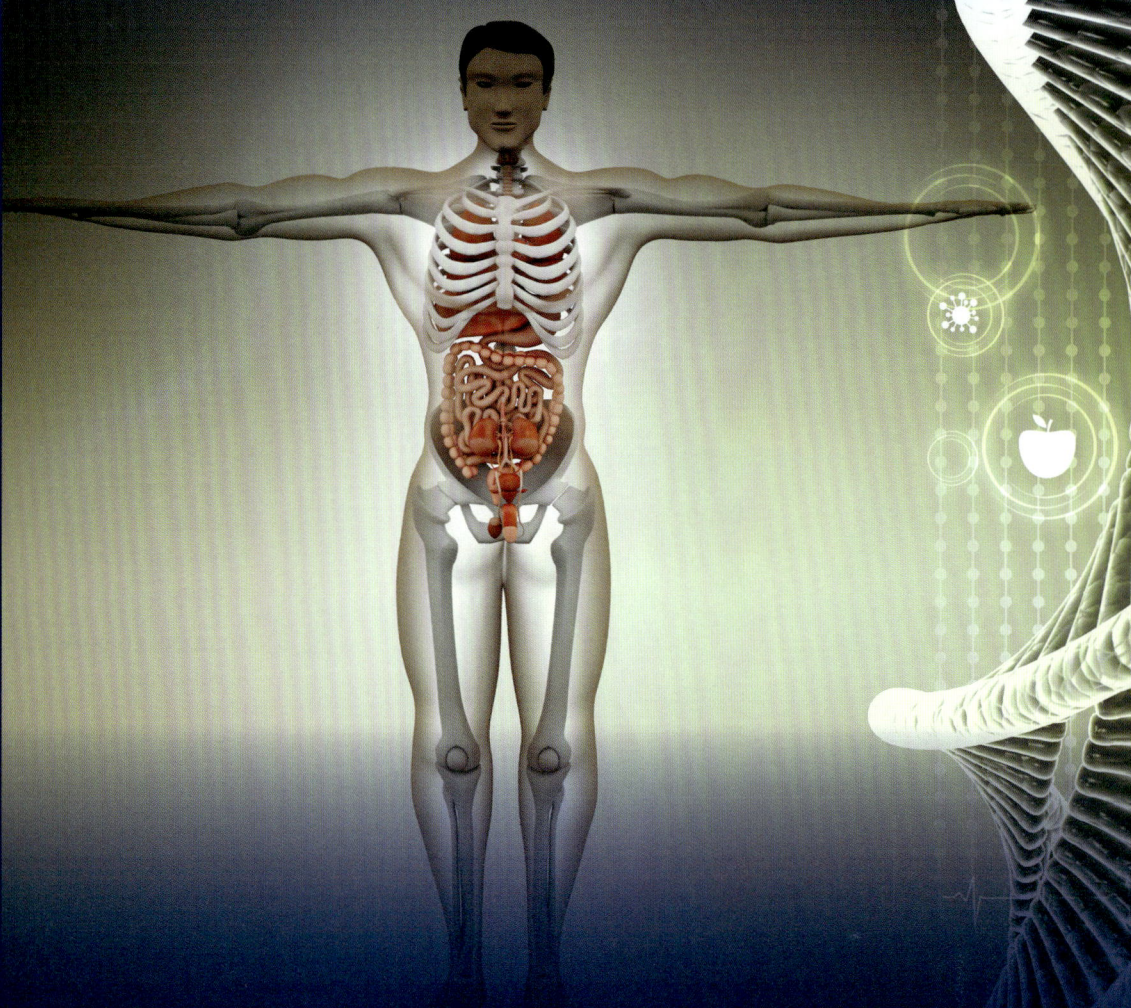

Chapter 9 ▸ Circulation: The Cardiovascular and Lymphatic Systems
第 9 章　循环：心血管与淋巴系统

Chapter 10 ▸ Blood and Immunity
第 10 章　血液与免疫

Chapter 11 ▸ The Respiratory System
第 11 章　呼吸系统

Chapter 12 ▸ The Digestive System
第 12 章　消化系统

Chapter 13 ▸ The Urinary System
第 13 章　泌尿系统

Chapter 14 ▸ The Male Reproductive System
第 14 章　男性生殖系统

Chapter 15 ▸ The Female Reproductive System; Pregnancy and Birth
第 15 章　女性生殖系统、妊娠与分娩

Chapter 16 ▸ The Endocrine System
第 16 章　内分泌系统

Chapter 17 ▸ The Nervous System and Behavioral Disorders
第 17 章　神经系统和行为障碍

Chapter 18 ▸ The Sensory System
第 18 章　感觉系统

Chapter 19 ▸ The Skeletal System
第 19 章　骨骼系统

Chapter 20 ▸ The Muscular System
第 20 章　肌肉系统

Chapter 21 ▸ The Integumentary System
第 21 章　皮肤

CHAPTER 9 循环：心血管与淋巴系统

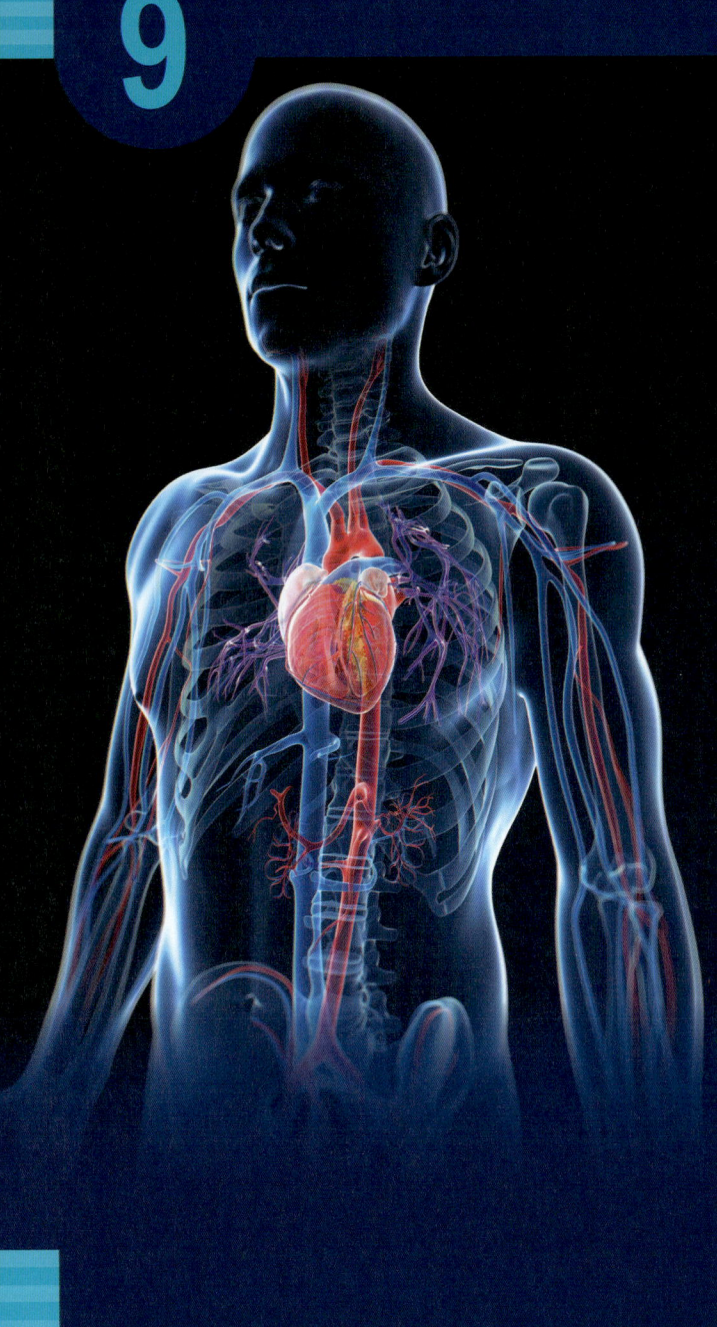

预测试

多项选择，选择正确的答案，在每个题号的左侧写出你选择的字母。

____1. The cardiovascular system includes the heart and
   a. lungs
   b. digestive organs
   c. blood vessels
   d. endocrine system

____2. The thick, muscular layer of the heart wall is the
   a. endocardium
   b. valve
   c. myocardium
   d. apex

____3. An upper chamber of the heart is a(n)
   a. ventricle
   b. atrium
   c. base
   d. systole

____4. A vessel that carries blood away from the heart is a(n)
   a. vein
   b. chamber
   c. lymph node
   d. artery

____5. The tonsils, spleen, and thymus are part of the
   a. digestive system
   b. endocrine system
   c. epicardium
   d. lymphatic system

____6. The medical term for a "heart attack" is
   a. cerebrovascular accident
   b. myocardial infarction
   c. aneurysm
   d. pneumonia

____7. The accumulation of fatty deposits in the lining of a vessel is called
   a. obesity
   b. stent
   c. atherosclerosis
   d. angiogenesis

____8. Phlebitis is inflammation of a
   a. vein
   b. heart
   c. blood cell
   d. nerve

学习目标

学完本章后，应该能够：

1. ▶ 描述心脏的结构。
2. ▶ 追踪心脏中血流的路径。
3. ▶ 追踪通过心脏的电传导的路径。
4. ▶ 识别心电图的组成部分。
5. ▶ 区分动脉、小动脉、毛细血管、小静脉和静脉。
6. ▶ 解释血压的成因，并描述如何测量血压。
7. ▶ 识别并使用与心血管系统和淋巴系统相关的词根。
8. ▶ 描述影响心血管系统和淋巴系统的主要疾病。
9. ▶ 定义与心血管系统和淋巴系统相关的医学术语。
10. ▶ 列出淋巴系统的功能及其组成部分。
11. ▶ 解释与循环相关的医学缩略语。
12. ▶ 分析涉及循环的案例研究中的医学术语。

Case Study: C. L.'s Arrhythmia during Army Boot Camp
案例研究：C. L. 在军队新兵训练营期间的心律失常

Chief Complaint

C. L., a 19-year-old man recently enlisted into the army, successfully passed the army physicals and reported to Fort Knox for basic training. The first two weeks were uneventful as C. L. became acclimated to the vigorous daily schedules of army life. As the physical training progressed, the platoon would go on long runs in full gear. C. L. passed out during two of these runs. The first time he was taken to the infirmary, where he was examined, cleared, and returned to duty. With the second incident, he was put on a sick leave and sent home for additional follow-up.

Examination

When C.L. came home, his family took him to see his primary care physician, who referred him to a cardiologist. C.L. explained to the physician that on some of the long, rigorous runs with full gear he would become short of breath and feel his heart start to race. He would then become dizzy and pass out. When he woke up, he would be lying on the ground with his sergeant standing over him.

The physician ordered some laboratory tests and also a Holter monitor that C. L. was to wear for a month. He explained to C. L. and his family that he suspected an abnormal heartbeat had caused the fainting spells. The monitor would record any arrhythmias that occurred during the month. He told C. L. to maintain normal activities, and the monitor would detect any abnormalities that might occur.

Clinical Course

At the conclusion of the month, C. L. saw the cardiologist again. The results of the Holter monitor indicated that he had an abnormal heart rhythm known as atrial fibrillation. The physician explained the two methods of treatment for the condition: a medical approach using anticoagulants to prevent blood clots and medication to slow the heart rate, and a surgical procedure called an ablation. It was decided after reviewing the test results and discussion with family on the pros and cons of the various treatment options that a pulmonary vein catheter ablation was the treatment of choice for C. L.

主诉

C. L. 是一名最近入伍的 19 岁男性，成功地通过了军队身体检查，并到诺克斯堡报到进行基本训练。前 2 个星期是平静的，C. L. 适应了军队生活中精力旺盛的日程表。随着身体训练的进行，C. L. 所在的排将进行满装长途行军训练。C. L. 在两次这样的行军中晕倒。第一次他被带到医务室（infirmary），在那里接受检查，清醒后重新归队。在第二次事件后，他因病假被送回家接受进一步随访。

检查

C. L. 回家后，他的家人带他去看初级保健医生，保健医生把他转诊给心脏科医生。C. L. 向医生解释说，在一些长距离满装行军训练中，他变得喘不上气，并感到心跳加快，然后会变得头昏并晕倒。当醒来时，他会躺在地上，他的军士站在他身边。

医生安排进行一些实验室检查，并要 C. L. 佩戴 1 个月的 Holter 监测器。他向 C. L. 及其家人说明怀疑是 C. L. 的心跳异常导致了昏厥。监测器将记录 1 个月期间发生的任何心律失常。他告诉 C. L. 要保持正常活动，监视器将会检测可能发生的任何异常。

临床病程

1 个月结束时，C. L. 再次来看心脏科医生。Holter 监测器的结果表明他有一种异常心律，称为房颤（atrial fibrillation）。医生解释了这种症状的两种治疗方法：使用抗凝剂防止血液凝块并用药物降低心率，和称为消融（ablation）的外科手术。在评估了测试结果和与家人讨论各种治疗选择的利弊后，决定 C. L. 的治疗选择是的肺静脉导管消融。

简介

血液（blood）在遍布全身的心血管系统（cardiovascular system）中循环，心血管系统由心脏（heart）和血管（blood vessel）组成（图 9-1）。该系统形成了一个不间断的回路，为所有细胞输送氧气并带走废物。淋巴系统（lymphatic system）也参与循环，它的管道将组织中存留的液体和蛋白质返回到血流之中。淋巴系统在免疫和消化过程中也起部分作用。本章详细讨论循环系统正常的临床表现，然后研究淋巴系统。

心脏

心脏位于两个肺之间，其尖端指向左下（图 9-2）。心脏壁有三层，其名称都带有词根 cardi，意为"心脏"。从最内层到最外层，它们是：

1．内心膜（endocardium）——覆盖心室和瓣膜的薄膜（前缀 endo- 意为"在……之内"）。

2．心肌（myocardium）——心壁绝大部分的厚厚的肌肉层（词根 my/o 意为"肌肉"）。

3．心外膜（epicardium）——包围心脏的薄膜（前缀 epi- 意为"在……之上"）。

一个纤维囊，心包膜（pericardium，前缀 peri- 意为"周围"）包围着心脏，并将心脏固定在其周围结构上。周围结构包括胸骨（sternum）和隔膜（diaphragm 等）。心脏的每个上接收室被称为心房（atrium，复数为 atria），每个下泵出室被称为心室（ventricle，复数为 ventricles），心房和心室之间由被称为隔膜（septum）的壁分开。室间隔（interventricular septum）分开两个心室，房间隔（interatrial septum）分开两个心房。在每一侧的心

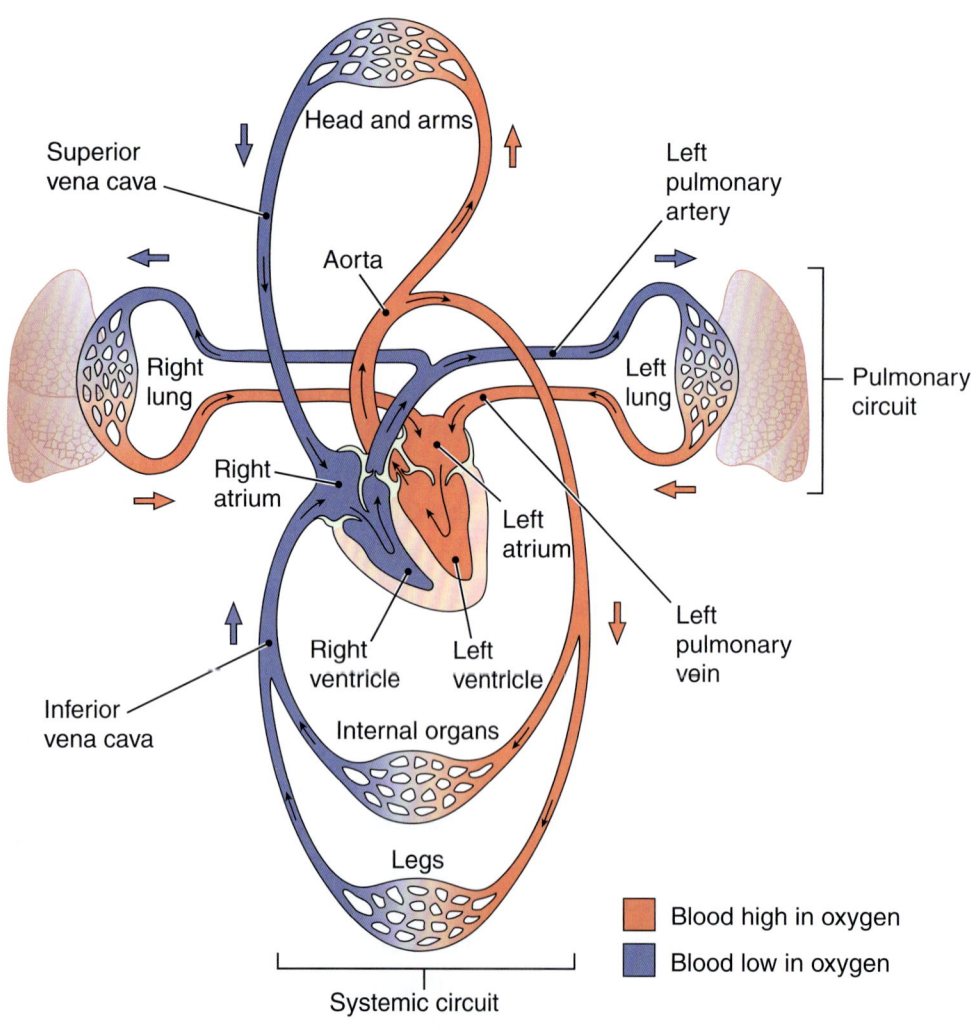

图 9-1　**心血管系统**。肺循环携带血液进入和离开肺；系统回路在身体的所有其他部分之间来回运送血液

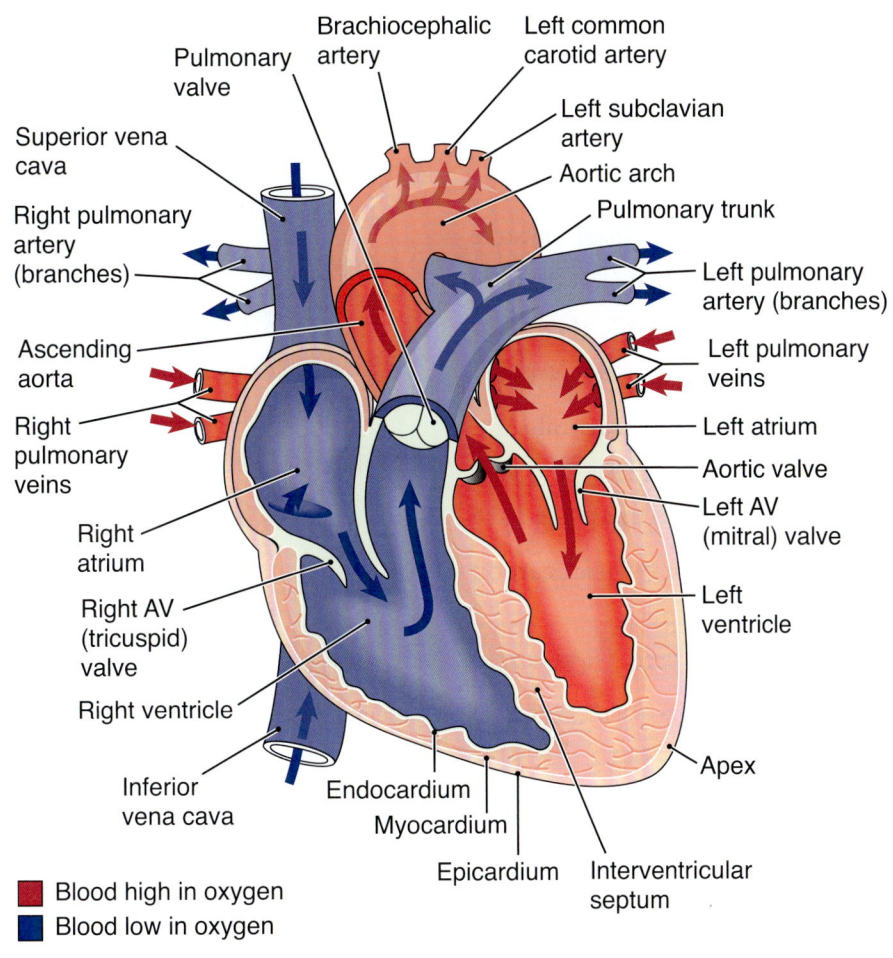

图 9-2　心脏和大血管。AV 代表房室

房与心室之间也有隔膜。

心脏通过两个回路泵出血液。右侧向肺泵出血液，通过肺循环（pulmonary circuit）使肺充满氧气；左侧通过系统回路（systemic circuit）向身体的其余部分供血（图 9-1）。

通过心脏的血流

通过心脏的血流如图 9-2 所示，其顺序为：

1. 右心房通过上腔静脉（superior vena cava）和下腔静脉（inferior vena cava）从身体的所有组织中接收低氧血；

2. 低氧血进入右心室，并通过肺动脉（pulmonary artery）泵入肺；

3. 高氧血从肺返回通过肺静脉（pulmonary veins）进入左心房；

4. 血液进入左心室，并被强力泵入分布在所有组织中的主动脉（aorta）。

心脏中的单向瓣膜（valve）保证血液向前流动。每一侧心房与心室之间的瓣膜是房室（atrioventricular，AV）瓣膜。右心房与右心室之间的右房室瓣膜也被称为三尖瓣（tricuspid valve），因为它有三个尖；左心房与左心室之间的左房室瓣膜被称为二尖瓣（bicuspid valve），因为它有两个尖，也被称为僧帽瓣（mitral valve，因其形状像主教的僧帽而得名）。

通向肺动脉和主动脉的瓣膜有三个尖，每个尖的形状都像半个月亮，所以它们也被称为半月瓣（semilunar valves，lunar 指月亮）。通向肺动脉的瓣膜被称为肺瓣（pulmonary valve），通向主动脉的瓣膜被称为主动脉瓣（aortic valve）。

心音（heart sounds）是伴随心脏功能而产生的。在胸壁上能够听到的最强的心音是瓣膜交替关闭而产生的。第一心音 S_1 是在心室和心房之间的瓣膜关闭时产生的，第二心音 S_2 是在通向主动脉和肺动脉的瓣膜关闭时产生的。心脏正常工作产生的任何声音都被称为功能性杂音（functional murmur）（murmur 与心脏一起使用表示异常的声音）。

心跳

心脏的每一次收缩被称为心缩期（systole ['sistəli]），紧接着是一个放松阶段心舒期（diastole [dai'æstəli]），在该阶段心房被充满。每次心跳（heartbeat）两个心房都收缩，紧接着两个心室收缩。心脏每分钟收缩的次数被称为心率（heart rate），心室每次收缩在血管中产生的压力波动被称为脉搏（pulse）。脉搏率一般通过外围动脉触诊进行计数，例如桡动脉（radial artery）或颈动脉（carotid artery）（图7-4）。

心脏收缩是由一个内置系统激发的，该系统有规律地向心脏发送电脉冲。这一传导系统的组成部分如图 9-3 所示。按照动作的顺序，它们包括：

1．窦房（sinoatrial，SA）结，位于右心房上部，因为它确定心跳的速率，所以被称为起搏器（pacemaker）。

2．房室（atrioventricular，AV）结，位于右心房下部，接近右心室。SA 和 AV 结间纤维传送贯穿两个心房的刺激脉冲。

3．窦房束（希氏束 bundle of His），位于室间隔的顶部。

4．左右束分支（bundle branche），沿隔膜的左右两侧分布。

5．浦肯野纤维（Purkinje fibers），传送贯穿两个心室壁的刺激脉冲（框 9-1）。

尽管心脏自己产生跳动，神经系统刺激、激素和药物因素都会影响心跳的速率和收缩的力度。

心电图

心电图（Electrocardiography，ECG）测量心脏在工作时的电活动（图 9-4），置于身体表面的电极（electrodes）检测电信号，然后将电信号放大并作为描记图像记录。发起于 SA 结，正常的或窦性心律（sinus rhythm）如图 9-4A 所示，图 9-4B 显示了一个完整周期的各个部分：

1．P 波代表心房肌肉电特性的改变，或去极化（depolarization）。

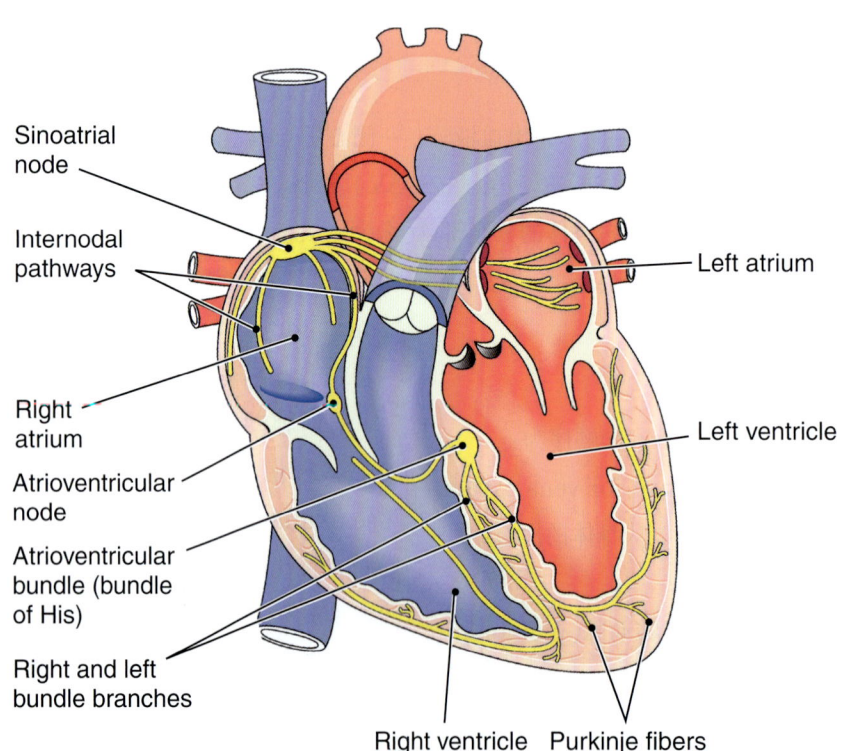

图 9-3　心脏的电传导系统。脉冲从窦房（SA）结到房室（AV）结，然后到房室束、束分支和浦肯野纤维。脉冲在贯穿整个心房的结间通路中传导

框 9-2

聚焦单词
心脏结构的命名

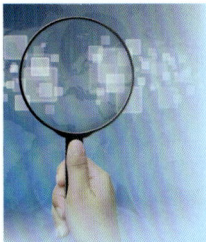

名祖词（eponym ['epənim]）是基于人名的名称，这个人通常是发现特殊的结构、疾病、原理或方法的人。心脏中的希氏束（bundle of His）和浦肯野纤维（Purkinje fibers）是电传导系统的组成部分，柯氏音（Korotkoff sounds）是在测量血压时在血管中听到的声音。用人名命名的心血管疾病包括法洛四联症（tetralogy of Fallot）——四种心脏先天缺陷的组合、小血管的雷诺病（Raynaud disease）和被称为沃-帕-怀综合征（Wolff-Parkinson-White syndrome）的心律不齐。在治疗中，多普勒超声心动描记术（Doppler echocardiography）是用 19 世纪物理学家的名字命名的。霍尔特心电动态监测仪（Holter monitor）和 Swan-Ganz 血流导向气囊导管（Swan-Ganz catheter）的名称向它们的开发者致敬。

在其他系统中，郎格罕氏岛（islets of Langerhans）是胰腺中分泌胰岛素的细胞团，卵巢中的格拉夫卵泡（graafian follicle）包围着一个成熟的卵细胞。欧氏管（eustachian tube）连接中耳和咽喉。

许多疾病的名称都是名祖词：帕金森和阿尔茨海默症（Parkinson and Alzheimer）影响大脑，格雷夫斯病（Graves）是一种甲状腺疾病，唐氏综合征（Down syndrome）是一种遗传疾病。微生物的属和种的名称通常是基于它们的发现者，例如埃希氏杆菌属（Escherichia）、沙门氏菌（Salmonella）、巴氏杆菌属（Pasteurella）和立克次氏体（Rickettsia）等。

许多试剂、设备、方法也是以开发者的名字命名的。X 线片的原始名称是 roentgenograph，以 X 线的发现者 Wilhelm Roentgen 命名。居里（curie）是衡量放射性的单位，源自于放射性的共同发现者之一的姓名 Marie Curie。

尽管名祖词向过去的医生和科学家致以敬意，但它们并不携带任何信息，还可能更难以学习、记忆。现在的趋势是用更具有描述性的名称取代它们，例如用咽鼓管（auditory tube）取代欧氏管，成熟卵泡（mature ovarian follicle）取代格拉扶卵泡，胰岛（pancreatic islets）取代郎格罕氏岛，21 三体综合征（trisomy 21）取代唐氏综合征。

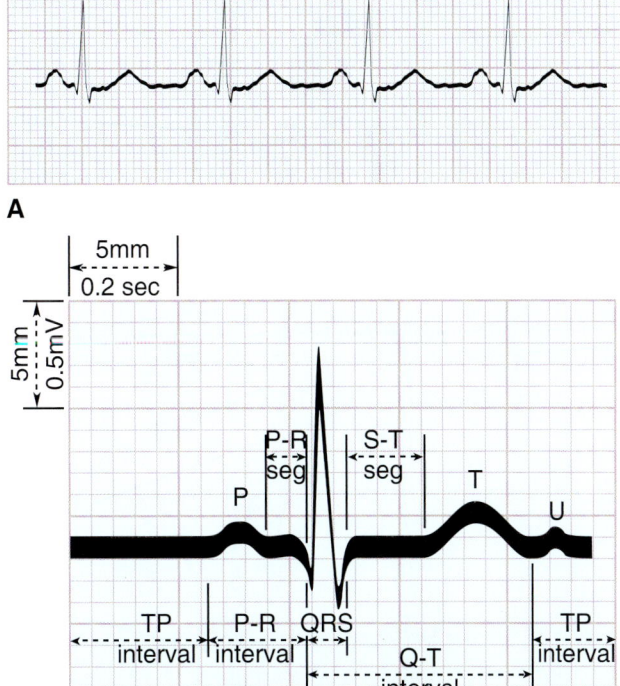

图 9-4　心电图（ECG）。A. 心电图追踪显示正常窦性心律。B. 正常心电图跟踪的组成部分，图中示出了 P、QRS、T 和 U 波，代表了心脏的不同部分中的电活动。间隔（interval）测量一个波到另一个波之间的距离，段（segment）是描记图像的一个较小的部分

2. QRS 部分显示心室的去极化。

3. T 波显示心室对其静息状态的回转，或复极化（repolarization），心房的复极化被 QRS 波隐蔽。

4. 小 U 波，如果存在的话，紧随 T 波出现。起源不确定。

间隔测量一个波到另一个波之间的距离，段（segment）是描记图像的一个较小的部分。许多心脏疾病在心电图中都会出现异常，其中一些会在本章后面讨论。

血管系统

血管系统（vascular system）由以下部分组成：

1. 动脉（artery），运输血液离开心脏（图 9-5）。
2. 小动脉（arteriole），通向毛细血管（capillary）的比动脉小的血管。
3. 毛细血管（capillary），最小的血管，血液和组织之间的交换都发生在毛细血管。
4. 小静脉（venule），从毛细血管接收血液并注入静脉的小血管。
5. 静脉（vein），将血液带回心脏（图 9-6）。

所有动脉，肺动脉（和胎儿的脐动脉）除外，都携带高氧血。动脉是厚壁的、有弹性的血管，在较高的压力下输送血液。所有静脉，肺静脉（和胎儿的脐静脉）除外，都携带低氧血。静脉血管壁比较薄，弹

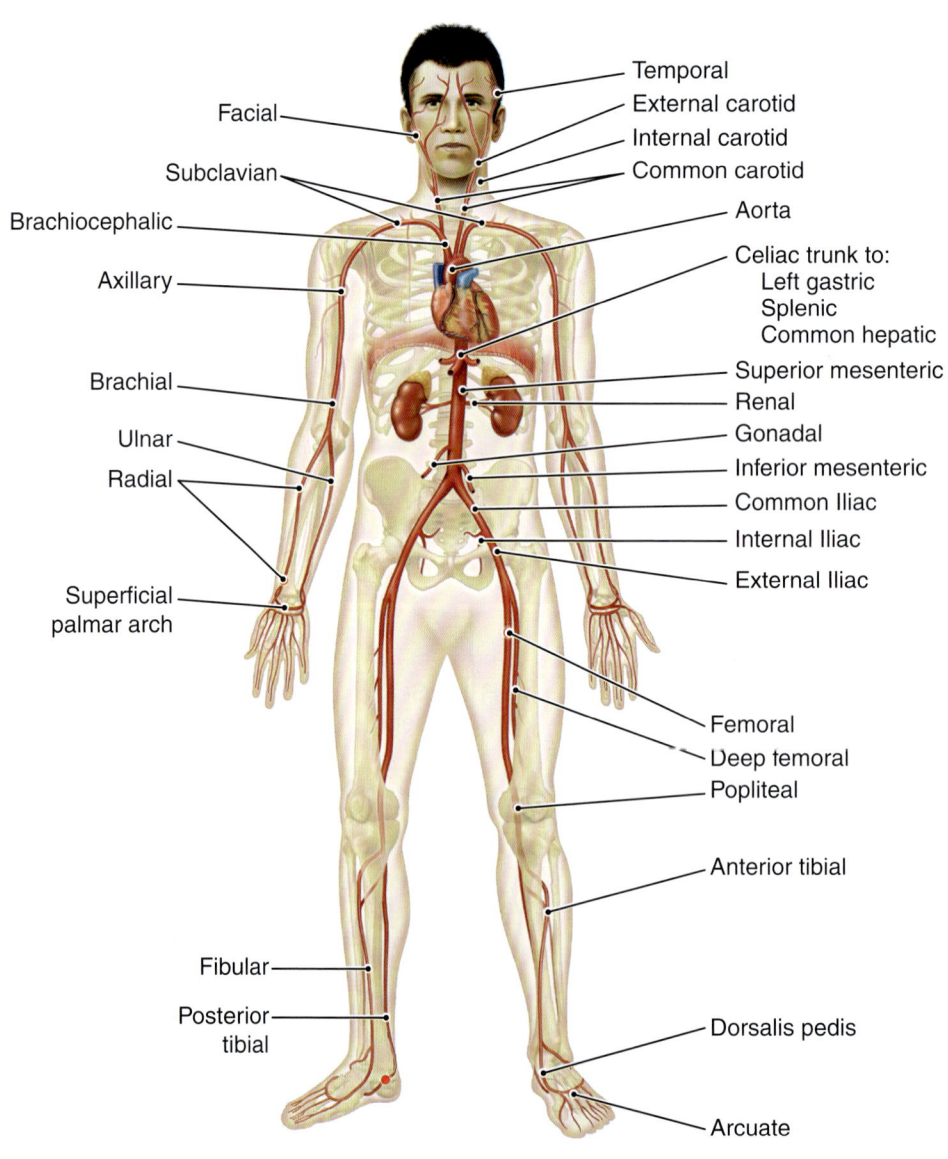

图 9-5　主要的全身动脉

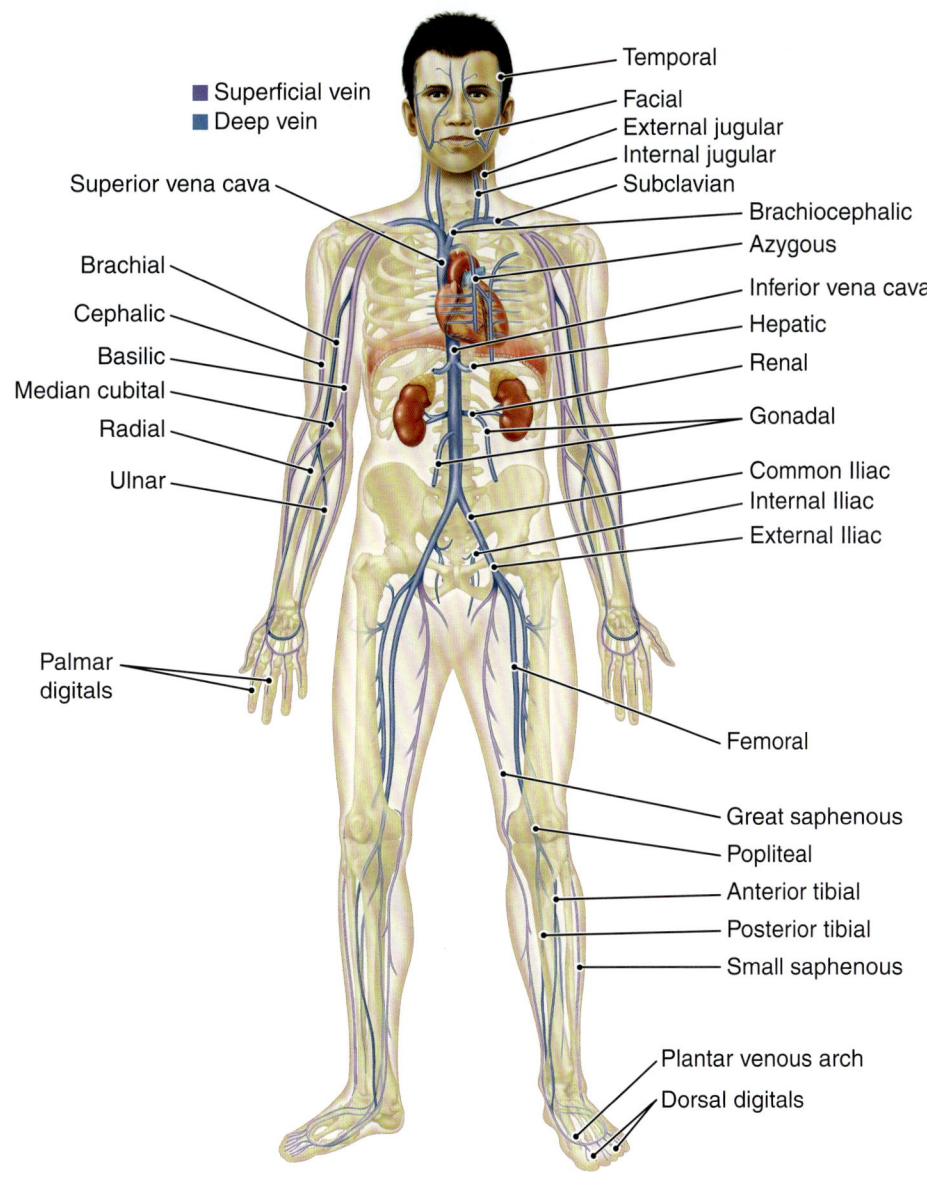

图 9-6　主要的全身静脉

性较小，倾向于在压力下后退。像心脏一样，静脉由单向瓣膜保持血液向前流动（图 9-6）。

神经系统刺激能够引起血管直径的扩大（血管舒张，vasodilation）或减小（血管收缩，vasoconstriction），这些变化会改变流向组织的血流，并影响血压。

血压

血压（blood pressure，BP）是血液对血管壁产生的压力。它随着血液离开心脏而降低，并受到多种因素的影响，包括心输出量、血管直径和血压总量。血管收缩会升高血压，血管舒张则会降低血压。

血压通常用一个被称为血压袖带或血压计的可充气袖带在主动脉处测量（图 9-7），血压计的学术名称为 sphygmomanometer。测量者给袖带充气阻止血液在血管中的流动，然后使用听诊器在气压缓慢释放过程中聆听血管中血液的流动。血液读数包括收缩压（systolic pressure）和舒张压（diastolic pressure），收缩压是心脏收缩时的血压，舒张压时心脏舒张时的血压（图 7-5）。报告时先报收缩压，再报舒张压，中间用一个斜线分开，例如 120/80。

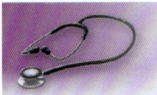

临床观点 〔框 9-2〕
心脏插管：从内部测量血压

因为动脉血压随着血液远离心脏而降低，使用包围上臂的简单充气袖带测量的血压只是心脏和肺动脉压力的反映。这些部位压力的精确测量对于特定心脏和肺部疾病的诊断是有帮助的。

更准确的读数能够通过直接向心脏和大血管插入导管来获得。常用的是肺动脉插管（也被称为 Swan-Ganz 导管），其顶部有一个充气囊。通过大静脉，这个装置被穿过心脏右侧。最常见的是通过右颈内静脉（right internal jugular vein），因为它是通向心脏最短、最直接的路径，但有时也会通过锁骨下静脉和股静脉（subclavian and femoral veins）。插入心脏的位置由胸部 X 线确定，一旦适当定位，就能记录心房和心室的血压。随着插管继续进入肺动脉，肺动脉血压即可获得。当气囊充气时，插管就卡在一个肺动脉分支，阻止血液流动。这时获得的读数被称为肺毛细血管楔压（pulmonary capillary wedge pressure，PCWP），它给出了心脏左侧压力和肺阻力的信息。与其他测试相结合，心脏插管可以用于诊断心脏和肺部疾病，例如休克、心包炎（pericarditis）、先天性心脏病和心脏衰竭等。

血压的单位用毫米汞柱（mmHg）表示，也就是血压能够推动水银在玻璃管中的高度。血压是一个易于获得的很有价值的诊断依据（血压测量的更多信息参见框 9-2）。

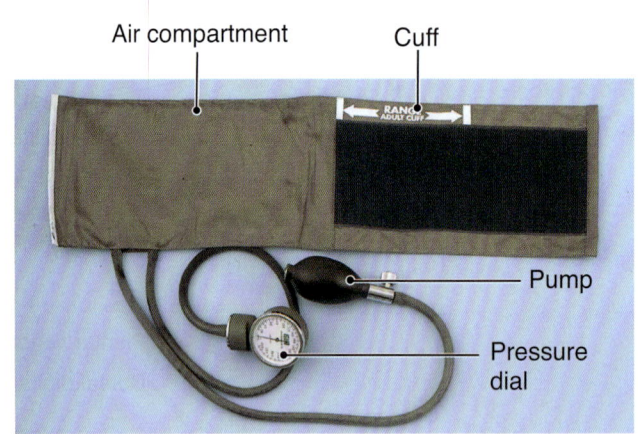

图 9-7 血压计袖带（血压计）。图中示出了袖带、用于使袖带充气的泵和用于测量血压的压力计

Terminology	心血管系统正常结构和功能
aorta [ei'ɔ:tə]	主动脉，最大的动脉，从左心室接收血液并分流到全身（词根：aort/o）
aortic valve [ei'ɔ:tik]	主动脉瓣，通向主动脉的瓣膜
apex ['eipeks]	顶部，锥形结构的尖端（复数：apical）。心脏的顶部由左心室构成，指向左下方
artery ['ɑ:təri]	动脉，将血液运出心脏的血管。除肺动脉和脐动脉外，所有动脉都携带高氧血（词根：arter、arteri/o）
arteriole [ɑ:'tiəriəʊl]	小动脉，将血液运输进入毛细血管的小血管（词根：arteriol/o）
atrioventricular (AV) node [ˌeitriəʊven'trikjələ]	房室结，在右心房下隔膜中的一小团物质，它将刺激脉冲从窦房结传导向心室

Terminology — 心血管系统正常结构和功能（续表）

术语	释义
atrioventricular (AV) valve	房室瓣，在心脏左右两侧心房与心室之间的瓣膜。右 AV 瓣是三尖瓣，左 AV 瓣是二尖瓣
atrium ['eitriəm]	心房，入口室，心脏的两个上接收室之一（词根：atri/o）
AV bundle	房室束，将刺激脉冲从房室结传送到心室间隔顶部的一束纤维。它分为左右两个束支，沿着隔膜的两侧下行；也被称为希氏束（bundle of His）
blood pressure	血压，血液对血管壁产生的压力
bundle branches	束支，AV 束在心室间隔左右两侧的分支
capillary [kəˈpiləri]	毛细血管，微小的血管，血液和组织通过毛细血管进行物质交换
cardiovascular system [ˌkɑːdiəʊˈvæskjələ(r)]	心血管系统，循环系统的一部分，由心脏和血管组成
depolarization ['diˌpəʊləraiˈzeiʃən]	去极化，神经或肌肉在静息状态下电荷的改变
diastole [daiˈæstəli]	舒张期，心跳周期中的放松阶段，形容词：diastolic
electrocardiography (ECG) [elektrəʊˈkɑːdiəʊgrəfi]	心电图，由置于身体表面的电极所探测到的心脏电活动的研究，也被缩写为 EKG，来自于德语 electrokardiography
endocardium [ˌendəʊˈkɑːdiəm]	心内膜，附于心脏内室和瓣膜上的薄膜
epicardium [ˌepiˈkɑːdiəm]	心外膜，心壁的最外层薄膜
functional murmur	功能性杂音，心脏正常工作时产生的任何声音
heart [hɑːt]	心脏，一个有四个腔室的肌肉器官，它周期性地收缩推动血液通过血管到达身体各个部分
heart rate	心率，心脏每分钟收缩的次数，记录为次/分钟
heart sounds	心音，心脏工作时产生的声音。两个最强的声音是由瓣膜交替关闭产生的，分别被称为 S_1 和 S_2
inferior vena cava [inˈfiəriə(r)]	下腔静脉，从下半身将低氧血流带回右心房的大静脉
left AV valve	左房室瓣，左心房与左心室之间的瓣膜，也叫僧帽瓣或二尖瓣
mitral valve [ˈmaitrəl]	僧帽瓣，左房室瓣或二尖瓣
myocardium [ˌmaiəˈkɑːdiəm]	心肌，由厚实的心脏肌肉构成的心壁中间层
pericardium [ˌperiˈkɑːdiəm]	心包膜，包围心脏的纤维囊
pulmonary artery [ˈpʌlmənəri]	肺动脉，将血液从心脏右部输送到肺的血管
pulmonary circuit	肺循环，将血液从心脏右部送到肺部充氧然后再返回心脏左侧的血管系统
pulmonary veins	肺静脉，将血液从肺输送到心脏左部的血管
pulse [pʌls]	脉搏，心室每次收缩在血管中产生的压力上升的波动

Terminology	心血管系统正常结构和功能（续表）
Purkinje fibers	浦肯野纤维，心传导系统的终端纤维，携带贯穿心室壁的脉冲
repolarization ['ri:pəʊləraɪ'zeɪʃən]	复极，神经或肌肉到达静息状态的电荷回复
right AV valve	右房室瓣，右心房与右心室之间的瓣膜；三尖瓣
septum ['septəm]	间隔，分开两个腔体的壁，例如心室间隔
sinus rhythm ['saɪnəs 'rɪðəm]	窦性心律，正常心律
sinoatrial (SA) node [saɪnəʊ'eɪtrɪəl]	窦房结，在右心室上部启动每次心跳脉冲的一小团物质；起搏器
sphygmomanometer [ˌsfɪgməʊmə'nɒmɪtɜ:]	血压计，测量动脉血压的仪器（词根：sphygm/o 意为"脉搏"）
superior vena cava	上腔静脉，从上半身将低氧血流带回右心房的大静脉
systemic circuit	体循环，将高氧血从心脏左部传送到除肺以外的所有组织，并将低氧血返回心脏右部的血管系统
systole ['sɪstəli]	收缩期，心跳周期的收缩阶段，形容词：systolic
valve [vælv]	瓣膜，保持液体向前流动的结构（词根：valv/o, valvul/o）
vein [veɪn]	静脉，将血液带回心脏的血管。除肺动脉和脐动脉以外，所有静脉都携带低氧血
ventricle ['ventrɪkl]	心室，两个心脏的泵出室之一（词根：ventricul/o）
venule ['venju:l]	小静脉，将血液从毛细血管带回静脉的小血管
vessel ['vesl]	管道，传送血液的管道或通道（词根：angi/o, vas/o, vascul/o）

与心血管系统相关的词根

参见表 9-1 和表 9-2

表 9-1 心脏的词根

词根	含义	示例	示例定义
cardi/o	心脏	cardiomyopathy* [ˌkɑ:dɪəʊmaɪ'ɒpəθɪ]	心肌症
atri/o	心房	atriotomy ['ɑ:trɪətəmɪ]	心房切开术
ventricul/o	腔，心室	supraventricular [sʌpreɪvent'rɪkjʊlə]	心室上的
valv/o, valvul/o	瓣膜	valvulotome [vælvjʊ'ləʊtəʊm]	瓣膜刀

* 优于 myocardiopathy（心肌病）

练习 9-1

填空

1. A valvuloplasty ［vælvjʊ'ləplæsti］ is plastic repair of a(n) _____.
2. Atriotomy ['ɑ:triətəmi] means surgical incision of a(n) _____.
3. Interventricular [ˌintəven'trikjulə] means between the _____.
4. The word cardiomegaly [kɑ:diəʊ'megəli] means enlargement of the _____.

写出下列定义的形容词，每个定义都给出了适当的后缀。

5. Pertaining to an atrium (-al) _____
6. Pertaining to the myocardium (-al) ending differs from adjective ending for the heart) _____
7. Pertaining to the heart (-ac) _____
8. Pertaining to a valve (-ar) _____
9. Pertaining to a ventricle (-ar) _____
10. Pertaining to the pericardium (-al) _____

按下列示例，写出下列与心脏组织相关定义的单词。

11. Inflammation of the fibrous sac around the heart _____pericarditis_____
12. Inflammation of the heart's lining (usually at a valve) _____
13. Inflammation of the heart muscle _____

写出下列定义的单词。

14. Originating (-genic) in the heart _____
15. Surgical incision of a valve _____
16. Pertaining to an atrium and a ventricle _____
17. Between (inter) the atria _____
18. Study (-logy) of the heart _____

表 9-2　血管的词根

词根	含义	示例	示例定义
angi/o*	血管	angiography [ˌændʒi'ɒgrəfi]	血管造影
vas/o, vascul/o	管道、通道	vasospasm ['væsəʊspæzm'veiz]	血管痉挛
arter/o, arteri/o	动脉	endarterial [endɑ:'tiəriəl]	动脉内的
arteriol/o	小动脉	arteriolar [ɑːˌtiəri'əʊlə]	小动脉的
aort/o	主动脉	aortoptosis [eiɔːtɒp'təʊsis]	主动脉下垂
ven/o, ven/i	静脉	venous ['vi:nəs]	静脉的

表 9-2　血管的词根（续表）

词根	含义	示例	示例定义
phleb/o	静脉	phlebotomy [fləˈbɒtəmi]	切开静脉放血

* 词根 angi/o 通常指血管，但也用于其他管道。hemangi/o 特指血管

练习 9-2

填空

1. Angioedema [ændʒiːəʊiːˈdiːmə] is localized swelling caused by changes in _____.
2. Vasodilation [ˌveɪzəʊdaɪˈleɪʃn] means dilation of a(n) _____.
3. Aortostenosis [eɪɔːtəʊsteˈnəʊsɪs] is narrowing of _____.
4. Endarterectomy [endɑːtəˈrektəmi] is removal of the inner lining of a(n) _____.
5. Arteriolitis [ˈɑːtɪəraɪəlaɪtɪz] is inflammation of a(n) _____.
6. Phlebectasia [flɪbekˈteɪʒə] is dilatation of a(n) _____.
7. The term microvascular [maɪkrəʊˈvæskjʊlə(r)] means pertaining to small _____.

定义下列单词。

8. arteriorrhexis [ɑːtɪəriəˈreksɪs] _____
9. intraaortic [ɪntrə eɪˈɔːtɪk] _____
10. angiitis [ənˈdʒaɪaɪtɪz] (note spelling); also angitis or vasculitis _____
11. phlebitis [fləˈbaɪtɪs] _____
12. cardiovascular [ˌkɑːdɪəʊˈvæskjələ(r)] _____

使用后缀 -gram 组成下列 X 线成像的单词。

13. vessels (use angi/o) _____
14. aorta _____
15. veins _____

使用词根 angi/o 写出下列含义的单词。

16. Plastic repair (-plasty) of a vessel _____
17. Any disease (-pathy) of a vessel _____
18. Dilatation (-ectasis) of a vessel _____
19. Formation (-genesis) of a vessel _____

使用适当的词根写出下列含义的单词。

20. Excision of a vein _____
21. Hardening (-sclerosis) of the aorta _____
22. Within (intra-) a vein _____
23. Incision of an artery _____

心血管系统的临床表现

动脉粥样硬化

动脉内壁脂肪沉积的积累被称为动脉粥样硬化（atherosclerosis [ˌæθərəʊskli'rəʊsis]）（图9-8）。当血管受到微小的损伤时，一种被称为斑块（plaque）的沉积开始形成，通常在分叉点上。随着纤维物质、细胞和其他沉积物的不断增加，斑块逐渐变厚、变硬，限制了血管管腔，减少了流向组织的血流，造成局部缺血（ischemia [is'ki:miə]）。导致动脉粥样硬化发展的主要危险因素是脂代谢异常（dyslipidemia），血液中的脂蛋白（lipoproteins）异常高或失调，尤其是高水平的含胆固醇的低密度脂蛋白（low-density lipoproteins，LDL），其他危险因素包括吸烟、高血压、不良饮食习惯、缺少运动、压力以及家族病史。动脉粥样硬化可能涉及任何动脉，但其影响主要体现在心脏的冠状动脉、主动脉、颈动脉和大脑的血管。后面介绍的治疗冠状动脉疾病（coronary artery disease，CAD）的技术也适用于这些血管。

动脉粥样硬化是一种被称为动脉硬化（arteriosclerosis）的更广泛的疾病的最常见表现形式，动脉硬化是任何原因引起的血管壁变硬。除斑块外，钙盐和瘢痕组织可能也对动脉硬化产生变化，使得动脉血管管腔变窄并失去弹性。

血栓形成和栓塞

动脉粥样硬化使人易患血栓症（thrombosis），也就是在血管中形成血凝块（图9-8）。血凝块被称为血栓（thrombus），会阻止该血管供给组织的血流，导致坏死（necrosis，组织死亡）。血管被血栓或其他血流中携带的团块阻塞被称为栓塞（embolism），导致栓塞的团块被称为栓塞物（embolus）。通常，栓塞物都是从血管壁上脱落的血凝块，但有可能是空气（来自于注射或外伤）、脂肪（骨折后留出的骨髓）、细菌或其他固体物质。静脉栓塞经常会穿过心脏，然后停在一个肺动脉中，导致威胁生命的肺栓塞。来自颈动脉的栓塞物经常会阻塞脑血管，导致脑血管伤害（cerebrovascular accident，CVA），通常被称为脑卒中（stroke）。

动脉瘤

被动脉粥样硬化、畸形、受伤或其他变化削弱的动脉可能会球囊性扩展，形成动脉瘤（aneurysm）。如果动脉瘤破裂，会造成大出血（hemorrhage）。脑动脉破裂是脑卒中的另一个起因。腹腔主动脉和颈动脉也是常见的动脉瘤发生地。在夹层动脉瘤（dissecting aneurysm）中（图9-9），出血进入动脉壁厚实的中间层，随着出血的扩散会切断肌肉，有时会使血管破裂。涉及主动脉的情况最为常见。通过手术移植可能修复夹层动脉瘤。

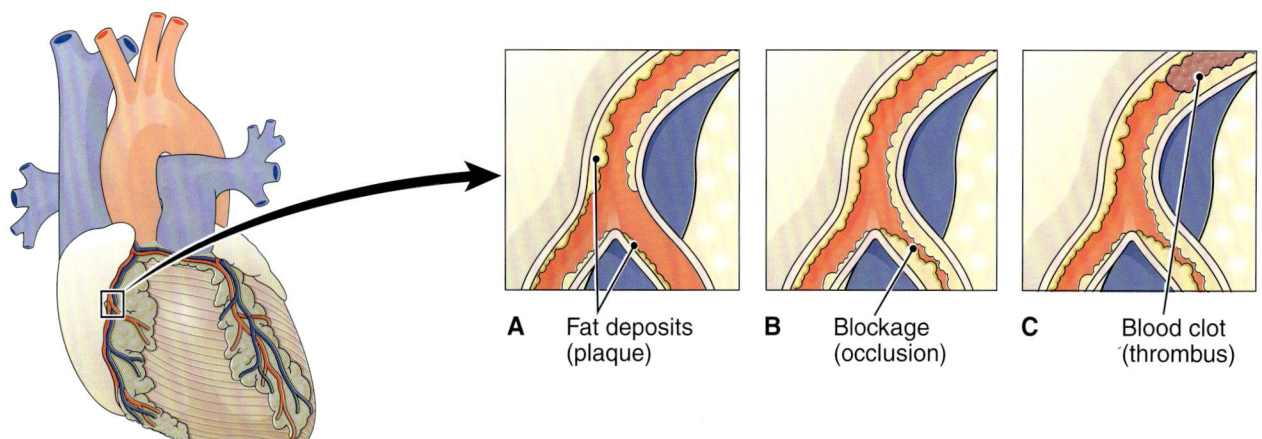

图9-8 冠状动脉粥样硬化。A. 脂肪沉积（Fat depocits）（斑块，Plaque）使动脉变窄，导致缺血（缺乏血液供应）；B. 斑块导致血管阻塞（Blockage）（闭塞，occlusion）；C. 血管中血凝块（Blood clot）（血栓，thrombus）的形成导致心肌梗死（myocardial infarction，MI）

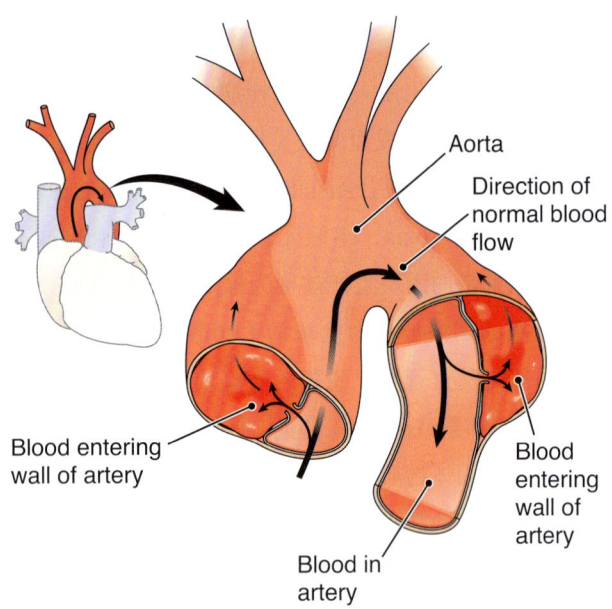

图 9-9　夹层主动脉瘤。血液分离了动脉壁的分层

高血压

高血压（hypertension，HTN）是所有上面所提及的疾病的一个促进因素。简单来说，收缩压高于 140mmHg 或舒张压高于 90mmHg 就被定义为高血压。高血压会引起左心室扩大（hypertrophy），这是工作量增加的结果。在一些病例中，高血压继发于其他疾病，例如肾功能障碍或内分泌失衡，但在大多数情况下，高血压的原发或实质病因不明。

饮食和生活习惯的改变是控制高血压的第一道防线。常用的药物包括排出液体的利尿剂（diuretics）、舒张血管的血管舒张药和阻止血管紧张素（angiotensin）生成或发生作用的药物。血管紧张素是血液中正常情况下起升高血压作用的物质（参见第 13 章）。

心脏疾病

冠状动脉疾病

冠状动脉疾病（coronary artery disease，CAD）是为心脏肌肉供血的血管发生粥样硬化的结果，在发达国家中是首要的致死因素（图 9-8）。CAD 的早期症状是被称为心绞痛（angina pectoris）的一种胸部疼痛。这是心脏周围收缩或疼痛的感觉，可能扩展到左臂或左肩，通常因劳累所致。一般还会带有焦虑、大汗（diaphoresis）和呼吸困难（dyspnea）。CAD 可以通过心电图、压力测试（stress test）、超声心动图（echocardiography）和冠状动脉造影术进行诊断。冠状动脉造影（coronary angiography）是一种介入性 X 线成像技术，需要插管通过血管进入心脏，向冠状动脉注入染色剂（图 9-10）。冠状动脉 CT 造影（coronary CT angiography，CTA）是非介入性的，在向上臂注入少量染色剂后使用计算机断层扫描，可以用于诊断心脏疾病。冠状动脉钙扫描（coronary calcium scan）能够显示冠状动脉壁上使血管变窄的钙沉积。研究人员还发现了一种与心血管系统健康相关的被称为 C 反应蛋白（C-reactive protein，CRP）的物质，这种蛋白质是在全身感染期间产生的，它可能会促进动脉粥样硬化。CRP 水平能够显示心血管疾病，并预测其预后（prognosis）。心脏病发作的特效测试是更为准确的高灵敏度 CRP（hs-CRP）测试。

CAD 可以通过控制锻炼和饮食治疗，也可以通过药物治疗，适当的时候还可以进行外科手术。像硝酸甘油（nitroglycerin）这样的药物可以用于扩张冠状动脉，其他药物可用于调节心率、加强心脏的力量、降低胆固醇（cholesterol）或阻止血栓的形成。

严重的 CAD 患者可能需要做血管清理术（angioplasty），或者使用球囊导管对阻塞的血管进行手术扩张，这种方法被称为经皮冠状动脉内成形术（percutaneous transluminal coronary angioplasty，PTCA）（图 9-10 和图 9-11）。血管清理术可能包括植入一个支架（一个小的网管），以保持血管的畅通

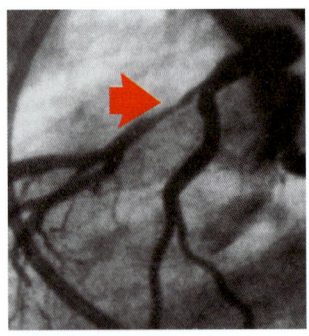
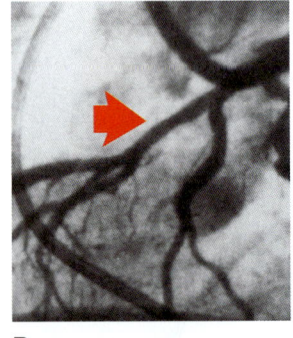

图 9-10　冠状动脉造影。在心脏导管插入术期间给予染色剂后，对冠状血管进行成像。A. 血管造影显示在左中前降支（LAD）动脉（箭头所示）变窄；B. 血管成形术后同一血管，血管成形术是扩张狭窄血管的手术。请注意通过动脉远端到修复端血流的改善

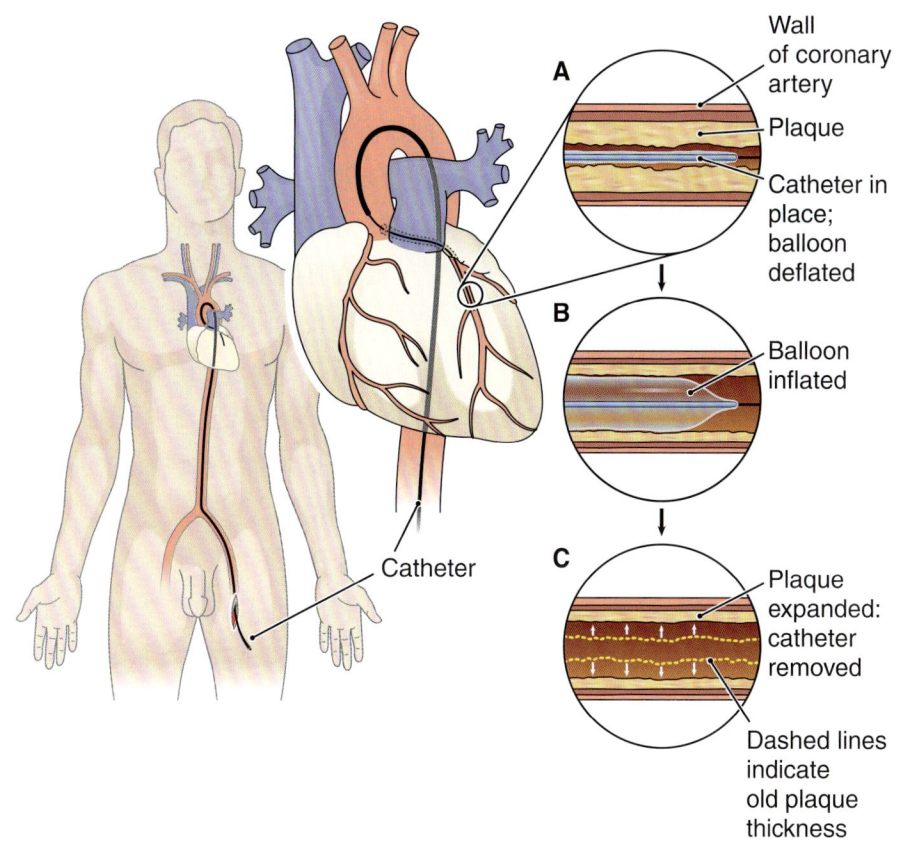

图 9-11　冠状动脉成形术（PTCA）。A. 引导导管穿入冠状动脉；B. 将气囊导管插入通过闭塞的部分；C. 使气囊充气和放气，直到斑块变平并打开血管

（图 9-12）。支架（stent）能够阻止血管的回弹，有多种形式可选。基本的类型是裸金属支架，另一种是药物涂层支架，可释放能够阻止血管再狭窄的药物。最新的支架是完全生物可吸收的，能够逐渐被代谢并被身体吸收。

如果需要进一步干预，可以通过手术用人工血管旁路受阻的血管（图 9-13），这种方法被称为冠状动脉旁路搭桥术（coronary artery bypass graft，CABG），另一段血管通常是左胸廓内动脉或小腿隐静脉（saphenous vein）被植入，将来自大动脉的血液运输到冠状动脉阻塞点之后。

心肌梗死

动脉的退行性变化使人易患血栓和冠状动脉突然闭合（occlusion）。心肌坏死的组合区域被称为梗死（infarct）（图 9-14），这一过程被称为心肌梗死（myocardial infarction，MI），"突发心脏病（heart attack）" 可能导致突然死亡。心肌梗死的症状包括心痛（心前区疼痛，precordial pain）或上腹部疼痛（上腹痛，epigastric pain），疼痛可能扩展到颚和上臂，面色苍白、大汗、恶心、疲劳、焦虑和呼吸困难，可能有类似于消化不良和胃灼热的烧痛感。对女性而言，因为退行性变化通常更多地会影响许多小血管，而不是主要的冠状通道，心肌梗死的症状常常会时间更长，

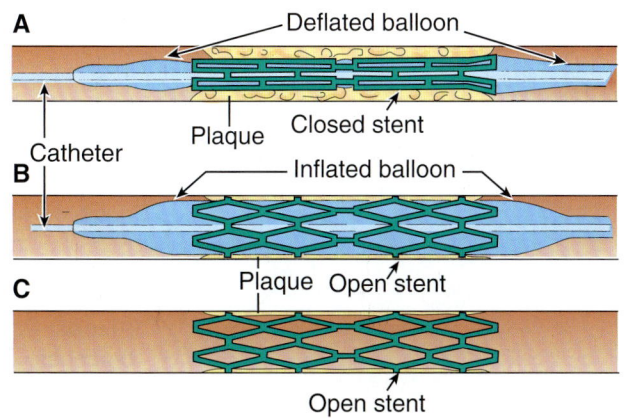

图 9-12　动脉支架。A. 支架闭合，气囊膨胀前；B. 支架打开，球囊充气，支架将在球囊放气和移除后保持扩张；C. 支架打开，球囊移除

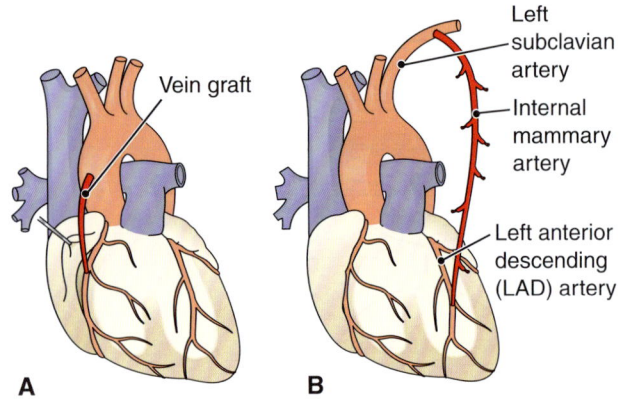

图 9-13 冠状动脉旁路移植术（CABG）。A. 隐静脉的一段将血液从主动脉运送到位于闭塞远端的右冠状动脉的一部分；B. 乳房动脉用于旁路左前降支（LAD）冠状动脉中的阻塞

比男性典型的强烈胸部疼痛更为敏感和弥散。

心肌梗死可以通过心电图和测定血液中特定的物质来诊断。肌酸激酶（creatine kinase，CK）是肌肉细胞中一种正常的酶，当肌肉组织受到损伤时释放量会增加。CK 针对心肌细胞的形态是肌酸激酶 MB（creatine kinase MB，CK-MB）。肌钙蛋白（troponin，Tn）是在肌肉细胞中调节收缩的蛋白质，血清中特殊形态的肌钙蛋白 TnT 和 TnI 的水平升高表明心肌梗死的可能。

患者的预后与损伤的程度和治疗溶栓与重建血流及心律的速度相关。

心律不齐

心律不齐（arrhythmia）是心律（heart rhythm）的任何异常，例如心率的变化、额外的心跳或跳动模式的改变。心动过缓（bradycardia）是低于正常的心率，心动过速（tachycardia）是高于正常的心率。

像心肌梗死这样的疾病给心脏组织带来的损伤可能导致心传导阻滞（heart block），是心脏电传导系统的中断，会导致心律不齐（图 9-15）。随着严重程度的升高，心传导阻滞被分为一级、二级和三级。束支的阻滞被命名为左或右束支阻滞（bundle branch block，BBB）。

无论任何原因，如果窦房结不产生正常的心跳或发生心传导阻滞，就需要植入人工起搏器（artificial pacemaker）以调节心率（图 9-16）。通常，起搏器被插在锁骨下的皮下，导线穿过静脉进入一个或两个右室腔。有些起搏器只在心脏不能正常工作时起作用，其他起搏器则根据活动需要调整心率的变化。

心肌梗死也是纤颤（fibrillation）的一个常见诱因，纤颤是极快速、无效的心跳，当它影响心室时尤其危险。心律转复术（cardioversion）是恢复正常心律的通用术语，可以采用药物和电击。医院的医护人员使用胸外电极进行紧急电除颤（defibrillation）。在购物中心、学校、教堂、飞机和体育场等公共场合的高危患者，除心肺复苏（cardiopulmonary

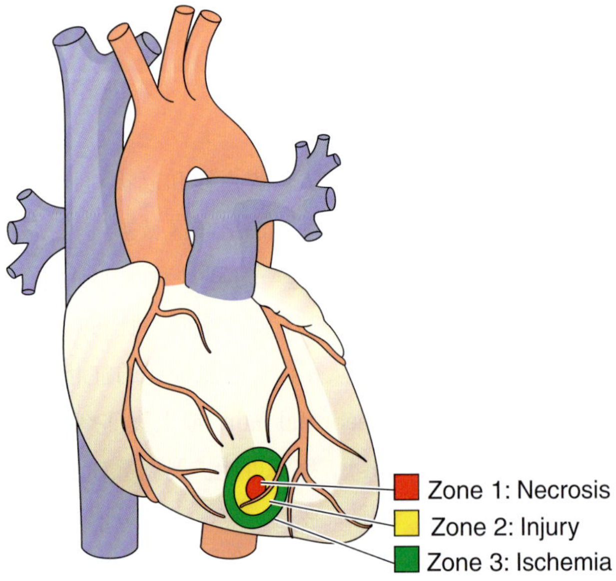

图 9-14 心肌梗死（MI）。血凝块（血栓）造成坏死区（组织死亡），周围组织遭受血液供应缺乏（缺血）

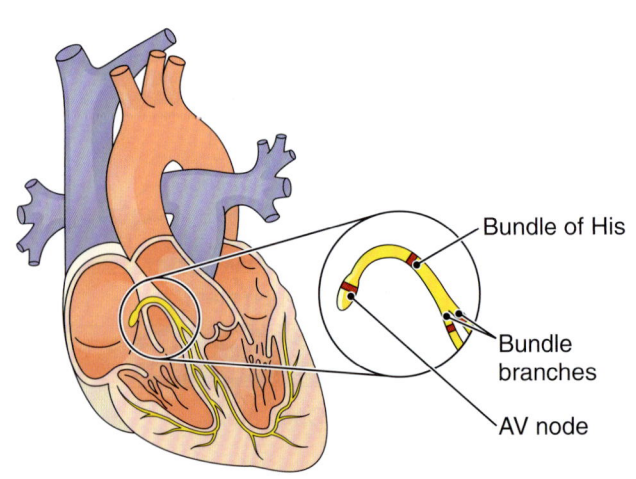

图 9-15 在心脏传导系统的房室（AV）部分中心脏阻塞的可能部位

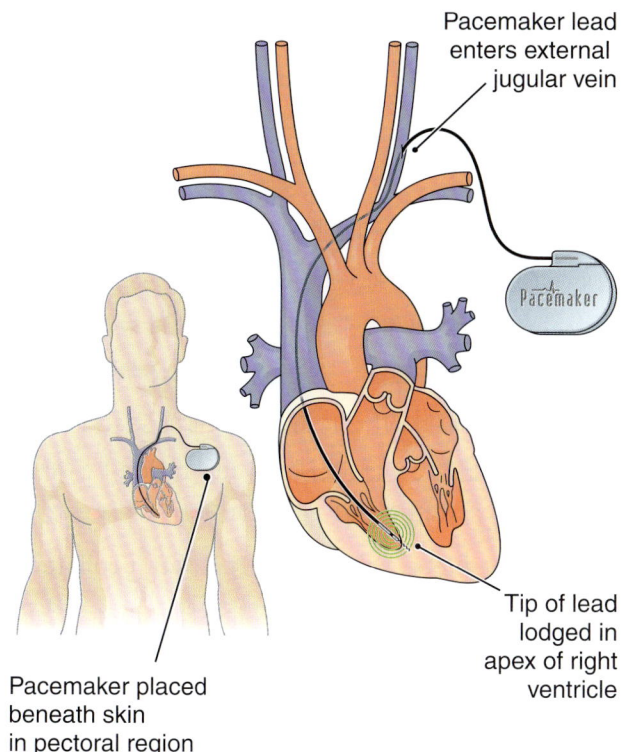

图 9-16 起搏器的放置。引线放置在心房或心室，通常在右侧。双腔起搏器在两个腔室中都有引线

resuscitation，CPR）外，自动体外除颤器（automated external defibrillators，AED）也能够帮助挽救生命。AED 能够检测致命的心律不齐，并自动发送一个正确的预编程电击。可植入的心脏复律除颤器（implantable cardioverter defibrillator，ICD）可以像起搏器那样应用，检测可能的纤颤，并自动电击心脏以恢复正常心律。

更新的治疗心律不齐方法是心脏射频消融术（cardiac ablation），将涉及心律不齐的部分传导通道破坏掉。电极导管消融术（electrode catheter ablation）使用高频声波、冻结（冷冻消融 cryoablation）或通过血管插管输送的电能消融失效的传导通道。

心力衰竭

心力衰竭（heart failure）这一通用术语是指心脏不能有效地排空的任何状况。其导致的压力上升会引起水肿，造成充血性心力衰竭（congestive heart failure，CHF）。左侧衰竭会导致可引起呼吸困难的肺水肿，右侧衰竭会引起伴有组织肿胀的周围性水肿，特别是在腿部，还会因为液体潴留（fluid retention）而体重增加。CHF 的其他症状包括紫绀（cyanosis）和晕厥（syncope）。

治疗心力衰竭需要休息，用药物加强心脏收缩，用利尿剂排出液体，并在饮食中限制盐的摄入。

心力衰竭是休克（shock）的一个诱因，休克是循环系统的严重失调，导致组织供血不足。根据诱因，休克被分类为：

- 心源性休克（cardiogenic shock），由心力衰竭所致。
- 低血容量性休克（hypovolemic shock），由失血所致。
- 感染性休克（septic shock），由细菌感染所致。
- 过敏性休克（anaphylactic shock），由严重过敏反应所致。

先天性心脏病

先天性缺陷（congenital defect）是出生时带有的任何缺陷。最常见的先天性心脏缺陷是间隔缺损（septal defect），在分开心房或心室的隔膜（壁）上有一个洞（图 9-17）。卵圆孔（foramen ovale）的存留通常会导致房间隔缺损，卵圆孔的左右是使胎儿血液循环绕过肺。间隔缺损会使血液从心脏的左侧分流到右侧并返回到肺，而不是流向全身，心脏不得不努力工作以满足组织对氧气的需求。间隔缺损的症状包括紫绀（cyanosis）、晕厥（syncope）和杵状指（clubbing）。

另一种因胎儿修正存留而导致的先天性缺陷是动脉导管未闭（patent ductus arteriosus，图 9-17D）。在这种情况下，肺动脉和主动脉之间的一个小旁路在出生时没有关闭，因而血液会从主动脉流向肺动脉并返回到肺。

心脏瓣膜畸形（heart valve malformation）是另一种先天性心脏缺陷。在心跳周期中能够听到杂音说明瓣膜不能正常开放或关闭。局部主动脉狭窄，或主动脉缩窄（coarctation of the aorta）是限制血液通过血管的先天性缺陷（图 9-17E）。上述大多数先天性缺陷都能够通过手术矫正。

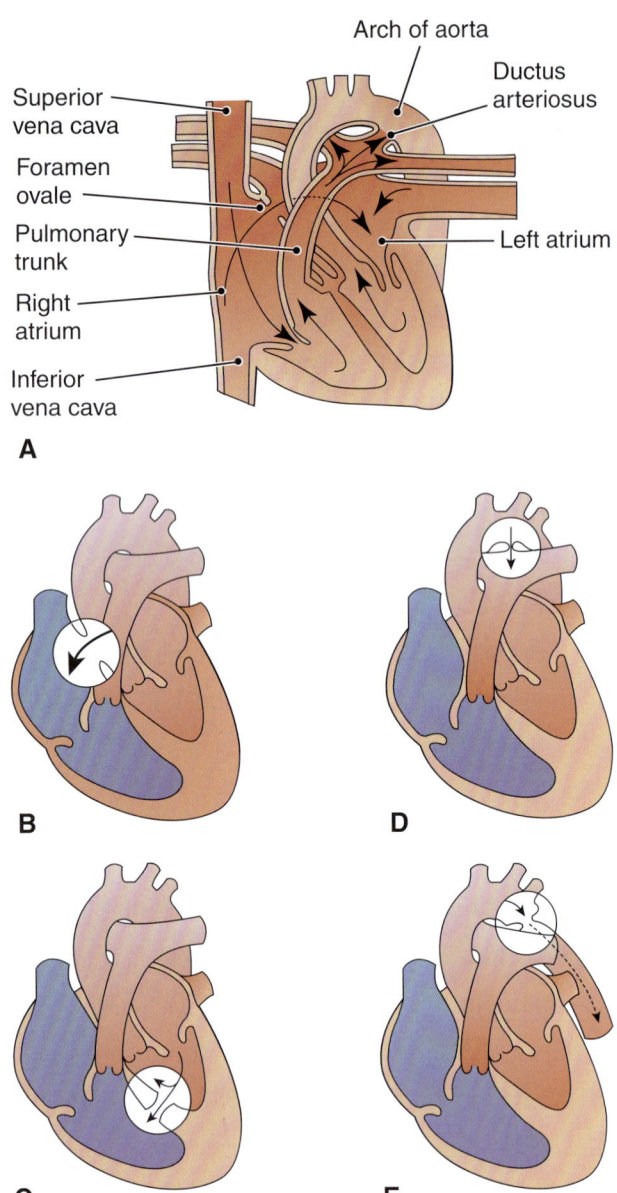

图 9-17 先天性心脏缺陷。A. 正常胎儿心脏显示卵圆孔和动脉导管；B. 卵圆孔的持续存在导致房间隔缺损；C. 心室间隔缺损；D. 动脉导管（动脉导管未闭）的持久存在迫使血液回到肺动脉；E. 主动脉的狭窄限制了主动脉中的外向血流

风湿性心脏病

在风湿性心脏病（rheumatic heart disease）中，特定类型链球菌感染建立的一种免疫反应会最终伤害心脏瓣膜。感染通常开始于"链球菌性喉炎"，大多数情况下都会涉及到二尖瓣。瘢痕组织在瓣膜的小叶上融合，引起干扰正常功能的狭窄（stenosis）。风湿性心脏病患者易于遭受重复性瓣膜感染，在介入性治疗和牙科治疗之前，可能需要预防性地使用抗生素。风湿性心脏病的严重病例需要手术矫正，甚至更换瓣膜。广泛使用抗生素以来，风湿性心脏病的发病呈下降趋势。

静脉病变

静脉瓣膜的损伤和这些血管的长期扩展会共同导致静脉曲张（varicose vein）（图 9-18）。静脉曲张表现为皮肤下扭曲和膨胀的血管，腿部最为常见。影响因素包括遗传、肥胖、长时间站立和怀孕，因为怀孕会增加骨盆静脉的压力。静脉曲张可能会阻碍血流，引起水肿、血栓、出血或溃烂（ulceration）。静脉曲张的治疗包括穿弹力袜和在某些情况下手术去除曲张的静脉，手术后自然会建立侧支循环（collateral circulation）。在直肠或肛管的静脉曲张被称为痔疮（hemorrhoid）。

静脉炎（phlebitis）是静脉的任何发炎，可能是由感染、受伤、循环不良或静脉瓣膜损伤引起的。这种发炎通常会引发血栓的形成，导致血栓静脉炎（thrombophlebitis）。任何静脉都可能患血栓静脉炎，但深层静脉比表层静脉的情况更严重，会形成深层静脉血栓（deep vein thrombosis，DVT）。最常发生 DVT 的是腿深层静脉，会引起这些区域静脉回流的严重减少。

血管技术员收集关于血管和循环的信息以协助诊断。有关这一职业的信息，请参见框 9-3。

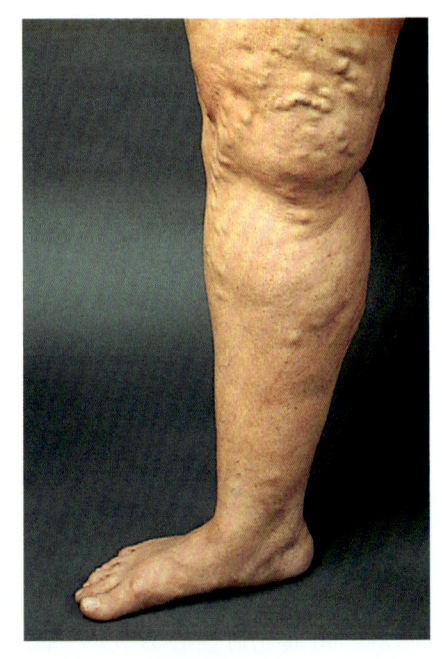

图 9-18 静脉曲张

健康职业
血管技术员

框 9-3

血管技术员（vascular technologist）执行非侵入性诊断研究，以评估头部、颈部、四肢和腹部的血管（动脉和静脉），帮助医生诊断血管疾病。血管技术员使用超声波获得血管的二维图像，并使用多普勒超声测量血流的速度和方向。他们使用其他仪器来测量血压、血容量的变化和血氧饱和度。

大多数血管技术员在医院工作，他们在那里准备患者的测试、记录临床病史、执行有限的身体检查、进行诊断测试并报告结果。他们也可以在办公室、诊所或实验室工作。虽然他们的大多数患者是老年人，但可能需要对任何年龄的患者进行血管研究。

与该领域的早期工作人员不同，这些人员通常接受过相关培训。血管技术员要完成由联合健康教育计划认证委员会（Commission on Accreditation of Allied Health Education Programs，CAAHEP）认证的 2 年或 4 年的教育项目。血管技术专门的认证可在美国诊断医学超声检查注册（American Registry for Diagnostic Medical Sonography）网站 www.ardms.org 和其他组织那里获得。认证需要适当的教育、临床经验、考试和继续教育。从 2017 年开始，在国际认可委员会（Intersocietal Accreditation Commission，IAC）认可的血管实验室工作的所有血管技术员都被要求获得认证。有关这个职业的更多信息，请访问血管超声协会（Society for Vascular Ultrasound）www.svunet.org。

Terminology 心血管病症

aneurysm [ˈænjərizəm]	动脉瘤，血管的局部异常扩张，通常是动脉，由脆弱的血管壁所致，最终可能会破裂
angina pectoris [ænˈdʒainəˈpektəris]	心绞痛，心脏周围的压缩感或疼痛，可能放射至左臂或左肩，通常是由劳累所致，因对心脏供血不足而引起
arrhythmia [əˈriθmiə]	心律不齐，心跳速率和节律的任何异常（从字面上看是"没用韵律"，请注意字面 r 要双写）。也被称为节律紊乱（dysrhythmia）
arteriosclerosis [ɑːˌtiəriəʊskləˈrəʊsis]	动脉硬化，动脉的硬化症（sclerosis），由于脂肪沉积（斑块，plaque）、钙盐沉积或瘢痕组织形成造成容量损失和弹性损失
atherosclerosis [ˌæθərəʊskliˈrəʊsis]	动脉粥样硬化，脂肪、纤维斑块在动脉内壁的发展，造成管腔狭窄和血管壁硬化。动脉粥样硬化是动脉硬化最常见的形式。词根 ather/o 意为"粥"或"麦片糊"
bradycardia [brædiˈkɑːdiə]	心动过缓，心率低于 60bpm
cerebrovascular accident（CVA）[ˌserəbrəʊˈvæskjələ]	脑血管意外，由于血流减少导致的大脑突然损伤。起因包括动脉粥样硬化、栓塞、血栓或破裂动脉瘤的出血，通常也被称为脑卒中
clubbing [ˈklʌbiŋ]	杵状指，由指甲周围软组织增生引起的手指或脚趾末端增大。在外围循环不良的很多疾病中可见
coarctation of the aorta [ˌkəʊɑːkˈteiʃən]	主动脉缩窄，主动脉局部变窄，限制血液流动
C-reactive protein (CRP)	C 反应蛋白，全身感染时产生的蛋白质，可能对动脉粥样硬化有影响；高 CRP 水平表明有心血管疾病及其预后
cyanosis [ˌsaiəˈnəʊsis]	紫绀，由缺氧所致的皮肤变紫

Terminology — 心血管系统正常结构和功能（续表）

术语	释义
deep vein thrombosis (DVT)	深层静脉血栓，涉及深层静脉的血栓静脉炎
diaphoresis [ˌdaiəfə'ri:sis]	发汗，大量出汗
dissecting aneurysm	夹层动脉瘤，血液进入动脉壁并将血管壁分层分离的动脉瘤；通常涉及主动脉
dyslipidemia [dislipi'demiə]	血脂异常，血清中脂类水平失调，是动脉粥样硬化发展的一个重要元素，包括高血脂（hyperlipidemia）、高胆固醇（hypercholesterolemia）和高甘油三脂（hypertriglyceridemia）
dyspnea [dis'pni:ə]	呼吸困难或吃力
edema [i'di:mə]	水肿，由于过量液体存在所致的身体组织肿胀。起因包括心血管失调、肾衰竭、发炎和营养不良
embolism ['embəlizəm]	栓塞，血管被血凝块或循环系统中输送的其他物体阻塞
embolus ['embələs]	栓塞物，循环系统中输送的物质，通常是血凝块，也可能是空气、脂肪、细菌或来自于体内或体外的固态物体
fibrillation [ˌfibri'leiʃən]	纤维性颤动，心房或心室自发的颤抖和肌纤维无效的收缩
heart block	心脏传导阻滞，心脏电传导系统的干扰，会导致心律不齐
heart failure	心力衰竭，心脏不能维持足够的血液循环所致的状况
hemorrhoid [ˌhemə'rɔid]	痔疮，直肠的静脉曲张
hypertension [ˌhaipə'tenʃn]	高血压，高于正常血压的状况。原发性（突发）高血压的原因不明
infarct [in'fɑ:kt]	梗死，由于为区域供血的动脉阻塞或变窄导致的局部组织坏死
ischemia [is'ki:miə]	局部缺血，由于循环阻塞引起的局部供血不足（词根：hem/o）
murmur	杂音，异常的心音
myocardial infarction (MI) [ˌmaiə'kɑ:diəl]	心肌梗死，由于为区域供血的冠状动脉阻塞或变窄所致的心肌组织局部坏死。通常是因为在血管中形成血栓所致。
occlusion [ə'klu:ʒn]	闭塞，血管的封闭或阻塞
patent ductus arteriosus ['pætnt 'dʌktəs ɑ:'tiəriəsəs]	动脉导管未闭，动脉导管在出生后继续存留。动脉导管是胎儿连接肺动脉与下行主动脉而使血流绕过肺的血管
phlebitis [flə'baitis]	静脉炎，静脉的任何炎症

Terminology　心血管系统正常结构和功能（续表）

plaque [plæk]	斑块，对心血管系统而言，斑块是血管壁上脂肪和其他物质的沉积，可能会阻塞血管
rheumatic heart disease [rʊ'mætik]	风湿性心脏病，特定类型链球菌（A 型溶血性链球菌）感染后对心脏瓣膜的损伤。应对感染所产生的抗体会产生瓣膜瘢痕，通常涉及二尖瓣
septal defect ['septl]	间隔缺损，心房或心室之间的隔膜上的开口；常见起因是卵圆孔（foramen ovale）的存留，卵圆孔是心房之间的开口，在胎儿的血液循环中的作用是使血流绕过肺
shock	休克，组织供血不足导致的循环衰竭
stenosis [sti'nəʊsis]	狭窄，开口收缩或变窄
stroke	脑卒中，参见脑血管意外
syncope ['siŋkəpi]	昏厥，因大脑供血不足引起的暂时意识丧失
tachycardia [ˌtæki'kɑ:diə]	心动过速，异常快的心率，一般高于 100bpm
thrombophlebitis [ˌθrɒmbəʊfli'baitis]	血栓静脉炎，带有血凝块形成的静脉炎
thrombosis [θrɒmˈbəʊsis]	血栓形成，血管中血凝块的发展
thrombus ['θrɒmbəs]	血栓，血管内形成的血凝块
varicose vein [ˌværikəʊs]	静脉曲张，由于瓣膜破损、血液淤积和长期血管扩张造成的扭曲、肿胀的静脉（词根：varic/o），也被称为 varix ['veəriks] 或 varicosity [ˌværi'kɒsiti]

Diagnosis and Treatment 诊断和治疗

ablation [ə'bleiʃn]	消融，去除或破坏。在心脏消融中，使用导管销毁心脏传导通道的一部分，以纠正心律不齐
angioplasty ['ændʒiəʊplæsti]	血管成形术，重新打开变窄的血管并恢复血流的一种方法。通常伴随手术去除斑块、为血管内的气囊充气或安装支架（stent）以保持血管通畅
artificial pacemaker	人工起搏器，一个能够产生电脉冲调节心跳的电池驱动的装置。可以外接或植入，可设计为根据需求响应，能够防止心动过速
cardiopulmonary resuscitation (CPR) [riˌsʌsi'teiʃn]	心肺复苏术，使用人工呼吸和胸部按压或心脏按摩在心脏骤停后恢复心脏输出和肺通气
cardioversion [kɑ:diə'vɜ:ʃən]	心脏复律，校正异常的心律。可能通过使用抗心律不齐的药物或使用电击（参见 defibrillation 除颤）
coronary angiography [ændʒi'ɒgrəfi]	冠状动脉造影术，使用导管通过血管插入心脏，向冠状动脉注入不透明的染色剂，然后进行 X 线造影检查
coronary artery bypass graft (CABG)	冠状动脉旁路搭桥术，通过手术建立分路，以绕过阻塞的冠状动脉

Terminology	心血管系统正常结构和功能（续表）
coronary calcium scan (heart scan)	冠状动脉钙扫描（心脏扫描），使冠状动脉内导致血管变窄的钙沉积可视化的一种方法。用于为中等风险患者或有未确诊胸痛患者诊断冠状动脉疾病
creatine kinase MB (CK-MB) [ˈkriːətin ˈkineis]	肌酸激酶MB，心肌梗死（myocardial infarction，MI）后心肌细胞增量释放的一种酶。血清化验能够帮助诊断心肌梗死并确定心肌损伤的程度
CT angiography (CTA)	CT血管造影，计算机断层扫描用于显示心脏和其他器官中的血管，只需要在上臂注入少量染色剂。能够为患有胸痛或异常压力测试结果的患者排除能够引起心肌梗死的冠状动脉阻塞
defibrillation [ˌdiːfibriˈleiʃn]	除颤，使用电子设备（除颤器）通过向心脏发送暂短的电击制止纤颤。电击可以通过胸部表面传送，如同自动外接除颤器（automated external defibrillator，AED）那样，或者使用可植入的心脏除颤器（implantable cardioverter defibrillator，ICD）通过导线直接传入心脏
echocardiography [ekəʊkɑːdiˈɒɡrəfi]	超声心动图，使用超声波显示内部心脏结构的非侵入式方法
lipoprotein [ˈlipəprəʊtiːn]	脂蛋白，蛋白质与脂肪的化合物。根据密度，脂蛋白被分类为非常低密度（VLDL）、低密度（LDL）和高密度（HDL）脂蛋白。相对高水平的HDL与心血管健康相关
percutaneous transluminal coronary angioplasty (PTCA)	经皮冠状动脉腔内成形术将气囊导管插入血管，然后充气向动脉壁压平斑块，扩张变硬的血管
stent	支架，一个放置在动脉内的线圈或缝管形状的小金属装置，用于在动脉内腔成形术之后保持血管的通畅
stress test	压力测试，通过在锻炼期间连续的心电图监视评估身体素质。在铊压力测试中，使用放射性同位素铊来追踪锻炼期间的心脏血流
troponin (Tn) [ˈtroʊpənin]	肌钙蛋白，肌肉细胞中调节收缩的一种蛋白质。血清中肌钙蛋白水平升高，主要是TnT和TnI形态的肌钙蛋白，显示最近可能发生过心肌梗死

淋巴系统

淋巴系统（lymphatic system）是具有多重功能的、广泛分布的系统（图9-19），它在循环中的作用是将过量的液体和蛋白质从组织中返回到血流。盲端毛细淋巴管从组织中提取这些物质，并将它们送入较大的血管（图9-20）。淋巴系统中携带的液体被称为淋巴液（lymph）。淋巴液从下半身和上半身左侧排出到胸导管（左淋巴导管，left lymphatic duct），向上穿过胸部流入靠近心脏的左锁骨下静脉（left subclavian vein）（图9-19）。右淋巴导管将上半身右侧的淋巴液汇入右锁骨下静脉。

淋巴系统的另一个主要功能是保护人体免受不洁物质和微生物的侵害（参见第10章免疫系统）。沿着淋巴管分布着很多小的淋巴组织团，即淋巴结（lymph nodes），它们的作用是过滤淋巴液（图9-21）。淋巴结集中在颈部（cervical）、腋窝（axillary）、胸部（mediastinal）和腹股沟（inguinal）区域。淋巴系统的其他保护性器官和组织包括：

- 扁桃腺（tonsils），位于喉部（pharynx）。它们过滤吸入或吞咽的物质，并在生命的早期协助免疫。
- 胸腺（thymus），位于胸部，心脏上方。它在免疫过程中处理并刺激淋巴细胞的活性。
- 脾脏（spleen），位于腹部的左上区域。它过滤血液，并摧毁衰老的红细胞。

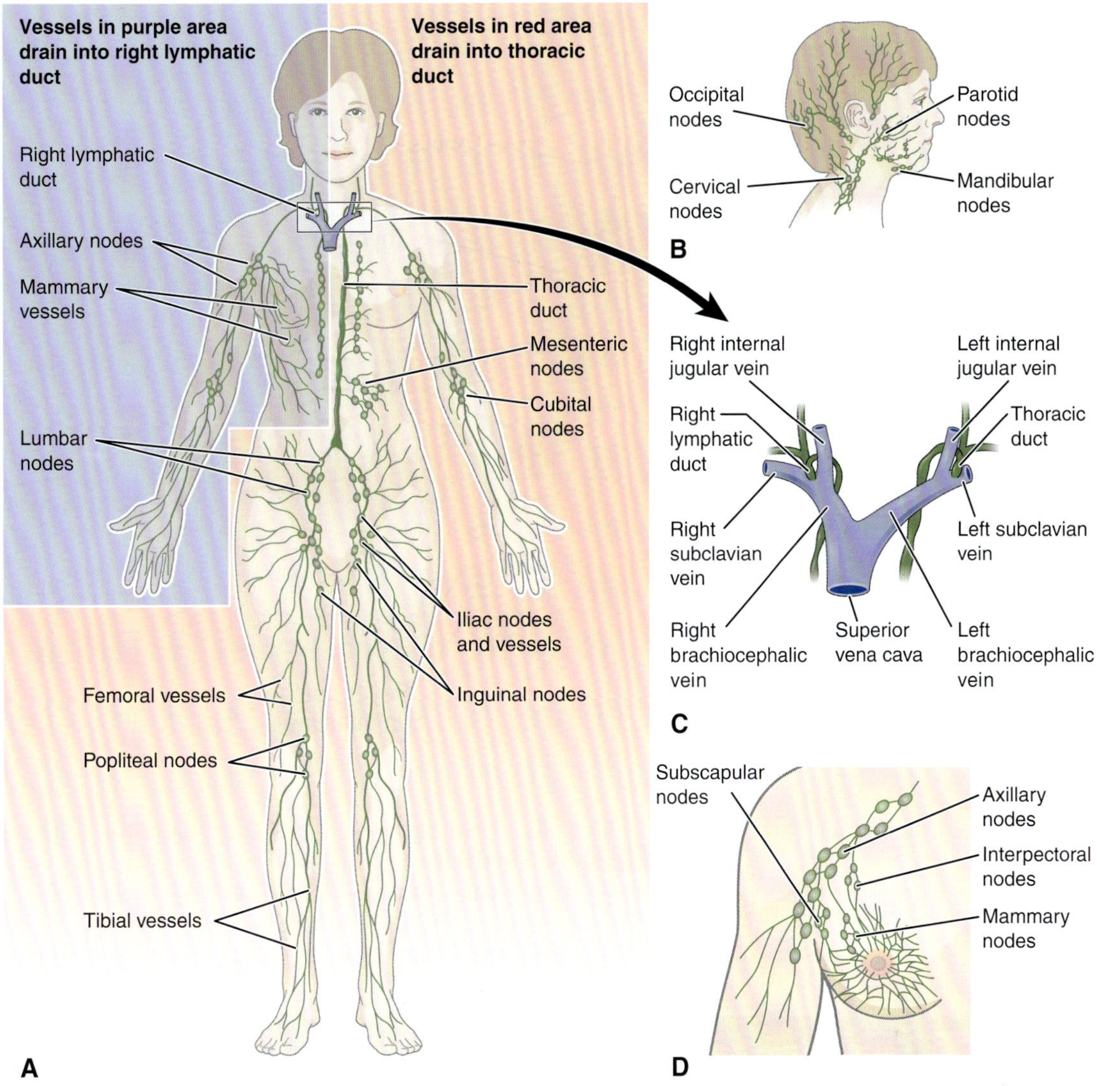

图 9-19 淋巴系统。A. 淋巴管几乎遍布身体的每个区域。淋巴结沿着血管的路径分布。排入右侧淋巴管的区域显示为紫色；排入胸导管的区域显示为红色；B. 淋巴结和头部的血管；C. 右淋巴管和胸导管流入锁骨下静脉；D. 乳房、乳腺和周围区域的淋巴结和血管

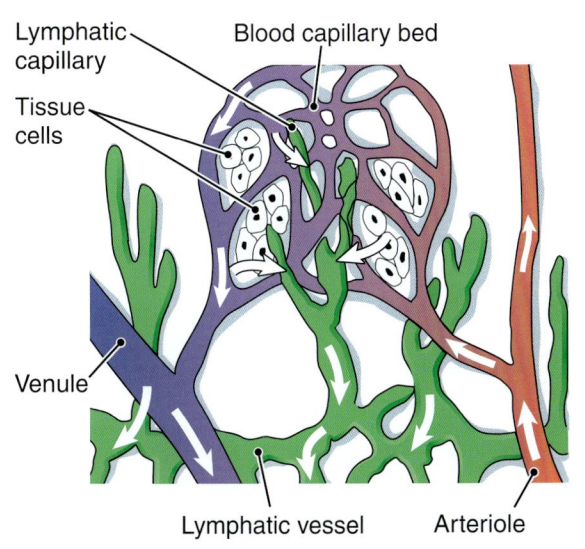

图 9-20 淋巴液流入组织中。毛细淋巴管吸收在组织中留下的液体和蛋白质，并将它们带回血流

- 阑尾（appendix），附着在大肠上。它可能协助免疫系统的发育。
- 派尔集合淋巴结（Peyer patches），在肠道内壁。它们帮助抵抗入侵的微生物。

淋巴系统的最后一个功能是从小肠吸收消化的脂肪。然后这些脂肪被流出胸导管的淋巴液加入到血液之中。

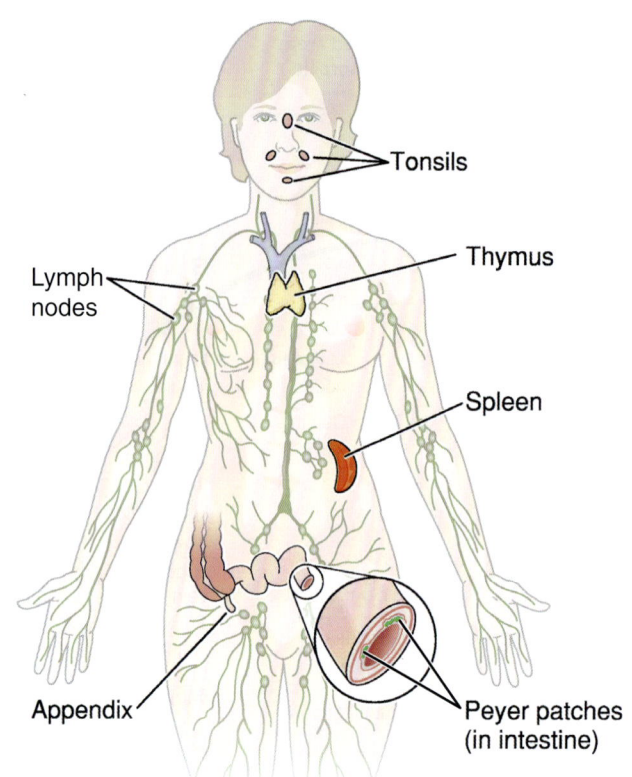

图 9-21 淋巴组织的位置

Terminology	淋巴系统正常结构和功能
appendix [əˈpendiks]	阑尾,附着于大肠前半部分的手指形的淋巴组织团
lymph [limf]	淋巴液,稀薄的、血浆样的液体,从淋巴组织中排出并在淋巴导管中输送(词根:lymph/o)
lymph node	淋巴结,沿着淋巴导管分布的的淋巴组织团,淋巴结过滤淋巴液(词根:lymphaden/o)
lymphatic system [limˈfætik]	淋巴系统,从组织中排出淋巴液和蛋白质,并将它们返回到血流系统。该系统也参与免疫,并帮助从消化道中吸收脂肪
Peyer patches	派尔集合淋巴结,小肠内壁的淋巴组织集合
right lymphatic duct	右淋巴导管,从人体上半身右侧排出淋巴液的淋巴导管
Spleen	脾脏,腹部左上区域的一个红褐色器官,它过滤血液并摧毁衰老的红细胞(词根:splen/o)
thoracic duct	胸导管,从上半身左侧和下半身排出淋巴液的淋巴导管,左淋巴导管
thymus [ˈθaiməs]	胸腺,位于胸部,心脏上方的淋巴器官,在免疫系统中发挥作用
tonsils [ˈtɒnsilz]	扁桃腺,位于喉部的小团淋巴组织

与淋巴系统相关的词根

参见表 9-3

表 9-3　淋巴系统的词根

词根	含义	示例	示例定义
lymph/o	淋巴液、淋巴系统	lymphoid ['lɪmfɔɪd]	淋巴的
lymphaden/o	淋巴结	lymphadenitis [lɪmˌfædɪ'naɪtɪs]	淋巴结炎
lymphangi/o	淋巴导管	lymphangiogram [lɪm'fændʒɪəgræm]	淋巴管造影
splen/o	脾脏	splenalgia [splɪ'nældʒɪə]	脾痛
thym/o	胸腺	athymia [ə'θɪmɪə]	无胸腺
tonsil/o	扁桃腺	tonsillar ['tɒnslə]	扁桃腺的

练习 9-3

填空。

1. Tonsillectomy [ˌtɒnsə'lektəmɪ] is surgical removal of a(n)_____.
2. Thymopathy ['θaɪməpəθɪ] is any disease of the_____.
3. Lymphadenectomy [lɪmfəd'nektəmɪ] is surgical removal of a(n)_____.
4. Lymphedema [lɪmfɪ'diːmə] means swelling caused by obstruction of the flow of_____.
5. A lymphangioma [lɪmˌfændʒɪ'əʊmə] is a tumor of_____.
6. Splenic ['splenɪk] means pertaining to the_____.

识别并定义下列单词的词根。

	Root	Meaning of Root
7. lymphangial [lɪm'fændʒɪəl]	_____	_____
8. perisplenitis [perɪsplɪ'naɪtɪs]	_____	_____
9. lymphadenography ['lɪmfədɪnəgrəfɪ]	_____	_____
10. tonsillectomy [ˌtɒnsə'lektəmɪ]	_____	_____
11. hypothymism [haɪpəʊ'θɪmɪzəm]	_____	_____

使用适当的词根写出下列含义的单词。

12. Enlargement (-megaly) of the spleen	_____	_____
13. Inflammation of a tonsil	_____	_____
14. Any disease (-pathy) of the lymph nodes	_____	_____
15. Inflammation of lymphatic vessels	_____	_____
16. Pertaining to (-ic) the thymus	_____	_____
17. A tumor (-oma) of lymphatic tissue	_____	_____

淋巴系统的临床表现

淋巴系统的变化通常与感染相关,包括被称为淋巴结炎(lymphadenitis)的淋巴结发炎与肿大和被称为淋巴管炎(lymphangitis)的淋巴导管炎症。因手术切开或感染造成的淋巴导管阻塞会导致组织水肿,被称为淋巴水肿(lymphedema,框9-4)。任何涉及淋巴结的肿瘤疾病都被称为淋巴瘤(lymphoma),这些肿瘤会影响淋巴系统中的白细胞。

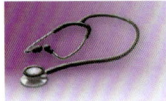

框 9-4 临床观点
淋巴水肿:当淋巴液停止流动时

人体的液体平衡需要液体在心血管系统、淋巴系统和组织中适当地分布。当平衡倒向组织中液体过量,就会发生水肿(edema)。通常,水肿是心力衰竭造成的。不过,淋巴导管的阻塞(导致液体在组织中积累)可能引起另一种水肿,被称为淋巴水肿(lymphedema)。淋巴水肿的临床特点是上臂或腿的长期水肿,而心力衰竭一般会引起双腿水肿。

淋巴水肿可能是原发的,也可能是继发的。原发性淋巴水肿是淋巴导管发育异常引起的罕见的先天性疾病,继发性淋巴水肿,或获得性淋巴水肿可能是肢体外伤、手术、放射疗法或淋巴导管发炎的结果。淋巴水肿最常见的起因是乳房切除术期间切除了腋下淋巴结,破坏了邻近上臂的淋巴液流动。前列腺手术后也可能发生淋巴水肿。

促进淋巴导管中液体流动的疗法有助于治疗淋巴水肿。这些疗法包括抬起被影响的肢体、通过按摩人工淋巴引流、轻微运动、紧裹肢体以提供压力等。另外,改变生活习惯也会减轻淋巴水肿的影响。例如,穿着宽松的衣服、用没有发生淋巴水肿的手臂携带随身提包、坐下时不要交叉双腿,这样能够防止进一步淋巴引流阻塞。淋巴管炎需要适当使用抗生素。及时治疗非常重要,因为除了水肿以外,还会有其他并发症,包括伤口愈合不良、皮肤溃疡和感染风险升高等。

Terminology 关键临床词汇

淋巴疾病

术语	解释
lymphadenitis [lim͵fædi'naitis]	淋巴结炎,淋巴结发炎并肿大,通常是感染所致
lymphangitis [limfən'dʒaitis]	淋巴管炎,细菌感染造成的淋巴导管炎症,表现为皮肤下疼痛的红色条纹(也拼写为 lymphangiitis,图9-22)
lymphedema [limfi'di:mə]	淋巴水肿,因淋巴导管阻塞或被切开造成的组织水肿(图9-22B 和框9-4)
lymphoma [lim'fəʊmə]	淋巴瘤,淋巴组织的任何肿瘤性疾病

Terminology 补充术语

正常结构和功能

术语	解释
apical pulse ['æpikəl]	心尖搏动,在心尖感觉到或听到的脉搏。可以在左侧第五肋间距中线8~9cm处测量
cardiac output	心输出量,每分钟从右心室泵到左心室的血量
Korotkoff sounds	柯氏音,用袖带测量血压时听诊器中听到的动脉搏动的声音

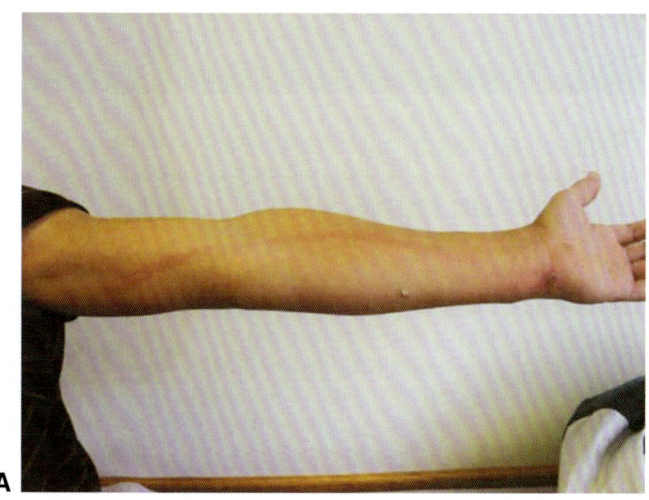 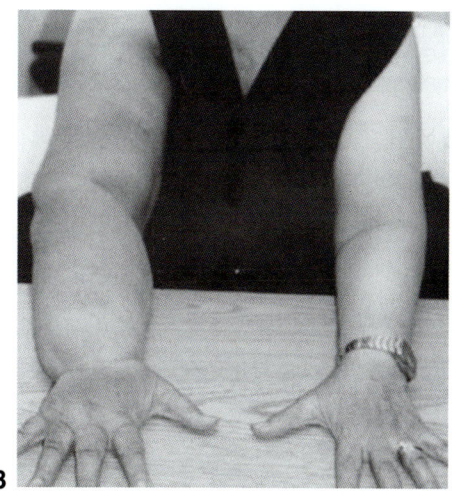

图 9-22 淋巴疾病。A. 淋巴管炎是淋巴管的炎症，请注意靠近皮肤感染的线性红色条纹；B. 去除腋窝淋巴结和淋巴液流阻塞后右上肢淋巴水肿

Terminology 补充术语（续表）

perfusion ［pə'fju:ʒən］	灌注，通过器官或组织的液体通道
precordium ［'pri:'kɔ:djəm］	心前区，胸廓下部心脏前面的区域，形容词：precordial
pulse pressure	脉压，收缩压与舒张压之差
stroke volume	心搏量，每次心跳从左心室喷出的血量
Valsalva maneuver	瓦尔萨尔瓦动作，屏气，如分娩和排便时，关闭鼻子和喉咙用力试图呼气。这一动作对心血管系统有作用
综合征和病症	
bruit ［bru:t］	杂音，听诊器中听到的异常声音
cardiac tamponade ［ˌtæmpə'neid］	心脏压塞，心包中液体的病理性积累，可能是心包炎或心脏和大血管受损所致
ectopic beat ［ek'tɒpik］	异位搏动，发自于窦房结之外的心脏某处的心跳
extrasystole ［ˌekstrə'sistəli:］	期前收缩，与正常心跳分开的过早的心脏收缩，发自于窦房结之外的心脏某处
flutter ［'flʌtə(r)］	振颤，心房或心室跳动非常快（200~300bpm），但是有规律的收缩
hypotension ［ˌhaipə'tenʃən］	低血压，比正常血压低的状态
intermittent claudication ［ˌklɔ:di'keiʃən］	间歇性跛行，锻炼时因供血不足引起的肌肉疼痛，休息时疼痛消失
mitral valve prolapse ［'prəʊlæps］	二尖瓣脱垂，心室收缩时二尖瓣的尖角进入左心房
occlusive vascular disease	闭塞性血管病，动脉硬化，通常是周围血管
palpitation ［ˌpælpi'teiʃən］	心悸，心跳异常快速或不规律的感觉

Terminology	补充术语（续表）
pitting edema	压凹性水肿，手指用力按压在皮肤后，水肿会保持手指的压痕（图 9-23）
polyarteritis nodosa	结节性多动脉炎，可能致命的胶原性疾病，会引起小内脏动脉发炎。症状取决于所影响的器官
Raynaud disease	雷诺病，以遇冷时四肢的周围血管异常收缩为特征的疾病
regurgitation [riˌɡɜːdʒiˈteiʃn]	反流，反向流动，例如血液通过有缺陷的瓣膜的反向流动
stasis [ˈsteisis]	淤积，正常流动的阻塞，如血液或尿液。血液淤积可能导致皮炎和溃疡
subacute bacterial endocarditis (SBE)	亚急性细菌性心内膜炎，细菌在以前被风湿热损伤的心脏或瓣膜上生长
tetralogy of Fallot [teˈtrælədʒi]	法洛四联症，四种先天性心脏异常的组合：肺动脉狭窄、室间隔缺陷、大动脉右位移和右心室肥大
thromboangiitis obliterans [θrɒmbəʊændʒiˈaitis]	血栓闭塞性脉管炎，炎症和血栓形成导致心血管闭塞，特别是在腿部。最常见于年轻人和相对重度吸烟者。腿部血管血栓性闭塞可能导致足坏疽，患者会烟草过敏。也被称为柏格氏症（Buerger disease）
vegetation [ˌvedʒəˈteiʃn]	赘生物，心脏瓣膜上异常的细菌生长，与风湿热相关
Wolff-Parkinson-White syndrome (WPW)	心脏功能缺陷预激综合征，由因替代性传导通道引起的心动过速和室性期前收缩构成的心律不齐

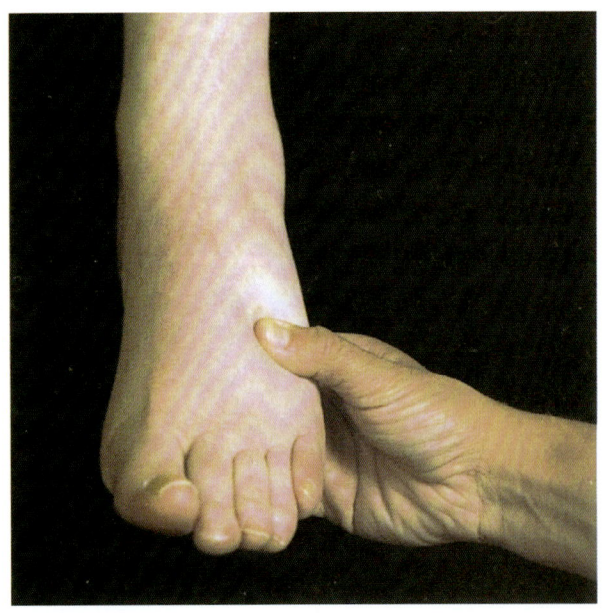
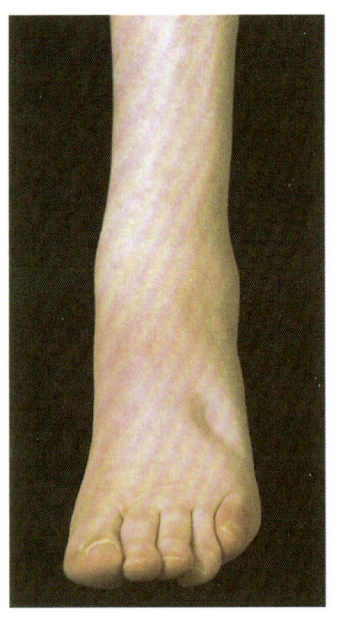

图 9-23 压凹性水肿。当用手指（A）紧紧按压皮肤时，移开手指（B）之后残留有凹坑

Terminology 补充术语（续表）

诊断

cardiac catheterization	心导管插入术，将导管通过血管插入心脏以注入造影剂，用于成像、诊断、获得样本或测量压力
central venous pressure (CVP)	中心静脉压，上腔大静脉的血压
cineangiocardiography [ˌsini'ænʤiəʊˌkɑːdi'ɒgrəfi]	心血管荧光电影照像术。利用动画技术摄影记录心脏和大血管的荧光图像
Doppler echocardiography [ekəʊkɑːdi'ɒgrəfi]	多普勒超声心动图，用于研究血流速度和模式的成像方式
Holter monitor	霍尔特氏心电动态监测仪，能够记录一个人正常活动 24 小时至 1 个月心电图的便携式设备
homocysteine [ˌhəʊməʊ'sistiːin]	同型半胱氨酸，血液中的一种氨基酸，高于正常水平会增加患心血管疾病的风险
phlebotomist [fli'bɒtəmist]	抽血者，专门抽血的技术人员
phonocardiography [fəʊnəkɑːdi'ɒgrəfi]	心音描记法，电子记录心音
plethysmography [pliθiz'mɒgrəfi]	体积描记法，基于获得或通过的血量测量器官或组织体积的变化。阻抗容积描记术测量电阻的变化，用于诊断深层动脉血栓
pulmonary capillary wedge pressure (PCWP)	肺毛细血管楔压，通过导管在肺动脉分支测量的血压，它是左心房血压的间接测量（框 9-2）
radionuclide heart scan	放射性核素心脏扫描，注射放射性同位素后的心脏成像。因为放射性同位素会被受损的组织占用，焦磷酸盐（pyrophosphate，PYP）扫描使用锝 -99m（99mTc）能够测试心肌梗死。平衡法多时闸心室造影（multigated acquisition，MUGA）能够给出心脏功能的信息
Swan-Ganz catheter	血流导向气囊导管，一种尖端带气囊的心脏导管，用于测量肺动脉压力。它被引导穿过静脉进入心脏右侧，然后进入肺动脉
transesophageal echocardiography (TEE)	经食管超声心动描记术，使用内窥镜将超声波换能器导入食管，以获得心脏成像
triglycerides [trig'lisəraidz]	甘油三酸酯，一种在血流中循环的简单的脂肪
ventriculography [ventrikjʊ'lɒgrəfi]	心室造影术，在通过导管注入不透明的染色剂后用 X 线研究心室

治疗和手术

atherectomy [æði'rektəmi]	粥样斑块旋切术，从血管内壁去除粥样斑块。可以通过开放手术，或者通过血管管腔进行
commissurotomy [kɒmiʃə'rɒtəmi]	连合部切开术，手术切开有瘢痕的二尖瓣，使瓣膜的开口增大
embolectomy [ˌembə'lektəmi]	栓子切除术，手术去除血栓

Terminology 补充术语（续表）

intraaortic balloon pump (IABP)	主动脉内球囊反搏泵，由可充气气囊泵构成的机械辅助装置，通过股动脉插入到胸部大动脉。在舒张期充气以改善冠状动脉循环，并在收缩期之后抽气使得血液能够从心脏中喷出
left ventricular assist device (LVAD)	左心室辅助装置，一个替代左心室功能的泵，将血液输送到体循环。这一装置用于协助等候心脏移植的患者或从心力衰竭中恢复的人
药物	
angiotensin-converting enzyme (ACE) inhibitor	血管紧张素转换酶抑制剂，通过阻止血管紧张素Ⅱ的生成降低血压的药物，血管紧张素的正常作用是提高血压
angiotensin receptor blocker (ARB)	血管紧张素受体拮抗剂，抑制组织对血管紧张素受体的药物
antiarrhythmic agent	抗心律不齐药，调节心跳速率和节律的药物
beta-adrenergic blocking agent	β-肾上腺素能阻断剂，降低心脏收缩速率和强度的药物，也叫β受体阻滞剂（beta-blocker）
calcium-channel blocker	钙通道阻滞剂，通过调节进入细胞的钙控制心脏收缩速率和强度的药物
digitalis [ˌdɪdʒɪˈteɪlɪs]	洋地黄，减缓并加强心肌收缩的药物
diuretic [ˌdaɪjʊˈretɪk]	利尿剂，通过增加肾排尿消除液体，降低的血容量会减少心脏的工作量
hypolipidemic agent	降血脂药，降低血清胆固醇的药物
lidocaine [ˈlɪdəkeɪn]	利多卡因，局部麻醉剂，用于静脉治疗心律不齐
loop diuretic	袢利尿剂，通过阻止肾单元对电解质的再吸收增加排尿量
nitroglycerin [ˌnaɪtrəʊˈglɪsərɪn]	硝酸甘油，用于治疗心绞痛的药物，扩张冠状动脉
statins [sˈteɪtɪnz]	他汀类药物，降低血脂的药物，它们的名称都带有-statin，例如洛伐他汀（lovastatin）、普伐他汀（pravastatin）、阿托伐他汀（atorvastatin）
streptokinase [ˌstreptəʊˈkaɪneɪs]	溶栓酶，一种用于溶解血栓的酶
tissue plasminogen activator (tPA)	组织型纤溶酶原激活剂，用于溶解血栓的药物，它激活血液中胞质素（plasmin）的产生，胞质素或溶解血栓
vasodilator [ˌvæsəʊdaɪˈleɪtə]	血管扩张剂，扩张血管并改善血流的药物

Terminology 缩略语

ACE	Angiotensin-converting enzyme	血管紧张素转换酶
AED	Automated external defibrillator	自动体外除颤器
AF	Atrial fibrillation	心房纤颤
AMI	Acute myocardial infarction	急性心肌梗死

Terminology 缩略语（续表）

APC	Atrial premature complex	房性期前收缩
AR	Aortic regurgitation	主动脉瓣关闭不全
ARB	Angiotensin receptor blocker	血管紧张素受体拮抗剂
AS	Aortic stenosis; arteriosclerosis	动脉硬化
ASCVD	Arteriosclerotic cardiovascular disease	动脉硬化性心血管疾病
ASD	Atrial septal defect	房间隔缺损
ASHD	Arteriosclerotic heart disease	动脉硬化性心脏病
AT	Atrial tachycardia	房性心动过速
AV	Atrioventricular	房室的
BBB	Bundle branch block (left or right)	束支传导阻塞（左或右）
BP	Blood pressure	血压
bpm	Beats per minute	每分钟心跳次数
CABG	Coronary artery bypass graft	冠状动脉旁路搭桥术
CAD	Coronary artery disease	冠状动脉疾病
CCU	Coronary/cardiac care unit	冠状动脉/心脏监护病房
CHD	Coronary heart disease	冠状动脉性心脏病
CHF	Congestive heart failure	充血性心力衰竭
CK-MB	Creatine kinase MB	肌酸激酶 MB
CPR	Cardiopulmonary resuscitation	心肺复苏
CRP	C-reactive protein	C 反应蛋白
CTA	Computed tomography angiography	CT 血管造影
CVA	Cerebrovascular accident	脑血管意外，脑卒中
CVD	Cardiovascular disease	心血管疾病
CVI	Chronic venous insufficiency	慢性静脉功能不全
CVP	Central venous pressure	中心静脉压
DOE	Dyspnea on exertion	运动性呼吸困难
DVT	Deep vein thrombosis	深静脉血栓形成
ECG (EKG)	Electrocardiogram, electrocardiography	心电图
HDL	High-density lipoprotein	高密度脂蛋白

Terminology 缩略语（续表）

hs-CRP	High-sensitivity C-reactive protein (test)		超敏 C 反应蛋白（测试）
HTN	Hypertension		高血压
IABP	Intraaortic balloon pump		主动脉内球囊反搏泵
ICD	Implantable cardioverter defibrillator		可植入心律转复除颤器
IVCD	Intraventricular conduction delay		心室内传导延迟
JVP	Jugular venous pulse		颈静脉搏动
LAD	Left anterior descending (coronary artery)		左前降支的（冠状动脉）
LAHB	Left anterior hemiblock		左前分支阻滞
LDL	Low-density lipoprotein		低密度脂蛋白
LV	Left ventricle		左心室
LVAD	Left ventricular assist device		左心室辅助装置
LVEDP	Left ventricular end-diastolic pressure		左室舒张末压
LVH	Left ventricular hypertrophy		左心室肥厚
MI	Myocardial infarction		心肌梗死
mmHg	Millimeters of mercury		毫米汞柱
MR	Mitral regurgitation, reflux		二尖瓣关闭不全，反流
MS	Mitral stenosis		二尖瓣狭窄
MUGA	Multigated acquisition (scan)		平衡法多时闸心室造影（扫描）
MVP	Mitral valve prolapse		二尖瓣脱垂
MVR	Mitral valve replacement		二尖瓣置换术
NSR	Normal sinus rhythm		正常窦性心律
P	Pulse		脉搏
PAC	Premature atrial contraction		房性期前收缩
PAP	Pulmonary arterial pressure		肺动脉压
PCI	Percutaneous coronary intervention		经皮冠状动脉介入治疗
PCWP	Pulmonary capillary wedge pressure		肺毛细血管楔压
PMI	Point of maximal impulse		最强（心尖）搏动点
PSVT	Paroxysmal supraventricular tachycardia		阵发性室上性心动过速
PTCA	Percutaneous transluminal coronary angioplasty		经皮腔内冠状动脉成形术

Terminology 缩略语（续表）

PVC	Premature ventricular contraction	室性期前收缩
PVD	Peripheral vascular disease	周围血管疾病
PYP	Pyrophosphate (scan)	焦磷酸盐（扫描）
S_1	First heart sound	第一心音
S_2	Second heart sound	第二心音
SA	Sinoatrial	窦房结
SBE	Subacute bacterial endocarditis	亚急性细菌性心内膜炎
SK	Streptokinase	链激酶
SVT	Supraventricular tachycardia	室上性心动过速
99mTc	Technetium-99m	锝-99m
TEE	Transesophageal echocardiography	经食管超声心动图
Tn	Troponin	肌钙蛋白
tPA	Tissue plasminogen activator	组织型纤溶酶原激活剂
VAD	Ventricular assist device	心室辅助装置
VF, v fib	Ventricular fibrillation	心室纤颤
VLDL	Very-low-density lipoprotein	极低密度脂蛋白
VPC	Ventricular premature complex	室性期前收缩复合波
VSD	Ventricular septal defect	室间隔缺损
VT	Ventricular tachycardia	室性心动过速
VTE	Venous thromboembolism	静脉血栓栓塞症
WPW	Wolff-Parkinson-White syndrome	心脏功能缺陷预激综合征

Case Study Revisited 案例研究再访

C. L.'s Follow-Up

C. L. underwent a successful ablation procedure without any complications, and he has not had a recurrence of the atrial fibrillation. C. L.'s preexisting heart condition prohibited him from performing required duties in the army, so he was not able to return to boot camp. He was released from the service and returned to civilian life.

C. L. 的随访

C. L. 经历了成功的消融手术，没有任何并发症，他的房颤没有复发。C. L. 先前的心脏病使他无法在军队中履行必要的职责，所以他不能回到训练营。他被解除了服役，并恢复了平民生活。

CHAPTER 9 复习

标记练习

心血管系统

在对应的下划线上写出每个编号部分的名称。

Aorta
Head and arms
Inferior vena cava
Internal organs
Left atrium
Left lung
Left pulmonary artery

Left pulmonary vein
Left ventricle
Legs
Right atrium
Right lung
Right ventricle
Superior vena cava

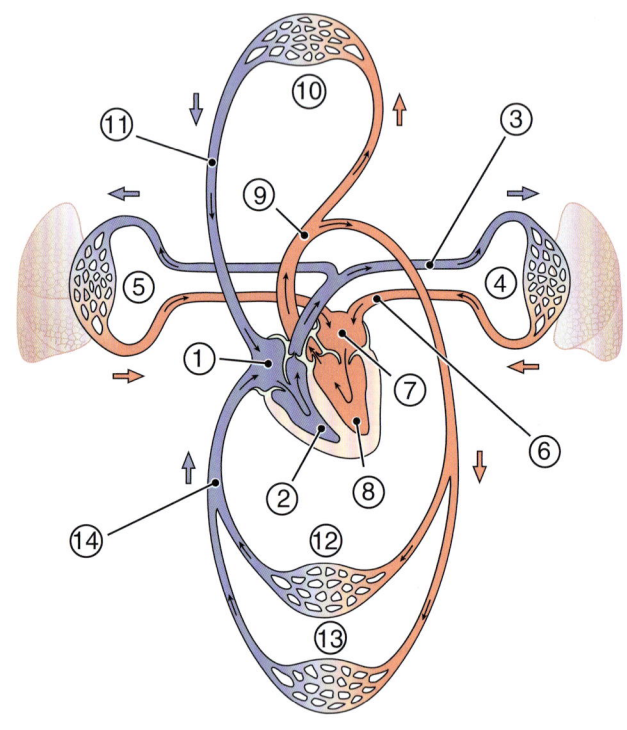

■ Blood high in oxygen
■ Blood low in oxygen

1. _____
2. _____
3. _____
4. _____
5. _____
6. _____
7. _____
8. _____
9. _____
10. _____
11. _____
12. _____
13. _____
14. _____

心脏和大血管

在对应的下划线上写出每个编号部分的名称。

Aortic arch
Aortic valve
Apex
Ascending aorta
Brachiocephalic artery
Endocardium
Epicardium
Inferior vena cava
Interventricular septum
Left atrium
Left AV (mitral) valve
Left common carotid artery
Left pulmonary artery (branches)
Left pulmonary veins
Left subclavian artery
Left ventricle
Myocardium
Pulmonary artery
Pulmonary valve
Right atrium
Right AV (tricuspid) valve
Right pulmonary artery (branches)
Right pulmonary veins
Right ventricle
Superior vena cava

1. _____
2. _____
3. _____
4. _____
5. _____
6. _____
7. _____
8. _____
9. _____
10. _____
11. _____
12. _____
13. _____
14. _____
15. _____
16. _____
17. _____
18. _____
19. _____
20. _____
21. _____
22. _____
23. _____
24. _____
25. _____

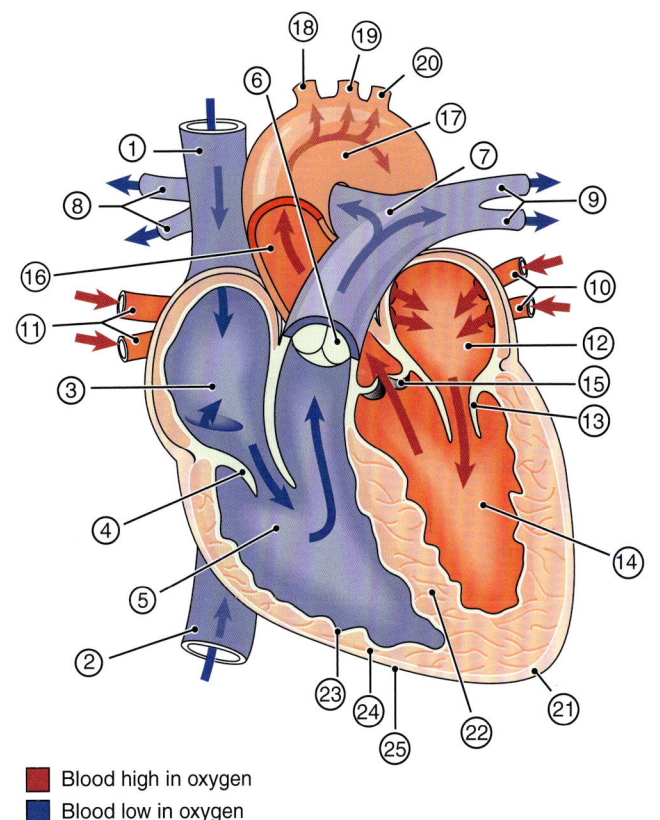

Blood high in oxygen
Blood low in oxygen

淋巴组织的位置

在对应的下划线上写出每个编号部分的名称。

Appendix　　　　　　　　Spleen
Lymph nodes　　　　　　Thymus
Peyer patches (in intestine)　Tonsils

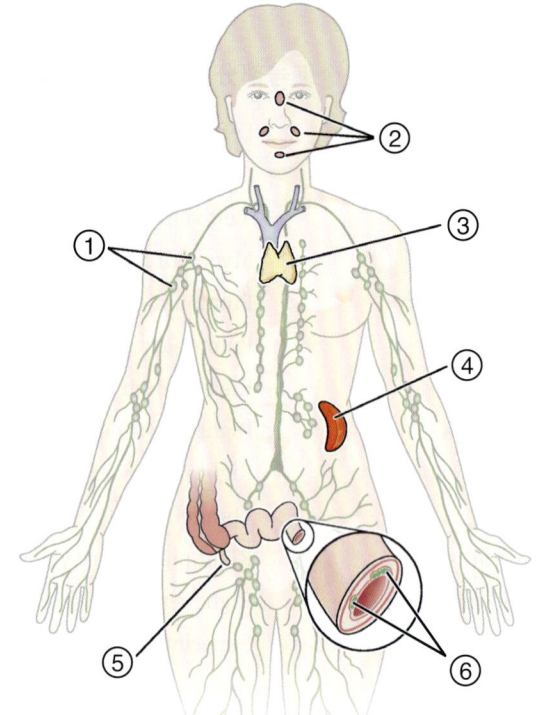

1. _____
2. _____
3. _____
4. _____
5. _____
6. _____

匹配

匹配下列术语，在每个题号的左侧写上适当的字母。

____ 1. atherosclerosis　　　　a. twisted and swollen vessel
____ 2. varix　　　　　　　　　b. blockage
____ 3. occlusion　　　　　　　c. absence of a heartbeat
____ 4. aneurysm　　　　　　　d. localized dilatation of a vessel
____ 5. asystole　　　　　　　　e. accumulation of fatty deposits

____ 6. thrombosis　　　　　　　a. ineffective quivering of muscle
____ 7. myocarditis　　　　　　　b. formation of a blood clot in a vessel
____ 8. infarction　　　　　　　　c. inflammation of the heart muscle
____ 9. fibrillation　　　　　　　d. local deficiency of blood
____ 10. ischemia　　　　　　　　e. local death of tissue

____ 11. lumen　　　　　　　　a. vessel that empties into the right atrium
____ 12. pericardium　　　　　　b. fibrous sac around the heart
____ 13. apex　　　　　　　　　c. structure that keeps fluid moving forward
____ 14. vena cava　　　　　　　d. central opening of a vessel
____ 15. valve　　　　　　　　　e. lower, pointed region of the heart

____ 16. HDL　　　　　　　　　a. stroke
____ 17. HTN　　　　　　　　　b. a type of blood lipid

____ 18. VT   c. rapid beat in the heart's lower chambers
____ 19. CVA   d. high blood pressure
____ 20. CABG   e. surgery to bypass a blocked vessel

补充术语

____ 21. diuretic   a. removal of plaque
____ 22. regurgitation   b. drug that increases urinary output
____ 23. streptokinase   c. premature contraction
____ 24. atherectomy   d. drug used to dissolve blood clots
____ 25. extrasystole   e. backward flow

填空

26. The heart muscle is the _____.
27. A microscopic vessel through which materials are exchanged between the blood and the tissues is a(n) _____.
28. Each upper receiving chamber of the heart is a(n) _____.
29. A sinus rhythm originates in the _____.
30. The largest artery is the _____.
31. A phlebotomist [fli'bɑtəmist] is one who drains blood from a(n) _____.
32. The term varicoid pertains to a(n) _____.
33. The lymphoid organ in the chest is the _____.
34. Blood returning to the heart from the systemic circuit enters the chamber called the _____.
35. At its termination in the abdomen, the aorta divides into the right and left（图 9-5）_____.
36. The large artery in the neck that supplies blood to the brain is the（图 9-5）_____.
37. The large vein that drains the lower body and empties into the heart is the（图 9-6）_____.
38. The right lymphatic duct and the thoracic duct drain into vessels called the（图 9-19）_____.
39. In C.L.'s case study, the device he wore to record his heart rhythm is called a(n) _____.
40. The abnormal heart rhythm that prevented C.L. from completing basic training is termed _____.
41. The catheterization technique used to correct C.L.'s arrhythmia is termed cardiac _____.

真假判断

检查以下语句。如果语句为真，则在第一个空白处写入 T；如果语句为假，则在第一个空格中写入 F，并通过在第二个空格中替换带下划线的单词来更正语句。

	True or False	Correct Answer
42. The left AV valve is the <u>aortic</u> valve.	_____	_____
43. The pulmonary vein carries blood to the <u>lungs</u>.	_____	_____
44. The brachial artery supplies blood to the <u>leg</u>.	_____	_____
45. <u>Diastole</u> is the relaxation phase of the heart cycle.	_____	_____
46. The <u>left ventricle</u> pumps blood into the aorta.	_____	_____
47. Blood returning from the lungs to the heart enters the <u>left atrium</u>.	_____	_____
48. The <u>systemic circuit</u> pumps blood to the lungs.	_____	_____
49. An <u>artery</u> is a vessel that carries blood back to the heart.	_____	_____

50. Peyer patches are in the intestine.
51. Bradycardia is a lower-than-average heart rate.
52. A beta-adrenergic blocking agent slows the heart rate.

排除

在下列每组中，为与其余不相配的单词加下划线，并解释你选择的理由。

53. SA node — Purkinje fibers — apex — AV node — AV bundle

54. murmur — systolic — sphygmomanometer — mmHg — diastolic

55. U — S1 — QRS — T — P

56. thymus — spleen — cusp — tonsil — Peyer patches

定义

定义下列术语。

57. avascular ［ə'vɑːskjʊlə］
58. atriotomy ［'ɑːtriətəmi］
59. splenectomy ［spli'nektəmi］
60. supraventricular ［sʌpreivent'rikjʊlə］
61. phlebectasis ［sʌpreivent'rikjʊlə］

写出下列定义的单词。

62. An instrument (-tome) for incising a valve
63. Suture (-rhaphy) of the aorta
64. Excision of a lymph node
65. Physician who specializes in study and treatment of the heart
66. Stoppage (-stasis) of lymph flow
67. Surgical fixation (-pexy) of the spleen

使用词根 aort/o 写出下列含义的单词。

68. Narrowing (-stenosis) of the aorta
69. Downward displacement (-ptosis) of the aorta
70. Radiograph (-gram) of the aorta
71. Before or in front of (pre-) the aorta

形容词

写出下列单词的形容词形式。

72. ventricle
73. septum

74. valve
75. thymus
76. sclerosis
77. spleen

复数

写出下列单词的复数形式。

78. thrombus
79. varix
80. stenosis
81. septum

缩略语

写出下列缩略语用于心血管系统时的含义。

82. AED
83. LVAD
84. DVT
85. VF
86. BBB
87. PTCA

单词构建

使用给出的单词组成部分写出下列定义的单词。

| -pathy | phleb | lymph/o | -oma | angi/o | -itis | aden/o | -plasty |

88. inflammation of a vein
89. any disease of a lymph node
90. neoplasm involving the lymphatic system
91. plastic repair of any vessel
92. inflammation of a lymphatic vessel
93. any disease of a vessel
94. inflammation of a lymph node
95. plastic repair of a vein
96. neoplasm of a lymph node
97. tumor involving any vessels

单词分析

定义下列单词，并给出每个单词组成部分的含义。如果需要，可以使用词典。

98. Phonocardiography [fəʊnəkɑːdiˈɒgrəfi]
    a. phon/o

    b. cardi/o＿＿＿＿＿＿＿＿＿＿＿＿＿＿＿＿＿＿＿＿＿＿＿＿＿＿＿＿＿＿＿＿＿＿＿＿＿

    c. –graphy＿＿＿＿＿＿＿＿＿＿＿＿＿＿＿＿＿＿＿＿＿＿＿＿＿＿＿＿＿＿＿＿＿＿＿＿

99. Endarterectomy ［endɑːtəˈrektɒmi］

    a. end/o＿＿＿＿＿＿＿＿＿＿＿＿＿＿＿＿＿＿＿＿＿＿＿＿＿＿＿＿＿＿＿＿＿＿＿＿＿＿

    b. arteri/o＿＿＿＿＿＿＿＿＿＿＿＿＿＿＿＿＿＿＿＿＿＿＿＿＿＿＿＿＿＿＿＿＿＿＿＿＿

    c. ecto-＿＿＿＿＿＿＿＿＿＿＿＿＿＿＿＿＿＿＿＿＿＿＿＿＿＿＿＿＿＿＿＿＿＿＿＿＿＿

    d. -tomy＿＿＿＿＿＿＿＿＿＿＿＿＿＿＿＿＿＿＿＿＿＿＿＿＿＿＿＿＿＿＿＿＿＿＿＿＿＿

100. Telangiectasia ［telˌændʒiˌekˈteiʒə］

    a. tel-＿＿＿＿＿＿＿＿＿＿＿＿＿＿＿＿＿＿＿＿＿＿＿＿＿＿＿＿＿＿＿＿＿＿＿＿＿＿＿

    b. angi/o＿＿＿＿＿＿＿＿＿＿＿＿＿＿＿＿＿＿＿＿＿＿＿＿＿＿＿＿＿＿＿＿＿＿＿＿＿＿

    c. -ectasia＿＿＿＿＿＿＿＿＿＿＿＿＿＿＿＿＿＿＿＿＿＿＿＿＿＿＿＿＿＿＿＿＿＿＿＿＿

101. Lymphangiophlebitis ［limphædʒaiɒfliˈbaitis］

    a. lymph/o＿＿＿＿＿＿＿＿＿＿＿＿＿＿＿＿＿＿＿＿＿＿＿＿＿＿＿＿＿＿＿＿＿＿＿＿＿＿

    b. angi/o＿＿＿＿＿＿＿＿＿＿＿＿＿＿＿＿＿＿＿＿＿＿＿＿＿＿＿＿＿＿＿＿＿＿＿＿＿＿

    c. phleb/o＿＿＿＿＿＿＿＿＿＿＿＿＿＿＿＿＿＿＿＿＿＿＿＿＿＿＿＿＿＿＿＿＿＿＿＿＿＿

    d. -itis＿＿＿＿＿＿＿＿＿＿＿＿＿＿＿＿＿＿＿＿＿＿＿＿＿＿＿＿＿＿＿＿＿＿＿＿＿＿＿

Additional Case Studies
补充案例研究

Case Study 9-1: PTCA and Echocardiogram
案例研究 9-1：经皮腔内冠状动脉成形术和超声心动图

A. L., a 68-year-old woman, was admitted to the CCU with chest pain, dyspnea, diaphoresis, syncope, and nausea. She had taken three sublingual doses of nitroglycerin tablets within a 10-minute time span without relief before dialing 911. A previous stress test and thallium uptake scan suggested cardiac disease.

Her family history was significant for cardiovascular disease. Her father died at the age of 62 of an acute myocardial infarction. Her mother had bilateral carotid endarterectomies and a femoral popliteal bypass procedure and died at the age of 72 of congestive heart failure. A. L.'s elder sister died from a ruptured aortic aneurysm at the age of 65. A.L.'s ECG on admission showed tachycardia with a rate of 126 bpm with inverted T waves. A murmur was heard at S1. Her skin color was dusky to cyanotic on her lips and fingertips. Her admitting diagnosis was possible coronary artery disease, acute myocardial infarction, and valvular disease.

Cardiac catheterization with balloon angioplasty (PTCA) was performed the next day. Significant stenosis of the left anterior descending coronary artery was shown and treated with angioplasty and stent placement. Left ventricular function was normal.

Echocardiography, two days later, showed normalsized left and enlarged right ventricular cavities. The mitral valve had normal amplitude of motion. The anterior and posterior leaflets moved in opposite directions during diastole. There was a late systolic prolapse of the mitral leaflet at rest. The left atrium was enlarged. The impression of the study was mitral prolapse with regurgitation. Surgery was recommended.

A. L. 是一名 68 岁的女性，因胸痛、呼吸困难、大汗、晕厥和恶心被送入 CCU。她在拨打 911 之前，在 10 分钟的时间间隔舌下服用了 3 次硝酸甘油片剂，症状没有得到缓解。先前的压力测试和铊摄取扫描提示有心脏病。

她的家族病史对心血管疾病很重要。她的父亲在 62 岁死于急性心肌梗死，母亲做过双侧颈动脉内膜切除术和股动脉旁路手术，并在 72 岁时死于充血性心力衰竭。她的姐姐在 65 岁时死于主动脉瘤破裂。A. L. 入院时心电图显示心动过速，T 波倒置，心率为 126bpm。在 S_1 听到一个杂音。她的嘴唇和指尖的皮肤颜色暗淡。她的入院诊断怀疑冠状动脉疾病、急性心肌梗死和瓣膜疾病。

第 2 天进行了气囊血管成形术（PTCA）的心导管插入术。发现左前降支冠状动脉显示狭窄，并用血管成形术和支架放置进行治疗。左心室功能正常。

2 天后，超声心动图显示左、右心室腔大小正常。二尖瓣运动幅度正常。在舒张期，前部和后部的瓣叶朝着相反的方向移动。在休息时，二尖瓣瓣叶有收缩期晚期脱垂，左心房扩大。该研究的意见是二尖瓣脱垂与反流。推荐手术。

Case Study 9-2: Mitral Valve Replacement Operative Report
案例研究 9-2：二尖瓣置换手术报告

A. L. was transferred to the operating room, placed in a supine position, and given general endotracheal anesthesia. The surgeon entered her pericardium longitudinally through a median sternotomy and found that her heart was enlarged, with a dilated right ventricle. The left atrium was dilated. Preoperative transesophageal echocardiography revealed severe mitral regurgitation with severe posterior and anterior prolapse. Extracorporeal circulation was established. The aorta was cross-clamped, and cardioplegic solution (to stop the heartbeat) was given into the aortic root intermittently for myocardial protection.

The left atrium was entered via the interatrial groove on the right, exposing the mitral valve. The middle scallop of the

A. L. 被转移到手术室，置于仰卧位，并给予气管插管全身麻醉。医生通过胸骨正中切口纵向进入她的心包，发现她的心脏增大，右心室扩张，左心房扩张。术前经食管超声心动图显示二尖瓣重度闭锁不全，伴有严重的后壁和前壁脱垂。建立体外循环，主动脉交叉夹紧，间断地向主动脉根部给与心脏停搏液（停止心跳）进行心肌保护。

通过右侧的房间沟槽进入左心房，暴露二尖瓣。切除后瓣叶的中间扇形，剩余的瓣叶移至缝合区，并被保

posterior leaflet was resected. The remaining leaflets were removed to the areas of the commissures and preserved for the sliding plasty. The elongated chordae were shortened to better anchor the valve cusps. The surgeon slid the posterior leaflet across the midline and sutured it in place. A No. 30 annuloplasty ring was sutured in place with interrupted No. 2–0 Dacron suture. The valve was tested by inflating the ventricle with NSS and proved to be competent. The left atrium was closed with continuous No. 4–0 Prolene suture. Air was removed from the heart. The cross-clamp was removed. Cardiac action resumed with normal sinus rhythm. After a period of cardiac recovery and attainment of normothermia, cardiopulmonary bypass was discontinued.

　　Protamine was given to counteract the heparin. Pacer wires were placed in the right atrium and ventricle. Silicone catheters were placed in the pleural and substernal spaces. The sternum and soft tissue wound was closed. A.L. recovered from her surgery and was discharged six days later.

存用于滑动成形术。细长的腱索被缩短以更好地锚定瓣尖。外科医生将后瓣叶滑过中线并缝合在适当位置。用中断的 2-0 号涤纶缝合线将 30 号瓣环成形环缝合在适当位置。 通过用 NSS 给心室充气来测试瓣膜，并证明是有能力的。左心房用连续的 4-0 号聚丙烯缝合线封闭。空气从心脏移除。除去交叉钳，心脏恢复正常窦性心律。在心脏恢复和达到正常体温后，停止心肺转流术。

　　给予鱼精蛋白以抵消肝素的作用。起搏器的导线被置于右心房和心室中，硅氧烷导管被置于胸膜和胸骨下空间，胸骨和软组织创伤被闭合。A.L. 从手术中恢复，6 天后出院。

案例研究问题

写出案例研究中下列含义的单词或短语。

1. Shortness of breath _____

2. An abnormal heart sound _____

3. Test of cardiac function during physical exertion _____

4. Pertaining to both the heart and blood vessels _____

5. Excision of the inner lining along with atherosclerotic plaque from an artery (plural) _____

6. Under the tongue _____

7. Bluish discoloration of the skin due to lack of oxygen _____

8. The state of profuse perspiration _____

9. Between the atria _____

10. Below the sternum _____

多项选择。选择正确的答案，并在每个题号的左侧写上你选择的字母。

____ 11. The word transluminal means

　　　a. across a wall

　　　b. between branches

　　　c. through a valve

　　　d. through a central opening

____ 12. The term that means backflow, as of blood, is

　　　a. infarction

　　　b. regurgitation

　　　c. amplitude

　　　d. prolapse

_____ **13.** The term for a narrowing of the bicuspid valve is

   a. atrial stenosis

   b. tricuspid prolapse

   c. mitral stenosis

   d. pulmonic prolapse

_____ **14.** Blowout of a dilated segment of the main artery is

   a. peritoneal infarction

   b. coarctation of the aorta

   c. cardiac tamponade

   d. ruptured aortic aneurysm

_____ **15.** Sternotomy is

   a. incision into the sternum

   b. removal of the sternum

   c. narrowing of the sternum

   d. surgical fixation of the sternum

_____ **16.** Extracorporeal circulation occurs

   a. within the brain

   b. within the pericardium

   c. outside the body

   d. in the legs

_____ **17.** Protamine was given to counteract the action of the heparin. This drug action is described as

   a. antagonistic

   b. synergy

   c. potentiating

   d. simulation

缩略语。定义下列缩略语。

18. ECG _____

19. AMI _____

20. CAD _____

21. LAD _____

22. CHF _____

23. TEE _____

24. MVR _____

25. CCU _____

CHAPTER 10

血液与免疫

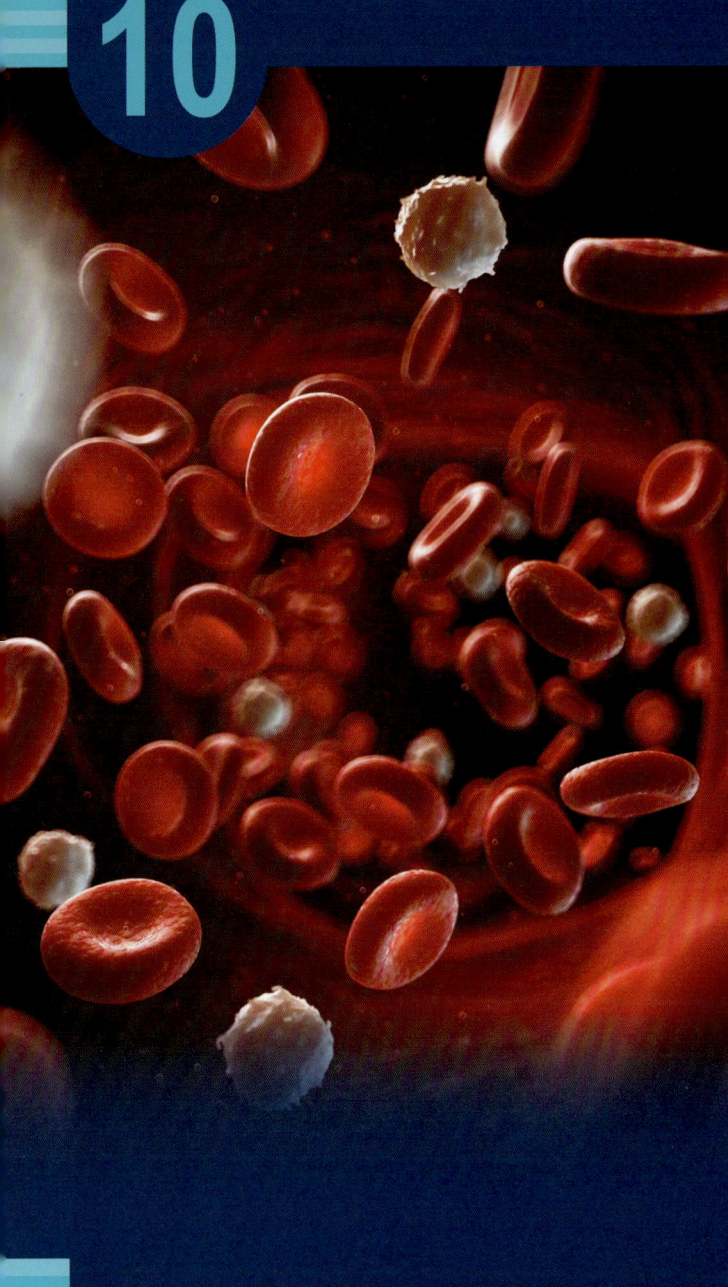

预测试

多项选择。选择正确的答案,并在每个题号的左侧写上你选择的字母。

____ 1. Erythrocyte is the scientific name for a
   a. white blood cell
   b. lymphocyte
   c. red blood cell
   d. muscle cell

____ 2. Platelets, or thrombocytes, are involved in
   a. digestion
   b. inflammation
   c. immunity
   d. blood clotting

____ 3. The white blood cells active in im munity are the
   a. chondrocytes
   b. lymphocytes
   c. adipose cells
   d. hematids

____ 4. Substances produced by immune cells that counteract microorganisms and other foreign materials are called
   a. antigens
   b. antibodies
   c. anticoagulants
   d. Rh factors

____ 5. A deficiency of hemoglobin results in the disorder called
   a. hypertension
   b. chromatosis
   c. anemia
   d. hemophilia

____ 6. A neoplastic overgrowth of white blood cells is called
   a. leukemia
   b. anemia
   c. fibrosis
   d. cystitis

▶ 学习目标

学完本章后，应该能够：

1. ▶ 描述血浆的构成。
2. ▶ 描述 3 种血液细胞并叙述它们的功能。
3. ▶ 区别不同类型的白细胞形态。
4. ▶ 解释构成血型的基础。
5. ▶ 定义免疫，并列出可能的免疫来源。
6. ▶ 识别并使用与血液和免疫相关的词根和后缀。
7. ▶ 识别并使用与血液化学相关的词根。
8. ▶ 列出并描述 3 种主要的血液疾病。
9. ▶ 描述血液研究使用的主要测试。
10. ▶ 列出并描述 3 种主要的免疫系统疾病。
11. ▶ 解释血压研究中使用的缩略语。
12. ▶ 分析几个案例研究中涉及血液的医学术语。

Case Study: Nurse Anesthetist M. R. with Latex Allergy
案例研究：护理麻醉师 M. R. 与乳胶过敏

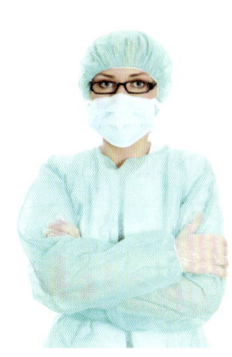

Chief Complaint

M. R., a 36-year-old certified registered nurse anesthetist (CRNA), noticed that her hands had a red patchy rash when she removed her gloves following cases in the OR. They began to itch after a few minutes of donning the gloves, so she figured she might have developed an allergy to the latex they contained. When she began to have a runny nose and itchy swollen eyes, she was worried and sought medical advice from her primary care physician, who referred her to an allergist.

Examination

The allergist examined M. R.'s hands and observed a localized red crusty rash that stopped at the wrists. There were a few blisters spread over the hand region. Along with the examination, a history indicated M. R. had noticed the contact dermatitis for a while when she wore powdered latex gloves in the OR, and she more recently had noted generalized allergic symptoms during surgical cases. During a recent case, she experienced some tachycardia, urticaria (hives) and rhinitis when she came in contact with latex gloves.

Clinical Course

M. R. was diagnosed with a type I hypersensitivity, IgE, T cell-mediated latex allergy, as shown by both immunologic and skin-prick tests. Although M.R. is a CRNA, she was educated on the course of latex allergies. She was reminded that there is no cure and that the only way to prevent an allergic reaction is to avoid coming into contact with latex.

This chapter describes the composition and characteristics of blood, the life-sustaining fluid that circulates throughout the body. A discussion of immunity is included because many components of the immune system are carried in the blood. M. R.'s case of allergy is an example of immunologic hyperactivity. One of the symptoms, tachycardia, was discussed in Chapter 9 and rhinitis will be introduced in the next chapter on the respiratory system.

主诉

M.R.是一名36岁的注册护理麻醉师（CRNA），在几个手术室病例后摘下手套时，她注意到手上有一个红色斑驳疹。戴上手套几分钟后斑疹开始瘙痒，所以她认为她可能对手套所含的乳胶过敏。当她开始出现流鼻涕和眼睛瘙痒肿胀时，她有些担心，并向她的初级保健医生寻求医疗建议，保健医生将她转诊给过敏症专科医生。

检查

过敏症专科医生检查了 M.R. 的手，观察到手腕上有一个局部的红色硬皮疹，在手部还有一些水泡。随着检查，病历显示在一段时间内，M.R.已经注意到当她在手术室戴加粉的乳胶手套时会产生接触性皮炎，近期她注意到在手术过程中出现了广泛的过敏症状。在最近的一个手术病例中，在接触乳胶手套时，她经历了心动过速、风疹（荨麻疹）和鼻炎。

临床病程

M. R. 被诊断为 I 型过敏反应、IgE 与 T 细胞介导的乳胶过敏，免疫学和皮肤穿刺测试结果都证明了诊断。虽然 M.R. 是一名注册护理麻醉师，她受过关于乳胶过敏课程的教育。她被提醒并没有治愈，防止过敏反应的唯一办法是避免接触乳胶。

本章讲述了在整个身体中循环的、维持生命的血液的组成和特性，也包括免疫的讨论，因为免疫系统的许多组成部分在血液中传输。M. R. 的过敏症是免疫亢进的一个例子，其中的一个症状心动过速，在第 9 章讨论过，鼻炎将在下一章呼吸系统中介绍。

简介

血液（blood）是通过血管循环的液体，为所有的细胞带来氧气和营养，并带走二氧化碳和其他废物。血液还为身体分配热量，并携带例如抗体与激素等特殊物质。特定的血液细胞是免疫系统（immune system）的主要组成部分，参与抵抗疾病。本章后面将讨论免疫系统。

血液

成年人体内血液总量大约是 5L。血液可以分为两个主要部分，液体部分，或血浆（plasma）占 55%，有形成分（formed elements），通常被称为血液细胞占 45%（图 10-1）。

血浆

血浆的 90% 是水，其余 10% 包含营养、电解质（electrolyte）、气体、白蛋白（albumin）（一种蛋白质）、凝血因子（clotting factor）、抗体、废物、酶（enzyme）以及激素。血浆的 pH 值稳定在 7.4 左右。

血液细胞

血液细胞（图 10-2）包括红细胞（erythrocyte，或红血球 RBC）、白细胞（leukocyte，或白血球 WBC）和血小板（platelet，或凝血细胞 thrombocyte）。所有血液细胞都是在红骨髓（red bone marrow）中产生的，某些白细胞在淋巴组织中也大量存在。框 10-1 给出了血液细胞的概要介绍，框 10-2 讨论了首字母缩写，例如 RBC 和 WBC。

红细胞

红细胞的主要功能是为细胞携带氧气，氧气被绑定细胞中在被称为血红蛋白（hemoglobin）的含铁色素上。红细胞很小、盘形，没有细胞核（图 10-3）。红细胞的浓度是每毫升 500 万，是血液中数量最多的血液细胞。每 100ml 血液平均含有 15g 血红蛋白。红细胞会有损耗，通常会在 120 天内死亡，所以必须不断补充。骨髓中红细胞的产生通过激素红细胞生成素（erythropoietin，EPO）调节，红细胞生成素由肾产生。

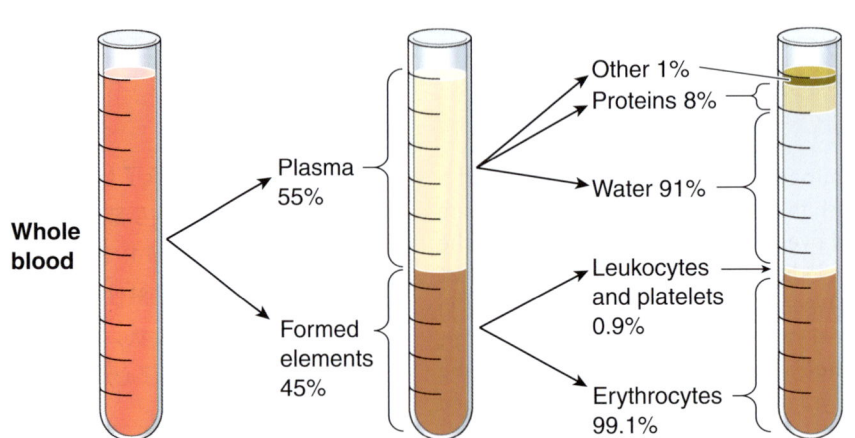

图 10-1 **全血的构成**。百分比显示了血浆和有形成分的不同组分的相对比例

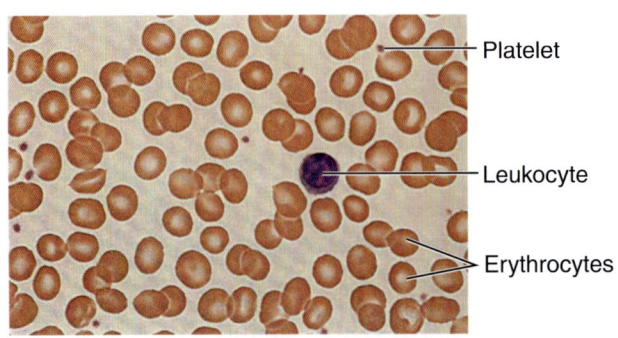

图 10-2 **血液细胞**。在使用显微镜观察时，所有三种有形成分都是可见的

框 10-1

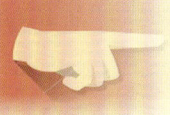

供你参考
血液细胞

细胞种类	每毫升数量	说明	功能
erythrocyte 红细胞（red blood cell）	500 万	极小（直径 7μm），没有核的双面凹盘	携带绑定在血蛋白上的氧气，也运送二氧化碳并缓冲血液
leukocyte 白细胞（white blood cell）	5 000~10 000	比红细胞大，有明显的分段的（粒性）或不分段的（无颗粒）核，根据染色特性分类	免疫。抵抗病原体并摧毁外来物质和碎片。存在于血液、组织和淋巴系统
platelet 血小板（thrombocyte）	150 000~450 000	大细胞（巨核细胞）的分段	止血。形成血小板堵塞并开始凝血

框 10-2

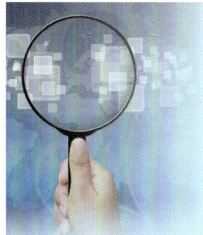

聚焦单词
首字母缩写

首字母缩写（acronym）是使用名称或短语中每个单词的第一个字母的缩写。因为在技术术语的数量和复杂性增加时节省时间和空间，它们变得非常受欢迎。适用于血液研究的一些示例是 CBC（全血细胞计数,complete blood count）以及 RBC（red blood cell）和 WBC（white blood cell）。一些其他常见的首字母缩略词包括 CNS（中枢神经系统,central nervous system 或临床护理专家 clinical nurse specialist）、ECG（心电图,electrocardiogram）、NIH（国立卫生研究院,National Institutes of Health）和 STI（性传播感染,sexually transmitted infection）等。

如果首字母缩写具有元音并且适合发音，它本身可以用作一个词，例如 AIDS（获得性免疫缺陷综合征，acquired immunodeficiency syndrome）、ELISA（酶联免疫吸附测定,enzyme-linked immunosorbent assay）、JAMA（美国医学协会杂志,Journal of the American Medical Association）、NSAID ［ensed］（非甾体抗炎药,nonsteroidal antiinflammatory drug）和 CABG（冠状动脉旁路移植术,coronary artery bypass graft），这不可避免地变成"卷心菜（cabbage）"。很少有人知道 LASER（激光）是首字母缩写，意思是"受激辐射的发射光放大 light amplification by stimulated emission of radiation"。

首字母缩略词通常是短语在文章中第一次出现时被引入，然后在没有解释的情况下使用。如果你要花费时间在一篇文章中沮丧地搜索一个首字母缩写的含义，你可能希望像其他读者一样，所有的首字母缩略词及其含义将会被列在每篇文章的开头。

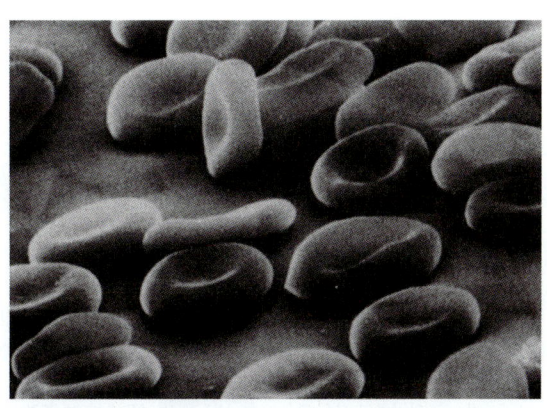

图 10-3 红细胞。在电子扫描显微镜下观察细胞，能够给出三维视图

供你参考

白细胞

框 10-3

细胞	相对百分比（成人）	功能
粒细胞		
neutrophils ['nju:trəfilz] 中性粒细胞	54%~62%	吞噬作用
eosinophils [i:əʊzi'nəfilz] 嗜酸性粒细胞	1%~3%	过敏反应，抵抗寄生虫
basophils ['bæsəfilz] 嗜碱性粒细胞	少于 1%	过敏反应
无粒白细胞		
lymphocytes ['limfəsaits] 淋巴细胞	25%~38%	免疫（T 细胞和 B 细胞）
monocytes [mɒnə'saits] 单核细胞	3%~7%	吞噬作用

白细胞

白细胞被染色后都会显示突出的核。白细胞的数量是每毫升 5 000~10 000 个，但在感染时数量会增加。有五种白细胞，它们所占的百分比和功能各异。白细胞的分类基于其大小和核的形状、染色特性以及在染色后细胞质中是否显示可见的颗粒，参见框 10-3。被分类为粒细胞（granulocytes）或无粒白细胞（agranulocytes）的有：

- 粒细胞或颗粒性白细胞在染色后细胞质中有可见的颗粒，具有分段的核。粒细胞分 3 种，根据颗粒吸收的颜色剂类型命名：
  - 弱酸性和弱碱性染色剂的中性粒细胞（neutrophils）
  - 强酸性染色剂的嗜酸性粒细胞（eosinophils）。
  - 碱性染色剂的嗜碱性粒细胞（basophils）。
- 无颗粒白细胞在染色后不显示可见的颗粒，它们的核较大，是圆的或弯曲的。有两种无颗粒白细胞：
  - 淋巴细胞（lymphocyte）是一种较小的无颗粒白细胞。

- 单核细胞（monocyte）是最大的白细胞。

白细胞抵抗外来物质的侵犯。某些通过吞噬作用（phagocytosis）吞噬外来物质（图 6-5），另一些在

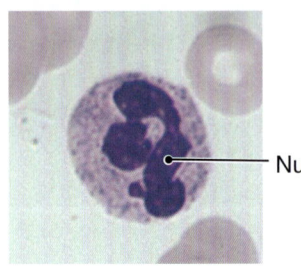

A Mature neutrophil

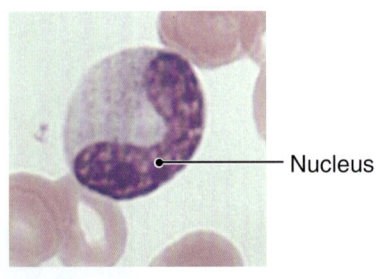

B Band cell (immature neutrophil)

图 10-4　**杆状核粒细胞。**A. 成熟嗜中性粒细胞；B. 杆状核粒细胞或杆状细胞是未成熟的中性粒细胞，具有粗的弯曲的核

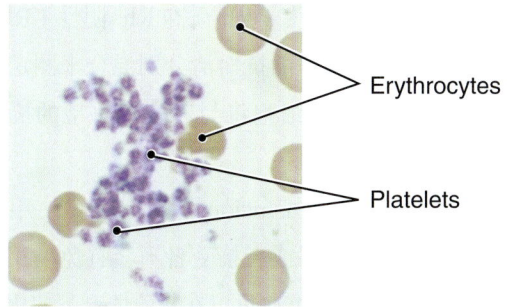

A Platelets

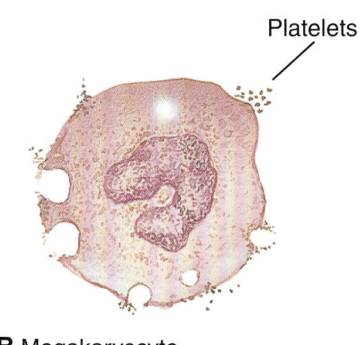

B Megakaryocyte

图 10-5　血小板。A. 在显微镜下在血液涂片中看到的血小板；B. 巨核细胞释放血小板

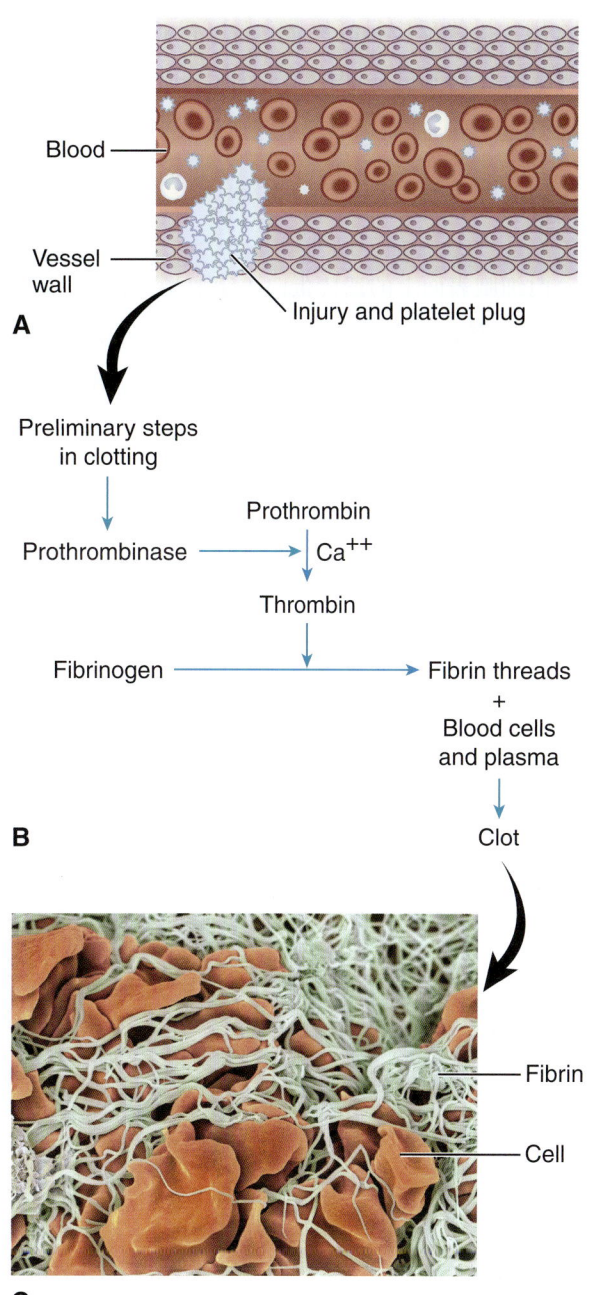

图 10-6　血液凝固（凝血）。血液凝固涉及导致纤维蛋白丝形成的复杂系列反应。纤维蛋白捕获血细胞以形成凝块。A. 从受损组织释放的物质开始凝血过程；B. 纤维蛋白形成的最后步骤，这些步骤之一需要钙（Ca^{2+}）；C. 血纤维蛋白捕获的血细胞的显微视图

免疫系统有不同的功能。在诊断中，不仅要了解白细胞的数量，还要了解每一类的相对数量，因为这些数字在不同的疾病中会有所变化。这些数字的实验室报告被称为白细胞分类计数（differential count Diff），是全血细胞计数（complete blood count，CBC）的一部分。大多数白细胞，嗜中性粒细胞被称为同质多形体（polymorphs），因为它们的核形状不同。它们也被称为分叶中性粒细胞（segs）、多形核白细胞（polys）或多形核白细胞（polymorphonuclear leukocytes，PMN）。杆状核粒细胞（band cell）也被称为杆状细胞（stab cell），是一种未成熟的带有固体弯曲的细胞核的嗜中性粒细胞（图 10-4），血液中杆状核粒细胞数量高表明有活动性感染。

血小板

血小板不是完整的细胞，而是一种被称为巨核细胞（megakaryocytes）的分段，巨核细胞也是在骨髓中生成的（图 10-5）。每 100ml 血液血小板的数量是 200 000~400 000。血小板能够凝结血液（coagulation），对止血（hemostasis）和防止血液流失非常重要。

当血管受伤时，血小板会聚集在一起，在受伤处形成堵塞。然后，血小板和受伤的组织释放的物质与血清中的凝血因子相互作用，产生一个封闭伤口的血凝块。凝血因子在受伤前是没有活性的。为了防止形成不需要的血凝块，十二种凝血因子在血液凝结前相

互作用，最终反应是纤维蛋白原（fibrinogen）转化为纤维蛋白（fibrin），困住血液细胞和血浆产生血凝块（图10-6）。血液凝结后剩余的血浆是血清（serum）。

血型

白细胞表面上的遗传蛋白决定血型。目前，超过20组的这种遗传蛋白质已被鉴定，最常见的是ABO和Rh血型。ABO系统包括类型A、B、AB和O血型，Rh类型是Rh^-阳性（Rh^+）和Rh^-阴性（Rh^-）。通过将样本与不同制备的抗血清分别混合来测定血液的血型。样本中的红细胞将与对应于血型的抗血清凝集（结块，图10-7）。

在输血（blood transfusions）时，必须使用与接受者相同血型的血液，或者接受者不会有免疫反应血型的血液。Rh阴性O型血可以在紧急情况下使用，因为这种血型的红细胞不会引起免疫反应。有时间的情

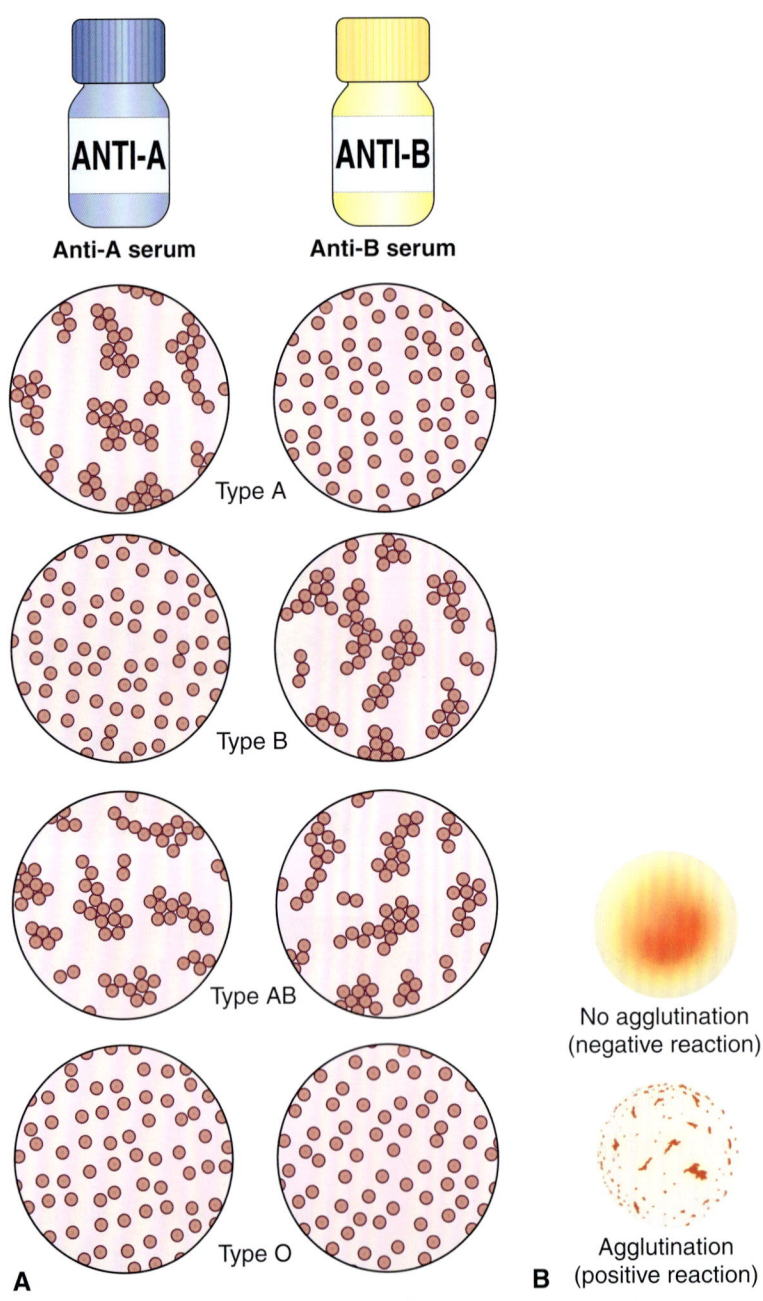

图10-7 血型。通过将样本与针对不同红细胞抗原制备的抗血清分别混合来测定血型，抗血清凝集表明存在相应的抗原。A. 每列顶部的标签表示添加到血液样品中的抗血清的种类，抗A血清凝集A型血液中的红细胞，但是抗B血清不凝集，抗B血清凝集B型血液中的红细胞，但抗A血清不凝集，两种血清都凝集AB型血细胞，但都不凝集O型血细胞；B. 血型分型反应的照片

况下，实验室要进行考虑额外血液蛋白的完全兼容性测试。在这种交叉匹配（cross-matching）过程中，要有供血者的红细胞与接受者的血清混合，以测试反应。

全血可以用于补充大量失血，但在大多数需要输血的情况下，只需要使用血液的一部分，例如压积红细胞（packed red cells）、血小板、血浆或特定的凝血因子（clotting factor）。

免疫

免疫（immunity）就是预防疾病，包括防御有害微生物及其产生物，还有任何外来物质。这些防御能力可能是天生的，也可能是生活中获得的（图10-8）。

先天免疫

先天防御机制（nonspecific defense mechanisms）抵抗任何入侵微生物或有害的外来物质，而不是特定的一种。这种防御是天生的（inborn）或先天的（innate），是基于个人的遗传基因构成的。这些保护能力大都是物理障碍或化学防御，包括：

- 完好的皮肤，起屏障作用。
- 纤毛（cilia），细小的细胞凸出物，将杂质扫出体外，例如呼吸道中的纤毛。
- 黏液（mucus），困住外来物质。
- 杀菌的（bactericidal）身体分泌物，如在眼睛、皮肤、消化道和生殖道的分泌物。
- 条件反射（reflex），例如咳嗽和打喷嚏，将杂质驱除。
- 淋巴组织，过滤血液和淋巴液中的杂质（参见第9章）。
- 吞噬细胞（phagocyte），攻击、吞噬并摧毁外来微生物。

适应性免疫

适应性或特异性免疫（specific or adaptive immunity）是在生命期间获得的，直接针对特定的致病微生物或其他外来物质。例如预防麻疹的免疫能力就不能预防水痘或任何其他疾病。

适应性免疫反应涉及淋巴系统与血液复杂的相互作用。任何外来物质，主要是蛋白质，都可能作为抗原（antigen），也就是触发免疫反应的物质。这种反应来自于在血液和淋巴系统中循环的两种淋巴细胞：

- T细胞（T淋巴细胞）在胸腺（thymus）中成熟，它们能够直接攻击外来细胞，产生细胞介导免疫。巨噬细胞（macrophages）是单核细胞的后代，对T细胞的功能非常重要。巨噬细胞吞噬并处理外来抗原，当在巨噬细胞表面接触到抗原与身体自身的蛋白质在一起时，T细胞就会被激活。
- B细胞（B淋巴细胞）在骨髓中成熟。当遇到外来抗原时，它们迅速繁殖并成熟为浆细胞（plasma cell）。这些浆细胞会产生抗体（antibody），也被称为免疫球蛋白（immunoglobulins，Ig），能够使抗原失活（图10-9）。抗体保留在血液中，通常会针对该特定的抗原提供长期免疫。基于抗体的免疫也被称为体液免疫（humoral immunity）。

适应性免疫的种类

特异性免疫可以通过自然后人工方式获得（图10-8）。另外，获得免疫的途径可能是主动或被动的。在主动免疫中，人在接触抗原时自己产生抗体；在被

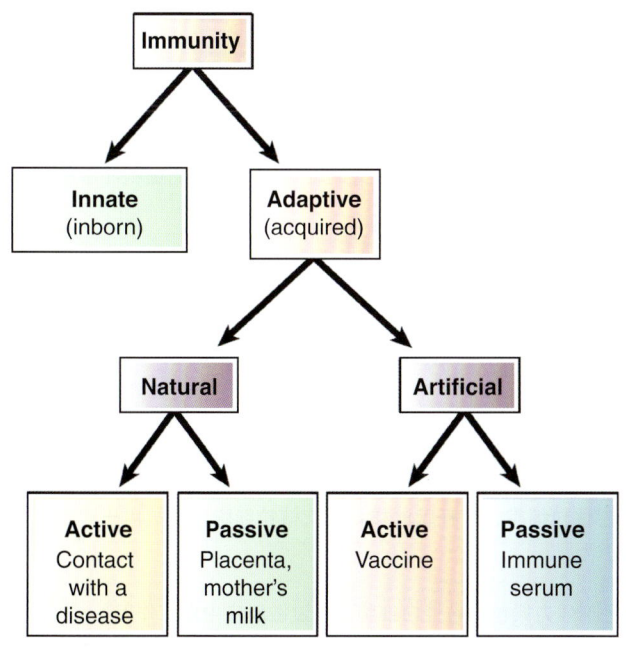

图10-8 免疫的类型

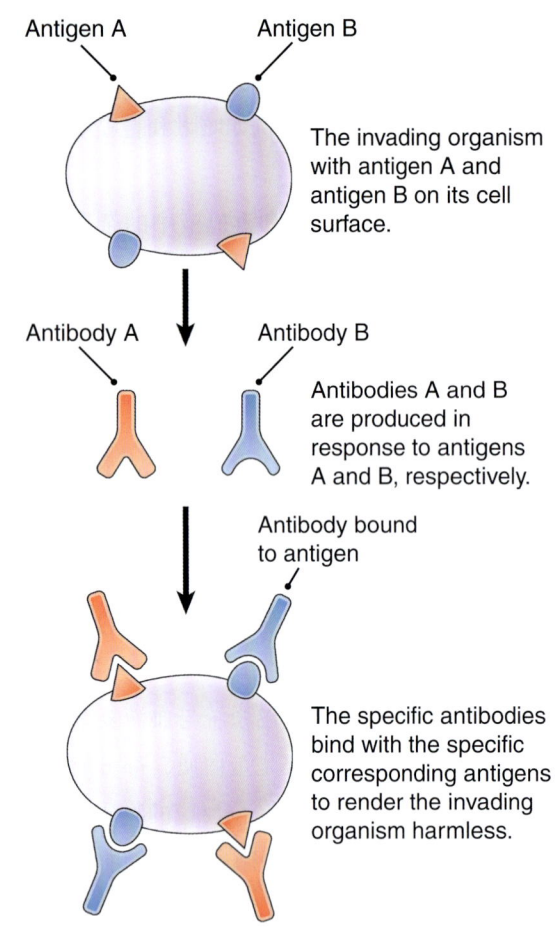

图 10-9 抗原-抗体反应。由免疫细胞产生的抗体与特异性抗原结合以使抗原消除

动免疫中，被称为免疫血清的抗体从外部传入体内。免疫血清可能来自他人或免疫的动物。包含抗体的部分血清是丙种球蛋白（gamma globulin）馏分。适应性免疫的种类有：

- 自然特异性免疫
  - 主动：来自于接触致病微生物或外来抗原；
  - 被动：来自于母亲通过胎盘（placenta）或母奶传送的抗体。

- 人工特异性免疫
  - 主动：通过使用疫苗（vaccine），疫苗可能是被杀死或削弱的微生物、微生物的一部分或被改变了的毒素（类毒素 toxoid）；
  - 被动：通过使用来自于他人或动物的免疫血清。

长期以来，免疫学（immunology）一直是一个活跃的研究领域。上述内容只是在免疫反应中所发生事件的最简单的概述，还有很多细节有待发现。一些研究领域包括对自身组织产生抗体的自身免疫病（autoimmune diseases）、遗传或获得性免疫缺陷（immunodeficiency）疾病、癌症与免疫的关系以及避免对移植组织排斥技术的发展。

Terminology 关键术语

正常结构和功能

agranulocyte [ei'grænjʊləʊsait]	无粒白细胞，细胞质中没有可见颗粒的白细胞。无颗粒白细胞包括淋巴细胞和单核细胞（框 10-3）
albumin [æl'bju:min]	白蛋白，血浆中的一种简单的蛋白质
antibody ['æntibɒdi]	抗体，与特定抗原响应与相互作用中产生的蛋白质
antigen ['æntidʒən]	抗原，引起抗体形成的物质
B cell	B 细胞，在淋巴组织中成熟的淋巴细胞，在生产抗体中发挥作用；也被称为 B 淋巴细胞
band cell	杆状核粒细胞，未成熟的中性粒细胞，有杆状的核。杆状核粒细胞计数被用于追踪感染和其他疾病（图 10-4）
basophil [bæsə'fil]	嗜碱性粒细胞，被碱性染色剂强力染色的粒性白细胞，在过敏反应中发挥作用
blood [blʌd]	血液，在心血管系统中循环的液体（词根：hem/o, hemat/o）

Terminology 关键术语（续表）

coagulation [kəuˌægjʊˈleiʃn]	凝结，血液凝结成块
cross-matching	交叉匹配，在输血准备工作中测试供血者与接受者血型的兼容性。供血者的红细胞与接受者的血清混合，观察是否有免疫反应。在组织移植前也要做类似的测试
electrolyte [iˈlektrəlait]	电解质，在溶液中分离成带电粒子（离子）的物质。这一术语也指体液中的离子
eosinophil [ˌi:əˈsinəfil]	嗜酸性粒细胞，被酸性染色剂强力染色的粒性白细胞，在过敏反应和防御寄生虫过程中发挥作用
erythrocyte [iˈriθrəsait]	红细胞，为人体组织供应氧气的血液细胞（词根：erythr/o, erythrocyt/o，图 10-2 和图 10-3）
erythropoietin (EPO) [iriθrəˈpɔiətin]	促红细胞生成素，肾产生的一种激素，能够刺激骨髓中红细胞的产生。现在，这种激素已经能够通过基因工程制造，在临床使用
fibrin [ˈfaibrin]	纤维蛋白，在血液凝结过程中形成血凝块的蛋白质
fibrinogen [faiˈbrinədʒən]	纤维蛋白原，纤维蛋白的非活性前体
formed elements	有形成分，血液中红细胞、白细胞和血小板的总称
gamma globulin	丙种球蛋白，包含抗体的部分血浆；用于被动免疫传送
granulocyte [ˈgrænjʊləsait]	粒细胞，细胞质中有可见颗粒的白细胞。粒性白细胞包含中性粒细胞、嗜碱性粒细胞和嗜酸性粒细胞（框 10-3）
hemoglobin (Hb, Hgb) [ˌhi:məʊˈgləʊbin]	血红蛋白，红细胞中传送氧气的含铁色素
hemostasis [ˌhi:məˈsteisis]	止血，阻止出血
immunity [iˈmju:nəti]	免疫，处于预防疾病的状态（词根：immun/o）
immunoglobulin (Ig) [iˈmju:nəʊˈglɒbjʊlin]	免疫球蛋白，一种抗体。免疫球蛋白有 5 种，每一种都用一个大写字母缩写：IgG, IgM, IgA, IgD, IgE
eukocyte [ˈlu:kəˌsait]	白细胞，能够抵御外来物质侵害的血液细胞（词根：leuk/o, leukocyt/o）
lymphocyte [ˈlimfəsait]	淋巴细胞，活跃在免疫系统的粒性白细胞（T 细胞和 B 细胞），存在于血液和淋巴组织之中（词根：lymph/o, lymphocyt/o）
megakaryocyte [megəˈkæriəʊsait]	巨核细胞，大骨髓细胞，分段后释放出血小板
macrophage [ˈmækrəfeidʒ]	巨噬细胞，源于单核细胞的噬菌细胞，通常存在于组织之中。巨噬细胞为 T 细胞处理抗原
monocyte [ˈmɒnəsait]	单核细胞，一种无颗粒噬菌白细胞
neutrophil [ˈnju:trəfil]	中性粒细胞，可被酸性和碱性染色剂弱染色的粒性白细胞。中性粒细胞是白细胞中数量最多的一种，是一种噬菌细胞
phagocytosis [ˌfægəsaiˈtəʊsis]	吞噬作用，白细胞吞噬外来物质
plasma [ˈplæzmə]	血浆，血液的液体部分

Terminology	关键术语（续表）
plasma cell	浆细胞，能够产生抗体的成熟的 B 细胞
platelet ［ˈpleitlət］	血小板，血液有形成分的一种，在凝血中发挥作用；凝血细胞（thrombocyte，词根：thrombocyt/o）
serum ［ˈsiərəm］	血清，血液凝结后血浆的剩余部分，相当于没有凝血因子的血浆（复数：sera）
T cell	T 细胞，在胸腺中成熟并直接攻击外来细胞的淋巴细胞
thrombocyte ［ˈθrɒmbəsait］	凝血细胞、血小板

与血液和免疫相关的单词组成部分

参见表 10-1 至表 10-3

表 10-1　与血液相关的后缀

与血液相关的后缀	含义	示例	示例定义
-emia,* -hemia	血液疾病	polycythemia ［pɒlisaiˈθi:mjə］	红细胞增多症
-penia	减少、缺乏	cytopenia ［ˌsaitəˈpi:niə］	血液细胞减少
-poiesis	形成、产生	hemopoiesis ［ˌhi:məpɔiˈi:sis］	造血作用

* 词根 hem 加后缀 -ia 的缩写形式

练习 10-1

定义下列术语。

1. thrombocytopenia ［θrɒmbəʊsaitəʊˈpi:niə］ _____
2. bacteremia ［bæktəˈrimiə］ _____
3. leukocytopenia ［lju:kəsaitəˈpi:niə］ _____
4. erythropoiesis ［iˌriθrəʊpɔiˈi:sis］ _____
5. toxemia ［tɒksˈi:miə］ _____
6. hypoproteinemia ［haipɒprəʊti:ˈni:miə］ _____
7. hyperalbuminemia ［haipəælbjʊmiˈni:miə］ _____

使用后缀 -emia 写出下列定义的单词。

8. Presence of viruses in the blood _____
9. Presence of excess white cells (leuk/o) in the blood _____
10. Presence of pus in the blood _____

许多与血液细胞相关的单词的构成包含词根 cyt/o，也可以没有这个词根，例如 erythropenia（红细胞减少）或 erythrocytopenia，leukopoiesis（白细胞生成）或 leukocytopoiesis。其余类型的血液细胞都有易于辨识的词根，例如 agranulocyt/o、monocyt/o、granul/o 等（表 10-2）。

表 10-2　与血液和免疫相关的词根

词根	含义	示例	示例定义
myel/o	骨髓	myelogenous [maiəˈlɒdʒənəs]	骨髓性的
hem/o, hemat/o	血液	hemopathy [hiːˈmɒpəθi]	血液病
erythr/o, erythrocyt/o	红细胞	erythroblast [iˈriθrəblæst]	成红细胞
leuk/o, leukocyt/o	白细胞	leukocytosis [ˌluːkəʊsaɪˈtəʊsɪs]	白细胞增多
lymph/o, lymphocyt/o	淋巴细胞	lymphocytic [ˌlɪmfəˈsaɪtɪk]	淋巴细胞的
thromb/o	血液凝结	thrombolytic [θrɒmbəʊˈlɪtɪk]	溶栓
thrombocyt/o	血小板	thrombopoiesis [θrɒmbəʊpɔɪˈiːsɪs]	血小板形成
immun/o	免疫、免疫系统	immunization [ˌɪmjʊnaɪˈzeɪʃn]	免疫接种

练习 10-2

识别并定义下列单词的词根。

　　　　　　　　　　　　　　　　　　　　　　Root　　Meaning of root

1. leukocytosis [ˌluːkəʊsaɪˈtəʊsɪs]　　　　____　　_____
2. ischemia [ɪsˈkiːmiə]　　　　　　　　　　____　　_____
3. preimmunization [preɪmjuːnaɪˈzeɪʃən]　____　　_____
4. hematology [ˌhiːməˈtɒlədʒi]　　　　　　____　　_____
5. prothrombin [prəˈθrɒmbɪn]　　　　　　 ____　　_____
6. panmyeloid [pænˈmiːlɔɪd]　　　　　　　____　　_____

填空。

7. Lymphokines [ˈlɪmfəkaɪnz] are chemicals active in immunity that are produced by_____.
8. A hematoma [ˌhiːməˈtəʊmə] is a swelling caused by collection of _____.
9. Hemorrhage [ˈhemərɪdʒ] is a profuse flow (-rhage) of _____.
10. Myelofibrosis [ˌmaɪələʊfaɪˈbrəʊsɪs] is formation of fibrous tissue in _____.
11. Erythroclasis [eriˈθrɒkləsɪs] is the breaking (-clasis) of _____.
12. An immunocyte [ɪˈmjuːnəʊsaɪt] is a cell active in _____.
13. The term thrombocythemia [θrɒmbəsɪˈθiːmiə] refers to a blood increase in the number of _____.
14. Leukopoiesis [ljuːkəpɔɪˈiːsɪs] refers to the production of _____.

练习 10-2 （续表）

写出下列定义的单词。

15. Decrease in white blood cells _____
16. Tumor of bone marrow _____
17. Immature lymphocyte _____
18. Dissolving (-lysis) of a blood clot _____
19. Formation (-poiesis) of bone marrow _____

后缀 -osis 加在一种血液细胞的词根上意为该类细胞数量的增加，使用该后缀写出下列含义的单词。

20. Increase in granulocytes in the blood _____
21. Increase in lymphocytes in the blood _____
22. Increase in red blood cells _____
23. Increase in monocytes in the blood _____
24. Increase in platelets in the blood _____

表 10-3　与血液化学相关的词根

词根	含义	示例	示例定义
azot/o	氮化合物	azoturia ［əˈzəʊtəriə］	氮尿（-uria）
calc/i	钙（Ca）	calcification ［ˌkælsifiˈkeiʃn］	钙化
ferr/o, ferr/i	铁（Fe）	ferrous ［ˈferəs］	含铁的
sider/o	铁	sideroderma ［saidˈrəʊdəmə］	铁色皮症
kali	钾（K）	hyperkalemia* ［haipəkəˈli:miə］	高钾血症
natri	钠（Na）	natriuresis ［neitrijʊˈri:sis］	尿钠排泄
ox/y	氧（O）	hypoxia ［haiˈpɒksiə］	缺氧

*词根中的 i 省略了

练习 10-3

填空。

1. A sideroblast ［ˈsidərəblɑ:st］ is an immature cell containing _____.
2. The term hypokalemia ［haipəʊkəˈli:mjə］ refers to a blood deficiency of _____.
3. The bacterial species Azotobacter is named for its ability to metabolize _____.
4. Hypoxemia ［ˌhaipɒkˈsi:miə］ is a blood deficiency of _____.

练习 10-3 （续表）

5. Ferritin ['ferɪtən] is a compound that contains_____.
6. A calcareous [kæl'keərɪəs] substance contains_____.

使用后缀 -emia 构成下列含义的单词。

7. Presence of sodium in the blood _____
8. Presence of nitrogenous compounds in the blood _____
9. Presence of potassium in the blood _____
10. Presence of calcium in the blood _____

血液疾病的临床表现

贫血

贫血（anemia）被定义为血液中血红蛋白异常偏低。贫血可能是红细胞太少或太小（microcytic），或者血红蛋白太低（hypochromic）的结果。诊断贫血的关键是测试全血细胞计数、平均红细胞体积（mean corpuscular volume，MCV）和平均红细胞血红蛋白浓度（mean corpuscular-hemoglobin concentration，MCHC）。框 10-4 介绍了各种血液测试。框 10-5 给出了血液学相关职业的信息。

贫血的一般症状包括乏力（fatigue）、呼吸急促、心悸（heart palpitations）、苍白（pallor）和易激动（irritability）。

供你参考
常用血液测试 框 10-4

测试	缩略语	说明
red blood cell count 红细胞计数	RBC	每毫升血液红细胞的数量
white blood cell count 白细胞计数	WBC	每毫升血液白细胞的数量
differential count 分类计数	Diff	不同类型白细胞的相对百分比
Hematocrit 血细胞比容（图 10-10）	Ht, Hct, crit	给定血容量压积红细胞的相对百分比
packed cell volume 红细胞压积	PCV	同上
Hemoglobin 血红蛋白	Hb, Hgb	每 100ml 血液血红蛋白的克数
mean corpuscular volume	MCV	平均红细胞体积
mean corpuscular hemoglobin	MCH	平均红细胞血红蛋白
mean corpuscular hemoglobin concentration	MCHC	平均红细胞血红蛋白浓度
erythrocyte sedimentation rate 红细胞沉降率	ESR	单位时间红细胞的沉降速率，用于检测感染或炎症
complete blood count 全血细胞计数	CBC	包括细胞计数、血细胞比容、血红蛋白和胞体积的测量

健康职业

血液学中的职业

框 10-5

血液学家（hematologist）是专门研究血液和血液病的医生和其他科学家。在医学实践中，血液学常常与血癌的研究和治疗相结合，称为血液肿瘤学（hematology-oncology）专科。

其他在血液学领域工作的医疗专业人员根据其学术准备而发挥不同的作用（框 2-2）。这些职业包括医疗技术专家、医疗技术员和抽血员（phlebotomist），他们在医院、诊所、门诊实验室和私人办公室工作。

医疗技术专家和技术员可以专门从事各种临床环境的工作，例如血库和微生物学与化学实验室。每个职位都需要先进的技能和电子设备、仪器仪表和计算机的工作知识。在血液学工作的人员测试血液异常或感染，并可以进行输血的交叉匹配测试。他们检查血液细胞的癌症和其他疾病的迹象。他们必须熟悉实验室安全政策和程序，并且在使用体液和组织时必须采取适当的预防措施。有关医学实验室技术职业的信息，请联系美国临床实验室科学学会（American Society for Clinical Laboratory Science），网址为 http://www.ascls.org。

抽血员是为测试、输血或研究进行抽血的医疗专业人士。抽血员在医院、实验室、私人医生办公室、诊所和血库工作。他们通常从静脉抽取血液（静脉穿刺），但也可以从动脉或通过皮肤穿刺，例如手指或足跟抽取血液。抽血员必须接受无菌技术和安全预防措施的培训，以防止传染病的传播。他们必须在不伤害患者或干扰医疗护理的情况下取样，并且必须准确地为样本贴标签并送到相应的实验室。各州的教育要求各不相同。通常，国家静脉切开术协会（National Phlebotomy Association）认证的内部培训是可以接受的（www.nationalphlebotomy.org）。

有许多不同类型的贫血，一些是红细胞的产生错误所致，另一些是红细胞损伤或破坏所致。

红细胞产生受损引起的贫血

- 再生障碍性贫血（aplastic anemia）是骨髓受损并影响所有血液细胞（pancytopenia）所致，可能是由药物、病毒、放射或骨髓癌引起的。再生障碍性贫血致死率较高，但通过骨髓移植可以成功治疗。
- 营养性贫血（nutritional anemia）是因为缺乏维生素 B_{12} 或叶酸（folic acid）所致，红细胞发育需要维生素 B。最常见的是因为缺乏生成血红蛋白所需的铁所致（图 10-11）。缺乏叶酸常见于那些饮食不良、怀孕及哺乳期的女性和酗酒的人群。缺铁性贫血是饮食不良、铁吸收不良或血液损失所致。缺乏叶酸和缺铁都可以通过饮食补充。
- 恶性贫血（pernicious anemia）是一种特定形式的维生素 B_{12} 缺乏，是缺少内因子（intrinsic factor，IF）所致。内因子是胃产生的一种帮助小肠吸收维生素 B_{12} 的物质。恶性贫血必须通过定期注射维生素 B_{12} 进行治疗。
- 铁粒幼细胞贫血（sideroblastic anemia），有足够的铁供应，但铁不能适当地用于生产血

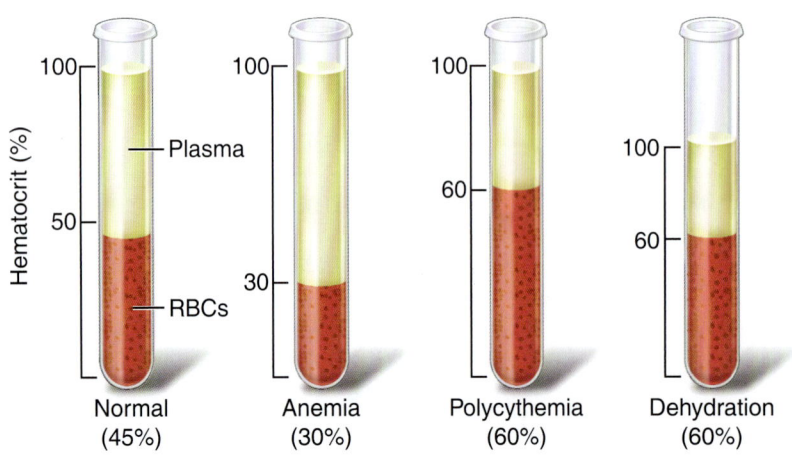

图 10-10 血细胞比容。血细胞比容测试全血中红细胞的体积百分比，最左侧的试管显示正常的血细胞比容，两个中间的试管显示异常血细胞比容，一个显示低的红细胞百分比，表明贫血，而另一个显示过高的红细胞百分比，如红细胞增多症。最右侧的试管显示脱水造成的相对高的红细胞百分比

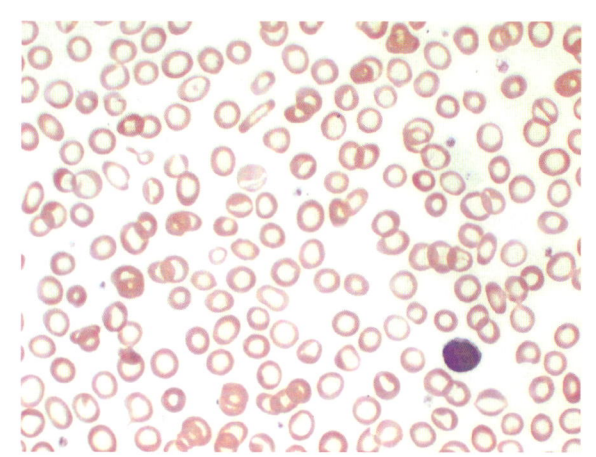

图 10-11 缺铁性贫血。红细胞小（小红细胞），缺乏血红蛋白（血红蛋白过低）

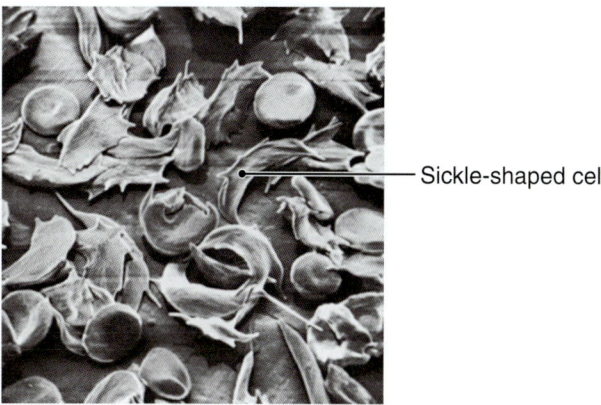

图 10-12 镰状细胞性贫血的血涂片。当异常细胞放出氧气时，其呈现新月形（镰刀形）

红蛋白。这种疾病可以是遗传性的，或者是获得性的，例如暴露于特定的毒素或药物所致。铁粒幼细胞贫血也可能继发于其他疾病。过量的铁会沉积于未成熟的红细胞（幼红细胞 normoblasts）。

红细胞损失或破坏引起的贫血

- 失血性贫血（hemorrhagic anemia）是因失血所致。可能是突然的失血，例如受伤，或者是长期内部出血，例如因溃疡或癌症引起的消化道出血。
- 地中海贫血（thalassemia）是一种遗传疾病，主要集中在地中海。一种基因变异引起血红蛋白生成异常和红细胞溶解（hemolysis）。根据血红蛋白分子被影响的部分，地中海贫血被分为 α 型和 β 型，严重的 β 型地中海贫血也被称为库利贫血（Cooley anemia）或重型地中海贫血（thalassemia major）。
- 镰状细胞性贫血（sickle cell anemia），血红蛋白分子发生了变化，释放出氧气后就会沉降，使红细胞变成镰状（图 10-12）。被改变的细胞会阻塞小血管并使组织缺氧，这被称为镰状细胞危机。变形的细胞很容易被破坏（溶血，hemolyzed），这种疾病主要发生于黑种人。带有基因缺陷的人有一个正常基因和一个异常基因，会显示镰状细胞特性。除了在高海拔氧气较少的情况下，镰状细胞性贫血通常没有症状。不过，患者会将有缺陷的基因遗传给后代。镰状细胞性贫血及其他许多遗传性疾病能够在胎儿出生前被诊断出来。

网织红细胞计数（reticulocyte counts）可以用于诊断贫血的原因。网织红细胞是未成熟的红细胞，通常只占全部红细胞很小的百分比。网织红细胞计数的上升表明红细胞的增加，这是对失血或细胞破坏的响应。网织红细胞数量下降表明红细胞生产不足，营养性贫血或再生障碍性贫血就会出现这种情况（框 10-6）。

凝血障碍

凝血（coagulation）问题的最常见原因是缺乏血小板，被称为血小板减少症（thrombocytopenia）。可能的起因包括再生障碍性贫血、骨髓癌和破坏骨髓的 X 线或特定药物。这种疾病会导致皮肤和黏膜出血，出现瘀点（petechiae）、瘀斑（ecchymoses）或紫癜（purpura）。

在弥散性血管内凝血（disseminated intravascular coagulation，DIC）中，血管中有广泛分布的血凝块，会阻塞组织循环。随着凝血因子的消失会出现发散性出血，凝血过程被损害。DIC 是很多原因所致的，包括感染、癌症、出血、受伤和过敏。

血友病（hemophilia）是一种缺乏特定凝血因子的遗传疾病，是一种母亲传给儿子的伴性遗传病。

> **框 10-6**
>
> ### 临床观点
> **在诊断中使用网织红细胞**
>
> 随着红细胞在骨髓中成熟，它们会经历几个阶段，在这期间会失掉细胞核和大部分细胞器，为血红蛋白提供最大的空间。在发育最后几个阶段之一，细胞内残留少量核糖体和糙面内质网（rough endoplasmic reticulum），在染色后呈现网状。这个阶段的红细胞被称为网织红细胞。网织红细胞离开骨髓并进入血流，在 24~48 小时内成熟。在任何给定时点，通过网织红细胞阶段进入成熟的红细胞平均数量是 1%~2%，这一数值的变化可用于诊断特定的血液疾病。
>
> 当红细胞损失或被破坏时，例如长期出血或一些形式的失血性贫血，红细胞的生产会加速，以补偿损失。大量的网织红细胞会在达到完全成熟之前释放到血液中，计数就会高于正常值。另一方面，循环中的网织红细胞数量的下降说明红细胞的生产有问题，例如缺乏性贫血和骨髓活性抑制。

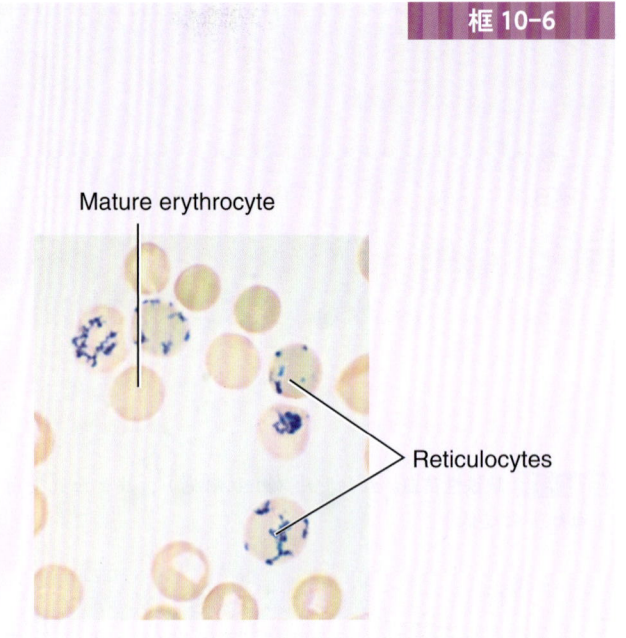

患者会发生组织出血，特别是在关节处（关节出血症 hemarthrosis）。血友病必须通过输入必要的凝血因子进行治疗。框 10-7 介绍了凝血障碍的相关测试。

肿瘤

白血病（leukemia）是白细胞的肿瘤（neoplasm）。快速分裂但无效的白细胞在组织中累积，并挤出其他血液细胞。白血病的症状包括贫血、乏力、容易出血、脾肿大（splenomegaly）以及有时肝肿大（hepatomegaly）。白血病起因不明，可能包括暴露于放射性或有害化学品、遗传因素和病毒感染。

基于始发处和涉及的细胞，白血病分为两类：
- 骨髓性（myelogenous）白血病始发于骨髓，主要涉及粒性白细胞。
- 淋巴性白血病影响 B 细胞和淋巴系统，导致淋巴结病（lymphadenopathy），反过来影响免疫系统。

基于临床进展，白血病被进一步分为急性和慢性。

> **框 10-7**
>
> ### 供你参考
> **凝血测试**
>
> | 名称 | 说明 | 功能 |
> | --- | --- | --- |
> | activated partial thromboplastin time 活化部分凝血活酶时间 | APTT | 测量血凝块形成所需的时间，用于评估凝血因子和监测肝素治疗 |
> | bleeding time 出血时间 | BT | 测量标准皮肤切开后血小板阻止出血的能力 |
> | partial thromboplastin time 部分凝血活酶时间 | PTT | 与 APTT 相似，用于评估凝血因子，但灵敏度稍差 |
> | prothrombin time 前凝血酶时间 | PT, pro time | 间接测量凝血酶原，用于监测抗凝血治疗，也被称为 Quick 测试 |
> | Thrombin time (thrombin clotting time) 凝血酶原时间（凝血酶凝血时间） | TT (TCT) | 测量血凝块形成的速度 |

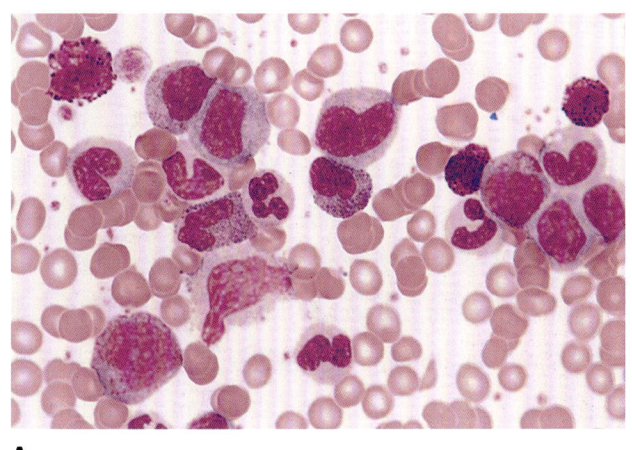 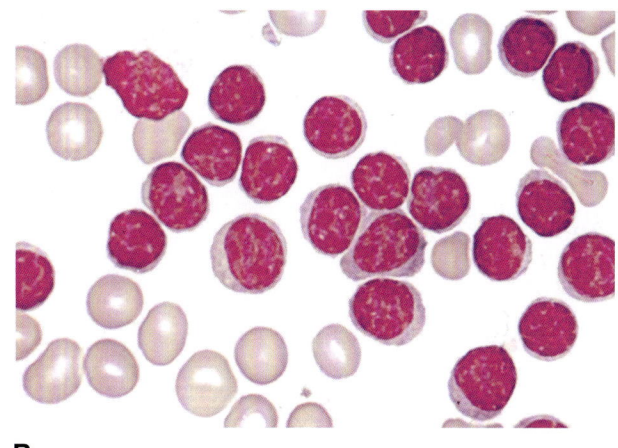

图 10-13 白血病。白血病是源自骨髓或淋巴系统的白细胞的恶性过度生长。A. 慢性骨髓性白血病显示所有类别的白细胞的过量产生，B. 慢性淋巴细胞白血病显示大量的淋巴细胞

急性白血病是幼儿最常见的癌症。急性白血病有：

- 急性髓细胞（粒细胞）白血病［acute myeloblastic (myelogenous) leukemia，AML］，儿童和成年患者的预后都不好。
- 急性成淋巴细胞（淋巴细胞）白血病［Acute lymphoblastic (lymphocytic) leukemia，ALL］，通过治疗，急性成淋巴细胞白血病的缓解率较高。
- 慢性白血病有：
- 慢性髓细胞白血病，也被称为慢性粒细胞白血病，影响青年和中年人群（图 10-13A）。大多数病例显示有费城染色体（Philadelphia chromosome，Ph），是一种遗传畸形，22 号染色体的一部分转移到了 9 号染色体（图 10-13B）。

- 慢性淋巴细胞白血病（chronic lymphocytic leukemia，CLL）只发生在老年人身上，是一种发展最缓慢的疾病。

白血病的治疗包括化疗、放疗和骨髓移植。骨髓移植的一个进步是使用脐带血（umbilical cord blood）代替骨髓中的造血细胞。脐带血比骨髓更容易获得，而且不必为避免排斥做匹配。

霍奇金病（Hodgkin disease）是一种可能扩散到其他组织的淋巴系统疾病。它起始于颈部增大但无痛的淋巴结，然后发展到其他淋巴结。霍奇金病的一个特征是淋巴结中被称为里-施细胞（Reed-Sternberg cell）的巨大细胞（图 10-14）。症状包括发热、盗汗、失重和皮肤瘙痒（pruritus）。任何年龄的人都可能患病，但主要影响年轻人和超过 50 岁的人群。大多数病例可通过放疗和化疗治愈。

非霍奇金淋巴瘤（non-Hodgkin lymphoma，NHL）也被称为淋巴结恶性增大，但没有里德-斯特恩伯格细胞。它比霍奇金病更为常见，并有较高的死亡率，病例的严重程度和预后有所不同，在老年人、艾滋病患者和其他形式的免疫缺陷患者中最为流行。NHL 涉及 T 细胞和 B 细胞，某些病例可能与特定病毒感染相关。这种疾病需要全身化疗，有时需要骨髓移植。

多发性骨髓瘤（multiple myeloma）是造血细胞的癌症，主要是出生抗体的浆细胞。该病会引起贫血、骨痛和骨质疏松。因为免疫缺陷，患者易受感

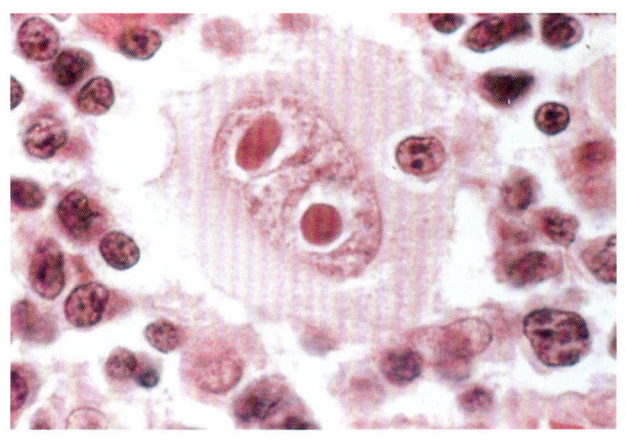

图 10-14 里德斯特恩伯格细胞

染。血液中钙和蛋白质水平异常高通常会导致肾衰竭（kidney failure）。多发性骨髓瘤需要进行放疗和化疗，但预后一般都不好。

免疫的临床表现

过敏症

过敏症（hypersensitivity）是免疫系统有害的过度反应，通常被称为过敏反应（allergy）。在过敏反应情况下，患者对特定抗原比一般人更为敏感，常见过敏原有花粉（pollen）、动物皮屑、灰尘、食品等，种类繁多。对吸入花粉的季节性过敏常被称为"花粉热（hay fever）"，反应可能包括发痒、发红、眼睛流泪（结膜炎 conjunctivitis）、皮疹、哮喘、流鼻涕（鼻炎 rhinitis）、打喷嚏、风疹（urticaria）和血管性水肿（angioedema），血管性水肿类似于皮疹（hives），但涉及更深层的组织。过敏性反应（anaphylactic reaction）是一种全身的过敏反应，由于休克和呼吸窘迫可能快速致死，必须立即使用肾上腺素并保持呼吸道畅通。也可以使用氧气、抗组胺药（antihistamines）和糖皮质激素（corticosteroids）。过敏性反应的常见起因是药物，特别是盘尼西林和其他抗生素、疫苗、诊断性化学品、食物和昆虫毒液（insect venom）。

迟发性超敏反应（delayed hypersensitivity reaction）涉及T细胞，发病需要至少12小时。常见的情况是接触植物刺激物，例如毒葛（poison ivy）和毒栎（poison oak）。

免疫缺陷

免疫缺陷（immunodeficiency）是指免疫系统的任何缺陷。这可能是先天性的或获得性的，可能涉及系统的任何组成部分，缺陷的严重性可能有差异，但总是显示为易患疾病。

艾滋病（获得性免疫缺陷综合征，acquired immunodeficiency syndrome，AIDS）是通过感染人类免疫缺陷病毒（human immunodeficiency virus，HIV）获得的，该病毒攻击T细胞。这些细胞对HIV有特定表面附着部位，CD4受体。HIV通过性接触、使用不洁的针头、输血和母婴进行传播，它使宿主易受机会性感染，如由真菌卡氏肺孢子虫（Pneumocystis jiroveci）引起的肺炎、由白色念珠菌（Candida albicans）引起的口腔真菌感染和感染能够引起绞痛和腹泻的隐孢子虫（Cryptosporidium），还会是患者易患一种曾经罕见的皮癌卡波西肉瘤（Kaposi sarcoma）。

艾滋病还会诱发自身免疫病或攻击神经系统。通过CD4+ T淋巴细胞计数可以诊断并监测艾滋病，这种测试可测量带HIV受体细胞的数量。低于每微升200的计数显示有严重的免疫缺陷。HIV抗体水平和直接的病毒血液计数也被用于跟踪疾病的发展。对艾滋病目前没有疫苗或治愈手段，药物只是延迟它的进展。

自身免疫病

针对自身组织免疫反应所导致的失调被划分为自免疫病（autoimmune disease），其原因可能是免疫系统失效，或者是对自身细胞的反应被变异或疾病轻微改变。确认由自身免疫，或者部分是因自身免疫引起的疾病清单很长，其中一些影响多个系统的组织，如系统性红斑狼疮（systemic lupus erythematosus，SLE）、系统性硬化症（systemic sclerosis）和干燥综合征（Sjögren syndrome）。另一些则只针对更确定的器官或系统，如恶性贫血（pernicious anemia）、类风湿性关节炎（rheumatoid arthritis）、甲状腺格雷夫斯病（Graves disease）、重症肌无力（myasthenia gravis）、纤维肌痛综合征（fibromyalgia syndrome）、风湿性心脏病和肾小球肾炎（glomerulonephritis）。

Terminology 关键术语

病症

AIDS (acquired immunodeficiency syndrome)	艾滋病（获得性免疫缺陷综合征），因为感染人类免疫缺陷病毒（HIV）引起的免疫系统失效。病毒影响 T 细胞，进而干扰免疫系统
allergen [ˈælədʒən]	过敏原，引起过敏反应的物质
allergy [ˈælədʒi]	过敏，过敏反应
anaphylactic reaction [ˌænəfiˈlæktik]	过敏性反应，对外来物质的极度过敏反应（词根：phylaxis 意为"保护"）。如果不治疗，可能因循环衰竭和呼吸窘迫导致死亡。
anemia [əˈniːmiːə]	贫血，血液中血红蛋白缺乏，可能是因血液流失、营养不良、遗传缺陷、环境因素和其他原因所致（图 10-11 和图 10-12）
angioedema [ændʒiːəʊiːˈdiːmə]	血管性水肿，带有大片荨麻疹的水肿，类似与风疹，但涉及更深层的皮肤和皮下组织
aplastic anemia [eiˈplæstik]	再生障碍性贫血，因骨髓功能衰竭导致血液细胞生产不足，特别是红细胞不足引起的贫血；全血细胞减少症（pancytopenia）
autoimmune disease	自身免疫病，一种免疫系统对自身组织产生抗体的状况（前缀 auto-，意为"自己"）
Cooley anemia	库利贫血，一种地中海贫血（遗传学贫血），影响 β 血红蛋白链；重型地中海贫血（thalassemia major）
delayed hypersensitivity reaction	迟发性超敏反应，涉及 T 细胞的过敏反应，发病至少需要 12 小时；结核素菌反应（tuberculin reaction）和移植组织排斥
disseminated intravascular coagulation (DIC)	弥散性血管内凝血，微血管中广泛形成血凝块，可能继发于凝血因子损耗所致的出血
ecchymosis [ˌekiˈməʊsis]	瘀斑，因小血管渗漏所致的皮下血液凝集（词根：chym，意为"果汁"）
hemolysis [hiˈmɒlisis]	溶血，血液细胞破裂和血红蛋白的释放（形容词：hemolytic）
hemophilia [ˌhiːməˈfiliə]	血友病，用于缺少凝血因子所致，并会导致异常出血的遗传学血液病
hemorrhagic anemia [ˈheməræzaik]	出血性贫血，因血液流失所致的贫血，血液流失的原因可能是受伤或内部出血
HIV (human immunodeficiency virus)	人类免疫缺陷病毒，引起艾滋病的病毒
Hodgkin disease	霍奇金病，一种起因不明的肿瘤疾病，涉及淋巴结、脾、肝和其他组织；特征是出现巨大的里-施细胞（ReedSternberg cells，图 10-14）
hypersensitivity [ˌhaipəˌsensəˈtivəti]	过敏反应，针对一种对其他大多数人都无害的物质的免疫反应；常用 allergy
immunodeficiency [ˌimjuːnəʊdiˈfiʃnsi]	免疫缺陷，先天性或获得性的免疫系统失效，无法防御疾病
intrinsic factor [inˈtrinsik]	内因子，在胃中产生的一种物质，能够帮助小肠吸收生产红细胞所必须的维生素 B_{12}，缺乏内因子会引起恶性贫血

Terminology 关键术语（续表）

Kaposi sarcoma [sɑːˈkəʊmə]	卡波西肉瘤，皮肤和其他组织的癌性损害，常见于艾滋病患者
leukemia [luːˈkiːmiə] 白血病	不成熟白细胞的恶性增生，可能是急性的或慢性的；可能影响骨髓（骨髓性白血病 myelogenous leukemia）或淋巴组织（淋巴细胞性白血病，lymphocytic leukemia）
lymphadenopathy [lɪmˌfædəˈnɒpəθi]	淋巴结肿大，一种淋巴结的疾病
multiple myeloma [ˌmaɪəˈləʊmə]	多发性骨髓瘤，骨髓中造血组织的肿瘤
non-Hodgkin lymphoma (NHL)	非霍奇金淋巴瘤，一种普遍的涉及淋巴细胞的恶性淋巴结疾病，与霍奇金病的差异是没有里德斯特恩伯格细胞
nutritional anemia	营养性贫血，饮食缺乏，通常是缺乏铁、维生素 B_{12} 或叶酸所致的贫血
Philadelphia chromosome (Ph)	费城染色体，在大多数慢性粒细胞（骨髓性）白血病患者细胞中发现的一种异常染色体
pernicious anemia [pəˈnɪʃəs]	恶性贫血，因为胃不能生产内因子所致的贫血；内因子是吸收维生素 B_{12} 所必须的物质，而维生素 B_{12} 是产生红细胞所必须的
petechiae [pəˈtekieɪt]	瘀点，皮下或黏膜上点状、平的、紫红色出血点（单数 petechia）
purpura [ˈpəpjʊrə]	紫癜，以皮下、黏膜、内部器官和其他组织出血为特征的一种状况（来自于希腊语，意为"紫色"）。血小板减少性紫癜（Thrombocytopenic purpura）是血小板缺乏所致
sickle cell anemia [ˈsɪkl]	镰状细胞性贫血，因出血异常血红蛋白所致的遗传学贫血。当释放氧气后红细胞变成镰状，并干扰血液正常流向组织（图 10-12），常见于西部非洲血统的黑种人
sideroblastic anemia [ˈsɪdərəblɑːstɪc]	铁粒幼细胞贫血，因不能将可用的铁生产血红蛋白所致的贫血。过量的铁沉积在铁粒幼细胞
Sjögren syndrome	干燥综合征，涉及外分泌腺功能障碍并影响眼泪、唾液和其他体液分泌的一种自身免疫病。会导致口干、龋齿、角膜损伤、眼睛感染和吞咽困难
splenomegaly [ˌspliːnəʊˈmegəli]	脾大，白血病的症状之一
systemic lupus erythematosus [ˈluːpəs ˌerəˌθiːməˈtəʊsəs]	系统性红斑狼疮，影响皮肤和多个器官的结缔组织炎症。患者对光线敏感，在鼻子和面颊有红色蝴蝶状皮疹
systemic sclerosis [skləˈrəʊsɪs]	系统性硬化症，可能涉及任何系统的分散性结缔组织疾病，会引起炎症、退化和纤维化。因为会引起皮肤变厚，也被称为硬皮病
thalassemia [θæləˈsiːmiə]	地中海贫血，在地中海人群中常见的一类遗传学贫血（来自于希腊语意为"海洋"的单词）
thrombocytopenia [θrɒmbəʊsaɪtəʊˈpiːniə]	血小板减少症，血液中缺乏血小板
urticaria [ˌɜːtɪˈkeərɪə]	荨麻疹，由瘙痒的圆形丘疹构成的皮肤反应；也常用 hives

诊断和治疗

adrenaline [əˈdrenəlɪn]	肾上腺素，参见 epinephrine
CD4+ T lymphocyte count	CD4+ T 淋巴细胞计数，带艾滋病毒 CD4 受体的 T 淋巴细胞计数。计数每微升低于 200 表明有严重免疫缺陷

Terminology 关键术语（续表）

epinephrine [ˌepiˈnefrin]	肾上腺素，由肾上腺和交感神经系统产生的强兴奋剂。能够激活需要应对压力的心血管系统、呼吸系统和其他系统。用于治疗严重过敏反应和休克，也被称为 adrenaline
reticulocyte counts [riˈtikjʊləsait]	网织红细胞计数，一种未成熟红细胞的计数，由于诊断说明红细胞生成的速率（框 10-6）
Reed-Sternberg cells	里-施细胞，巨大细胞，霍奇金病的特征，它们通常有两个大核，由一个孔环包围（图 10-14）

Terminology 补充术语

正常结构和功能

agglutination [əˌgluːtinˈeiʃən]	凝集，细胞或颗粒由于特定抗体存在而聚集
bilirubin [ˌbiliˈruːbin]	胆红素，血红蛋白破裂后产生的色素，由胆汁在肝脏中消除
complement [ˈkɒmplimənt]	补体，与抗体相互作用的一组血浆酶
corpuscle [ˈkɔːpʌsl]	小体，血液中的小体就是血液细胞
hemopoietic stem cell [ˌhiːməpɔiˈiːtik]	造血干细胞，能够产生所有种类血液细胞的原始骨髓细胞
heparin [ˈhepərin]	肝素，存在于全身的阻止血液凝固的物质；抗凝剂
plasmin [ˈplæzmin]	纤溶酶，一种溶解血凝块的酶，也被称为溶纤维蛋白酵素（fibrinolysin）
thrombin [ˈθrɒmbin]	凝血酶，源自于凝血酶原的酶，能够将纤维蛋白原转化为纤维蛋白

病症和状况

agranulocytosis [eiˌgrænjələsaiˈtəʊsis]	粒细胞缺乏症，涉及血液中粒细胞减少的一种状况，也被称为粒细胞减少症（granulocytopenia）
Erythrocytosis [iriθrəʊsaiˈtəʊsis]	红细胞增多症，血液中红细胞增多，可能是正常的，例如对生活在高海拔地区的补偿；也可能是异常的，例如肺或心脏疾病
Fanconi syndrome	范科尼综合征，先天性再生障碍性贫血，发生于初生到 10 岁之间；可能是遗传性的，或者是出生前受病毒等的伤害所致
graft versus host reaction (GVHR)	移植物抗宿主反应，移植的淋巴细胞反抗宿主组织的免疫反应；一种常见的骨髓移植并发症
hairy cell leukemia	多毛细胞白血病，一种形式的白细胞，细胞会出现微丝，看起来像（毛发状）
hematoma [ˌhiːməˈtəʊmə]	血肿，局部血液聚集，通常是血凝块，因血管破裂所致
hemolytic disease of the newborn (HDN)	新生儿溶血病，因目前与胎儿的血液不兼容所致的疾病，通常涉及 Rh 因子。在怀孕后期，Rh 阴性的母亲会对 Rh 阳性的胎儿产生抗体，将会破坏胎儿的红细胞。治疗方法是用抗体消除目前的 Rh 抗原

Terminology	补充术语（续表）
hemosiderosis ['hi:məʊsidə'rəʊsis]	含铁血黄素沉积，涉及含铁色素（血铁黄素，hemosiderin）只要在肝和脾沉积的状况。色素来源于被分解的红细胞释放的血红蛋白
idiopathic thrombocytopenic purpura (ITP)	原发性血小板减少性紫癜，因血小板破坏所致的凝血疾病，通常继发于病毒感染。会引起皮肤和黏膜的瘀斑和出血
infectious mononucleosis [ˌmɒnəʊˌnju:kli'əʊsis]	传染性单核细胞增多，由艾普斯登·巴尔病毒（Epstein-Barr virus，EBV）引起的急性传染病。特征是发热、虚弱、淋巴结肿大、肝脾肿大和非典型淋巴细胞（类似单核细胞，图10-15）
lymphocytosis [ˌlimfəʊsai'təʊsis]	淋巴细胞增多，循环中的淋巴细胞数量增多
myelodysplastic syndrome [maiələʊdi'spleiztik]	骨髓增生异常综合征，骨髓功能障碍导致贫血和中性粒细胞和血小板缺乏。可能发展为白血病；白血病前期（preleukemia）
myelofibrosis [ˌmaiələʊfai'brəʊsis]	骨髓纤维变性，骨髓被纤维组织替代的状况
neutropenia [ˌnju:trə'pi:niə]	中性粒细胞减少，易受感染。起因包括药物、放射和感染。可能是恶性肿瘤治疗的不良反应
pancytopenia [pænsaitə'pi:niə]	全血细胞减少，所有血液细胞数量都下降，如再生障碍性贫血
polycythemia [pɒlisai'θi:mjə]	红细胞增多，红细胞比在所有血液细胞中的比例相对上升的任何状况。可能是因为缺氧使红细胞产生过量所致，原因包括高海拔、呼吸阻塞、心力衰竭或特定的毒素。相对红细胞增多可能是血液浓缩所致，如脱水
polycythemia vera	真性红细胞增多，过于活跃的骨髓细胞产生太多红细胞的结果。过多的红细胞会干扰循环，并导致血栓形成和出血。治疗方法是放血，也被称为 erythremia
septicemia [ˌsepti'si:miə]	败血症，血液中出现微生物
spherocytic anemia [sfərə'sitik]	溶血性贫血，一种遗传学贫血，其红细胞是圆的而不是盘形，且过度破裂
thrombotic thrombocytopenic purpura (TTP)	血栓性血小板减少性紫癜，一种通常会致命的疾病，血管中有很多血凝块

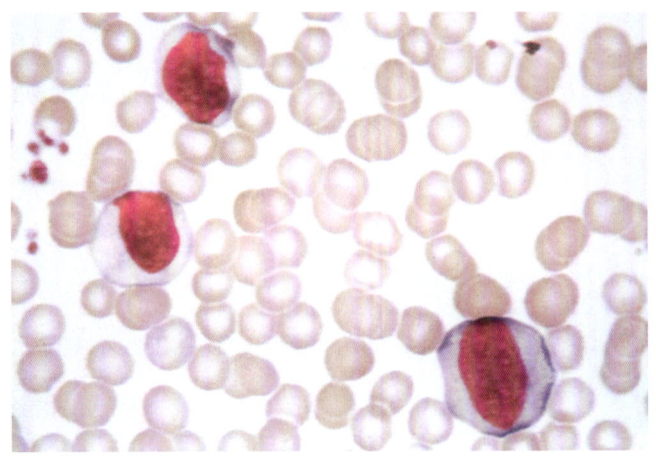

图10-15 **传染性单核细胞增多症。**非典型淋巴细胞是这种病毒性疾病的特征

Terminology 补充术语（续表）

von Willebrand disease	血管性血友病，因缺少凝血所需的冯·维勒布兰德因子所致的遗传性出血疾病，

诊断

Bence Jones protein	本周蛋白，多发性骨髓瘤患者尿液中出现的一种蛋白质
Coombs test	库姆斯实验，一种检测针对红细胞抗体的测试，例如在自身免疫溶血性贫血出现的抗体
electrophoresis [iˌlektrəʊfəˈriːsis]	电泳疗法，通过使用电场分离液体中的离子；用于分离血液成分
Enzyme-linked immunosorbent assay (ELISA)	酶联免疫吸附试验，高灵敏度免疫测试，用于诊断 HIV 感染、肝炎和莱姆病（Lyme disease）
monoclonal antibody [ˌmɒnəʊˈkləʊnəl]	单克隆抗体，实验室生产的纯抗体，用于诊断和治疗
Schilling test	维生素 B_{12} 吸收试验，通过测量尿液中放射性维生素 B_{12} 的排泄量测定维生素 B_{12} 的吸收
seroconversion [siərəʊkənˈvɜːʒən]	血清转化，血清对疾病或免疫接种出现抗体
Western blot assay	蛋白印迹法，一种特别灵敏的测试，检测血液中少量的抗体
Wright stain	瑞特染液，一种常用血液染色

治疗

anticoagulant [ˌæntikəʊˈægjələnt]	抗凝剂，阻止血液凝固的药物
antihistamine [ˌæntiˈhistəmiːn]	抗组胺药，抵抗组胺反应的药物，用于治疗过敏反应
apheresis [ˌəˈferisis]	分离技术，一种抽血后分离并保留一部分，剩余部分再返回供血者的方法。Apheresis 可用作后缀，与一个词根一起表示被保留的部分，如血浆置换（plasmapheresis）和白细胞取出法（leukapheresis）
autologous blood [ɔːˈtɒləgəs]	自体血，一个人自己的血液。如果需要，可以事先为手术或输血捐献
cryoprecipitate [kraiəpriˈsipiteit]	冷沉淀，通过冷却获得的沉淀物。通过冷却血浆获得的部分包含凝血因子
desensitization [ˌdiːˌsensətaiˈzeiʃn]	脱敏，通过注射少量侵犯抗原治疗过敏。这会增加抗体，反过来快速消灭抗原
homologous blood [həˈmɒləgəs]	异体血，来自于同物种动物的血液，例如一个人给另一个人输的血。用于输血的血液必须与接受者的血液兼容
immunosuppression [ˌimjunəʊsəˈpreʃn]	免疫抑制，免疫系统的抑制。可能与疾病相关，也可能是由避免组织移植排斥的治疗引发的
protease inhibitor [ˈprəʊtieiz]	蛋白酶抑制剂，抗 HIV 药物，抑制病毒繁殖所需要的酶

Terminology 缩略语

Ab	Antibody	抗体
Ag	Antigen, also silve	抗原，也是银的化学符号
AIDS	Acquired immunodeficiency syndrome	获得性免疫缺陷综合征
ALL	Acute lymphoblastic (lymphocytic) leukemia	急性成淋巴细胞（淋巴细胞）白血病
AML	Acute myeloblastic (myelogenous) leukemia	急性髓细胞（粒细胞）白血病
APTT	Activated partial thromboplastin time	活化部分凝血活酶时间
BT	Bleeding time	出血时间
CBC	Complete blood count	全血细胞计数
CGL	Chronic granulocytic leukemia	慢性粒细胞白血病
CLL	Chronic lymphocytic leukemia	慢性淋巴细胞白血病
CML	Chronic myelogenous leukemia	慢性髓细胞性白血病
crit	Hematocrit	血液细胞容积率
DIC	Disseminated intravascular coagulation	弥散性血管内凝血
Diff	Differential count	白细胞分类计数
EBV	Epstein-Barr virus	艾普斯登·巴尔病毒
ELISA	Enzyme-linked immunosorbent assay	酶联免疫吸附试验
EPO, EP	Erythropoietin	促红细胞生成素
ESR	Erythrocyte sedimentation rate	血红细胞沉降率
FFP	Fresh frozen plasma	新鲜冷冻血浆
Hb, Hgb	Hemoglobin	血红蛋白
Hct, Ht	Hematocrit	血细胞比容
HDN	Hemolytic disease of the newborn	新生儿溶血病
HIV	Human immunodeficiency virus	人类免疫缺陷病毒
IF	Intrinsic factor	内因子
Ig	Immunoglobulin	免疫球蛋白
ITP	Idiopathic thrombocytopenic purpura	特发性血小板减少性紫癜
lytes	Electrolytes	电解质
MCH	Mean corpuscular hemoglobin	平均红细胞血红蛋白
MCHC	Mean corpuscular hemoglobin concentration	平均红细胞血红蛋白浓度

Terminology 缩略语（续表）

mcL	Microliter	微升
mm	Micrometer	毫米
MCV	Mean corpuscular volume	平均红细胞体积
MDS	Myelodysplastic syndrome	骨髓发育异常综合征
mEq	Milliequivalent	毫当量
NHL	Non-Hodgkin lymphoma	非霍奇金淋巴瘤
PCV	Packed cell volume	红细胞压积
pH	Scale for measuring hydrogen ion concentration (acidity or alkalinity)	离子浓度（酸性或碱性）测量尺度
Ph	Philadelphia chromosome	费城染色体
PMN	Polymorphonuclear (neutrophil)	中性粒细胞
poly	Neutrophil	中性粒细胞
PT	Prothrombin time; pro time	凝血酶原时间
PTT	Partial thromboplastin time	部分凝血活酶时间
RBC	Red blood cell; red blood (cell) count	红细胞计数
seg	Neutrophil	中性粒细胞
SLE	Systemic lupus erythematosus	全身性红斑狼疮
T(C)T	Thrombin (clotting) time	凝血酶（凝血）时间
TTP	Thrombotic thrombocytopenic purpura	血栓性血小板减少性紫癜
vWF	von Willebrand factor	冯·维勒布兰德因子
WBC	White blood cell; white blood (cell) count	白细胞计数

Case Study Revisited 案例研究再访

M. R.'s Case Study Follow-Up

M. R. avoids all contact with any natural rubber latex in her home and at work. She can work only in a pediatric OR, as they are latex-free, because many children with congenital disorders are allergic to latex. She wears a medical alert bracelet, uses a bronchodilator inhaler at the first symptom of bronchospasm, and carries a syringe of epinephrine at all times.

M. R. 案例研究的随访

M. R. 避免在家和工作中与任何天然橡胶、胶乳的物品接触。她只能在儿科手术室中工作，那里是无乳胶的，因为许多患有先天性疾病的儿童对乳胶过敏。她穿着医疗警戒手镯，在支气管痉挛的最初症状发生时使用支气管扩张吸入器，并且随时携带肾上腺素注射器。

CHAPTER 10 复习

标记练习

血细胞

在对应的下划线上写出每个编号部分的名称。

Erythrocyte
Leukocyte
Platelet

1. _____
2. _____
3. _____

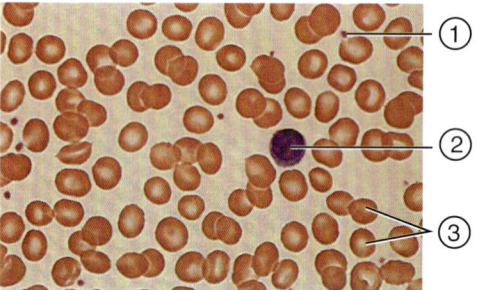

白细胞（白血球）

在对应的下划线上写出每个编号部分的名称。

Basophil   Monocyte
Eosinophil   Neutrophil
Lymphocyte

1. _____
2. _____
3. _____
4. _____
5. _____

Leukocytes (white blood cells)

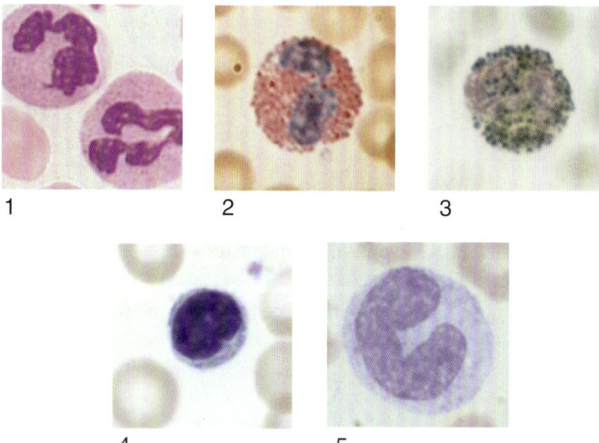

匹配

匹配下列术语，在每个题号的左侧写上适当的字母。

____ 1. anemia   **a.** substance active in blood clotting
____ 2. thrombolytic   **b.** cell that produces platelets
____ 3. antibody   **c.** deficiency in the amount of hemoglobin in the blood
____ 4. megakaryocyte   **d.** able to dissolve a blood clot
____ 5. prothrombin   **e.** substance active in an immune response

____ 6. hypokalemia   **a.** condition involving iron deposits
____ 7. natriuresis   **b.** deficiency of potassium in the blood
____ 8. ferric   **c.** urinary excretion of sodium
____ 9. siderosis   **d.** urinary excretion of nitrogenous compounds
____ 10. azoturia   **e.** pertaining to iron

____ 11. hemophilia   **a.** allergy
____ 12. hemostasis   **b.** hereditary form of anemia
____ 13. hypersensitivity   **c.** stoppage of blood flow
____ 14. thalassemia   **d.** hereditary clotting disorder
____ 15. purpura   **e.** bleeding into the tissues

____ 16. pH   **a.** laboratory test of blood
____ 17. HIV   **b.** a form of leukemia
____ 18. ALL   **c.** hematocrit
____ 19. PCV   **d.** virus that causes an immunodeficiency disease
____ 20. CBC   **e.** scale for measuring acidity or alkalinity

补充术语

____ 21. erythrocytosis   **a.** separation of blood and use of componentswww
____ 22. heparin   **b.** increase in the number of RBCs in the blood
____ 23. apheresis   **c.** anticoagulant
____ 24. ELISA   **d.** method for separating components of a solution
____ 25. electrophoresis   **e.** sensitive immunologic test

填空

26. The engulfing of foreign material by white cells is called_____.
27. The iron-containing pigment in red blood cells that carries oxygen is called_____.
28. A substance that separates into ions in solution is a(n) _____.
29. The cell fragments active in blood clotting are the _____.
30. A hemocytometer is used to count _____.
31. Oxyhemoglobin is hemoglobin combined with_____.
32. A hematoma is a localized collection of_____.
33. A disorder involving lack of hemoglobin in the blood is_____.

34. A myeloma is a neoplasm that involves the _____.
35. The abbreviation Ig means _____.

多项选择

参照本章开头的 M.R. 的案例研究，选择正确的答案，在每个题号的左侧写上你选择的字母。

____ 36. Anaphylaxis, a life-threatening physiologic response, is an extreme form of
    a. remission
    b. hemostasis
    c. hypersensitivity
    d. homeostasis

____ 37. Urticaria is commonly called
    a. hives
    b. dermatitis
    c. rhinitis
    d. congenital

____ 38. The cells involved in a T cell-mediated allergic response are
    a. basophils
    b. monocytes
    c. lymphocytes
    d. B cells

____ 39. The natural latex protein in latex gloves may act as a(n)
    a. antibody
    b. allergen
    c. purpura
    d. immunocyte

____ 40. The common name for epinephrine is
    a. cortisone
    b. adrenaline
    c. heparin
    d. antihistamine

真假判断

检查以下语句。如果语句为真，则在第一个空白处写上 T；如果语句为假，则在第一个空格中写上 F，并在第二个空格中通过替换带下划线的单词来更正语句。

	True or False	Correct answer
41. A leukocyte is also called a <u>platelet</u>.	_____	_____
42. A plasma cell produces <u>antibodies</u>.	_____	_____
43. The liquid that remains after blood coagulates is called <u>serum</u>.	_____	_____
44. Blood that does not react with either A or B antiserum is <u>type O</u>.	_____	_____
45. A band cell is an immature <u>monocyte</u>.	_____	_____
46. The root kali- pertains to <u>potassium</u>.	_____	_____

定义

后缀 -ia、-osis 和 -hemia 都表示词根所指类型的细胞数量上升。请定义下列术语。

47. leukocytosis ［ˌlukosai'tosis］ _____
48. eosinophilia ［ˌiəˌsinə'filiə］ _____
49. erythrocytosis ［iˌriθrəusai'təusis］ _____
50. thrombocythemia ［ˌθrɔmbəusau'θi:miə］ _____

51. neutrophilia [ˌnjuːtrəˈfiliə] _____

52. monocytosis [ˌmɑnəsaiˈtosis] _____

写出下列定义的单词。

53. An immature red blood cell _____

54. A decrease in the number of platelets (thrombocytes) in the blood _____

55. Presence of pus in the blood _____

56. Specialist in the study of immunity _____

定义下列单词。

58. hemolysis _____

59. neutropenia _____

60. myelotoxin _____

61. autoimmunity _____

62. viremia _____

形容词

使用后缀 -ic 写出下列单词的形容词形式。

63. hemolysis _____

64. leukemia _____

65. basophil _____

66. septicemia _____

67. thrombosis _____

68. lymphocyte _____

排除

在下列各组中，为与其余不相配的单词加下划线，并接受你选择的理由。

69. fibrin — thrombin — thrombolysis — prothrombin — fibrinogen

70. Diff — Hct — MCV — EPO — MCH

71. eosinophil — reticulocyte — monocyte — basophil — lymphocyte

72. allergy — hypersensitivity — gamma globulin — urticaria — anaphylaxis

单词构建

使用给出的单词组成部分写出下列定义的单词。

| -penia | -blast | leuk/o | -oid | -poiesis | myel/o | gen- | -emia | erythr/o | -ic | -oma | cyt/o |

73. pertaining to a red blood cell _____

74. an immature white blood cell _____
75. pertaining to bone marrow _____
76. originating in bone marrow _____
77. an immature bone marrow cell _____
78. neoplastic overgrowth of white cells in the blood _____
79. deficiency of white cells in the blood _____
80. cancer of bone marrow _____
81. formation of red blood cells _____
82. pertaining to bone marrow cells _____

单词分析

定义下列单词，并给出每个单词组成部分的含义。如果需要，可以使用词典。

83. Pancytopenia [pænsaitə'pi:niə] _____
  a. pan- _____
  b. cyt/o _____
  c. -penia _____

84. Polycythemia [pɒlisai'θi:mjə] _____
  a. poly- _____
  b. cyt/o _____
  c. hem/o _____
  d. -ia _____

85. Anisochromia [ənisək'rəʊmiə] _____
  a. an- _____
  b. iso- _____
  c. chrom/o _____
  d. -ia _____

86. Myelodysplastic [maiələʊdi'spleitik] _____
  a. myel/o _____
  b. dys- _____
  c. plast(y) _____
  d. –ic _____

Additional Case Studies
补充案例研究

Case Study 10-1: Blood Replacement
案例研究 10-1：血液置换

C. L., a 16-year-old girl, sustained a ruptured liver when she hit a tree while sledding. Emergency surgery was needed to stop the internal bleeding. During surgery, the ruptured segment of the liver was removed, and the laceration was sutured with a heavy, absorbable suture on a large smooth needle. Before surgery, her hemoglobin was 10.2 g/dL, but the reading decreased to 7.6 g/dL before hemostasis was attained. Cell salvage, or autotransfusion, was set up. In this procedure, the free blood was suctioned from her abdomen and mixed with an anticoagulant (heparin). The RBCs were washed in a sterile centrifuge with NS and transfused back to her through tubing fitted with a filter. She also received six units of homologous, leukocyte-reduced whole blood, five units of fresh frozen plasma, and two units of platelets. During the surgery, the CRNA repeatedly tested her Hgb and Hct as well as prothrombin time and partial thromboplastin time to monitor her clotting mechanisms.

C. L. is B-positive. Fortunately, there was enough B-positive blood in the hospital blood bank for her surgery. The laboratory informed her surgeon that they had two units of B-negative and six units of O-negative blood, which she could have received safely if she needed more blood during the night. However, her hemoglobin level increased to 12 g/dL, and she was stable during her recovery. She was monitored for DIC and pulmonary emboli.

C. L. 是一名 16 岁的女孩，当她的雪橇撞到树时，肝脏破裂了。她需要紧急手术来止住内出血。在手术期间，破碎的肝被清除，并且用粗的可吸收缝合线和光滑的大缝针缝合了伤口。手术前，她的血红蛋白为 10.2 g / dl，但在止血前降至 7.6 g / dl。为她建立了细胞补救（cell salvage），或称为自体输血（autotransfusion）。在该过程中，从她的腹部抽吸游离的血液，并与抗凝血剂（heparin，肝素）混合。白细胞在具有生理盐水（NS）的无菌离心机中洗涤，并通过装配有过滤器的管道输送回她的身体。她还接受了 6U 的同源、白细胞减少的全血、5U 的新鲜冷冻血浆和 2U 的血小板。在手术期间，CRNA 重复测试她的血红蛋白（Hgb）和血细胞比容（Hct）以及凝血酶原时间和部分凝血活酶时间，以监测她的凝血机制。

C. L. 的血液为 B 型。幸运的是，医院血库中有足够的 B 型血用于她的手术。实验室告诉她的外科医生，他们有 2U 的 B 型血和 6U 的 O 型血，她可以安全地接受，如果在夜间她需要更多的血液的话。然而，她的血红蛋白水平增加到 12 g / dl，她在恢复期间是稳定的。还监测了她的弥漫性血管内凝血（disseminated intravascular coagulation，DIC）和肺栓塞。

Case Study 10-2: Myelofibrosis
案例研究 10-2：骨髓纤维化

A.Y., a 52-year-old kindergarten teacher, had myelofibrosis that had been in remission for 25 years. She had seen her hematologist regularly and had had routine blood testing since the age of 27. After several weeks of fatigue, idiopathic joint and muscle aching, weakness, and a frightening episode of syncope, she saw her hematologist for evaluation. Her hemoglobin was 9.0 g/dL and her hematocrit was 29 percent. Concerned that she was having an exacerbation, her doctor scheduled a bone marrow aspiration, and the results were positive for myelofibrosis.

A.Y. went through a six-month therapy regimen of iron supplements in the form of ferrous sulfate tablets and received weekly vitamin B12 injections. Interferon was given every other week in addition to erythropoiesis therapy, which was unsuccessful. She was treated for presumed aplastic anemia. During treatment, splenomegaly developed, which compromised her abdominal organs and pulmonary

A.Y. 是一名 52 岁的幼儿园老师，患有骨髓纤维化（myelofibrosis），已缓解 25 年。她经常去看到她的血液学医生，并从 27 岁开始进行常规的血液检查。经过几个星期的疲劳、突发性关节和肌肉疼痛、乏力以及可怕的晕厥发作后，她找到血液学医生进行评估。她的血红蛋白是 9.0 g / dl，血细胞比容是 29%。关注到她病情发生了恶化（exacerbation），医生安排了骨髓抽吸，结果为骨髓纤维化阳性。

A.Y. 经历了 6 个月的硫酸亚铁片剂形式的铁补充剂治疗，并且每周接受维生素 B_{12} 注射。除了红细胞生成治疗之外，每隔 1 周服用干扰素（interferon），但并不成功。她被按照再生障碍性贫血进行治疗，在治疗期间，发生了脾肿大，损害了她的腹部器官和肺功能。她的体重持续降低，血红蛋白降至 6.0 g / dl。每周输注浓缩红

function. She continued to lose weight, and her hemoglobin dropped as low as 6.0 g/dL. Weekly transfusions of packed RBCs did not improve her hemoglobin and hematocrit.

After a regimen of high-dose chemotherapy to shrink the fibers in her bone marrow and a splenectomy, A.Y. received a stem cell transplant. The stem cells were obtained from blood donated by her brother, who was a perfect immunologic match. After a six-month period of recovery in a protected environment, required because of her immunocompromised state, A.Y. returned home and has been free of disease symptoms for over one year.

细胞不能改善她的血红蛋白和血细胞比容。

在大剂量化疗以收缩其骨髓中的纤维和脾切除术完成之后，A.Y. 接受干细胞移植。干细胞从她的兄弟捐献的血液中获得，其是完美的免疫学匹配。在受保护的环境中恢复 6 个月后，由于免疫受损状态的需要，A.Y. 返回家中，在超过 1 年的时间中没有疾病症状。

案例研究问题

多项选择，选择正确的答案，在每个题号的左侧写上你选择的字母。

____ 1. The unit for hemoglobin measurement (g/dl) means

    a. grams in decimal point

    b. grains in a deciliter

    c. drops in 50 mL

    d. grams in 100 Ml

____ 2. Heparin, an anticoagulant, is a drug that

    a. increases the rate of blood clotting

    b. takes the place of fibrin

    c. makes blood thinner than water

    d. interferes with blood clotting

____ 3. The RBCs were washed with NS. This means the _____ were washed with_____.

    a. reticulocytes, heparin

    b. red blood cells, nutritional solution

    c. erythrocytes, normal saline

    d. red blood cells, heparin

____ 4. Autotransfusion is transfusion of autologous blood, that is, the patient's own blood. Homologous blood is taken from

    a. another human

    b. synthetic chemicals

    c. plasma with clotting factors

    d. IV fluid with electrolytes

____ 5. Patients who lose significant amounts of blood may lose clotting ability. Effective therapy in such cases would be replacement of

    a. IV solution with electrolytes

    b. packed RBCs

    c. platelets

    d. heparin

____ 6. C.L.'s blood type is B-positive. The best blood for her to receive is

    a. A-negative

    b. AB-positive

    c. B-negative

    d. B-positive

____ 7. Myelofibrosis, like aplastic anemia, is a disease in which there is

    a. overgrowth of RBCs

    b. destruction of the bone marrow

    c. dangerously high hemoglobin and hematocrit

    d. absence of bone marrow

____ 8. Erythropoiesis is

    a. production of blood

    b. production of red cells

    c. destruction of platelets

    d. destruction of white cells

____ 9. The "ferrous" in ferrous sulfate represents
   a. electrolytes
   b. B vitamins
   c. iron
   d. oxygen

____ 10. Hemoglobin and hematocrit values pertain to
   a. leukocytes
   b. fibrinogen
   c. granulocytes
   d. red blood cells

____ 11. Splenomegaly is
   a. prolapse of the spleen
   b. movement of the spleen
   c. enlargement of the lymph glands
   d. enlargement of the spleen

____ 12. The stem cells A.Y. received were expected to develop into new
   a. spleen cells
   b. bone marrow cells
   c. hemoglobin
   d. cartilage

____ 13. A.Y.'s health was compromised because the high-dose chemotherapy caused
   a. immunodeficiency
   b. electrolyte imbalance
   c. anoxia
   d. autoimmunity

定义下列缩略语。

14. PT _____

15. PTT _____

16. FFP _____

17. Hgb _____

18. Hct _____

19. DIC _____

CHAPTER 11

呼吸系统

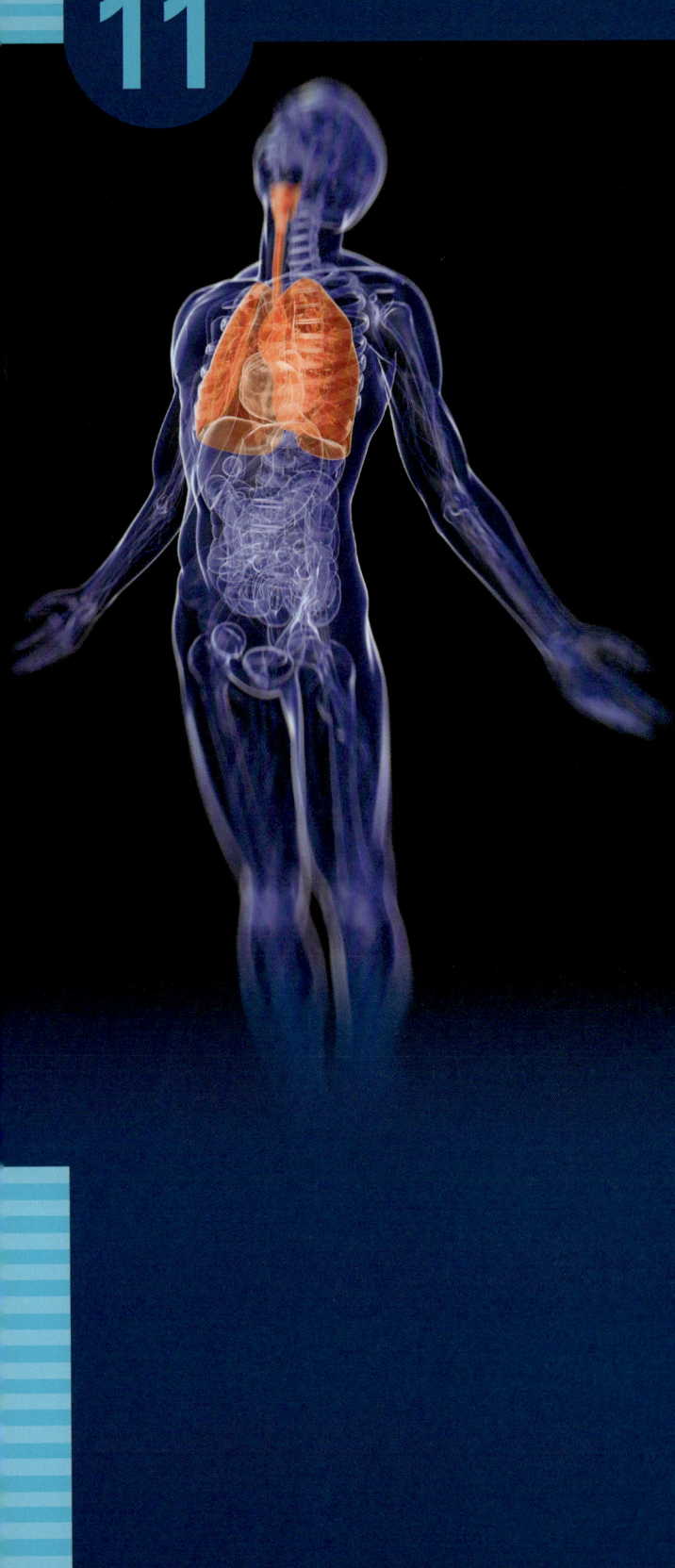

预测试

多项选择。选择正确的答案,在每个题号左侧写上你选择的字母。

_____ 1. The gas that is supplied to tissues by the respiratory system is
   a. sulfur
   b. neon
   c. oxygen
   d. carbon dioxide

_____ 2. The gas that is eliminated by the respiratory system is
   a. chlorine
   b. carbon dioxide
   c. hydrogen
   d. fluoride

_____ 3. The air sacs through which gases are exchanged in the lungs are the
   a. trachea
   b. bronchi
   c. bursae
   d. alveoli

_____ 4. The structure that holds the vocal folds is the
   a. larynx
   b. tongue
   c. uvula
   d. tonsils

_____ 5. The tubes that carry air from the trachea into the lungs are the
   a. arteries
   b. nares
   c. veins
   d. bronchi

_____ 6. The domeshaped muscle under the lungs is the
   a. palate
   b. hiatus
   c. diaphragm
   d. esophagus

_____ 7. The membrane around the lungs is the
   a. peritoneum
   b. mucosa
   c. pleura
   d. mediastinum

_____ 8. A term for inflammation of the lungs is
   a. bronchitis
   b. pneumonia
   c. pleurisy
   d. laryngitis

学习目标

学完本章后，应该能够：

1. ▶ 比较外部和内部的气体交换。
2. ▶ 描述呼吸道的结构，并了解它们的功能。
3. ▶ 描述呼吸的机制，包括隔膜和膈神经的作用。
4. ▶ 说明氧气和二氧化碳是如何在血液中运送的。
5. ▶ 识别并使用与呼吸系统相关的单词组成部分。
6. ▶ 讨论呼吸系统的九种疾病。
7. ▶ 列举出影响呼吸系统的三种微生物类型，并给出每种类型的示例。
8. ▶ 列出并定义测量肺功能使用的 10 种流量和容量。
9. ▶ 解释呼吸系统中常用的缩略语。
10. ▶ 分析案例研究中关于呼吸的医学术语。

Case Study: Preoperative Respiratory Testing for A. D., a Young Girl with Asthma
案例研究：一名患有哮喘的女孩 A. D. 的手术前呼吸测试

Chief Complaint

A. D., a 13yearold girl, was seen in the preadmission testing unit in preparation for her elective spinal surgery for scoliosis. She has a history of mild asthma since age 4 with at least one attack a week. In an acute attack, she will have mild dyspnea, diffuse wheezing, yet an adequate air exchange that responds to bronchodilators. She was sent to pulmonary health services for a consult with a pulmonologist and pulmonary function studies to clear her for the upcoming spinal surgery.

主诉

A. D. 是一名 13 岁的女孩，在入院前试验病房为她矫正脊柱侧凸的选择性脊柱外科手术做准备。她从 4 岁起就有轻度哮喘病史，每周至少发作一次。在急性发作中，她会有轻微的呼吸困难和弥漫性喘息，但有足够的气体交换对支气管扩张剂做出反应。她被送到肺部健康服务部门咨询胸内科医生，并做肺功能分析，以便她进行即将到来的脊柱手术。

Examination

Her physical examination was unremarkable except for her respiratory status. Her prebronchodilator spirometry showed a mild reduction in vital capacity but with a moderate to severe decrease in FEV1 and FEV1/FVC ratio. After bronchodilator administration, there was a mild but insignificant improvement in FEV1. The postbronchodilator FEV1 was 55 percent of predicted value and was considered moderately abnormal. The flow volume loops and spirographic curves were consistent with airflow obstruction.

检查

除了呼吸状况外，她的身体检查无明显异常。她的呼吸支气管扩张剂肺活量测定显示肺活量的轻微降低，但 FEV1 和 FEV1 / FVC 比值中度至重度降低，在给予支气管扩张剂后，FEV1 有轻度但不明显的改善。支气管扩张剂 FEV1 为预测值的 55%，被认为是中度异常。流量环路和螺旋曲线与气流阻塞一致。

Clinical Course

The anesthesiologist reviewed the pulmonologist's report. A. D.'s respiratory status was compromised for the surgical procedure and would require medical intervention prior to going to the OR. When the FEV1 was acceptable, he spoke with A. D. and the family and explained that her respiratory status would be closely monitored during and after surgery. Additional medications would be needed to maintain optimal airflow and oxygenation.

临床病程

麻醉师评估了胸内科医生的报告。A. D. 的呼吸状态危及外科手术，在进入手术室之前需要医疗干预。在 FEV1 是可接受状态时，他向 A. D. 及其家人说明她的呼吸状态将在手术期间和之后进行密切监测，需要额外的药物来维持最佳的气流和氧合。

简介

呼吸系统（respiratory system）的主要功能是为全身的细胞提供氧气以进行新陈代谢（metabolism），并排除新陈代谢的副产品二氧化碳（carbon dioxide）。因为这些气体必须从细胞中送入血液，呼吸系统与心血管系统紧密合作，以完成气体交换（图11-1）。这一活动有两个阶段：

- 发生在外部空气与血液之间的外部气体交换。
- 发生在血液与组织之间的内部气体交换。

外部交换发生在位于胸腔的肺（lung）。呼吸道的其余部分由一系列引导空气进入和流出肺部的通道构成，在这些通道内并不发生气体交换。图11-2给出了呼吸系统的构成。

上呼吸道

上呼吸道（upper respiratory passageways）由鼻子和咽（pharynx）构成。空气也可以通过口腔进行交换，但针对通过该途径吸进的空气的清洁机制比较少。

鼻子

空气由鼻子（nose）进入，纤毛和黏膜覆盖的鼻腔会将空气加温、过滤和湿润。纤毛（cilia）——覆盖鼻腔内部细胞的微小毛发状突起——将灰尘和外来物质扫向喉咙，以便清除。通过咳嗽或清理喉咙被呼吸道清除的物质被称为痰（sputum）。嗅觉受体位于鼻腔骨侧突起，被称为鼻甲骨（turbinate bones）或鼻甲（conchae）。

颅骨与鼻子附近的脸部是充气的腔体，该腔体内附黏膜，引流到鼻腔。这些腔体能够减轻骨骼，并在说话时产生共振，这些被称为窦的腔体分别根据它们所位于的骨骼命名，例如额（frontal）窦、蝶（sphenoidal）窦、筛（ethmoidal）窦和上颌

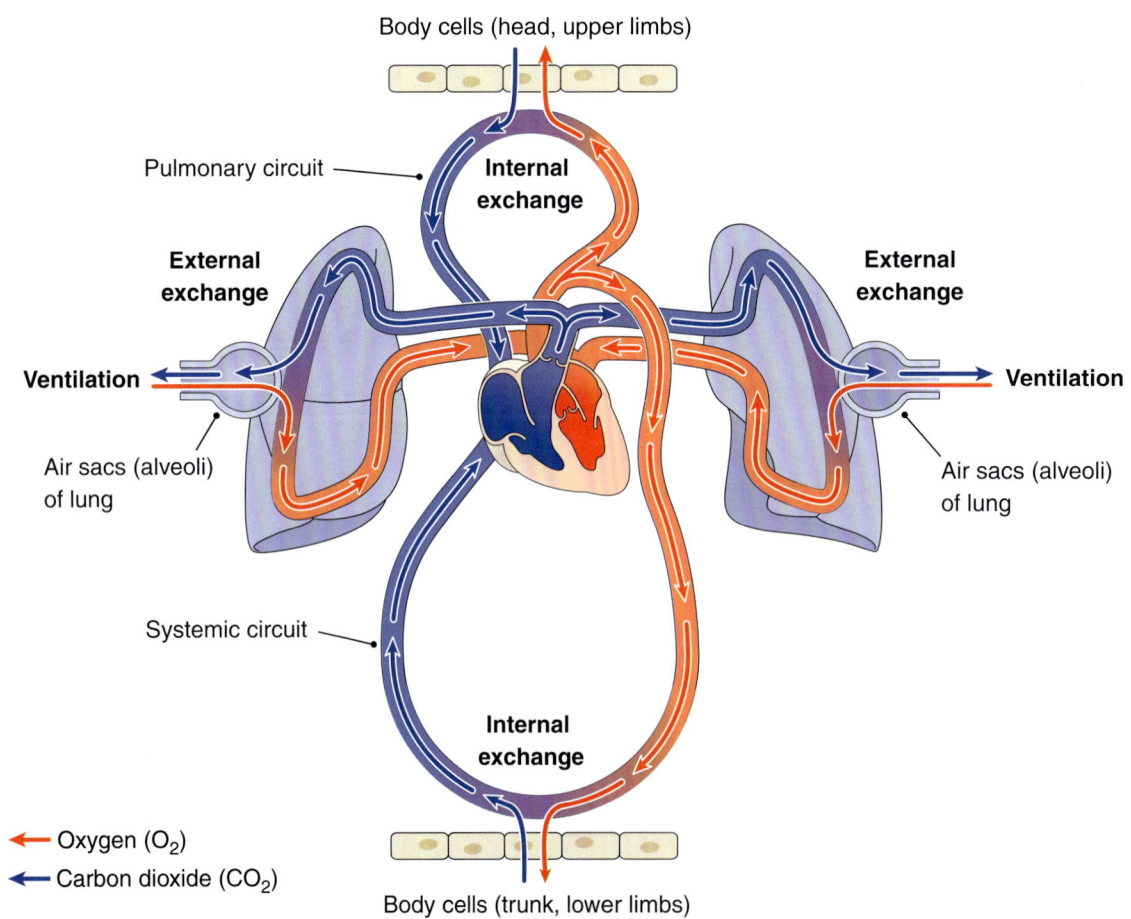

图11-1 呼吸。在通气中，气体进入和并流出肺。在外部交换中，气体在肺的气囊（肺泡）和血液之间流动。在内部交换中，气体在血液和体细胞之间流动。体内循环输送血液中的气体

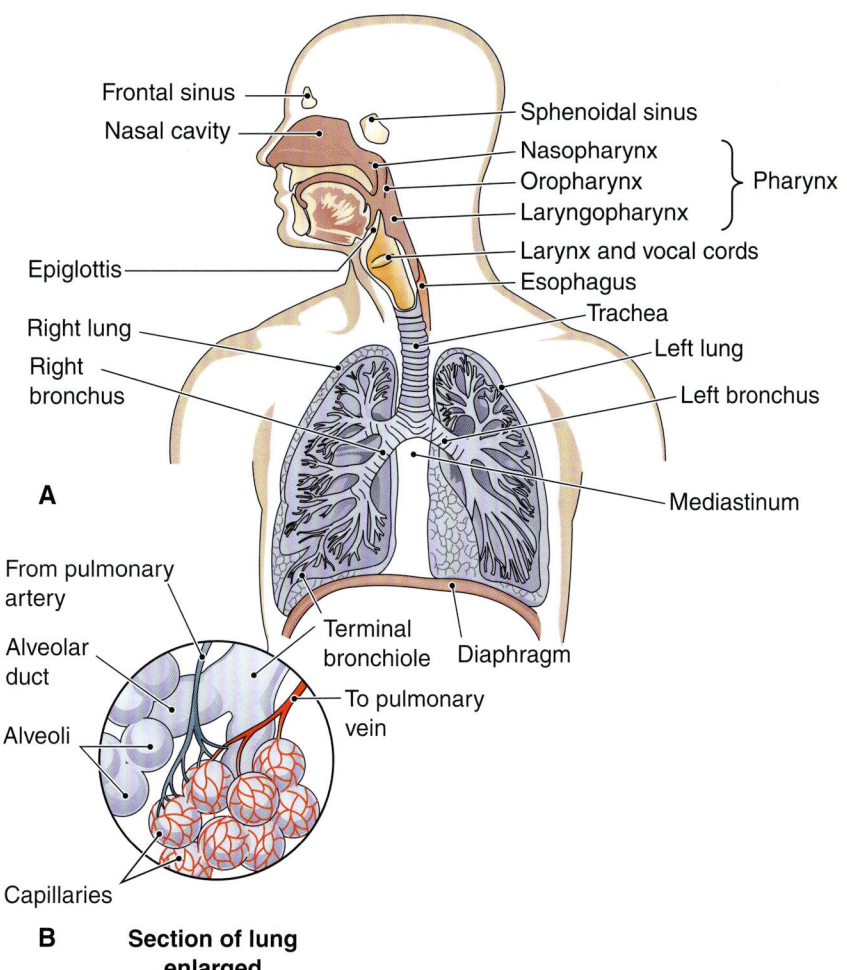

图 11-2 呼吸系统。A. 概貌；B. 肺组织的放大部分，显示肺泡（气囊）和毛细血管之间的关系

（maxillary）窦。因为它们靠近鼻子，这些腔体一起被称为鼻窦（paranasal sinuses）。图 11-2 显示了额叶和蝶状窦的位置。

咽

吸入的空气通过喉咙，或咽（pharynx），与通过口进入的空气和要进入消化道的食物混合在一起。咽有三个部分，如同 11-2 所示：

- 鼻咽（nasopharynx），咽喉的上部，位于鼻腔后面。
- 口咽（oropharynx），咽喉的中部，位于口腔的后面。
- 喉咽（laryngopharynx），咽喉的下部，位于喉的后面。

第 9 章描述的扁桃腺（tonsils）是位于咽的淋巴组织（图 11-3）：

- 腭扁桃腺（palatine tonsil），口咽两侧的软腭。
- 单咽扁桃腺（single pharyngeal tonsil），常被称为腺状体（adenoid），位于鼻咽。
- 舌扁桃腺（lingual tonsil），舌后部的小淋巴组织丘。

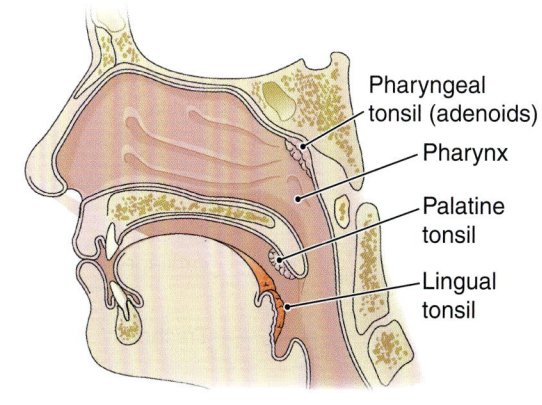

图 11-3 扁桃腺。所有扁桃腺都位于咽（咽喉）附近

框 11-1

临床观点
扁桃腺切除术：一种被反思的治疗方法

扁桃腺炎是扁桃腺的细菌感染，是一种儿童常见病。在过去，手术切除被感染的扁桃腺是一种标准治疗方法，扁桃腺切除术（tonsillectomy）被用于防止类似脓毒性咽喉炎等严重感染。因为扁桃体被认为没有什么功能，手术通常会切掉感染的扁桃腺——甚至是健康的扁桃腺，以便防止扁桃炎。随着扁桃腺被发现有很重要的免疫功能，在美国被执行的扁桃腺切除术数量急剧下降，在 1980 年降到最低。

现在，尽管许多扁桃腺炎能够用适当的抗生素成功治疗，但扁桃腺切除术却越来越多。如果发生感染或扁桃腺肿大使吞咽或呼吸困难，就会考虑手术。许多儿童扁桃腺行切除术是为了治疗阻塞性睡眠呼吸暂停（obstructive sleep apnea），有这种状况的儿童在睡眠期间会有几秒钟停止呼吸。最近的研究显示，扁桃腺切除术对患有中耳炎（otitis media）的儿童也有益处，因为扁桃腺细菌感染可能会传到耳朵的这一区域。

大多数扁桃腺切除术通过电烙术（electrocautery）完成，这是一种使用电流将扁桃腺烧掉的技术。现在又开发出了新技术，低温消融扁桃体切除术（coblation tonsillectomy）使用无线电波分解扁桃腺组织。研究表明，与电烙术相比，这种方法恢复快、并发症少、术后疼痛下降。

关于切除扁桃腺的相关看法随时间而变（框 11-1）。

下呼吸道和肺

空气从咽进入喉（larynx）。喉位于气管（trachea，windpipe）的顶部，气管将空气导入通向肺的支气管系统（bronchial system）。

喉

喉（larynx）是由九块软骨（cartilage）构成的，最主要的是形成喉结（Adam's apple）的前甲状软骨（anterior thyroid cartilage）（图 11-4）。喉顶部的小叶状软骨是会厌软骨（epiglottis），在吞咽时，会厌软骨盖住喉的开口，并协助防止食物进入呼吸道。

喉包含声带（vocal cords），是对发声非常重要的组织褶皱（图 11-5）。空气通过声带产生的震动是产生语音的基础，不过喉咙和口腔都是清晰的语音发音所必须的。声带之间的开口是声门（glottis），会厌软骨在声门之上。

气管

气管（trachea）是被 C 形软骨环加强了的管

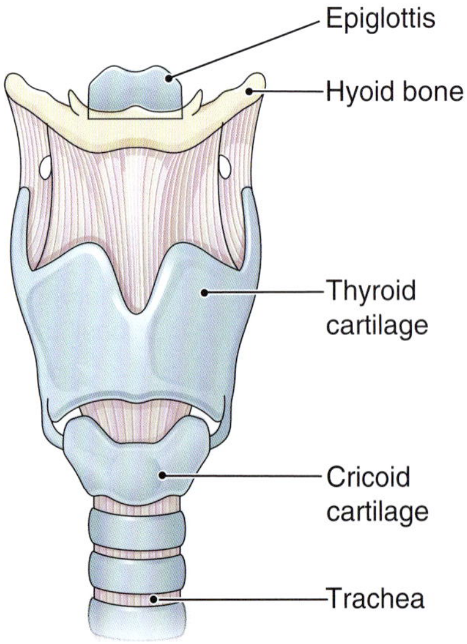

图 11-4 喉前视图

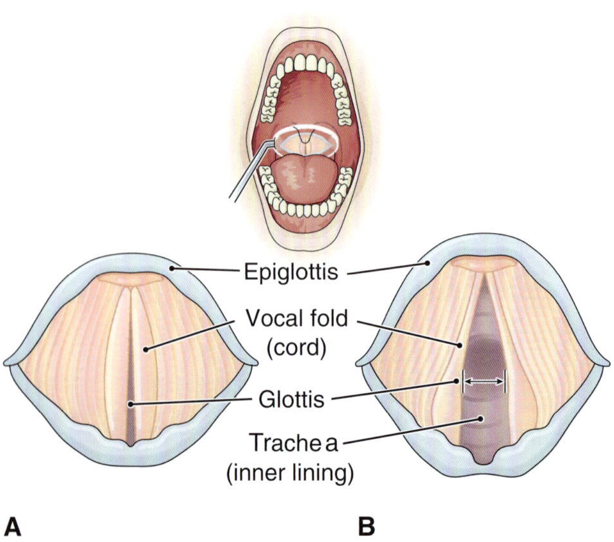

图 11-5 声带，上部视图。A. 声门处于关闭位置；B. 声门处于打开位置

道，加强是为了避免塌陷（如果你用手指轻按喉咙，能够感觉到这些软骨环）。气管内壁上的纤毛能够将杂质移到喉咙，在那里它们被通过吞咽、吐痰（expectoration）或咳嗽排出。

气管在一个被称为纵隔腔（mediastinum）的区域，该区域由肺之间的空间和在这个空间里的器官组成（图 11-2）。除气管外，纵隔腔还包括心脏、食管（esophagus）、大血管和其他组织。

支气管系统

气管在自身的下端分为进入肺的左右两侧主支气管（bronchus）。右支气管比较短粗，在右肺分为三根次支气管；左支气管在左肺分为两根次支气管。进一步的分叉产生数量不断增加的更小的气管为更小的肺组织供应空气。随着空气进入肺，气管壁上的软骨环逐渐消失，并被平滑肌取代。

最小的气管是细支气管（bronchiole），将空气送入微小的气囊——肺泡（alveolus，复数alveoli），肺与血液在肺泡中进行气体交换。通过肺泡极薄的壁及其周围的毛细血管，氧气被释放到血液中，血液中的二氧化碳被排出（图 11-2）。

肺

锥形的肺（lung）占据了胸腔的主要部分。右肺比较大，分为三个肺叶（lobe）。左肺比较小以便为心脏留出空间，分为两个肺叶。肺叶进一步细分到对应的支气管系统。

胸膜（pleura）是双层的隔膜，覆盖肺并内衬整个胸腔（图 11-6）。胸膜的两层是：

- 壁层胸膜（parietal pleura），胸膜的外层，附着在胸腔壁。
- 脏层胸膜（visceral pleura），胸膜的内层，附着在肺的表面。

在两层胸膜之间非常狭窄、充满液体的是胸膜腔。湿润的胸膜可以在胸腔内彼此滑过，使得肺能够在呼吸期间膨胀。

呼吸

通过呼吸（breathing）过程，空气进入并流出肺。这一过程被技术性地称为肺通气（pulmonary ventilation），包含一个稳定的吸气（inspiration）（吸入，inhalation）和呼气（expiration，呼出，exhalation）周期，中间有一个间隔。呼吸通常是由脑干中心无意识地调节。这些中心根据血液成分的变化，特别是二氧化碳的浓度调节呼吸的速率和节奏。

吸气

当膈神经（phrenic nerve）刺激膈肌（diaphragm）

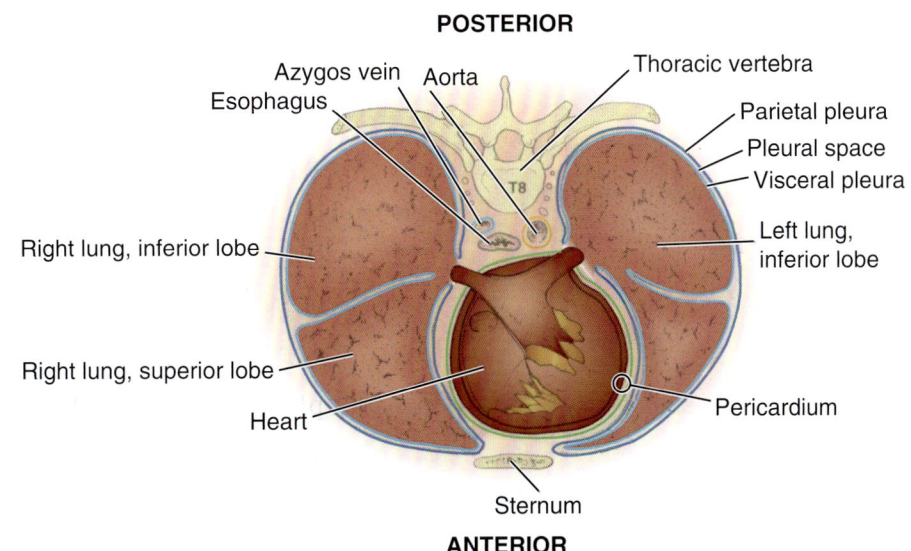

图 11-6 胸膜。通过肺的横截面显示胸膜的腔壁和内脏层以及纵隔的结构

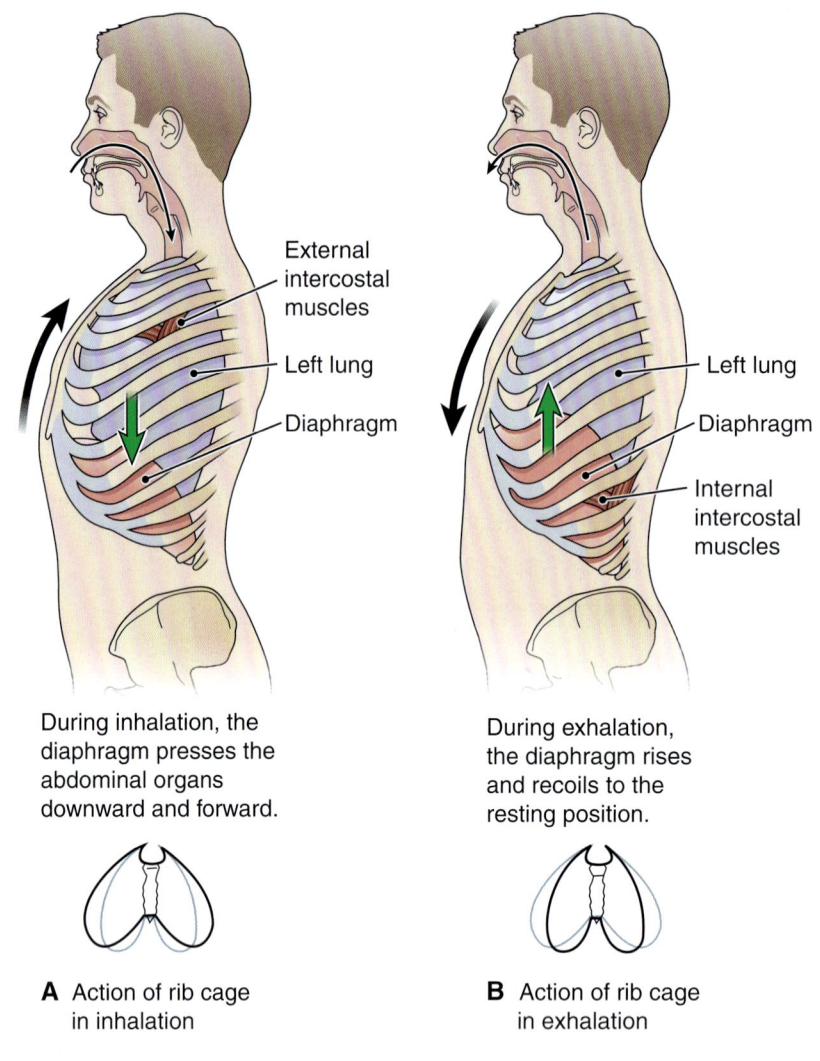

图 11-7 肺通气。A. 吸入时，隔膜下降，外肋间肌抬高胸廓；B. 呼气时，呼吸肌松弛，膈肌上升，肺恢复原来的大小。内肋间肌在有力的呼气时向下拉动胸廓

收缩变平，扩张胸腔，吸气（inspiration）就开始了。同时，肋骨之间的外部肋间肌提升并扩大胸廓（rib cage），导致胸腔内部压力下降，使空气流入肺中（图 11-7）。颈部和胸部的肌肉被用于加强吸入的力度。

肺在压力下扩张的度量是依从性（compliance）。肺产生的被称为表面活性剂（surfactant）的液体，通过降低肺泡内的表面张力协助这一依从性。

呼气

随着呼吸肌放松，有弹性的肺恢复到原来的大小，呼气（expiration）开始发生。较小的胸腔内升高的压力使得空气从肺中流出。在有力的呼出过程中，内部肋间肌收缩胸廓缩小，腹部肌肉收缩，将内部器官推向膈肌。

气体输送

氧气（oxygen）由红细胞中的血红蛋白（hemoglobin）携带，释放给需要氧气的细胞。二氧化碳（carbon dioxide）以几种不同的方式运送，主要是转化为碳酸（carbonic acid），基于碳酸的形成量，二氧化碳的呼出量对调节身体的酸碱度非常重要。血液 pH 值的偏离可能是呼出太多或太少的二氧化碳所致。

Terminology 关键术语

正常结构和功能

术语	释义
adenoids ['ædənɔidz]	腺状体，位于鼻咽的淋巴组织；咽扁桃腺
alveoli [æl'vi:əlai]	肺泡，肺中微小的气囊，在呼吸过程中，空气与血液在肺泡中进行气体交换（单数：alveolus）
bronchiole ['brɒŋkiəʊl]	细支气管，比较小的支气管分支（词根：bronchiol）
bronchus ['brɒŋkəs]	支气管，通向肺的较大的空气通道。支气管起始于气管的两个分支，进而在肺中细分（复数：bronchi；词根：bronch）
carbon dioxide (CO_2)	二氧化碳，细胞中能量新陈代谢产生的气体，通过肺排出
carbonic acid	碳酸，二氧化碳在水中分解产生的一种酸；H_2CO_3
compliance [kəm'plaiəns]	依从性，肺在压力下扩张的度量。在许多种呼吸疾病中，依从性都有下降
diaphragm ['daiəfræm]	膈肌，肺之下的圆顶形肌肉，在吸气期间变平（词根：phren/o）
epiglottis [ˌepi'glɒtis]	会厌软骨，在吞咽期间覆盖喉部以防止食物进入气管的叶形软骨
expectoration [ikˌspektə'reiʃn]	咳痰，将杂质（痰）咳出呼吸道的动作
expiration [ˌekspə'reiʃn]	呼气，将空气从肺中排出的动作；exhalation glottis ['glɒtis] 呼气声门、声带之间的开口
inspiration [ˌinspə'reiʃn]	吸气，将空气吸入肺中的动作；inhalation 吸入
larynx ['læriŋks]	喉，气管扩大的上部，其中包含声带（词根：laryng/o）
lung [lʌŋ]	肺，锥形海绵状呼吸器官，在胸腔之内（词根：pneum, pulm）
mediastinum [ˌmi:diæs'tainəm]	纵隔腔，两肺之间的空间和该空间中包含的器官
nose [nəʊz]	鼻子，面部用于呼吸和容纳嗅觉受体的器官；包括外部和内部鼻腔（词根：nas/o, rhin/o）
oxygen (O_2) ['ɒksidʒən]	氧气，细胞在新陈代谢过程中需要的用于从食物中释放能量的气体
palatine tonsils ['pælətain 'tɒnsilz]	腭扁桃腺，位于口咽两侧成对的淋巴组织团
pharynx ['færiŋks] 咽	喉咙，食物进入食管和空气进入喉的公用通道（词根：pharyng/o）
phrenic nerve ['frenik]	膈神经，触发膈肌的神经（词根：phrenic/o）
pleura ['plʊərə]	胸膜，内衬胸腔（壁层胸膜 parietal pleura）并覆盖肺（脏层胸膜 visceral pleura）的双层隔膜（词根：pleur/o）
pleural space ['plʊrə]	胸膜腔，两层胸膜之间的狭窄、充满液体的空间；也称作 pleural cavity
pulmonary ventilation ['pʊlməˌneri: ˌventl'eiʃən]	肺通气，空气进出肺的运动
sinus ['sainəs]	窦，腔体或沟道；鼻窦（paranasal sinuses）位于鼻子附近，引流进入鼻腔

Terminology	关键术语（续表）
sputum ['spju:təm]	痰，通过咳嗽或清洁喉咙排出的物质；可能包含来自呼吸道的多种物质
surfactant [sɜːˈfæktənt]	表面活性剂，肺泡中降低表面张力、促使肺扩张的一种物质
trachea [trəˈkiːə]	气管，从喉延伸到支气管的气体通道（词根：trache/o）
turbinate bones ['tɜːbinit]	鼻甲骨，鼻腔的骨骼突起，包含嗅觉受体
vocal cords	声带，喉两侧的膜褶皱，对发声非常重要。也被称为 vocal folds

与呼吸系统相关的单词组成部分

参见表 11-1 至表 11-3

表 11-1　与呼吸相关的后缀

后缀	含义	示例	示例定义
-pnea	呼吸	orthopnea [ɔːˈθɒpnjə]	端坐呼吸
-oxia*	氧气水平	hypoxia [haɪˈpɒksiə]	组织缺氧
-capnia*	二氧化碳水平	hypercapnia [ˌhaɪpəˈkæpniə]	高碳酸血症
-phonia	语音	dysphonia [dɪsˈfəʊniə]	发音障碍

* 在指血液中氧气和二氧化碳的水平时，使用后缀 -emia，例如 hypoxemia, hypercapnemia

练习 11-1

使用后缀 -pnea 构成下列含义的单词。

1. breathing difficulty that is relieved by assuming an upright position (ortho)
2. slow (brady-) rate of breathing
3. easy, normal (eu-) breathing
4. painful or difficult breathing

使用后缀 -pneic 写出上面单词的形容词形式。

5.
6.
7.
8.

练习 11-1　（续表）

使用表 11-1 中的后缀写出下列含义的单词。

9. difficulty speaking　　　　　　　　　　_____
10. decreased carbon dioxide in the tissues　_____
11. lack of (an-) oxygen in the tissues　　　_____
12. increased levels of carbon dioxide in the tissues　_____

表 11-2　呼吸道的词根

词根	含义	示例	示例定义
nas/o	鼻子	intranasal [ˌintrəˈneizəl]	鼻内的
rhin/o	鼻子	rhinoplasty [ˈrainəˌplæsti]	鼻成形术
pharyng/o*	咽	pharyngeal [fəˈrindʒiəl]	咽部的
laryng/o*	喉	laryngospasm [lærinˈgɒspæzəm]	喉痉挛
trache/o	气管	tracheotome [tˈrækiɒtəʊm]	气管刀
bronch/o, bronch/i	支气管	bronchogenic [brɒnkədˈʒenik]	源于支气管的
bronchiol	细支气管	bronchiolectasis [brɒntʃiːəʊˈlektəsis]	细支气管扩张

*在形容词结尾 -al 前词根要加一个 e

练习 11-2

写出下列定义的单词。

1. discharge from the nose　　　　　　　　　_____
2. pertaining to the larynx（表 11-2）　　　　_____
3. inflammation of the bronchi　　　　　　　_____
4. endoscopic examination of the pharynx　_____
5. plastic repair of the larynx　　　　　　　_____
6. surgical incision of the trachea　　　　　_____
7. narrowing of a trachea　　　　　　　　　_____
8. inflammation of the bronchioles　　　　　_____

定义下列单词（请注意形容词结尾）。

9. bronchiolar [ˌbrɒnkiˈəʊlə]　　_____
10. paranasal [pærəˈneizəl]　　　_____

练习 11-2 （续表）

11. peribronchial ［ˌperaib'rɒnkjəl］
12. endotracheal ［ˌendəʊ'treikiəl］
13. nasopharyngeal ［ˌneizəʊfə'rindʒiəl］
14. bronchiectasis ［brɒŋki'ektəsis］

表 11-3　肺和呼吸的词根

词根	含义	示例	示例定义
phren/o	膈肌	phrenic ［'frenik］	膈肌的
phrenic/o	膈神经	phrenicectomy ［freni'sektəmi］	膈神经切除术
pleur/o	胸膜	pleurodesis ［plʊə'rəʊdi:sis］	胸膜固定术
pulm/o, pulmon/o	肺	extrapulmonary ［ikstræ'pʌlmənəri］	肺外的
pneumon/o	肺	pneumonitis ［nju:məʊ'naitis］	肺炎，pneumonia
pneum/o, pneumat/o	空气，气体	pneumothorax ［ˌnju:mə'θɔ:ræks］	气胸
spir/o	呼吸	spirometer ［ˌspaiə'rɒmitə］	肺活量计

练习 11-3

定义下列单词。

1. pleuralgia ［plʊə'rældʒiə］
2. intrapulmonary ［intrə'pʌlmənəri］
3. pneumonectomy ［ˌnju:mə'nektəmi］
4. pneumoplasty ［ˌnju:mə'plæsti］
5. pulmonology ［pʌl'mənɒlədʒi］
6. apneumia ［æp'nju:miə］
7. phrenicotomy ［freni'kətəmi］

写出下列定义的单词。

8. within the pleura
9. above the diaphragm
10. surgical puncture of the pleural space
11. any disease of the lungs (pneumon/o)
12. crushing of the phrenic nerve
13. record of breathing volumes

呼吸系统的临床表现

任何影响空气进入呼吸道或限制胸部扩张的疾病都会影响肺功能。这些疾病可能直接涉及呼吸系统，例如感染、受伤、过敏、吸入外来物体或癌症；也可能源于其他系统，例如骨骼、肌肉、心血管或神经系统。

如上所述，通气的变化可能影响血液的 pH 值（酸碱度）。如果通气过度（hyperventilation）呼出太多的二氧化碳，血液就会偏碱性，造成碱中毒（alkalosis）。如果通气过（hypoventilation）低导致呼出二氧化碳过少，血液就会偏酸性，造成酸中毒（acidosis）。

感染

很多种微生物都会感染呼吸道，框 11-2 中给出了其中的一些，并列出了它们会引起的疾病。儿童免疫接种（immunization）急剧地减少了某些感染性呼吸疾病的发生，例如白喉（diphtheria）和百日咳

框 11-2

供你参考
感染呼吸系统的微生物

微生物	疾病
细菌	
Streptococcus pneumoniae 肺炎链球菌	最常见的肺炎起因，streptococcal pneumonia
Haemophilus influenzae 流感嗜血杆菌	肺炎，特别是对虚弱的患者
Klebsiella pneumoniae 肺炎克雷伯菌	老年和虚弱患者的肺炎
Mycoplasma pneumoniae 肺炎支原体	轻症肺炎，常见于青年和儿童
Legionella pneumophila 嗜肺军团菌	军团病（legionellosis），一种通过水源，例如空调、游泳池和加湿器等传播的呼吸系统疾病
Chlamydia psittaci 鹦鹉热衣原体	鹦鹉热（psittacosis），一种会传染给人的鸟病
Streptococcus pyogenes 酿脓链球菌	链球菌性喉炎（strep throat）；猩红热（scarlet fever）
Mycobacterium tuberculosis 结核杆菌	肺结核
Dordetella pertussis 百日咳鲍特菌	百日咳
Corynebacterium diphtheriae 白喉棒状杆菌	白喉
病毒	
Rhinoviruses 鼻病毒	一般感冒的主要起因
Influenzavirus 流行性感冒病毒	流行性感冒
Respiratory syncytial virus (RSV) 呼吸道合胞病毒	婴儿呼吸疾病常见起因
SARS coronavirus SARS 冠状病毒	严重的急性呼吸综合征；高传染性疾病，出现于 2003 年，由小型哺乳动物传染给人类
Hantavirus 汉坦病毒	汉坦病毒肺综合征（Hantavirus pulmonary syndrome，HPS）；通过吸入干燥动物粪便中的病毒传播

> 续框 11-2
>
> **供你参考**
> **感染呼吸系统的微生物**
>
> **真菌**
>
> | | |
> |---|---|
> | Histoplasma capsulatum 荚膜组织胞浆菌 | 组织胞浆菌病（histoplasmosis）；由空气中的孢子传播 |
> | Coccidioides immitis 粗球孢子菌 | 球孢子菌病（coccidioidomycosis，山谷热，圣华金热）；出现在干燥碱性土壤 |
> | Blastomyces dermatitidis 皮炎芽生菌 | 芽生菌病（blastomycosis）；罕见但通常会致死的真菌性疾病 |
> | Pneumocystis jiroveci 耶氏肺孢子虫 | 肺孢子虫性肺炎（pneumocystis pneumonia，PCP）；见于免疫功能受损的宿主 |

（pertussis）[百白破疫苗（DTaP），D 代表白喉，P 代表百日咳，T 代表破伤风（tetanus）]。下面详细介绍一些感染性呼吸疾病。

肺炎

肺炎（pneumonia）是由许多不同的微生物引起的，通常是细菌或病毒。最常见的细菌是肺炎链球菌（streptococcus pneumoniae）和肺炎克雷伯菌（Klebsiella pneumoniae）。病毒性肺炎更具扩散性，通常是由流感病毒和腺病毒引起的，少儿多是由呼吸道合胞病毒（respiratory syncytial virus，RSV）引起的（图 11-8）。

- 支气管肺炎（bronchopneumonia），起始于被渗出物阻塞并已形成固态斑块的支气管末端。
- 大叶性肺炎（lobar pneumonia），涉及一个或多个肺叶。

对原本健康的人，肺炎通常能够被成功治疗，但对虚弱的患者，肺炎是致死的首要原因。免疫功能受损患者，例如艾滋病患者，通常会感染一种被称为卡氏肺孢子虫肺炎（Pneumocystis pneumonia，PCP）的真菌性肺炎。

肺炎这一术语也用于非传染性肺炎，例如因哮喘、过敏或吸入刺激物所致的肺部感染。不过，在这些情况下，通常会使用更宽泛的术语局限性肺炎（pneumonitis）。

结核病

随着艾滋病的增加和致病微生物结核分支杆菌（mycobacterium tuberculosis，MTB）出现抗生素耐药性，结核病（tuberculosis，TB）的发生近年来有所增加。因为结核分支杆菌的染色特性，它也被称为 AFB，意为抗酸杆菌（acid-fast bacillus）。结核病的命名是源于感染部位出现的结核状损害。结核的中心能够液化，随后破裂，在血流中释放细菌。一般的结核病被称为粟粒性结核病（miliary tuberculosis），因为感染组织中许多结核的大小都像小米种子（图 11-9）。

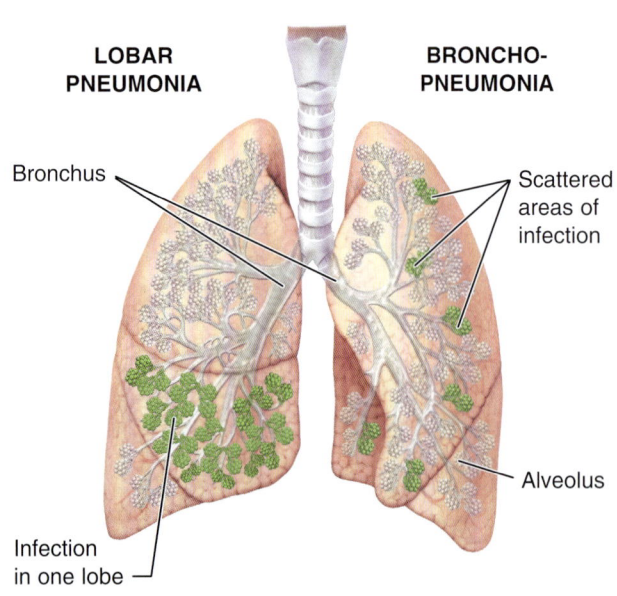

图 11-8 **肺炎。** 在肺叶性肺炎（左肺）中，整个肺叶发生实变。在支气管肺炎（右肺）中，斑片区域的实变发生在整个肺中

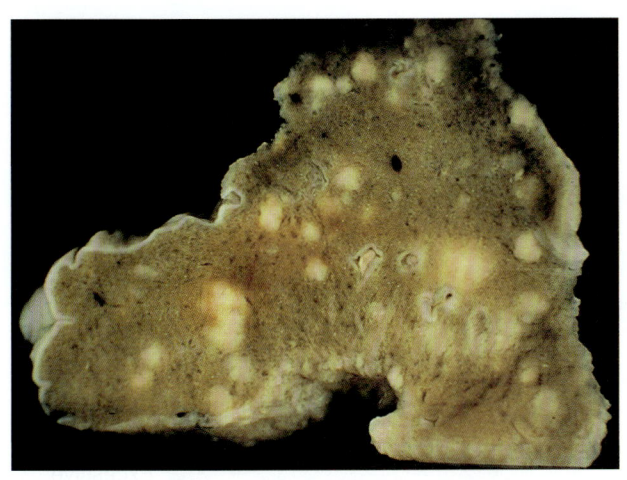

图 11-9 结核病。在粟粒性结核病中，肺切面显示有很多白色结节

肺结核的症状包括发热、体重减轻、虚弱、咳嗽和咯血（hemoptysis），咳出含血的痰，肺泡中渗出物的积累会导致肺组织硬化。活动性结核病可以通过胸部 X 线透视和痰样本的实验室培养离心分析、染色并确认致病微生物来诊断。如果在培养中发现致病微生物，可以进行药敏（drug susceptibility）试验。引起结核病的致病微生物生长非常缓慢，实验室研究可能需要 8 周的时间，所以临床医生也使用一些快速测试来确认结核病感染。这些测试包括：

- 结核菌素试验（tuberculin test），一种皮肤测试，也被称为芒图测试（Mantoux test）。测试材料结核菌素是由结核杆菌的副产品制成的。纯蛋白衍生物（purified protein derivative，PPD）是结核菌素的常用形式。在皮下注射结核菌素 48~72 小时内，已经被结核杆菌感染的人会出现凸起的肿块。该测试不能区别活动性和非活动性病例。
- 干扰素释放测试（interferon-gamma release assay，IGRA），一种诊断肺结核的快速血液测试，被用于对高结核病风险人群确定阴性皮肤测试结果。
- 核酸增扩测试（nucleic acid amplification，NAA test），一种痰测试，可在 24 小时内确定结核病阳性诊断。

BCG 疫苗被广泛用于预防结核病，用于疫苗的菌株（bacillus B）是用发现无毒的结核分枝杆菌菌株的 Calmette (C) 和 Guérin (G) 的名字命名的。

流感

流感（流行性感冒，influenza，flu）是一种病毒性呼吸疾病，有发冷、发热、头痛、肌肉痛和类似感冒的症状。流感通常会在几天内缓解，但严重的流感曾引起致命的大流行，最近的发生于 1918、1957 和 1968 年。病毒会快速变异，并在例如鸟或猪等动物和人群中传播。

因为流感病毒变化太快，科学家必须针对在任意给定年份最可能引起流行的菌株准备疫苗。流感病毒菌株被分为 A、B、C 三类，A 类最严重，C 类最不严重。它们还被进一步指定了带数字的 H 和 N，例如 H3N2 和 H5N1。H 和 N 代表病毒用于感染宿主的表面蛋白。

医护人员用疫苗、隔离感染人群、消灭感染动物和抗病毒治疗来对抗流感。

普通感冒

已知有两百多种病毒会引起感冒，大约一半是鼻病毒（rhinovirus），其他的包括呼吸系统病毒（adenovirus）和冠状病毒（coronavirus）。众所周知的感冒症状包括打喷嚏、急性鼻炎（acute rhinitis）（鼻通道感染，有大量的水样黏液分泌物）、眼睛流泪和充血。感染可能会从鼻子扩散到喉咙和鼻窦、中耳和下呼吸道。

感冒病毒大多是通过被感染的患者咳嗽和打喷嚏排出的充满病毒的液滴传播的。经常洗手和不要用手接触患者的脸部是良好的预防措施。感冒可能会持续几周，因为是病毒引起的，抗生素没有治疗作用。最好多休息、多喝水、对症治疗。感冒病毒数量多，变异快，使得开发有效疫苗难以实现。

框 11-3 给出了关于呼吸道感染和其他疾病术语的一些历史。

肺气肿

肺气肿（emphysema）是一种与肺泡过度扩张和破坏的慢性疾病（图 11-10A），常见起因是长期吸烟和暴露于其他污染中导致慢性感染。肺气肿是慢性阻塞性肺疾病（chronic obstructive pulmonary disease，

Chronic Bronchitis

Normal bronchial tube — Healthy Bronchi — Lumen — Mucus — Cilia — Mucus glands

Narrowed bronchial tube — Chronic Bronchitis — Lumen — Excessive mucus retention — Bacteria — Damaged cilia — Enlarged mucous glands

Emphysema

Normal alveoli — Damaged alveoli — Loss of lung tissue

A B

图 11-10 慢性阻塞性肺疾病（COPD）的类型。A. 肺气肿导致肺泡的扩张和破坏；B. 慢性支气管炎包括气道炎症、对纤毛的损害和过多的黏液分泌物

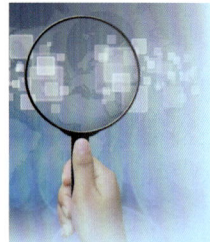

聚焦单词
不要说非专业术语

框 11-3

一些关于呼吸道的症状和病症的外行术语是如此古老和优雅，今天你只能在维多利亚时代的小说中看到它们。catarrh［kəˈtɑː(r)］（黏膜炎）是表示有许多黏液产生的上呼吸道感染的一个古老单词，quinsy［ˈkwinzi］（扁桃腺炎）指的是喉咙痛或扁桃体脓肿，consumption（消耗性疾病）是结核病，dropsy 是指全身性水肿。grippe 则意为流感，常被缩写为"flu"。

一些不科学的单词仍在使用中。包括把百日咳（pertussis）称为 whooping cough，把喉痉挛（laryngeal spasm）称为 croup，把疱疹病变（herpes lesion）称为 cold sore 或 fever blister，以及把痰（sputum）称为 phlegm。

许多人使用非正式术语而不是科学词语来描述他们的症状。健康专业人员应该熟悉患者可能使用的俚语或口语，以便能够更好地与他们沟通。

COPD，或 chronic obstructive lung disease，COLD）中的主要病症，其他病症包括哮喘（asthma）、支气管扩张（bronchiectasis）和慢性支气管炎（bronchitis）（图 11-10B）。

哮喘

哮喘（asthma）是支气管变窄所致。这种狭窄与支气管内壁水肿、感染和黏液积累共同导致气喘、极度呼吸困难（dyspnea）和紫绀（cyanosis）。

哮喘常见于儿童。尽管起因不明，过敏所致的刺激是一个主要因素，遗传也有一定的作用。哮喘的治疗包括：

· 消除过敏原。

· 使用支气管扩张剂（bronchodilators）扩张空气通道。

· 使用糖皮质激素（corticosteroids）减少感染。

尘肺病

由吸入粉尘所致的慢性刺激和严重被称为肺尘埃沉着病（pneumoconiosis），这是一种常见于矿工

和石材加工行业的职业危害。基于吸入粉尘的类型，肺尘埃沉着病分别被命名为矽肺病（silicosis，吸入硅或石英）、煤肺病（anthracosis，吸入煤尘）和石棉肺（asbestosis，吸入石棉纤维）。

尽管肺尘埃沉着病这一术语局限于吸入无机粉尘所致的病症，肺刺激也可能是吸入有机粉尘所致，例如纺织物或粮食粉尘。

肺癌

肺癌（lung cancer）是人类与癌症相关死亡的首要原因。肺癌的发生在过去50年稳步上升，特别是在女性人群。吸烟是主要的风险因素，当然还有其他因素。肺癌最常见的形式是鳞状细胞癌（squamous carcinoma），发源于支气管的内壁（支气管原的 bronchogenic）。肺癌一般无法早期发现，但转移迅速。总体长期生存率比较低。

诊断肺癌的方法有X线造影研究、计算机断层扫描和痰液检查癌细胞。医生使用支气管窥镜（bronchoscope）检查呼吸道，并收集研究样本，也可能通过手术或穿刺活检采集样本。

呼吸窘迫综合征

新生儿呼吸窘迫综合征（respiratory distress syndrome，RDS）发生于早产婴儿，是这个人群最常见的致死原因。它是由于缺乏肺表面活化剂，降低了呼吸依从性所致。急性呼吸窘迫综合征（ARDS）也被称为休克肺（shock lung），可能是外伤、过敏反应、感染或其他原因所致。ARDS会引起水肿，如果不能及时治疗，会导致呼吸衰竭（respiratory failure）和死亡。

囊性纤维化

囊性纤维化（cystic fibrosis，CF）是白人儿童最常见的致命遗传性疾病。导致囊性纤维化的缺陷基因通过改变跨细胞膜氯化物的传送影响腺体分泌。浓稠的支气管分泌物会造成感染和其他呼吸疾病。其他黏液分泌腺、汗腺和胰腺都会涉及，引起电解质失衡（electrolyte imbalance）和消化功能紊乱（digestive disturbance）。

汗液中钠和氯含量的增加可以用于诊断囊性纤维化，遗传学家通过DNA分析也能够确认引起囊性纤维化的基因。目前，囊性纤维化无法治愈，治疗只能是缓解患者的症状，例如通过体位引流、气溶胶囊（aerosol mists）、支气管扩张剂（bronchodilator）、抗生素和化痰剂（mucolytic agent）等。

婴儿猝死综合征

婴儿猝死综合征（sudden infant death syndrome，SIDS）也被称为"摇篮病（crib death）"，是看起来健康的1岁以下婴儿不明原因的死亡。死亡通常发生在睡眠期间，没有任何迹象。尸体解剖和家庭病史及环境的认真调查均不能提供任何线索。

怀孕期间母亲的特定状况与婴儿猝死综合征的风险升高相关，但没有肯定的预测。可能包括吸烟、20岁以下年龄怀孕、低体重、贫血、非法使用毒品和生殖道或尿路感染。

一些做法可能能够减少婴儿猝死综合征的发生：

- 让婴儿仰卧睡眠；
- 让婴儿远离吸烟的环境；
- 使用结实、平坦的婴儿睡垫；
- 不要使婴儿过热。

胸膜疾病

胸膜炎（pleurisy或pleuritis）是胸膜的炎症，通常与感染有关。胸膜炎的常见症状是疼痛，因为呼吸或咳嗽时发炎的胸膜会移动，会加剧疼痛，呼吸会变得快而浅。止痛药和抗感染药物被用于治疗胸膜炎。

胸膜受伤、感染或衰弱的结果是在两层胸膜之间可能会有物质积累，当空气或气体在这一空间聚集时，就会发生气胸（pneumothorax，图11-11）。压力可能会引起肺塌陷，被称为肺不张（atelectasis）。

在胸腔积液中，会积累其他物质（图11-12）。根据所涉及的物质，分别被描述为脓胸（empyema或pyothorax）、血胸（hemothorax或）水胸（hydrothorax）。这些病症的原因包括受伤、感染、心力衰竭和肺栓塞（pulmonary embolism）。可能需要胸腔穿刺术（thoracentesis）消除积液（图11-13）

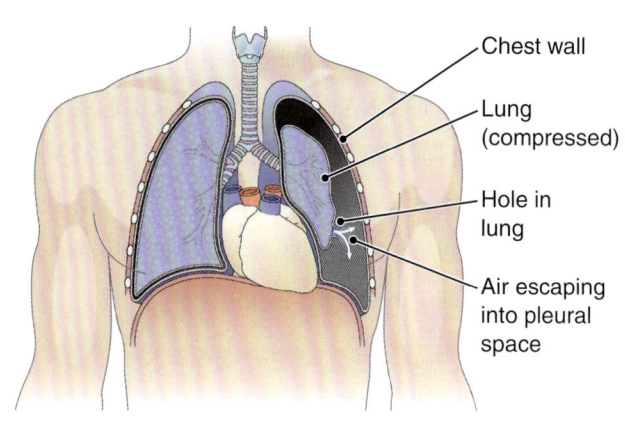

图 11-11 气胸。肺组织损伤使得空气进入胸膜腔中并对肺产生压力

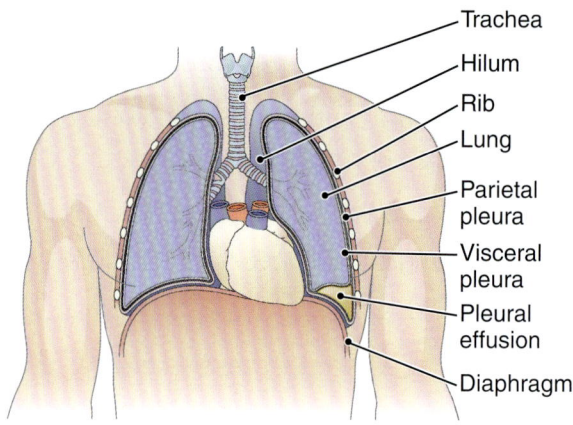

图 11-12 胸腔积液。异常的液体量聚集在胸膜腔中

或进行胸膜粘合术（pleurodesis），还可能要插入胸管排出胸膜之间的空气和液体。

呼吸疾病的诊断

除了胸部 X 线、CT 扫描和核磁共振扫描，诊断呼吸疾病的方法还有肺扫描（lung scans）、支气管窥镜（bronchoscopy）、通过胸腔穿刺术获得的胸膜积液测试等。动脉血气分析（Arterial blood gases ABGs）通过测量动脉血液样本中二氧化碳、氧气、碳酸氢盐和 pH 值，用于评估肺中的气体交换。血氧饱和度测试（pulse oximetry）一般用于测量动脉血的氧气饱和度，测量要使用一个血氧计（oximeter），是一个放置于身体比较细小部位（通常是手指或耳朵）的简单装置（图 11-14）。

肺功能测试（pulmonary function test）被用于评估呼吸状况，通常使用肺活量计（spirometer），测量在不同程度的努力下进出肺部的空气量。肺功能测试常被用于过敏、哮喘、气肿（emphysema）和其他呼吸疾病治疗的监测，也被用于测量戒烟的进展。框 11-4 汇总了测试得出的主流量和容量，容量是两个或多个流量之和（图 11-15）。

框 11-5 给出了呼吸治疗师的信息，这些人执行许多上述测试。

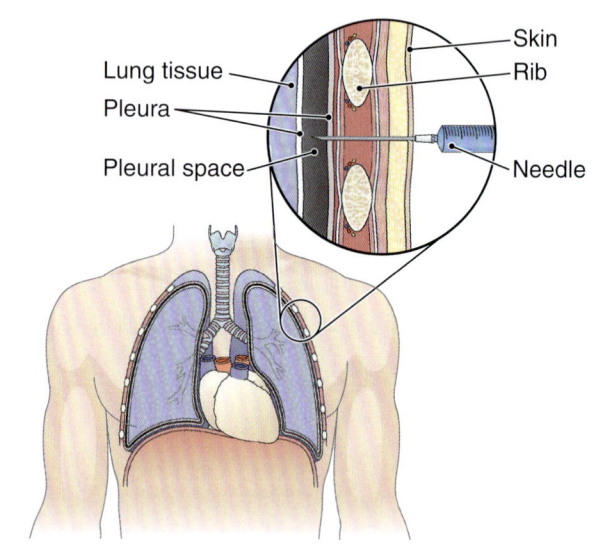

图 11-13 穿刺。将针插入胸膜间隙中

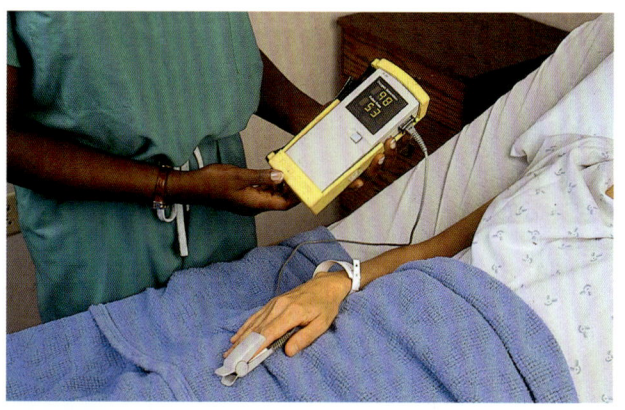

图 11-14 脉搏血氧饱和度。血氧计测量动脉血的氧饱和度

框 11-4

供你参考
用于肺功能测试的流量和容量

流量或容量	定义
tidal volume (TV) 潮气量	在平静、放松呼吸中进出肺部的空气量
residual volume (RV) 残气量	最大呼出后肺中剩余的空气量
expiratory reserve volume (ERV) 补呼气量	正常呼出后能够呼出的空气量
inspiratory reserve volume (IRV) 补吸气量	正常吸入之上能够吸入的空气量
total lung capacity (TLC) 肺总量	在最大吸入后肺所能包含的空气总量
inspiratory capacity (IC) 吸气容量	正常呼出后能够吸入的空气量
vital capacity (VC) 肺活量	肺在最大吸入后通过最大呼出所能排出的空气量
functional residual capacity (FRC) 功能残气量	正常呼出后肺中剩余的空气量
forced expiratory volume (FEV) 用力呼气量	在给定时间间隔内用最大力量能够呼出的空气量;时间用下标显示,如 FEV1(1秒)和 FEV3(3秒)
orced vital capacity (FVC) 最大肺活量	在一次完全吸入后尽可能快速且完全呼出的空气量

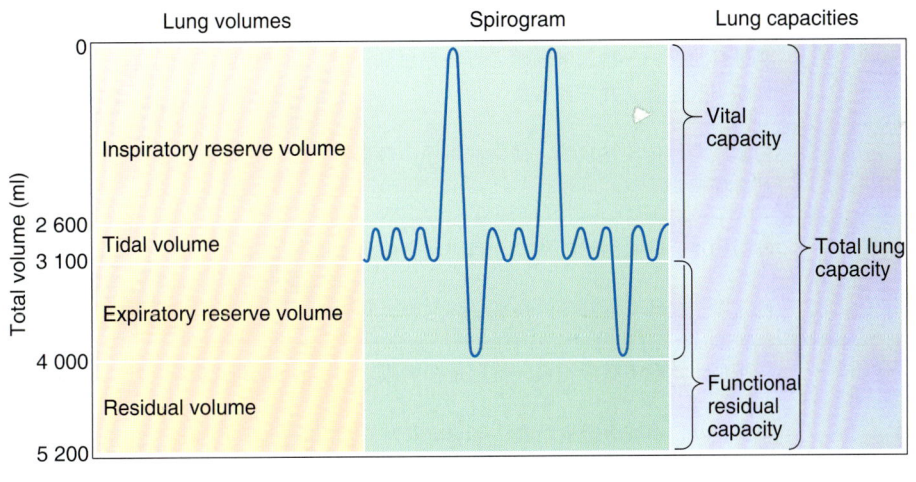

图 11-15 肺活量图。肺活量计产生肺流量和容量(流量的总和)的追踪记录

框 11-5

健康职业
呼吸治疗职业

呼吸治疗师(respiratory therapist)和呼吸治疗技术员(respiratory therapy technician)专门评估和治疗呼吸障碍。呼吸治疗师通过记录完整的病史和使用专门设备测试呼吸功能来评估患者病情的严重程度。基于他们的发现并与医生协商,治疗师设计和实施个性化治疗计划,可能包括氧疗(oxygen therapy)和胸部理疗(chest physiotherapy)。他们还教育患者使用呼吸机(ventilator)和其他医疗设备。呼吸治疗技术员协助进行评估和治疗。

为了履行职责,这两种类型的从业者都需要有全面的科学背景。大多数美国的呼吸治疗师都接受来自认可的学院或大学的培训,并参加国家许可考试。呼吸治疗师和技术员在各种环境中工作,例如医院、护理机构和私人诊所。有关呼吸治疗职业的其他信息,请访问美国呼吸保健协会(American Association for Respiratory Care)网站 www.aarc.org。

Terminology 关键术语

疾病

acidosis [ˌæsiˈdəʊsis]	酸中毒，体液异常酸性。呼吸酸中毒是由异常高水平的二氧化碳所致
acute respiratory distress syndrome (ARDS)	急性呼吸窘迫综合征，能够快速导致致命呼吸衰竭的肺水肿；原因包括外伤、肺吸入异物、病毒性肺炎和药物反应；休克肺
acute rhinitis [raiˈnaitis]	急性鼻炎，鼻黏膜发炎，会打喷嚏、流泪和大量的水样黏液，常见于一般感冒
alkalosis [ˌælkəˈləʊsis]	碱中毒，体液异常碱性。呼吸碱中毒是由异常低水平的二氧化碳所致
aspiration [ˌæspəˈreiʃn]	吸入，食物或异物被意外吸入肺，也指通过吸引将液体抽出体腔
asthma [ˈæsmə]	哮喘，以呼吸困难和喘息为特征的疾病，由支气管痉挛或黏膜肿胀所致
atelectasis [ˌætəˈlektəsis]	肺不张，肺或肺的一部分不能完全扩张，肺塌陷。可能在婴儿出生时发生（呼吸窘迫综合征）或由支气管阻塞或肺组织压迫所致（前缀 atel/o 意为"不完全"）
bronchiectasis [brɒŋkiˈektəsis]	支气管扩张，支气管或细支气管慢性扩张
bronchitis [brɒŋˈkaitis]	支气管炎，支气管的炎症
chronic obstructive pulmonary disease (COPD)	慢性阻塞性肺疾病，任何慢性、进行性和虚弱性呼吸疾病的组合，包括肺气肿、哮喘、支气管炎和支气管扩张（图 11-10）
cyanosis [ˌsaiəˈnəʊsis]	紫绀，因血液缺氧所致的皮肤变色发青（形容词：cyanotic）（图 3-4）
cystic fibrosis (CF) [ˌsistik faiˈbrəʊsis]	囊性纤维化，一种影响胰腺、呼吸系统和汗腺的遗传性疾病。特征是支气管中黏液累积引起阻塞，并导致感染
diphtheria [difˈθiəriə]	白喉，急性传染性疾病，通常局限于下呼吸道，特征是形成由细胞和凝结物质构成的表面假膜
dyspnea [disˈpni:ə]	呼吸困难，呼吸困难或费力，有时伴有疼痛；"空气饥饿"
emphysema [ˌemfiˈsi:mə]	肺气肿，一种慢性肺病，特征是肺泡肿大和破坏
empyema [ˌempaiˈi:mə]	积脓症，体腔中脓液积累，特别是在胸膜之间；pyothorax 脓胸
hemoptysis [hiˈmɒptisis]	咯血，从口中或呼吸道吐血（-ptysis 意为"吐"）
hemothorax [ˌhi:məˈθɔ:ræks]	血胸，胸膜之间出现血液
hydrothorax [ˌhaidrəˈθəʊræks]	胸腔积液，胸膜之间出现液体
hyperventilation [ˌhaipəˌventiˈleiʃn]	通气过度，呼吸速率和深度提高；进入肺泡的空气量增加
hypoventilation [ˌhaipəʊventiˈleiʃən]	通气不足，呼吸速率和深度降低；进入肺泡的空气量减少
influenza [ˌinfluˈenzə]	流感，一种急性、传染性呼吸疾病，会引起发热、发冷、头痛和肌肉疼痛；简写为 flu
pertussis [pəˈtʌsis]	百日咳，一种急性传染性疾病，特征是咳嗽结束时发出"嗬嗬"的吸气声音

Terminology 关键术语（续表）

术语	释义
pleural effusion ['plʊərə]	胸腔积液，胸膜之间液体积累。液体中可能包含血（hemothorax，血胸）或脓（pyothorax，脓胸，图 11-12）
pleurisy ['plʊərəsi]	胸膜炎，胸膜炎症，也拼写为 pleuritis。胸膜炎的一个症状是呼吸时剧痛
pneumoconiosis [ˌnjuːməkəʊni'əʊsis]	尘肺，由吸入粉尘颗粒所致的呼吸道疾病。根据所吸入粉尘的种类命名；例如矽肺（silicosis）、煤肺（anthracosis）、石棉肺（asbestosis）
pneumonia [njuːˈməʊniə]	肺炎，一般因感染引起的肺部炎症。可能涉及支气管和肺泡（支气管肺炎，bronchopneumonia）或者一个或多个肺叶（肺叶肺炎，lobar pneumonia，图 11-8）
pneumonitis [njuːməʊ'naitis]	局限性肺炎，肺部炎症，可能是由感染、哮喘、过敏或吸入刺激物所致
pneumothorax [ˌnjuːmə'θɔːræks]	气胸，胸膜之间空气或气体积累。可能是受伤或疾病所致，可能人工产生肺塌陷（图 11-11）
pyothorax [paiəʊ'θɔːræks]	脓胸，胸膜之间脓液积累
respiratory distress syndrome (RDS)	呼吸窘迫综合征，影响缺乏肺表面活性剂的早产婴儿的呼吸疾病。使用呼吸支持和表面活性剂治疗
sudden infant death syndrome (SIDS)	婴儿猝死综合征，表面健康婴儿突然且不明原因的死亡
tuberculosis [tjuːˌbɜːkjuˈləʊsis]	结核病，一种由结合分支杆菌引起的传染性疾病。通常涉及肺，但也会涉及身体其他部分。粟粒性肺结核（miliary tuberculosis）是结核病最常见的形式，感染组织中会出现小米种子大小的结核损伤（图 11-9）

诊断

术语	释义
arterial blood gases (ABGs)	动脉血气，气体，特别是氧气和二氧化碳在动脉血液中的浓度。报告结果是气体在动脉（a）血液中的分气压（P），例如 PaO_2 或 $PaCO_2$，这些结果对测量酸碱平衡非常重要
bronchoscope [b'rɒntʃəskəʊp]	支气管镜，用于检查气管和支气管通道的内窥镜，也被用于活组织检查采样或去除外来异物（图 11-16）
lung scan	肺扫描，基于放射性同位素在肺组织中积累的研究。换气扫描测量吸入放射性物质后的换气，灌注扫描测量注射放射性物质后的血液供应，也被称为肺闪烁扫描（pulmonary scintiscan）
pulse oximetry [ɒk'simitri]	脉搏血氧饱和度，通过光电装置（血氧测量仪，oximeter）确定动脉血氧饱和度；报告结果是 SpO_2 百分比（图 11-14）
pulmonary function tests	肺功能测试，用于评估呼吸功能的测试，通常使用呼吸量测定法来做。
spirometer [ˌspaiə'rɒmitə]	肺活量计，用于测量呼吸流量和容量的装置，测试报告被称为呼吸图（spirogram，图 11-15）
thoracentesis [θɔːrəsen'tiːsis]	胸腔穿刺术，胸腔外科穿孔，以去除手术后或因受伤、感染或心血管问题所致的空气或液体积累（图 11-13）
tuberculin test [tjuːˈbɜːkjulin]	结核菌素测试，结核病皮肤测试。结核菌素（tuberculin PPD）是由结核杆菌生产的测试材料，被皮下注射后，48~72 小时内出现的凸起硬肿块表明有活动性或非活动性结核杆菌感染。也被称为芒图测试（Mantoux test）

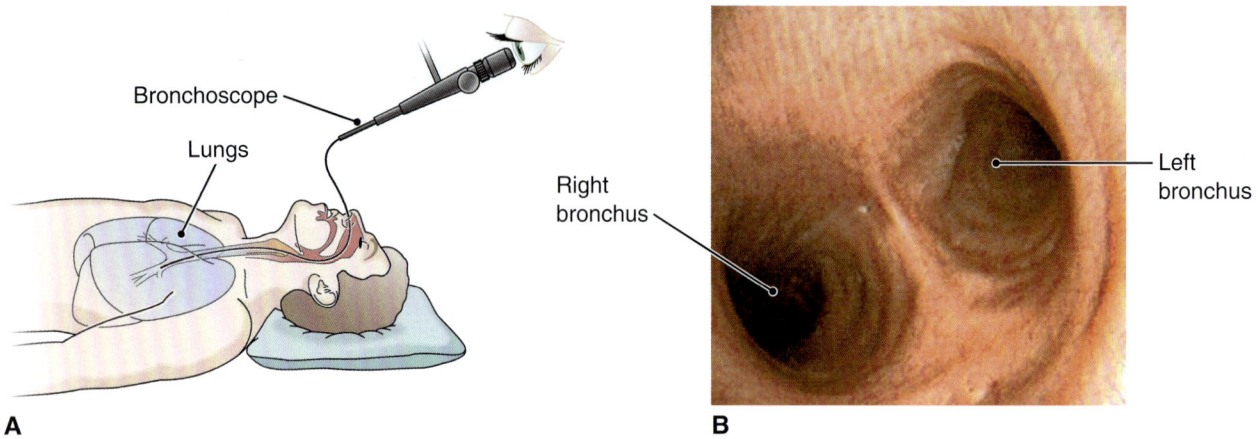

图 11-16 使用支气管镜。A. 支气管镜是用于检查支气管、采集样本和去除异物的发光的导管；B. 通过支气管镜观察支气管开口，请注意较大的右支气管

Terminology　补充术语

正常结构和功能

carina [kəˈrainə]	隆起，形成两根支气管之间的山脊形状的最低的气管软骨凸起。任何山脊或山脊形结构（源自于拉丁语意为"龙骨"的单词）
hilum [ˈhailəm]	门，器官的一个解剖凹陷，血管和神经从那里进入器官
nares [ˈneiriːz]	鼻孔，鼻子的外部开口，也拼写为 nostrils（单数：naris）
nasal septum	鼻中隔，将鼻腔分为两部分的隔壁（词根：sept/o 意为隔壁，隔膜）

症状和状况

anoxia [æˈnɒksiə]	缺氧症，组织中缺乏或没有氧气；常被误指组织缺氧（hypoxia）
asphyxia [æsˈfiksiə]	窒息，氧气摄入不足所致的状况；也常用 suffocation（字面含义时"没有脉搏"）
Biot respirations	比奥呼吸，被突然的暂停中断的深度、快速的呼吸；常见于脊膜炎和其他中枢神经系统疾病
bronchospasm [ˈbrɒŋkəˌspæzəm]	支气管痉挛，平滑肌痉挛引起的支气管狭窄，在哮喘和支气管炎中常见
Cheyne-Stokes respiration	潮式呼吸，逐渐增强，然后逐渐变弱，接着一段呼吸暂停的周期性重复，由脑干中的呼吸中枢受压迫所致；常见于昏迷和临终患者
cor pulmonale [ˈkɔː ˌpuməˈnæli]	肺源性心脏病，由肺或肺血管疾病所致的右心室扩大
coryza [kəˈraizə]	鼻炎，有大量鼻涕的鼻腔急性炎症；急性鼻炎
croup [kruːp]	义膜性喉炎，涉及上呼吸道感染和阻塞所致的儿童疾病，特征是犬吠样咳嗽、呼吸困难和喉痉挛
deviated septum	鼻中隔偏曲，鼻中隔偏离中线；可能需要手术矫正

Terminology 关键术语

epiglottitis [epiglɒˈtaitis]	会厌炎，会厌软骨炎症，可能导致上呼吸道阻塞；常见于义膜性喉炎（也拼写为 epiglottiditis）
epistaxis [ˌepiˈstæksis]	鼻出血，鼻腔出血（nosebleed）（希腊语后缀 -staxis 意为"滴下"）
fremitus [ˈfremitəs]	震颤，震动，特别是触诊时在胸壁上感到的
Kussmaul respiration	库斯莫尔呼吸，快速、深度、不停歇的喘息式呼吸；严重酸中毒的特征
pleural friction rub	胸膜摩擦音，听诊时听到的由两层胸膜摩擦产生的声音；胸膜炎的常见体征
rales [ˈrɑːlz]	罗音，空气进入小气管或含有液体的肺泡时产生的异常胸音，通常在吸气时听到。也被称为爆裂音（crackles）
rhonchi [ˈrɒŋki]	干罗音，有积液的呼吸道产生的异常胸音；在呼气时更明显（单数：rhonchus）
stridor [ˈstraidə]	喘鸣，上呼吸道阻塞引起的刺耳、尖厉的声音
wheeze [wiːz]	喘息，呼吸道狭窄引起的呼啸或叹息声

病症

byssinosis [bisiˈnəʊsis]	棉尘肺，由对未加工的植物纤维的反应所致的呼吸道阻塞性疾病
sleep apnea	睡眠呼吸暂停，睡眠期间间断性呼吸停止。中枢性睡眠呼吸暂停是因脑干不能刺激呼吸引起的，阻塞性睡眠呼吸暂停是深睡眠期间呼吸道阻塞所致，如肥胖或扁桃腺肿大
small cell carcinoma [ˌkɑːsiˈnəʊmə]	小细胞癌，高度恶性支气管肿瘤，涉及小的未分化细胞

诊断

mediastinoscopy [mediəsˈtinɒskəpi]	纵隔镜检查，通过在胸骨上部切口插入内窥镜的方式检查胸腔纵隔
plethysmograph [pləˈθizməgrɑːf]	体积描记器，测量呼吸期间气体流量和压力变化的仪器
pneumotachometer [njuːməʊˈtækɒmitər]	呼吸速度测定器，测量空气流量的仪器
thoracoscopy [θɔːrəˈkɒskəpi]	胸腔镜，通过内窥镜检查胸腔；也拼写为 pleuroscopy

治疗

aerosol therapy [ˈeərəsɒl]	雾化疗法，通过吸入雾状药物或水进行治疗
continuous positive airway pressure (CPAP)	持续气道正压通气，使用呼吸机为自发呼吸的患者在整个呼吸周期维持压力
extubation [ikstjʊˈbeiʃn]	拔管，除去已插入的导管
intermittent positive pressure breathing (IPPB)	间歇正压呼吸，吸入期间使用呼吸机在正压力下间隔为肺充气

Terminology 关键术语（续表）

intermittent positive pressure ventilation (IPPV)	间歇正压通气，使用呼吸机强迫气体进入肺，同时允许被动呼出
nasal cannula [ˈkænjʊlə]	鼻插管，双塑料管装置，插入鼻孔输送氧气（图 11-17）
orthopneic position [əθɒpˈniːk]	端坐呼吸体位，帮助呼吸的直立或半直立体位
positive end-expiratory pressure (PEEP)	呼气末正压通气，使用呼吸机在呼气末端增加进入肺的空气量，以改善气体交换
postural drainage	体位引流，利用体位通过重力将分泌物引出肺部
thoracic gas volume (TGV, VTG)	胸腔气体容量，通过人体体积描记器的测量值计算的胸腔气体容量
手术	
adenoidectomy [ˌædinɔiˈdektəmi]	腺样体切除术，手术切除腺样体
intubation [ˌintjʊˈbeiʃn]	插管，向中空的器官插入导管，例如向喉或气管插管使空气进入（图 11-18）。在手术麻醉期间或为保持呼吸道畅通，患者可能需要插管。气管内插管可能由于呼吸道阻塞的紧急情况
lobectomy [ləʊˈbektəmi]	叶切除术，手术切除肺或气体器官的一叶
tracheotomy [ˌtrækiˈɒtəmi]	气管切开术，通过颈部切开气管，通常是在器官阻塞情况下建立空气通道
tracheostomy [ˌtreikiˈɒstəmi]	气管造口术，在气管上手术建立开口，以便形成空气通道或准备换气插管（图 11-19），也指被建立的开口
药物	
antihistamine [ˌæntiˈhistəmiːn]	抗组胺药，防止组胺介导的反应的药物，过敏和炎症反应就是由组胺介导的
antitussive [ˌæntiˈtʌsiv]	止咳药，预防或缓解咳嗽的药物
asthma maintenance drug	哮喘维持药，用于防止哮喘发作和长期治疗哮喘的药物
bronchodilator [ˌbrɒŋkəʊdaiˈleitə]	支气管扩张剂，缓解支气管痉挛并扩张支气管的药物
corticosteroid [ˌkɒtikəʊˈstiərɔid]	糖皮质激素，来自于肾上腺皮质的激素；用于降低感染
decongestant [ˌdiːkənˈdʒestənt]	解充血药，降低充血或水肿的药物
expectorant [ikˈspektərənt]	祛痰剂，协助消除支气管肺分泌物的药物
isoniazid [ˌaisəʊˈnaiəzid]	异烟肼，治疗结核病的药物
leukotriene antagonist [ˌluːkəˈtraiiːn ænˈtægənist]	白三烯拮抗剂，通过阻止白三烯预防或降低感染的药物，白三烯是白细胞制造的促进感染的一种物质；能够压缩支气管并增加黏液的产生；用于治疗哮喘
mucolytic [ˌmjʊkəʊˈlitik]	化痰剂，稀释痰液以利于排出的药物
rifampin [raiˈfæmpin]	利福平，抗结核药，也拼写为 rifampicin [rifæmˈpaisin]

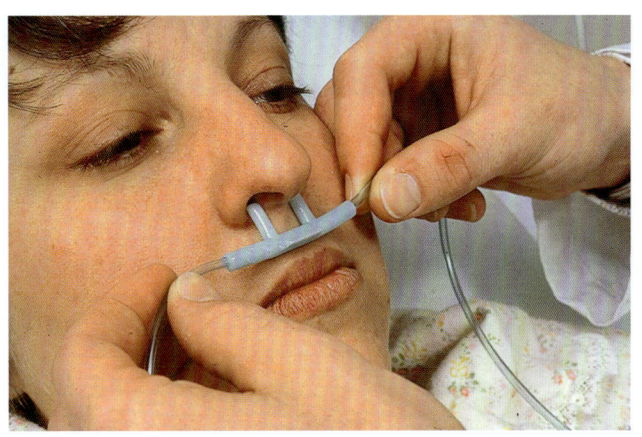

图 11-17 鼻插管

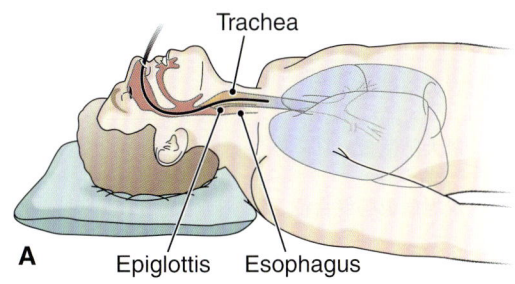

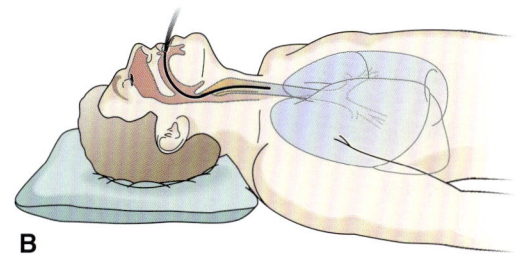

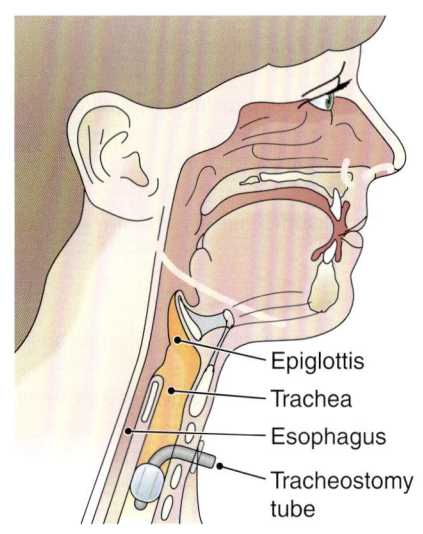

图 11-18 气管内插管。A. 鼻气管内导管在正确的位置；B. 口腔气管内插管

图 11-19 在适当位置的气管造口管

Terminology　缩略语

ABG(s)	Arterial blood gas(es)	动脉血气
AFB	Acid-fast bacillus (usually Mycobacterium tuberculosis)	抗酸杆菌（通常是结核分支杆菌）
ARDS	Acute respiratory distress syndrome; shock lung	急性呼吸窘迫综合征；休克肺
ARF	Acute respiratory failure	急性呼吸衰竭
BCG	Bacillus Calmette-Guérin (tuberculosis vaccine)	卡介苗（结核病疫苗）
BS	Breath sounds	呼吸音
C	Compliance	依从性

Terminology 缩略语（续表）

CF	Cystic fibrosis	囊性纤维化
CO_2	Carbon dioxide	二氧化碳
COLD	Chronic obstructive lung disease	慢性阻塞性肺疾病
COPD	Chronic obstructive pulmonary disease	慢性阻塞性肺疾病
CPAP	Continuous positive airway pressure	持续气道正压通气
CXR	Chest radiograph, chest x-ray	胸部 X 线检查
DTaP	Diphtheria, tetanus, pertussis (vaccine)	百白破疫苗
ERV	Expiratory reserve volume	补呼气量
FEV	Forced expiratory volume	用力呼气量
FRC	Functional residual capacity	有效余气量
FVC	Forced vital capacity	最大肺活量
HPS	Hantavirus pulmonary syndrome	汉坦病毒肺综合征
IC	Inspiratory capacity	深吸气量
IGRA	Interferon-gamma release assay (test for TB)	干扰素释放反应（结核病测试）
INH	Isoniazid	异烟肼
IPPB	Intermittent positive pressure breathing	间歇性正压呼吸
IPPV	Intermittent positive pressure ventilation	间歇性正压换气
IRV	Inspiratory reserve volume	补吸气量
LLL	Left lower lobe (of lung)	左下肺叶
LUL	Left upper lobe (of lung)	左上肺叶
MEFR	Maximal expiratory flow rate	最大呼气流速
MMFR	Maximum midexpiratory flow rate	最大呼气中段流速
NAA	Nucleic acid amplification (test) (for TB)	核酸扩增（测试）（结核病测试）
O_2	Oxygen	氧气
$PaCO_2$	Arterial partial pressure of carbon dioxide	二氧化碳动脉分压
PaO_2	Arterial partial pressure of oxygen	氧气动脉分压
PCP	Pneumocystis pneumonia	卡氏肺孢子虫肺炎
PEEP	Positive end-expiratory pressure	呼气末正压
PEFR	Peak expiratory flow rate	呼气峰值流速
PFT	Pulmonary function test(s)	肺功能测试

Terminology 缩略语（续表）

PIP	Peak inspiratory pressure	吸气峰值压力
PND	Paroxysmal nocturnal dyspnea	阵发性夜间呼吸困难
PPD	Purified protein derivative (tuberculin)	纯化蛋白衍生物（结核菌素）
R	Respiration	呼吸
RDS	Respiratory distress syndrome	呼吸窘迫综合征
RLL	Right lower lobe (of lung)	右下肺叶
RML	Right middle lobe (of lung)	右中肺叶
RSV	Respiratory syncytial virus	呼吸道合胞病毒
RUL	Right upper lobe (of lung)	右上肺叶
RV	Residual volume	残气量
SARS	Severe acute respiratory syndrome	严重急性呼吸综合征
SIDS	Sudden infant death syndrome	婴儿猝死综合征
SpO_2	Oxygen percent saturation	氧饱和度
T & A	Tonsils and adenoids; tonsillectomy and adenoidectomy	扁桃体和腺样体；扁桃腺切除术和腺样体切除术
TB	Tuberculosis	结核病
TGV	Thoracic gas volume	胸腔气体容量
TLC	Total lung capacity	肺总量
TV	Tidal volume	潮气量
URI	Upper respiratory infection	上呼吸道感染
VC	Vital capacity	肺活量
VTG	Thoracic gas volume	胸腔气体容量

Case Study Revisited 案例研究再访

A. D.'s Follow-Up to Surgery

A. D.'s surgery went well and there were no complications. The anesthesiologist closely monitored her respiratory status to make certain it was not compromised. He administered additional medications to maintain optimal airflow. Postoperatively, A. D.'s asthma was kept under control. The postoperative spirometry was adequate. Her discharge instructions were to resume preoperative medications and to follow up with her pulmonologist if there were any problems.

A. D. 的手术随访

A. D. 的手术进展很好，没有并发症。麻醉师密切监视她的呼吸状态，以确保它不受损伤。他给予额外的药物以保持最佳气流。术后，A. D. 的哮喘保持在控制之下，术后肺功能是足够的。她的出院指示是恢复使用手术前的药物，如果有任何问题，联系胸内科医生。

CHAPTER 11 复习

标记练习

呼吸系统

在对应的下划线上写出每个编号部分的名称。

Alveolar duct	Left lung
Alveoli	Mediastinum
Capillaries	Nasal cavity
Diaphragm	Nasopharynx
Epiglottis	Oropharynx
Esophagus	Right bronchus
Frontal sinus	Right lung
Laryngopharynx	Sphenoidal sinus
Larynx and vocal folds	Terminal bronchiole
Left bronchus	Trachea

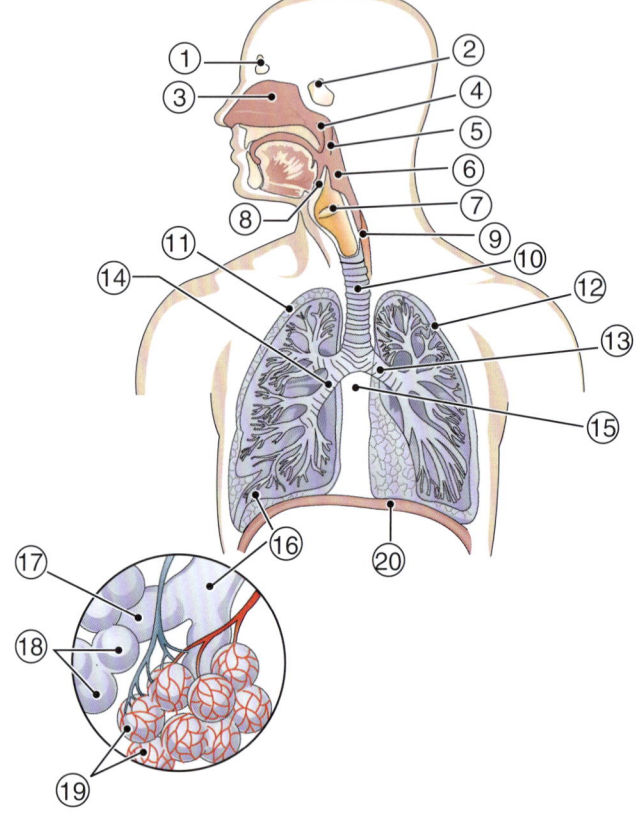

1. _____
2. _____
3. _____
4. _____
5. _____
6. _____
7. _____
8. _____
9. _____
10. _____
11. _____
12. _____
13. _____
14. _____
15. _____
16. _____
17. _____
18. _____
19. _____
20. _____

匹配

匹配下列术语，在每个题号左侧写上适当的字母。

____ 1. atelectasis   a. pulmonary disease with destruction of alveoli
____ 2. emphysema   b. increased carbon dioxide in the blood
____ 3. hypercapnemia   c. decreased rate and depth of breathing
____ 4. hypopnea   d. whooping cough
____ 5. pertussis   e. incomplete expansion of lung tissue

____ 6. mediastinum   a. accidental inhalation of foreign material into the lungs
____ 7. aspiration   b. space between the lungs
____ 8. sputum   c. substance that reduces surface tension
____ 9. surfactant   d. a measure of how easily the lungs expand
____ 10. compliance   e. expectoration

____ 11. PCP   a. childhood vaccine
____ 12. DTaP   b. tuberculosis vaccine
____ 13. CF   c. hereditary disease that affects respiration
____ 14. IPPB   d. pneumonia seen in compromised patients
____ 15. BCG   e. a form of respiratory treatment

补充术语

____ 16. epistaxis   a. suffocation
____ 17. intubation   b. nosebleed
____ 18. asphyxia   c. insertion of a tube into a hollow organ
____ 19. stridor   d. harsh, high-pitched respiratory sound
____ 20. expectorant   e. agent that helps remove bronchial secretions

____ 21. mucolytic   a. irregular respiration seen in terminally ill patients
____ 22. Cheyne–Stokes   b. agent that loosens mucus to aid in its removal
____ 23. rales   c. acute rhinitis
____ 24. orthopneic   d. pertaining to an upright position
____ 25. coryza   e. abnormal chest sounds

填空

26. The trachea divides into a right and a left primary_____.
27. The phrenic nerve activates the_____.
28. The gas produced in the tissues and exhaled in respiration is_____.
29. The double membrane that covers the lungs and lines the thoracic cavity is the_____.
30. The small air sacs in the lungs through which gases are exchanged between the atmosphere and the blood are the_____.
31. The turbinate bones contain receptors for the sense of_____.
32. A pneumotropic virus is one that invades the_____.

33. The term acid-fast bacillus (AFB) is commonly applied to the organism that causes_____.
34. The apparatus used to measure A.D.'s breathing volumes in the opening case study is called a(n)_____.
35. The amount of air that A.D. could expel from her lungs by maximum exhalation after maximum inhalation is termed the _____.

补充术语

36. A thoracoscopy is an examination of the through an endoscope_____.
37. An antitussive agent prevents_____.
38. A mucolytic agent dissolves_____.
39. Intermittent periods of not breathing during sleep are termed sleep_____.
40. A.D. was given a drug to widen the bronchi. This type of drug is called a(n) _____.

真假判断

检查下列语句。如果语句为真，则在第一个空白处写入 T；如果语句为假，则在第一个空格中写入 F，并通过在第二个空格中替换带下划线的单词来更正语句。

	True or False	Correct Answer
41. The pharynx is the throat.	_____	_____
42. The diaphragm flattens during exhalation.	_____	_____
43. The vocal folds are located in the pharynx.	_____	_____
44. The right lung has three lobes.	_____	_____
45. The opening between the vocal folds is the glottis.	_____	_____
46. The adenoids are in the nasopharynx.	_____	_____

定义

写出下列定义的单词。

47. incision of the phrenic nerve _____
48. decrease in rate and depth of breathing _____
49. inflammation of the throat _____
50. inflammation of the bronchioles _____
51. creation of an opening into the trachea _____

单词 thorax 被用于组合单词的结尾，意为物质在胸腔积累。定义下列术语。

52. pneumothorax_____
53. hydrothorax_____
54. pyothorax_____
55. hemothorax_____

定义下列单词。

56. tracheostenosis_____
57. hemoptysis_____
58. hypoxia_____

59. pneumonopathy _____

60. tachypnea _____

61. bronchiectasis _____

62. rhinoplasty _____

63. pleurodynia _____

识别并定义下列单词的词根。

	Root	Meaning of Root
64. rhinoplasty	_____	_____
65. pulmonologist	_____	_____
66. respiration	_____	_____
67. phrenicotomy	_____	_____
68. pneumatic	_____	_____

反义词

写出下列含义的反义词。

69. bradypnea _____

70. hypocapnia _____

71. expiration _____

72. extrapulmonary _____

73. extubation _____

形容词

写出下列单词的形容词形式。

74. larynx _____

75. alveolus _____

76. nose _____

77. trachea _____

78. pleura _____

79. bronchus _____

复数

写出下列单词的复数形式。

80. naris _____

81. pleura _____

82. alveolus _____

83. concha _____

84. bronchus _____

排除

在下列每组中，为与其余不相配的单词加下划线，并解释你选择的理由。

85. turbinates — septum — nares — tonsil — conchae

86. sinus — thyroid cartilage — epiglottis — cricoid cartilage — vocal folds

87. diphtheria — tuberculosis — asthma — common cold — influenza

88. RUL — URI — LUL — LLL — RML

89. TLC — FRC — FEV — TV — RDS

单词构建

使用给出的单词组成部分写出下列定义的单词。

| -pnea | -ia | ox/I | a- | -metry | phon/o | hyper- | dys- | capn/o | hypo- | eu- | tachy |

90. loss of voice
91. increased levels of carbon dioxide
92. difficulty in speaking
93. increased rate and depth of breathing
94. measurement of oxygen levels
95. difficulty in breathing
96. low levels of oxygen in the tissues
97. normal, regular breathing
98. rapid breathing
99. excessive voice production

单词分析

定义下列单词，并给出每个单词组成部分的含义。如果需要，可以使用词典。

100. pneumotachometer ［nju:məʊˈtækɒmitər］ _____
    a. pneum/o _____
    b. tach/o _____
    c. -meter _____

101. atelectasis ［ˌætəˈlektəsis］ _____
    a. atel/o- _____
    b. -ectasis _____

102. pneumatocardia ［nju:mætəˈkɑ:diə］ _____
    a. pneumat/o _____
    b. cardi _____
    c. -ia _____

103. pneumoconiosis [ˌnjuːməkəʊniˈəʊsɪs] _____

    a. pneum/o _____

    b. coni/o _____

    c. –sis _____

Additional Case Studies
补充案例研究

Case Study 11-1: Giant Cell Sarcoma of the Lung
案例研究 11-1：肺巨细胞肉瘤

L. E., a 68 y/o man, was admitted to the pulmonary unit with chest pain on inspiration, dyspnea, and diaphoresis. He had smoked one and a half packs of cigarettes per day for 52 years and had quit three months ago. L. E. was retired from the advertising industry and admitted to occasional alcohol use. He was treated for primary giant cell sarcoma of the left lung three years ago with a lobectomy of the left lung followed by radiation and chemotherapy.

Physical examination was unremarkable except for a thoracotomy scar in the left hemithorax, decreased breath sounds, and dullness to percussion of the left base. There was no hemoptysis. Chest and upper abdomen CT scan showed findings compatible with recurrent sarcoma of the left hemithorax. Abnormal mediastinal nodes were evident. A thoracentesis was attempted but did not yield fluid. L.E. was scheduled for a left thoracoscopy, mediastinoscopy, and biopsy.

L. E. 是一名 68 岁的男性，因胸部吸气时痛、呼吸困难和发汗住入肺科病房。他在过去的 52 年中每天吸一包半香烟，3 个月前戒烟。L. E. 从广告业退休，并承认偶尔喝酒。3 年前，他治疗了左肺原发性巨细胞瘤，左肺叶切除术，然后放射和化疗。

体格检查无明显异常，除了左胸胸廓切开的瘢痕，呼吸音减弱，左侧基底叩击浊音。没有咯血，胸部和上腹部 CT 扫描显示与左半胸的复发性肉瘤相符的结果。纵隔节点异常明显。试图进行胸腔穿刺，但没有产生液体。L.E. 被安排进行左胸腔镜检查、纵隔镜检查和活组织检查。

Case Study 11-2: Terminal Dyspnea
案例研究 11-2：终末期呼吸困难

N. A., a 76-year-old woman, was in the ICU in the terminal stage of multisystem organ failure. She had been admitted to the hospital for bacterial pneumonia, which had not resolved with antibiotic therapy. She had a 20-year history of COPD. She was not conscious and was unable to breathe on her own. Her ABGs were abnormal, and she was diagnosed with refractory ARDS. The decision was made to support her breathing with endotracheal intubation and mechanical ventilation. After one week and several unsuccessful attempts to wean her from the ventilator, the pulmonologist suggested a permanent tracheostomy and discussed with the family the options of continuing or withdrawing life support. Her physiologic status met the criteria of remote or no chance for recovery. N. A.'s family discussed her condition and decided not to pursue aggressive life-sustaining therapies.

N. A. was assigned DNR status. After the written orders were read and signed by the family, the endotracheal tube, feeding tube, pulse oximeter, and ECG electrodes were removed, and a morphine IV drip was started with prn boluses ordered to promote comfort and relieve pain. The family sat with her for many hours, providing comfort and support. After a while, they noticed that her breathing had become shallow with Cheyne–Stokes respirations. N.A. died quietly in the presence of her family and the hospital chaplain.

N. A. 是一名 76 岁的女性，在多系统器官功能衰竭的终末阶段住进 ICU。她因细菌性肺炎而住院，但仍未接受抗生素治疗。她有 20 年的 COPD 病史。她没有意识，不能自己呼吸，ABG 异常，被诊断为难治性 ARDS。决定用气管插管和机械通气辅助她呼吸。在 1 周时间的几次不成功地尝试摆脱呼吸机后，呼吸科医生建议永久气管造口术，并与家人讨论继续或撤消生命支持的选择。她的生理状态满足恢复机会渺茫或根本不能恢复。N. A. 的家人讨论了她的病情，决定不采取积极的维持生命疗法。

N. A. 被指定为 DNR 状态。在家庭阅读和签署书面医嘱后，取出了气管内导管、胃管、脉搏血氧计和 ECG 电极，并开始吗啡静脉滴注，且在需要时加大剂量以促进舒适和缓解疼痛。家人坐在她身边几个小时，提供安慰和支持。过了一会儿，他们注意到她的呼吸已变浅，呈切斯氏呼吸。N.A. 在她的家人和医院牧师面前静静地死了。

案例研究问题

多项选择。选择正确的答案，并在每个题号左侧写上你选择的字母。

____ 1. 1. The root pulmon, as in pulmonary, means

    a. chest

    b. air

    c. lung

    d. breath sound

____ 2. Hemoptysis is

    a. drooping eyelids

    b. discoloration of skin

    c. blue nail beds

    d. spitting of blood

____ 3. Dyspnea could NOT be described as

    a. difficulty breathing

    b. eupnea

    c. air hunger

    d. Cheyne–Stokes respirations

____ 4. Pulse oximetry is used to measure

    a. forced expiratory volume

    b. tidal volume

    c. positive end-expiratory pressure

    d. oxygen saturation of blood

____ 5. An endotracheal tube is placed

    a. within the trachea

    b. beyond the carina

    c. within the bronchus

    d. under the trachea

写出补充案例研究中下列含义的单词。

6. Removal of a lobe_____

7. Profuse sweating_____

8. Surgical incision of the chest_____

9. Endoscopic examination of the chest cavity_____

10. Half of the chest_____

11. Endoscopic examination of the space between the lungs_____

12. Movement of air into and out of the lungs_____

缩略语。定义下列缩略语。

13. COPD_____

14. ABG_____

15. ARDS_____

16. DNR_____

17. BS_____

CHAPTER 12 消化系统

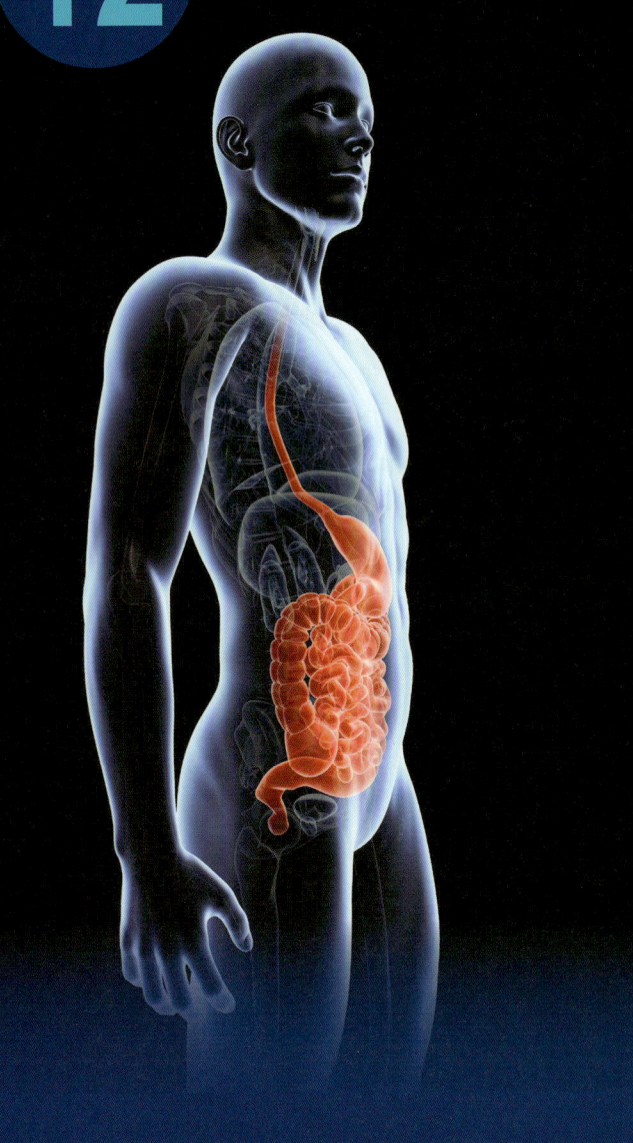

预测试

多项选择。选择正确的答案,并在每个题号左侧写上你选择的字母。

____1. An organic catalyst is a(n)
 a. enzyme
 b. sugar
 c. nucleic acid
 d. saliva

____2. The organ that carries food from the pharynx to the stomach is the
 a. trachea
 b. larynx
 c. esophagus
 d. intestine

____3. The word root for the stomach is
 a. hepat/o
 b. ren/o
 c. gastr/o
 d. cardi/o

____4. The word root enter/o refers to the
 a. gallbladder
 b. intestine
 c. kidney
 d. heart

____5. The wave-like action that moves substances through an organ is called
 a. pulmonary
 b. peristalsis
 c. parotid
 d. mastication

____6. The process of moving digested nutrients from the intestine into the circulation is called
 a. lymphedema
 b. digestion
 c. egestion
 d. absorption

____7. The organ that secretes bile is the
 a. kidney
 b. spleen
 c. liver
 d. stomach

____8. Cholecystitis is inflammation of the
 a. gallbladder
 b. throat
 c. diaphragm
 d. small intestine

学习目标

学完本章后，你应该能够：

1 ▶ 描述消化道的器官，给出它们的功能。
2 ▶ 描述附属器官，并说明它们在消化中的作用。
3 ▶ 识别并使用与消化系统和附属器官相关的词根。
4 ▶ 描述消化系统的主要疾病。
5 ▶ 定义用于消化系统的医学术语。
6 ▶ 解释用于胃肠系统的缩略语。
7 ▶ 分析案例研究中与消化系统相关的医学术语。

Case Study: B. F.'s Gastroesophageal Reflux Disease (GERD) and Erosive Esophagitis
案例研究：B. F. 的胃食管反流病（GERD）和侵蚀性食管炎

Chief Complaint

B. F. is a 51-year-old African American businessman with complaints of epigastric pain. He has a 10-year history of heartburn that he notes has become worse over the last year. The heartburn occurs both after meals and at bedtime. His sleep has been interrupted by nighttime symptoms, and he feels generally fatigued. Intermittently he says he feels that things come back up into his throat, but he lacks clear signs of aspiration into the respiratory tract. He is aware that gastroesophageal reflux disease (GERD) is a chronic condition and may be associated with a risk for complications that include serious morbidity and mortality. Due to his required travel for business, he has put off making a doctor's appointment but realizes he needs to see his physician. The heartburn has increased in frequency (daily now) and severity, so he finally schedules an office visit.

Examination

B. F. is seen by his primary care physician and describes his daily episodes of discomfort. B. F. is 6-foot-1-inch and weighs 230 pounds. The physician reviews a colonoscopy from last year with him that was normal. His blood pressure and other physical examination findings at this visit are within normal ranges. Results of a complete blood count, chemistry profile, and lipid profile are all within normal limits. He describes his self-medication by taking over-the-counter (OTC) drugs including antacids, histamine-2 receptor antagonists (H2 blockers), and the OTC proton pump inhibitor (PPI) omeprazole. He notes the latter helped "a little bit," but he discontinued use after two weeks, as noted in the packaging instructions. He has no history of smoking or alcohol abuse. He has an unremarkable past medical and family history.

Clinical Course

The physician explained to B. F. that he is experiencing classic esophageal symptoms that are highly specific to GERD, heartburn, and regurgitation. The physician also informed him that GERD might be associated with erosive esophagitis, which is best diagnosed on endoscopy via esophagogastroduodenoscopy (EGD). Because B.F. is 51 and has been experiencing heartburn for more than 10 years with daily symptoms for the past year, he should be evaluated by endoscopy. He has been referred for the procedure, but the appointment is not for seven weeks. He is prescribed a PPI and is instructed to return to the office in approximately four weeks while still on therapy for assessment of symptoms prior to his appointment.

主诉

B. F. 是一名51岁的非裔美国商人，主诉上腹痛。他有10年的胃灼热病史，过去1年中他注意到胃灼热变得更严重。胃灼热发生在饭后和就寝时，他的睡眠被夜间症状终止，他常常感觉疲劳。他说他断续地感觉有东西反流到他的喉咙，但没有吸入呼吸道的明显迹象。他知道胃食管反流病（GERD）是一种慢性疾病，可能有病情严重的并发症和死亡的风险。由于他需要出差，他推迟了与医生的约会，但意识到他需要看医生。胃灼热的频率（每天的现在）和严重性正在上升，所以他终于安排到医生办公室看病。

检查

B. F. 被他的初级保健医生检查，他描述了每天不适的发作。B. F. 身高6英尺1英寸（1.86m），体重230磅（104.3kg）。医生审查了去年的结肠镜检查结果，他是正常的，他的血压和其他体格检查结果都在正常范围内。全血细胞计数、化学检查和血脂检查结果正常。他描述了自己使用的非处方药（OTC），包括抗酸药、H₂ 受体拮抗剂（H₂ 受体阻滞剂）和OTC质子泵抑制剂（PPI）奥美拉唑。他注意到后者有一点帮助，但他按包装说明的要求在2个星期后停止使用。他没有吸烟史或酗酒史，有一个不值得的注意的既往病史和家庭病史。

临床病程

医生向B. F. 说明他正在经历GERD、胃灼热和反流的高度特异的典型食管症状。医生还告诉他，GERD 可能与侵蚀性食管炎相关，诊断最好通过食管胃十二指肠内镜检查（EGD）进行。因为B.F. 已经51岁，已经经历了超过10年的胃灼热，而且过去1年中每日都有症状，他应该做内窥镜检查。他的内窥镜检查已被提交预约，但7周内都约不上。医生给他开了PPI，并指示他在大约4周内返回医生办公室，在治疗的同时对其症状进行评估，以确定是否预约内窥镜检查。

简介

消化系统（digestive system）的功能是为人体细胞摄入准备食物，营养必须通过机械和化学的方法分解为小到足以能够被吸收的分子。在细胞内，营养被用于制造能量和重建重要的细胞成分。

消化

消化（digestion）发生在消化道内，消化道从口腔延伸至肛门。蠕动（peristalsis）是器官壁波动样的收缩，将食物在消化道内移动，并将不能消化的废物移出体外。对消化有贡献的还有几个向消化道释放分泌物的附属器官（accessory organ）。整个消化过程都需要酶（enzyme），这些酶是能够加速食物化学分解的生物催化剂（organic catalyst），它们的名称大都带有后缀 -ase。

消化道

消化道（digestive tract，alimentary canal）也被称为胃肠道［gastrointestinal (GI) tract］，本质上是一根很长的管道，在不同的位置改变成为具有特殊功能的独立器官（图 12-1）。框 12-1 总结了每个消化器官的功能。一个大的浆膜——腹膜（peritoneum）覆盖着腹腔内的器官，支撑并分开它们。

从口到胃

消化起始于嘴（图 12-2），也被称为口腔，食物在这里被牙齿咀嚼成小块。成人有 32 颗牙齿，包括切咬食物的切齿（incisor）和犬齿（canine）以及磨

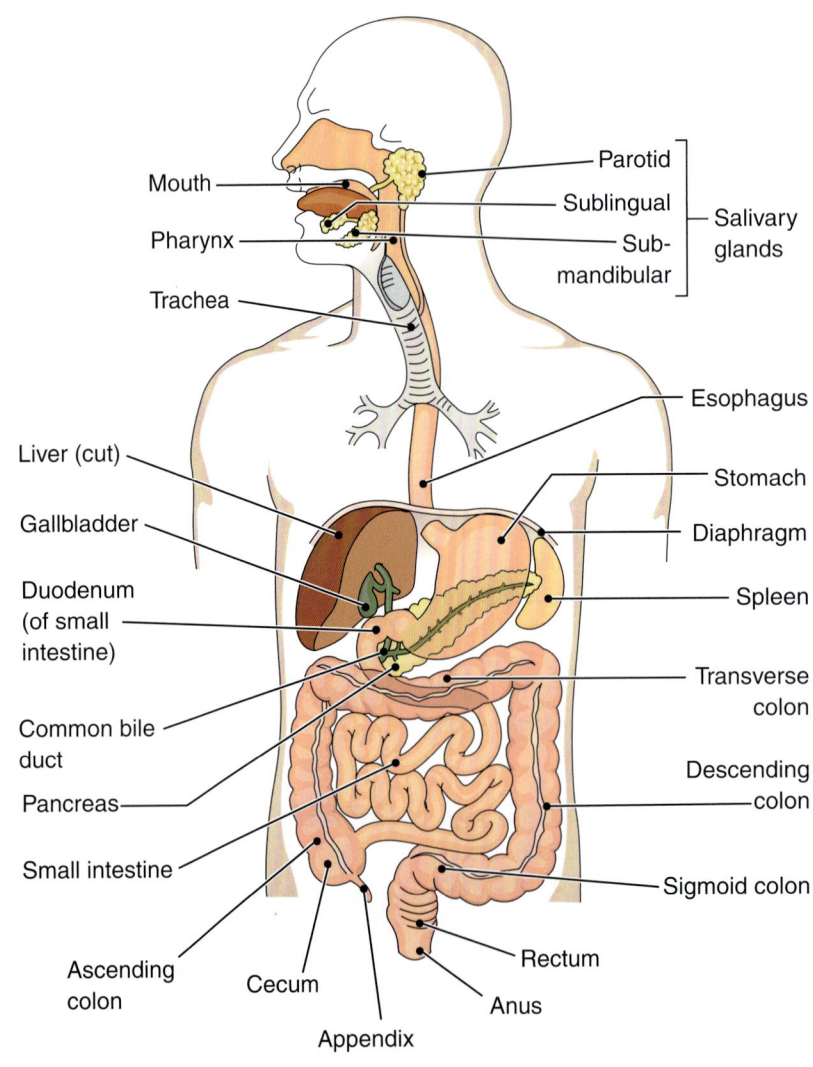

图 12-1 **消化系统。** 图中示出了小肠和大肠的一些分段。附属器官是唾液腺、肝、胆囊和胰腺。显示出了气管、隔膜和脾供参考

供你参考
消化道的器官

框 12-1

器官	消化活动
Mouth 口	切咬并咀嚼食物。将食物与唾液混合，唾液含有唾液淀粉酶，能够开始消化淀粉。将食物粉碎，由舌推向咽
Pharynx 咽	通过反射作用吞咽食物，并移入食管
Esophagus 食管	通过蠕动将食物移入胃
Stomach 胃	储存食物；将食物与水合消化液搅拌混合。分泌消化蛋白质的盐酸（hydrochloric acid, HCl）和胃蛋白酶
Small intestine 小肠	分泌酶。接收来自附属器官消化并中和食物的分泌物。是大多数营养被消化和吸收进入循环的场所
Large intestine 大肠	形成、存储并排出不能消化的废物

碎食物的臼齿（molar）。臼齿的结构特征及其周围组织如图12-3所示。腭（palate）是口腔的顶部，前半部（硬腭）由骨骼构成，后半部（软腭）由软组织构成，用于发声的肉质悬雍垂（uvula）悬在软腭上。牙齿保健师帮助照顾口腔和牙齿，框12-2有关于牙齿卫生职业的信息。

在咀嚼（chewing，mastication）过程中，舌（tongue）、唇（lip）、面颊（cheek）和腭也协助粉碎食物，并将食物与唾液混合。唾液（saliva）是一种能够湿润食物并开始淀粉（starch）消化的分泌物。唾液腺（salivary gland）向口中分泌唾液（图12-1），是附属消化器官。

湿润的食物被移向咽部（喉咙），在那里吞咽反射（swallowing reflex）会将它们推进食管，蠕动使食物沿着食管进入胃。在食管的末端连接着胃，食管具有能够收缩防止胃内容物反流的肌肉组织。这个食

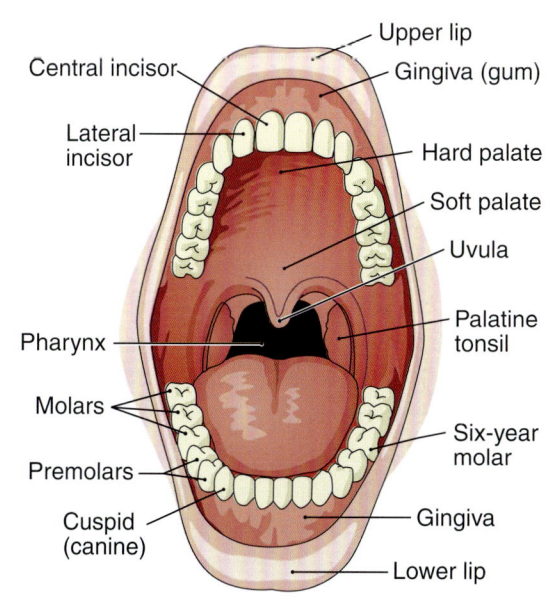

图12-2 口。图中示出了口腔中的牙齿、咽、扁桃体和其他结构

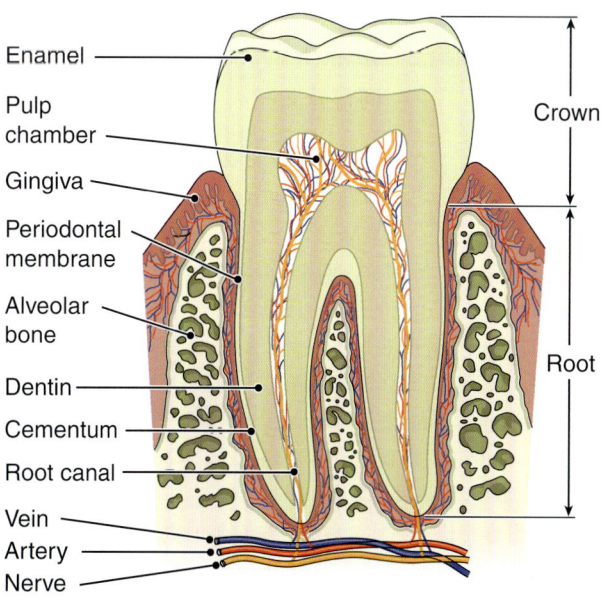

图12-3 臼齿。图中示出了骨槽、齿龈、血管和神经供应以及牙齿的其他部分

框 12-2

健康职业
牙科保健员

牙科保健员（dental hygienist）主要关注牙齿健康维护和预防性牙科护理。他们检查患者的牙列和牙周（牙齿的支撑结构），拍摄X线片，并用手和超声波仪器进行口腔预防治疗（oral prophylaxis），以除去沉积物，例如结石、污渍和斑块。他们还会使用氟化物防止龋齿（caries）。他们独立工作或与牙医一起进行局部麻醉和一氧化二氮镇静，并进行口腔筛查、磨光修复、拆除缝线、应用牙科保护胶，并执行牙周手术。牙科保健员必须了解关于X线设备的安全性、麻醉和传染性疾病。他们佩戴安全眼镜、手术口罩和手套，以保护自己和他们的患者。牙科保健员工作的主要组成部分之一是维持良好口腔健康的患者教育。他们可以指导营养和适当的口腔护理，如刷牙、牙线和使用抗菌漱洗剂。

大多数牙齿健康项目授予副学士学位，一些提供学士或硕士学位。在公共或学校保健机构中进行研究、教学或执业，需要更高的学位。专业课程需要1年的大学水平的预修课程。课程包括放射学、牙科解剖学、药理学、头颈解剖学以及其他健康与牙科相关科学课程。

项目培训包括有关于口腔健康执业的法律和伦理方面的补充内容，以及广泛的临床培训。毕业后，牙科保健员必须在其所在的州通过由美国牙科协会（American Dental Association, ADA）国家牙科检查联合委员会（Joint Commission on National Dental Examinations）管理的临床和书面考试，获得执照。

几乎所有的保健员都在牙科诊所工作。该领域的一个优点是调度灵活性和兼职工作的机会。工作前景好，牙齿健康是增长最快的职业之一。福利因工作地点而异。更多有关信息，请联系美国牙科保健员协会（American Dental Hygienists' Association）www.adha.org。

管下端括约肌（lower esophageal sphincter，LES）也被称为贲门括约肌（cardiac sphincter），因为它位于胃贲门（cardia）之上，是胃的上开口。

在胃中，随着被与含有能够分解蛋白质的胃蛋白酶（pepsin）和强力的盐酸（hydrochloric acid，HCl）的搅拌与混合，食物被进一步分解。随后，部分消化的食物进入胃的下半部幽门（pylorus），然后进入小肠。

小肠

食物离开胃进入十二指肠（duodenum），十二指肠是小肠的最初部分。随着食物进入小肠的其余部分——空肠和回肠（jejunum and ileum），消化就完成了（ileum 的发音与 ilium 相似，ilium 是骨盆

框 12-3

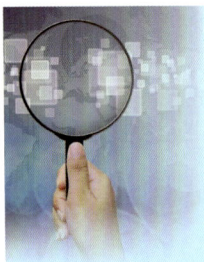

聚焦单词
同音异义词

同音异义词（homonym）是有相似发音，但有不同含义的单词。要理解实际意义，必须了解它们被使用的上下文。例如，骨盆的上半部是髂骨（ilium ['iliəm]），小肠的最后一段是回肠（ileum ['iliəm]），它们的形容词形式是不同的，前一个是 iliac，后一个是 ileal。单词 meiosis [mai'əʊsis]（减数分裂）是指染色体数量减半以形成配子（gametes）的细胞分裂类型，miosis [mai'əʊsis] 是指瞳孔的异常收缩。两个单词都源自于希腊语意为减少的单词。

发音相似的名称会导致一些有趣的拼写错误。上臂的肱骨 humerus 经常被写成 "humorous（幽默）"。迷走神经（vagus ['veigəs] nerve）是由意为 "迷路" 的词根命名的，因为这根神经分叉到许多内部器官。一些人书写这个名称时常常会联想到著名的赌城 Las Vegas ['veigəs]。同音异义词可能还有更严肃的一面。一些药物名称的发音或看起来太过相似，以至于临床医生可能混淆它们，会导致危险的潜在致命的并发症。例如，一位50岁的妇女在服用 Flomax 而不是 Volmax 之后被送进医院，Flomax 被用于治疗前列腺肥大的症状，而 Volmax 被用于缓解支气管痉挛。另一个例子涉及两种治疗神经分裂症（schizophrenia）的药物氯氮平（clozapine）和奥氮平（olanzapine），一位青年人被给错了药，导致了严重的并发症。美国食品和药物管理局（FDA）和美国采用名称委员会（United States Adopted Names Council）负责监管发音相似或看起来相似的药物名称。世界卫生组织（World Health Organization，WHO）拒绝了许多拟议名称，甚至在一些药物上市后更改了它们的名称，因为导致了用药错误。

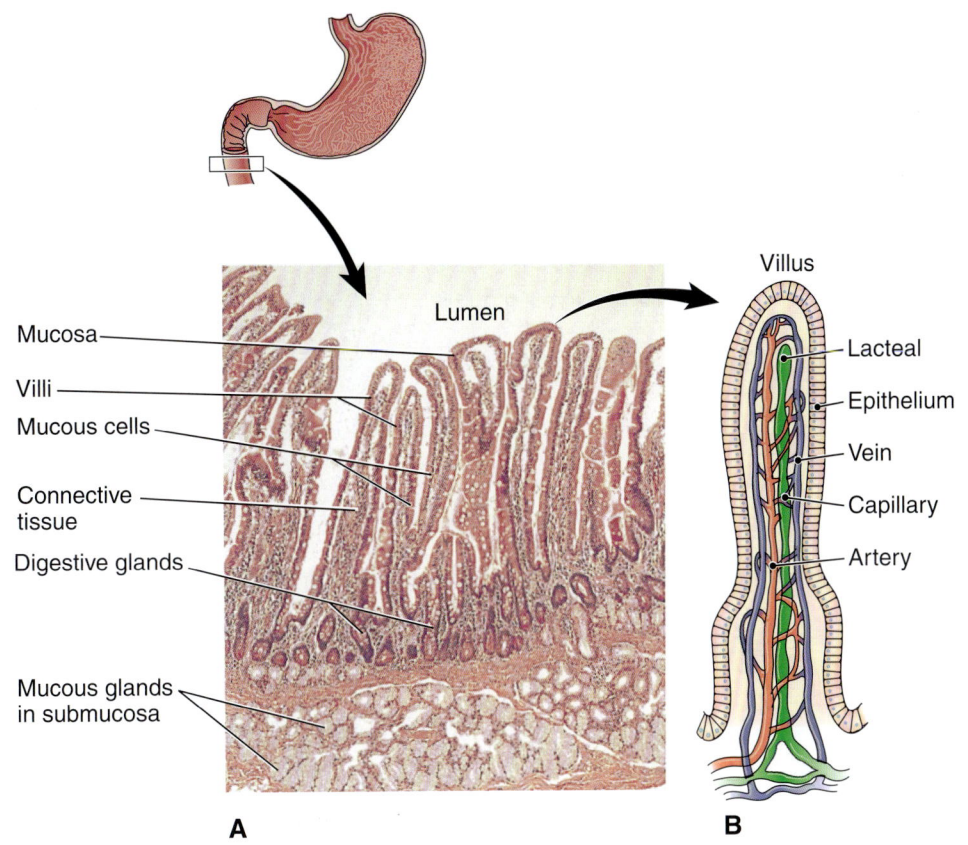

图 12-4 小肠绒毛。A.小肠内壁的显微镜观察显示分泌黏液和消化液的绒毛和腺体,管腔(lumen)是小肠的中心开口。B.小肠绒毛。每跟绒毛具有血管和用于吸收营养的乳头(淋巴毛细管)

中的一块大的骨骼。关于同音词的信息,请参见框 12-3。在小肠中活跃的消化性物质包括来自小肠自身的酶和附属器官分泌进入十二指肠的产物。

被消化的营养,包括水、矿物质和维生素,在小肠内壁被称为绒毛(villus,复数为 villi)的细小的凸起的帮助下,被吸入进入人体循环(图 12-4)。每根绒毛都有吸收营养进入血流的毛细血管和吸收已消化的小分子脂肪进入淋巴液的毛细淋巴管,或者称为乳糜管(lacteal)。当淋巴液流入心脏附件的血流时,这些脂肪就加入到血液之中。

大肠

任何尚未消化的食物与水和消化液一起进入大肠。这部分消化道起始于腹部右下区域,带有一个小囊——盲肠(cecum),阑尾(appendix)就附在其上(阑尾并不帮助消化,但它包含淋巴组织,在可能具有免疫功能)。大肠的下一部分是结肠(colon),通常用来表示大肠的名称,因为结肠构成了这个器官的很大一部分。结肠的升结肠(ascending colon)部分向上穿过腹部右侧,横结肠(transverse colon)部分跨过胃下,降结肠(descending colon)部分继续穿过腹部左侧。随着食物被推进结肠,水被再吸收,并形成粪便(stool, feces)。这些废物通过 S 形的乙状结肠(sigmoid colon)被储存在直肠(rectum),直到通过肛门(anus)排出。

附属器官

唾液腺(salivary glands)将体液分泌到口中,是参与消化的第一个附属器官,它们分泌一种开始消化淀粉的酶(salivary amylase,唾液淀粉酶)。其余的附属器官都位于腹部,并向十二指肠(duodenum)提供分泌物(图 12-5)。肝脏(liver)是一个大的腺体,具有许多功能,主要活动是处理血液,消除毒素并将营养转化为新的成分。一个特殊的循环途径是肝门静脉系(hepatic portal system),将血液从肝脏送到其他腹部器官。肝脏在消化中的功能是分泌胆

> **供你参考**
> **附属器官**
>
> 框 12-1
>
> | 器官 | 消化作用 |
> |---|---|
> | Salivary glands 唾液腺 | 分泌唾液，唾液湿润食物，并含有能够开始消化淀粉的唾液淀粉酶 |
> | Liver 肝脏 | 分泌胆汁，能够分解（乳化）脂肪 |
> | Gallbladder 胆囊 | 存储胆汁，需要时释放进入消化道 |
> | Pancreas 胰腺 | 分泌多种消化酶，还分泌碳酸氢盐中和胃酸，稀释食物 |

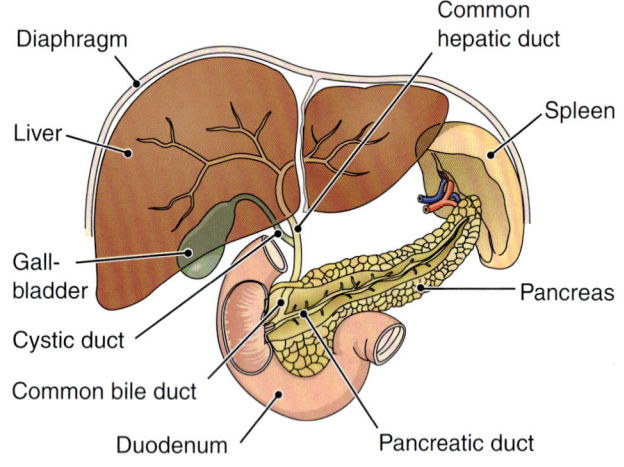

汁（bile），使脂肪乳化，分解为更小的单元。胆囊（gallbladder）存储胆汁，直至消化需要释放。来自于肝脏的肝总管（common hepatic duct）和来自于胆囊的胆囊管（cystic duct）合并形成胆总管（common bile duct），排入十二指肠。

胰腺（pancreas）产生消化酶混合物，通过胰管（pancreatic duct）送入十二指肠。胰腺还分泌大量碳酸氢盐（bicarbonate），中和强烈的胃酸。框12-4总结了附属器官的功能。

图 12-5 消化附属器官。图中示出了器官和管道，显示了隔膜和脾作为参考

Terminology 关键术语

正常结构和功能

anus [ˈeinəs]	肛门，消化道的末端开口（词根：an/o）
appendix [əˈpendiks]	阑尾，一个附属器官，附在盲肠上的一个淋巴组织管
bile [bail]	胆汁，肝脏分泌的一种液体，能够雾化脂肪并协助脂肪的吸收（词根：chol/e, bili）
cecum [ˈsiːkəm]	盲肠，大肠起始段的一个盲袋
colon [ˈkəʊlən]	结肠，大肠的主要部分；从盲肠延伸到直肠，包括升结肠、横结肠和降结肠部分（词根：col/o, colon/o）
common bile duct	胆总管，将胆汁送入十二指肠的导管，由胆管和肝总管合并形成（词根：choledoch/o）
duodenum [ˌdjuːəˈdiːnəm]	十二指肠，小肠的最初部分（词根：duoden/o）
enzyme [ˈenzaim]	酶，生物催化剂，加速化学反应

Terminology 关键术语（续表）

术语	释义
esophagus [iˈsɒfəgəs]	食管，将食物从咽输送到胃的肌肉管道
feces [ˈfiːsiːz]	粪便，从肠道排出的废物（形容词：fecal）
gallbladder [ˈgɔːlˌblædə]	胆囊，位于肝脏下表面的储存胆汁的囊（词根：cholecyst/o）
hepatic portal system	肝门静脉系，一个特殊的循环途径，将血液从腹部器官直接送入肝脏进行处理（也被简称为门静脉系）。进入肝脏的血管是肝门静脉（门静脉）
ileum [ˈiliəm]	回肠，小肠的末段（词根：ile/o）
intestine [inˈtestin]	肠道，胃与肛门直接的消化道，由小肠和大肠组成，其功能是消化、吸收和排出废物（词根：enter/o），也称为 bowel
jejunum [dʒiˈdʒuːnəm]	空肠，小肠的中段（词根：jejun/o）
lacteal [ˈlæktiəl]	乳糜管，小肠绒毛上的毛细淋巴管。乳糜管吸收脂肪进入淋巴液
large intestine	大肠，消化道的末段，有盲肠、结肠、直肠和肛门组成。大肠存储并排出未消化的废物（粪便）
liver [ˈlivə(r)]	肝脏，位于右上腹部的大腺体。除许多其他功能外，肝脏还分泌消化和吸收脂肪所需的胆汁（词根：hepat/o）
lower esophageal sphincter (LES) [ˈsfiŋktə(r)]	食管下括约肌，食管末端的肌肉组织（胃食管连接部，gastroesophageal junction），能够防止胃容物反流到食管，也被称为贲门括约肌（cardiac sphincter）
mastication [ˌmæstiˈkeiʃn]	咀嚼，也常用 chewing
mouth [maʊθ]	口，口腔，包括舌与牙齿。用于摄入并咀嚼食物，与唾液混合，并将食物移到喉咙吞咽
palate [ˈpælət]	腭，口腔的顶部，口腔与鼻腔的分割。由骨骼构成的前部硬腭和软组织构成的软腭组成（词根：palat/o）
pancreas [ˈpæŋkriəs]	胰腺，一个位于胃前面大而长的腺体。胰腺产生调节糖新陈代谢好激素，并产生消化酶（词根：pancreat/o）
peristalsis [ˌperiˈstælsis]	蠕动，器官壁波动样的收缩，将物质移动通过一个器官或通道
peritoneum [ˌperitəˈniəm]	腹膜，覆盖腹腔并支撑腹部器官的大浆膜
pharynx [ˈfæriŋks]	咽，喉咙；食物进入食管和空气进入后的公共通道（词根：pharyng/o）
pylorus [paiˈlɔːrəs]	幽门，胃进入十二指肠的末端开口（词根：pylor/o）。幽门由一个肌肉环——幽门括约肌控制
rectum [ˈrektəm]	直肠，大肠的末段部分，储存并排除未消化的废物（词根：rect/o, proct/o）
saliva [səˈlaivə]	唾液，释放到口腔的透明的分泌物，能够湿润食物，并含有淀粉消化酶（词根：sial/o）。唾液由三对腺体产生，分别是腮腺（parotid [pəˈrɒtid]）、下颌下腺（submandibular [sʌbmænˈdibjʊlə(r)]）和舌下腺（sublingual [sʌbˈliŋgwəl] glands）（图 12-1）
sigmoid colon [ˈsigmɔid]	乙状结肠，大肠末端的 S 形部分，位于降结肠和直肠之间

Terminology 关键术语（续表）

small intestine	小肠，胃与大肠之间的肠道，由十二指肠、空肠和回肠组成。附属器官的分泌物都进入小肠，大部分消化和吸收都发生在这里
stomach ['stʌmək]	胃，位于纵隔膜之下的囊状肌肉器官，能够储存食物，并分泌消化蛋白质的液体（词根：gastr/o）
uvula ['juːvjələ]	悬雍垂，悬在软腭上的肉质组织团，协助发声（字面含义时"小葡萄"，词根：uvul/o）
villi ['vilai]	绒毛，小肠内壁微小的凸起，能够将已消化的食物吸收进入循环（单数：villus）

与消化系统相关的词根

参见表 12-1 到表 12-3

表 12-1　与口腔相关的词根

词根	含义	示例	示例定义
bucc/o	面颊	buccoversion [bʌkʌ'vɜːʃn]	颊向错位
dent/o, dent/i	牙齿	edentulous [iː'dentʃələs]	缺齿的
odont/o	牙齿	periodontics [ˌperiəʊ'dɒntiks]	牙周病学
gingiv/o	牙龈	gingivectomy [dʒindʒi'vektəmi]	牙龈切除术
gloss/o	舌	glossoplegia [glɒ'səpliːdʒə]	舌麻痹
lingu/o	舌	orolingual [əʊrə'lɪŋwəl]	口舌的
gnath/o	颌	prognathous ['prɒgnəθəs]	下巴突出的
labi/o	唇	labium ['leibiəm]	唇或唇状结构
or/o	口	circumoral [ˌsɜːkəm'ɔːrəl]	口周
stoma, stomat/o	口	xerostomia [ˌziərə'stəʊmjə]	口干症
palat/o	腭	palatine ['pælətain]	腭的
sial/o	唾液、唾液腺、唾液管	sialogram [sjəlɒg'ræm]	唾液腺或管的 X 线造影
uvul/o	悬雍垂	uvulotome [juː'vjʊ'ləʊtəʊm]	悬雍垂切除刀

练习 12-1

使用形容词后缀 -al 写出下列含义的单词。

1. pertaining to the gums   gingival
2. pertaining to the tongue
3. pertaining to the teeth
4. pertaining to the cheek
5. pertaining to the lip
6. pertaining to the mouth

填空。

7. Dentistry ['dentistri] is the profession that studies, diagnoses, and treats the_____.
8. Micrognathia [maikrɒg'næθiə] is excessive smallness of the_____.
9. An orthodontist [ˌɔ:θə'dɒntist] specializes in straightening (ortho-) of the_____.
10. The oropharynx [əʊrə'færiŋks] is the part of the pharynx that is located behind_____.
11. Stomatoplasty [stə'mætəplæsti] is any plastic repair of the_____.
12. Hemiglossal [he'miglɒsl] means pertaining to one half of the_____.
13. A sialolith [sai'æləliθ] is a stone formed in a(n)_____ gland or duct.

定义下列单词。

14. buccopharyngeal [bʌkəfə'rindʒi:əl]
15. gingivoplasty [dʒigivɒ'plæsti]
16. sublingual [sʌb'liŋgwəl]
17. labiodental [ˌleibiəʊ'dentl]
18. uvuloptosis [juːvjʊlɒp'təʊsis]
19. hypoglossal [ˌhaipə'glɒsəl]
20. palatorrhaphy [pælei'tɒrəfi]

表 12-2　与消化道（口除外）相关的词根

词根	含义	示例	示例定义
esophag/o	食管	esophageal* [ˌiːsə'fædʒiəl]	食管的
gastr/o	胃	gastroparesis ['gæstrəʊpæeəisis]	胃轻瘫
pylor/o	幽门	pyloroplasty [pai'lɔ:rəplæsti]	幽门成形术
enter/o	肠道	dysentery ['disəntri]	肠道感染疾病
duoden/o	十二指肠	duodenostomy [djʊədi'nɒstəmi]	十二指肠切除术
jejun/o	空肠	jejunectomy [ˌdʒidʒuː'nektəmi]	空肠切除术
ile/o	回肠	ileitis [ˌili'aitis]	回肠炎
cec/o	盲肠	cecoptosis [siːkɒp'təʊsis]	盲肠下垂

续表 12-2　与消化道（口除外）相关的词根

词根	含义	示例	示例定义
col/o, colon/o	结肠	coloclysis [kə'lɒklisis]	结肠灌洗
sigmoid/o	乙状结肠	sigmoidoscope [sig'mɔidəskəʊp]	乙状结肠镜
rect/o	直肠	rectocele ['rektəsi:l]	脱肛
proct/o	直肠	proctopexy [prɒktɒ'peksi]	直肠固定术
an/o	肛门	perianal [peri'einəl]	肛周

* 注意 -al 前添加的

练习 12-2

使用形容词后缀 -ic 写出下列定义的单词。

1. pertaining to the pylorus　_____
2. pertaining to the colon　_____
3. pertaining to the stomach　_____
4. pertaining to the intestine　_____

使用形容词后缀 -al 写出下列定义的单词。

5. pertaining to the rectum　_____
6. pertaining to the jejunum　_____
7. pertaining to the ileum　_____
8. pertaining to the cecum　_____
9. pertaining to the anus　_____

写出下列定义的单词。

10. pertaining to the stomach and duodenum　_____
11. inflammation of the esophagus　_____
12. surgical creation of an opening in the intestine　_____
13. study of the stomach and intestines　_____
14. endoscopic examination of the stomach　_____
15. downward displacement of the pylorus　_____
16. inflammation of the jejunum and ileum　_____
17. excision of the ileum　_____
18. pertaining to the anus and rectum　_____

练习 12-2

使用词根 col/o 写出下列定义的单词。

19. inflammation of the colon _____
20. surgical creation of an opening into the colon _____
21. surgical fixation of the colon _____
22. surgical puncture of the colon _____

使用词根 colon/o 写出下列定义的单词。

23. any disease of the colon _____
24. endoscopic examination of the colon _____

消化道的两个器官或甚至同一器官的两个部分可在移除受损组织后用一个通道（吻合）手术连接（吻合术，anastomosis）。这种手术以连接的器官加上结尾 -stomy 命名。使用两个词根加上后缀 -stomy 写出下列定义的单词。

25. surgical creation of a passage between the esophagus and stomach _____esophagogastrostomy_____
26. surgical creation of a passage between the stomach and intestine _____
27. surgical creation of a passage between two portions of the jejunum _____
28. surgical creation of a passage between the duodenum and the ileum _____
29. surgical creation of a passage between the sigmoid colon and the rectum (proct/o) _____

表 12-3　与附属器官相关的词根

词根	含义	示例	示例定义
hepat/o	肝	hepatocyte ['hepətəsait]	肝细胞
bili	胆汁	biliary ['biliəri]	胆汁或胆管的
chol/e, chol/o	胆汁，胆囊	cholestasis [ˌkɒlə'stɑːsis]	胆汁淤积
cholecyst/o	胆囊	cholecystogram ['kəʊlsistəgræm]	胆囊造影
cholangi/o	胆管	cholangioma [kəʊ'lændʒiəʊmə]	胆管瘤
choledoch/o	胆总管	choledochal ['kəʊldɒtʃəl]	胆总管的
pancreat/o	胰腺	pancreatotropic [pæŋkriætət'rɒpik]	促胰腺的

练习 12-3

使用形容词后缀 -ic 写出下列定义的单词。

1. pertaining to the liver _____
2. pertaining to the gallbladder _____
3. pertaining to the pancreas _____

练习 12-3

使用后缀 -graphy 写出下列定义的单词。

4. radiographic study of the liver _____
5. radiographic study of the gallbladder _____
6. radiographic study of the bile ducts _____
7. radiographic study of the pancreas _____

使用后缀 -lithiasis 写出下列定义的单词。

8. condition of having a stone in the common bile duct _____
9. condition of having a stone in the pancreas _____

填空。

10. Inflammation of the liver is called _____.
11. The word biligenesis ['bilidʒnisis] means the formation of _____.
12. A cholelith ['kɒləliθ] is a(n) _____.
13. Choledochotomy [kəledə'kɒtəmi] is incision of the _____.
14. Cholecystectomy [ˌkɒlisis'tektəmi] is removal of the _____.
15. Hepatomegaly [hepətəʊ'megəli] is enlargement of the _____.
16. Cholangitis [kəʊlæn'dʒaitis] is inflammation of a(n) _____.
17. Pancreatolysis [pæŋkriæ'tɒləsis] is dissolving of the _____.

消化系统的临床表现

消化道

感染

很多微生物能够引起消化道感染，从病毒、细菌到原虫和蠕虫。在口中，细菌感染会造成龋齿（caries），引起牙龈感染（牙龈炎 gingivitis）甚至扩展到更深的组织和牙齿的骨质支持（牙周炎 periodontitis）。一些胃和肠道的感染可能产生胃肠炎（gastroenteritis）、恶心、腹泻和呕吐（emesis）等短期不适。还有一些胃肠道感染，例如伤寒（typhoid）、霍乱（cholera）和痢疾（dysentery）则非常严重，甚至致命。

阑尾炎（appendicitis）是阑尾感染所致，通常继发于阑尾阻塞。为避免阑尾破裂和腹膜炎（peritonitis），手术是必要的。

溃疡

溃疡（ulcer）是炎症和组织损伤造成的皮肤或黏膜损害。由胃液（gastric juices，peptic juices）的伤害作用在胃肠道内壁引起的溃疡被称为胃溃疡（peptic ulcers）。大多数胃溃疡发生在十二指肠的初段，起因不完全清楚，虽然幽门螺旋杆菌（Helicobacter pylori）感染曾被认为是主要原因。影响因素可能包括遗传和压力，还有慢性炎症和暴露于有害药物或饮食中的刺激物等。

目前，溃疡的治疗包括使用抗生素消除幽门螺旋杆菌感染和使用抑制胃酸分泌的药物。溃疡可能会导致出血或消化道穿孔。

溃疡通过内窥镜或胃肠道造影诊断（图 12-6，框 12-5），胃肠道造影要使用对比剂，通常是硫酸钡（barium sulfate）。钡餐检查（barium study）能够揭示多种胃肠道病症，出溃疡外，还包括肿瘤和梗阻。钡吞咽造影（barium swallow）被用于检查咽和食管，上胃肠道系列造影用于检查食管、胃和小肠。

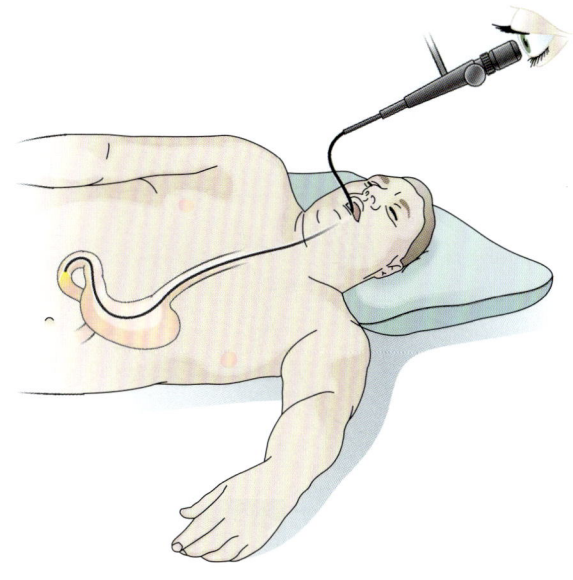

图 12-6　**内窥镜检查**。图中示出了正在做胃镜检查的患者

癌症

口腔的癌症通常涉及唇和舌，吸烟是主要的风险因素。黏膜白斑病（Leukoplakia）通常是因吸烟或其他刺激所致，在 25% 的情况下是癌症的早期迹象。胃肠道癌症的最常见所在是结肠和直肠，这些大肠癌症时美国癌症死亡的最常见死因。低纤维、低钙高脂肪饮食是大肠癌症的主要风险因素，遗传也是一个因素，例如像慢性结肠炎（colitis）。肠道息肉（polyp）经常可能转变为癌症，应该被切除。息肉可以通过内窥镜确认，甚至切除。

大肠癌症的一个迹象是肠道出血，可以通过大便化验检测。因为出血量可能很小，被描述为看不见的出血。根据杜克分类法（Dukes classification），大肠癌症可以根据严重性分为 A、B、C 三类。

检查者可以使用不同的内窥镜观察肠道的内部，这些内窥镜根据其被使用的特定区域命名，例如直肠镜（proctoscope）、乙状结肠镜（sigmoidoscope）和结肠镜（colonoscope）（图 12-7）。

在某些癌症病例中或因其他原因，可能需要手术切除部分胃肠道，并在腹壁上建立一个开口（stoma）以排除废物。这种造口（ostomy）手术基于其涉及的器官命名（图 12-8），例如回肠造口术（ileostomy）或结肠造口术（colostomy）。两个器官通道之间所执行做吻合术（anastomosis）要用两个器官命

框 12-5

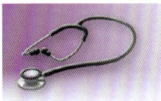

临床观点
内窥镜

现代医学在不用手术而观察人体内部方面取得了巨大的进展。内窥镜（endoscope）是一个插入人体开口或切口的装置，能够允许非介入性地检查通道、中空器官和体腔。最初的内窥镜是一个刚性的发光的望远镜，只能插入人体很浅的深度。现在，医生们使用光纤（fiberoptic）内窥镜能够在蜿蜒曲折的消化道内运行自如。

医生们能够用内窥镜检查胃肠道的结构异常、溃疡、炎症和肿瘤。另外，他们还利用内窥镜去除积液或采集测试样本。一些手术也可以用内窥镜完成，例如切除结肠息肉等。

内窥镜还可以用于关节（关节镜，arthroscopy）、膀胱（膀胱镜，cystoscopy）、呼吸道（支气管镜，bronchoscopy）和腹腔（腹腔镜，laparoscopy）的检查和手术。

"虚拟结肠镜（virtual colonoscopy）"使用计算机控制的 X 线产生结肠的细致图像，这一方法可用于大多数人的排查，不过少数人仍然需要用标准结肠镜做进一步的检查或手术。一个最新的技术进展是胶囊内窥镜（capsular endoscopy），能够更简单地进行胃肠道检查。它使用一个患者可以吞咽进去的胶囊大小的摄像机，随着在消化道移动，摄像机向置于患者腰带上的数据接收器传送视频图像。

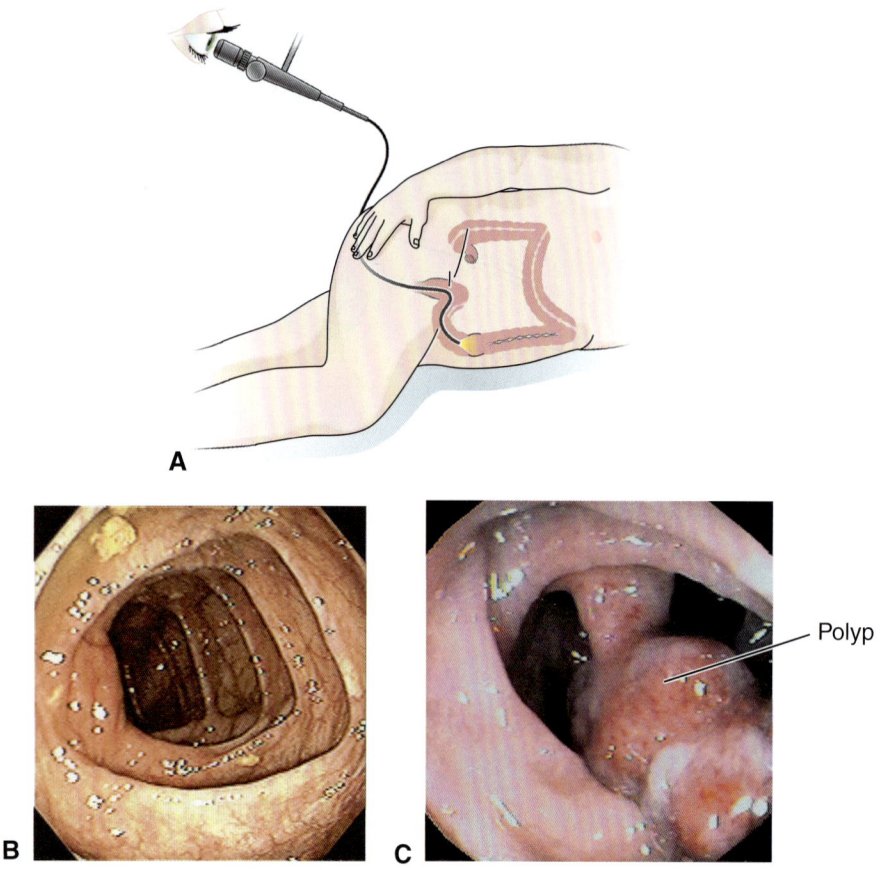

图 12-7 结肠镜检查。A. 乙状结肠镜检查。柔性光纤内窥镜前进通过近侧乙状结肠，然后进入降结肠；B. 盲肠的内窥镜图像，盲肠是大肠的第一部分；C. 结肠息肉的内窥镜图像

名，例如胃与十二指肠吻合术或结肠与直肠吻合术（coloproctostomy）。

阻塞

疝（hernia）是器官通过腹部开口向外突出，最常见的是腹股沟（inguinal）疝，将在第 14 章讨论（图

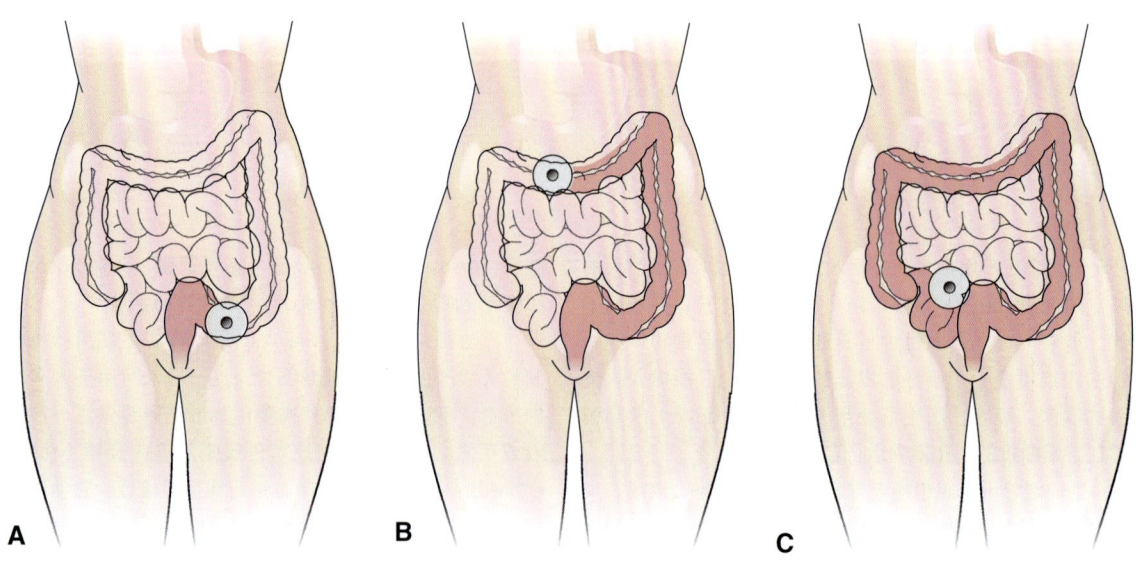

图 12-8 造口术。图中示出了各种位置，阴影部分代表已被移除或不活动的肠段，A. 乙状结肠造口术，B. 横向结肠造口术，C. 回肠造口术

14-7)。在食管裂孔疝（hiatal hernia）中，胃的一部分通过食管所通过的横隔膜空间向上移动到胸腔（图6-7）。通常这种情况不产生任何症状，但可能会引起胸痛、吞咽困难（dysphagia）和胃容物向食管反流。

在幽门狭窄（pyloric stenosis）病例中，胃与小肠之间的开口过小，多发于婴儿，而且男婴多于女婴。幽门狭窄的一个迹象是喷射性呕吐（projectile vomiting），可能需要手术矫正。

其他类型的阻塞包括肠套叠（intussusception）（图12-9A）、肠扭转（volvulus）和肠梗阻，肠套叠是一段肠道滑入其下部分（图12-9B），肠道阻塞通常是因缺乏蠕动所致。

痔疮（hemorrhoid）是直肠的静脉曲张，伴有疼痛、出血，某些情况会出现直肠脱垂（rectal prolapse）。

胃食管反流病

胃食管反流病（Gastroesophageal reflux disease，GERD）是指由于胃肠结合部，特别是食管下括约肌衰弱引起的胃液反流到食管（图12-10）。这些酸性分泌物如果通过反流向上推进，会刺激食管内壁，甚至喉咙和口腔。GERD 的症状俗称胃灼热

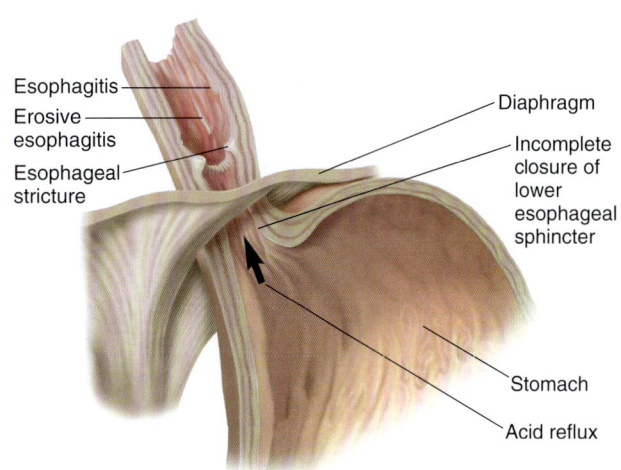

图12-10 胃食管反流病（GERD）。弱的食管下括约肌使得酸性胃内容物反流进入食道的下部，引起疼痛和刺激

（heartburn），是胸骨以下向上放射性灼痛感，并不涉及心脏，但疼痛区域处于心脏附近。

GERD 症状在胃内压力上升时更容易发生，例如餐后胃中饱满、躺下或弯腰时，以及肥胖或怀孕的人。食管裂孔疝也会导致胃肠道反流。治疗包括降低体重、将床头抬高 10~15cm、避免刺激性的食物和用药减少胃酸的分泌。如果需要，可以手术修复无力的食管下括约肌。

持续的食管反流可能会伤害食管内壁，导致巴瑞特综合征（Barrett syndrome）或巴瑞特食管。在这种病症中，食管黏液膜逐渐被与胃或肠道一样的皮膜所取代。巴瑞特综合征一般没有早期症状，可能的并发症包括食管痉挛、形成瘢痕组织、食管狭窄和癌症风险上升。

炎症肠道疾病

炎症性肠道疾病（inflammatory bowel disease，IBD）包括两种相似的疾病：

- 克罗恩病（Crohn disease）是一种慢性肠道壁炎症，通常在回肠和结肠，会引起疼痛、腹泻、脓肿（abscess）以及形成异常通道——瘘管（fistula）。
- 溃疡性结肠炎（ulcerative colitis）涉及结肠内壁连续性发炎，起始于直肠，并向近侧延伸（图12-11）。

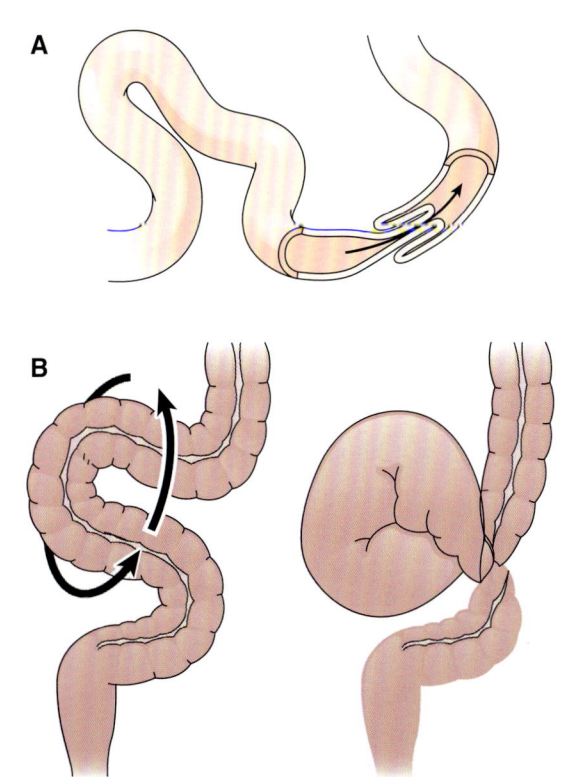

图12-9 肠梗阻。A.肠套叠；B.肠扭转，显示逆时针扭转

两种形式的炎症性肠道疾病主要发生于青春期儿童和年轻人，并显示有遗传特征。它们始发于一种异常免疫反应，也许是对正常肠道菌群（normal intestinal flora）的反应，还伴有自身免疫反应。治疗要使用抗炎药物、免疫抑制剂和反复手术切除受损的部分结肠。

乳糜泄（celiac disease）的特征是不能吸收含有麸质（gluten）的食物，麸质是小麦和一些其他粮食中含有的蛋白质。乳糜泄会影响小肠的上半部，始发于对麸质的过度免疫反应。黏膜炎症（mucosal inflammation）会减少肠道绒毛，并干扰吸收。乳糜泄要通过不含麸质的饮食进行治疗。

憩室炎（diverticulitis）通常会影响结肠。憩室（diverticula）是肠道壁上的小囊，会随着年龄的增加和出现。这些小囊的出现被称为憩室病（diverticulosis），是由低纤维饮食引起的。这些囊中的废物和细菌的积累会导致憩室炎，会伴随疼痛，有时会有出血。通过使用钡造影剂的下胃肠道造影研究能够发现憩室（图12-12）。尽管没有能够治愈的方法，憩室炎可以用高纤维饮食、大便柔软剂和降低胃动力的药物（antispasmodics）进行治疗。憩室感染可以用抗生素治疗。

附属器官

肝炎

肝炎（hepatitis）通常是由病毒感染所引起的。已经有多于五种的肝炎病毒被确认，针对甲型肝炎和

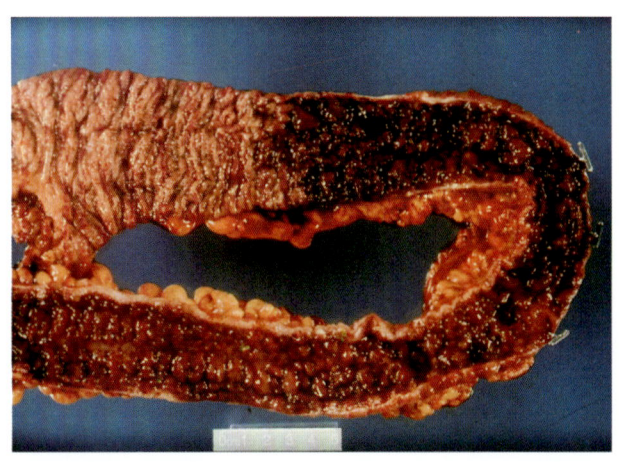

图 12-11 溃疡性结肠炎。结肠的突出红斑和溃疡开始于升结肠，并且在直肠乙状结肠区域最严重

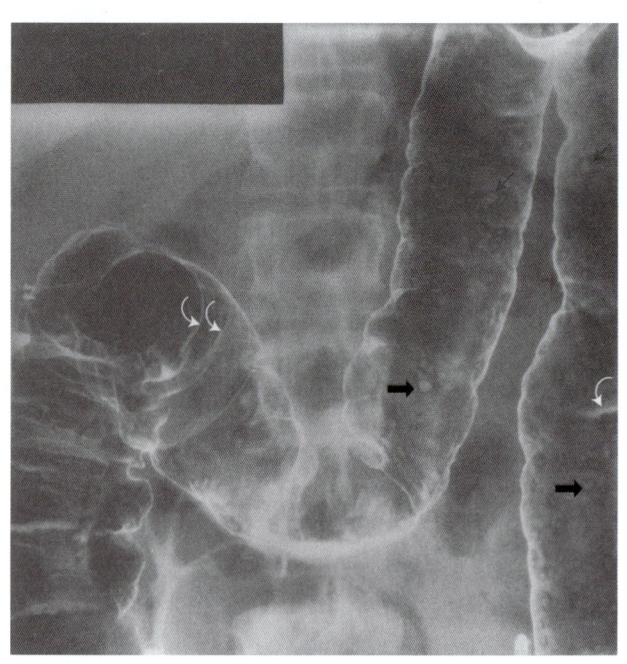

图 12-12 下胃肠道（GI）系列。钡灌肠显示肠炎（直箭头）和增厚的黏膜（曲线箭头）的病变

乙型肝炎有疫苗。

- 甲型肝炎病毒（hepatitis A virus，HAV）是最常见的肝炎病毒，它通过粪口污染（fecal-oral contamination）传播，通常是由食物处理和拥挤不洁的环境所致。也可以通过食用被污染的食物，特别是海鲜食物，受到感染。
- 乙型肝炎病毒（hepatitis B virus，HBV）是通过血液和其他体液传播的，它可能通过性传播，通常是共用注射针头和亲密接触。被感染的个人可能成为疾病携带者。大多数患者能够康复，但乙型肝炎可能会非常严重，可能导致肝癌，甚至致命。
- 丙型肝炎（hepatitis C）通过血液和血液制品或与被感染人密切接触传染。
- 丁型肝炎（hepatitis D）三角洲病毒（delta virus）是高致病性病毒，但只感染乙型肝炎患者。
- 戊型肝炎（hepatitis E），与甲型肝炎病毒相似，通过受污染的食物和水传播。曾在亚洲、非洲和墨西哥引起流行。

肝炎这一名称只是简单地意为"肝的炎症"，但是这一疾病也会引起肝细胞坏死。药物和毒素等其他感染也会引发肝炎。血清肝功能测试对诊断非常重要。

（splenomegaly）和食管末段静脉曲张，还可能会有出血。肝硬化的主要原因是过度饮酒。

胆结石

胆石病（cholelithiasis）是指胆囊（图12-14）或胆管中出现结石，通常伴随有胆囊炎（cholecystitis）。胆石病的特征是右上腹部的胆绞痛（biliary colic）、恶心和呕吐。

大多数胆结石（gallstones）是由胆固醇（cholesterol）构成的，胆固醇是胆汁的组成部分。胆结石更多发于女性人群，雌性激素（estrogen）的增加会促进胆结石的形成，因为雌性激素会提升胆汁中胆固醇的水平。诱发条件包括怀孕、使用口服避孕药和肥胖。奇怪的是，因为胆汁产量的变化和胆汁中胆固醇水平跌落，治疗病态肥胖的缩胃手术（stomach reduction surgery）后的快速体重下降通常会导致胆结石。药物能够分解胆结石，但彻底治愈的方法一般是通过胆囊切除术去除胆结石。以前这种手术需要很大的切口，但现在可以通过腹部的小切口用腹腔镜切除胆囊。胆囊切除以后，胆汁会通过胆总管直接流入十二指肠。

超声造影、X线造影和核磁共振成像被用于诊断胆结石（图12-14）。内镜逆行胰胆管造影术（endoscopic retrograde cholangiopancreatography，ERCP）可以观察胰腺和胆管（图12-15），并可用于

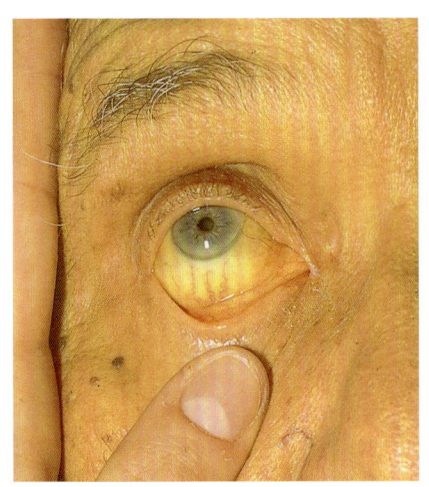

图12-13 黄疸。在眼睛中看到由于血液中的胆汁色素导致的黄色变色

黄疸症（jaundice或icterus）是肝炎和其他肝胆系统疾病的症状（图12-13）。由于血液中有胆汁色素，主要是胆红素（bilirubin），皮肤、眼白和黏膜发黄。

肝硬化

肝硬化（cirrhosis）是以肝肿大（hepatomegaly）、水肿、腹水（ascites）和黄疸为特征的慢性肝脏疾病。肝硬化的发展会导致因血液成分改变引起的内部出血和大脑损伤。肝硬化的一个并发症是门静脉血压过高（portal hypertension），门静脉是将血液从肝输送到腹部其他器官的血管。门静脉血压过高会引起脾大

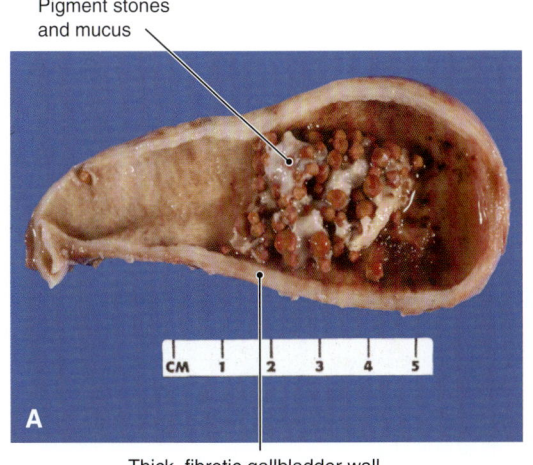
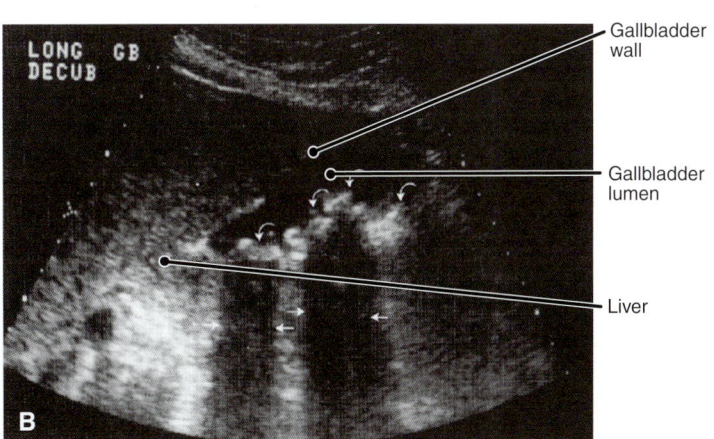

图12-14 胆石病（胆结石）。A.胆结石的形成（胆石病）引起胆囊炎症（胆囊炎）和胆汁阻塞。在该图中，由慢性炎症引起的大量胆结石和增厚的胆囊壁是明显的；B.超声图显示致密的胆结石（弯曲的箭头）。阴影出现（在直箭头之间），因为声波不能穿透石头（结石）

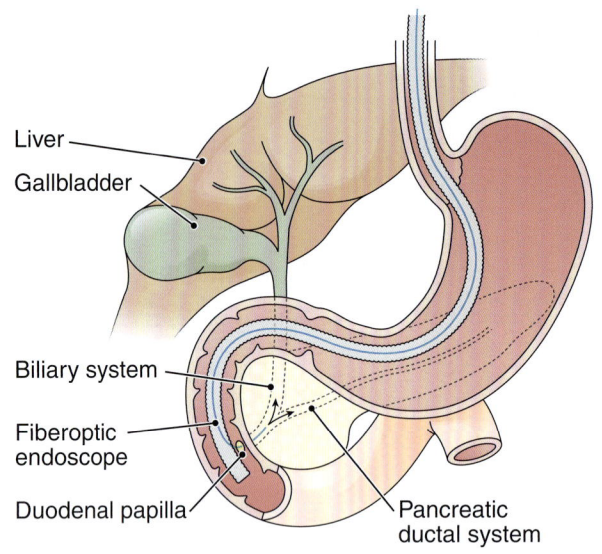

图 12-15 内镜逆行胰胆管造影（ERCP）。将造影剂注射到胰和胆管中以准备进行 X 线照相

执行特定的功能来缓解阻塞。

胰腺炎

胰腺炎（pancreatitis）可能是由酗酒、药物毒素、胆汁阻塞、感染或其他原因所致。急性胰腺炎的血液测试显示淀粉酶（amylase）和脂肪酶（lipase）水平升高，葡萄糖和胆红素水平也可能上升。对症治疗（symptomatic treatment）通常能够使该疾病消退。

Terminology	关键术语
病症	
appendicitis [əˌpendəˈsaitis]	阑尾炎，阑尾的炎症
ascites [æˈsaits]	腹水，腹腔液体积累，是一种形式的水肿。可能是由心脏疾病、淋巴或静脉阻塞、肝硬化或血清成分变化所致
Barrett syndrome	巴瑞特综合征，慢性食管炎症所致的病症，是由胃食管反流引起的。炎症伤害能够导致食管痉挛、瘢痕、狭窄和癌症风险上升
biliary colic [ˈbiljəri ˈkɔlik]	胆绞痛，由胆管结石引起的急性腹痛
bilirubin [ˌbiliˈru:bin]	胆红素，红细胞血红蛋白分解释放的色素；主要由肝脏分泌的胆汁排放
caries [ˈkɛəri:z]	龋齿，牙齿腐烂
celiac disease [ˈsi:liˌæk]	乳糜泻，不能吸收含有麸质的食物，由对麸质过度的免疫反应所致。麸质是小麦和其他一些粮食中含有的蛋白质
cholecystitis [ˌkɔlisisˈtaitis]	胆囊炎，胆囊的炎症
cholelithiasis [kəʊliliˈθaiəsis]	胆石病，胆囊中出现结石的病症；也指胆总管结石
cirrhosis [səˈrəʊsis]	肝硬化，肝组织变性的慢性肝病
Crohn disease	克罗恩病，胃肠道慢性炎症，通常涉及回肠和结肠

Terminology 关键术语（续表）

diarrhea [ˌdaɪəˈriə]	腹泻，频繁排泄水样粪便
diverticulitis [ˌdaɪvətɪkjʊˈlaɪtɪs]	憩室炎，消化道壁上，特别是结肠壁上的憩室（小囊）的炎症
diverticulosis [ˌdaɪvətɪkjʊˈləʊsɪs]	憩室病，消化道，特别是结肠上出现憩室
dysphagia [dɪsˈfeɪdʒɪə]	吞咽困难，食物从口腔至胃、贲门，运送过程中受阻而产生咽部、胸骨后或食管部位的梗阻或停滞的感觉
emesis [ˈeməsɪs]	呕吐，常用 vomiting
fistula [ˈfɪstjʊlə]	瘘管，两个器官或器官与身体表面之间的异常通道，例如直肠与肛门之间（肛门直肠瘘，anorectal fistula）
gastroenteritis [ˌgæstrəʊˌentəˈraɪtɪs]	胃肠炎，胃和肠道的炎症
gastroesophageal reflux disease (GERD) [ˈgæstrəʊɪsɒfəˈdʒiːəl]	胃食管反流，胃酸反流进入食管引起胃灼热、反流（regurgitation）、炎症和食管伤害的病症；因食管下括约肌（lower esophageal sphincter，LES）虚弱所致（图12-10）
heartburn [ˈhɑːtbɜːn]	烧心，胸骨以下的一种温暖或烧灼感，并向上辐射。通常伴有胃食管反流。医学专业术语是胃灼热 pyrosis [paɪˈrəʊsɪs]（pyr/o 意为"热"）
hemorrhoids [ˈhemərɔɪdz]	痔疮，直肠的静脉曲张，伴有疼痛、出血，有时会发生直肠脱垂
hepatitis [ˌhepəˈtaɪtɪs]	肝炎，肝脏的炎症，通常由病毒感染所致
hepatomegaly [hepətəʊˈmegəlɪ]	肝大，肝脏肿大，是肝硬化的特征之一
hiatal hernia [haɪˈeɪtəl]	食管裂孔疝，胃通过横膈膜开口突出，该开口是食管向下的通道（图6-7）
icterus [ˈɪktərəs]	黄疸，也常用 jaundice [ˈdʒɔːndɪs]
ileus [ˈɪlɪəs]	肠梗阻，肠道阻塞，可能是缺乏蠕动（麻痹，麻痹性肠梗阻）或收缩（动力性肠梗阻）所致。肠道内的物质或气体可以通过插入引流管排出
intussusception [ˌɪntəsəˈsepʃən]	肠套叠，一段肠道滑入其下的部分。主要发生于男婴的回盲区（图12-9A）。超过1天不能获得治疗就可能致命
jaundice [ˈdʒɔːndɪs]	黄疸症，由于血液中有胆汁色素引起的皮肤、黏膜和眼白出现黄色（源自于法语 jaune 意为"黄色"）。主要的胆汁色素是胆红素，是红细胞分解的副产品（图12-13）
leukoplakia [luːkəˈpleɪkɪə]	黏膜白斑病，舌黏膜上出现白斑，通常是吸烟或其他刺激所致；可能是癌症前期症状
nausea [ˈnɔːzɪə]	恶心，上腹部一种不适的感觉，常常会出现在呕吐之前。通常发生于消化不良、晕动症和怀孕早期
occult blood [əˈkʌlt]	隐血，只能用显微镜或化学方法检测到的极小量的出血；如果出现在大便中，是肠道出血的指征（occult 意为"隐藏"）
pancreatitis [ˌpæŋkrɪəˈtaɪtɪs]	胰腺炎，胰腺的炎症
peptic ulcer [ˌpeptɪk ˈʌlsə(r)]	胃溃疡，由胃液活动引起的食管、胃或十二指肠黏膜损伤

Terminology 关键术语

peritonitis [ˌperitəˈnaitis]	腹膜炎，腹膜的炎症，可能是由溃疡穿孔、阑尾破裂或生殖道感染以及其他原因所致
polyp [ˈpɒlip]	息肉，黏膜发育异常而形成的像肉质的突起部分
portal hypertension	门静脉高压，肝门静脉系统的异常压力升高，可能是由肝硬化、感染、血栓或肿瘤所致
pyloric stenosis [paiˈlɔːrik stiˈnəusis]	幽门狭窄，胃与十二指肠之间开口狭窄，也拼写为 pylorostenosis
regurgitation [riˌgɜːdʒiˈteiʃn]	反流，反向流动，如未消化食物的反流
ulcerative colitis [ˌʌlsərətiv kəˈlaitis]	溃疡性结肠炎，直肠或结肠的慢性溃疡，原因不明，可能与自身免疫有关
volvulus [ˈvɒlvjʊləs]	肠扭转，肠道扭转导致阻塞。通常涉及乙状结肠，儿童和老年人易发，可能是由先天畸形、外来异物或粘连所致。如不能立即治疗可能导致死亡（图 12-9B）
诊断和治疗	
anastomosis [ənæstəˈməusis]	吻合，两个血管或器官之间的通道。可能是正常的或病态的，也可能是手术建立的
barium study [ˈbeəriəm]	钡餐，在消化道荧光镜检查或X线造影中使用硫酸钡作为液体造影剂。能够显示阻塞、肿瘤、溃疡、食管裂孔疝、运动障碍，以及其他病症
cholecystectomy [ˌkɒlisisˈtektəmi]	胆囊切除术，手术切除胆囊
Dukes classification	杜克分类法，根据肠道壁侵入深度和所涉及的淋巴结对结直肠癌的分级系统；按严重性分为 A、B、C 级
endoscopic retrograde cholangiopancreatography (ERCP)	内镜逆行胰胆管造影，检查胰胆管并执行特定功能缓解阻塞的技术。X 线造影前要将造影剂从十二指肠注射进入胆管系统（图 12-15）
endoscopy [enˈdɒskəpi]	内窥镜检查，使用光纤内窥镜进行直接视觉检查。胃肠道检查包括食道、胃、十二指肠镜检查（esophagogastroduodenoscopy），直肠乙状结肠镜检查（proctosigmoidoscopy）和结肠镜检查（图 12-6 和图 12-7）
ostomy [ˈɒstəmi]	造口术，进入身体的开口，一般指为排出体内废物建立的开口。也指建立这样的开口的手术
stoma [ˈstəumə]	造口，手术建立的通向身体表面或两个器官之间的开口

Terminology 补充术语

正常结构和功能	
bolus [ˈbəuləs]	小而圆的物块，一团物质，例如吞咽下去的一团食物
cardia [ˈkɑːdiə]	贲门，胃接近食管的部分，因为其靠近心脏而得名
chyme [kaim]	食糜，从胃运动到小肠的半流体部分消化的食物

Terminology 补充术语（续表）

defecation [ˌdefə'keiʃən]	排便，从直肠排出粪便
deglutition [ˌdi:glu:'tiʃən]	吞咽，常用 swallowing
duodenal bulb	十二指肠球部，十二指肠靠近幽门的部分；十二指肠的第一个弯曲（褶皱）部分
duodenal papilla	十二指肠乳头，十二指肠上凸起的区域，胆总管和胰管在此进入（图 12-15）
greater omentum [əʊ'mentəm]	大网膜，从胃延伸至腹部器官的一圈腹膜
hepatic flexure [hi'pætik 'flekʃə]	结肠右曲，结肠右转弯部分，形成升结肠与横结肠的连接（图 12-1）
ileocecal valve [iliəʊ'si:kəl]	回盲瓣，回肠与小肠和盲肠与大肠之间的瓣状结构
mesentery ['mesəntəri]	肠系膜，折叠在肠道之上并支撑肠道的部分腹膜
mesocolon [ˌmezə'kəʊlən]	结肠系膜，折叠在结肠之上并支撑结肠的部分腹膜
papilla of Vater	十二指肠乳头，同 duodenal papilla
ruga ['ru:gə]	褶皱，胃内壁的大褶皱，胃空时可见
sphincter of Oddi	肝胰壶腹括约肌，胆总管进入十二指肠处的肌肉环
splenic flexure	结肠左曲，结肠的左转弯部分，形成横结肠与降结肠的连接（图 12-1）
病症	
achalasia [ˌækə'leiʒə]	失弛缓症，平滑肌不能放松，特别是食管下括约肌
achlorhydria [ˌeiklɔ:'haidriə]	胃酸缺乏，胃中缺乏盐酸，与胃酸过多（hyperchlorhydria）相反
anorexia [ˌænəˈreksiə]	厌食症，食欲丧失，神经性厌食症是心理诱导的拒绝或不能吃食物（形容词：anorectic, anorexic）
aphagia [æ'feigə]	吞咽不能，不能吞咽或吞咽困难；拒绝或不能吃食物
aphthous ulcer ['æfθəz]	口疮性溃疡，口腔黏膜溃疡
bruxism [b'ru:ksizəm]	磨牙症，牙齿紧咬并磨合，通常在睡眠期间
bulimia [buˈlimiə]	暴食症，过度、不满足的食欲。病症的特征是过量饮食，然后是诱导性的呕吐、腹泻或禁食
cachexia [kə'keksiə]	恶病质，严重的不健康、营养不良和消瘦
cheilosis [kai'ləusis]	唇干裂，嘴角开裂，通常是因维生素 B 缺乏所致（词根：cheil/o 意为"唇"）
cholestasis [ˌkɒlə'stɑ:sis]	胆汁淤积，胆汁停止流动
constipation [ˌkɒnsti'peiʃn]	便秘，排便很少或困难，排出干硬的粪便
dyspepsia [dis'pepsiə]	消化不良，消化能力差或有疼痛
eructation [ˌi:rʌk'teiʃən]	打嗝，也常用 belch

Terminology 补充术语（续表）

术语	释义
familial adenomatous polyposis (FAP)	家族性腺瘤性息肉病，一种遗传学疾病，在结肠和直肠中多发息肉，易患结直肠癌
flatulence ['flætjʊləns]	气胀，胃肠道中有空气或气体的病症
hematemesis [ˌhiːməˈteməsis]	咯血，从口中呕吐出血液
irritable bowel syndrome (IBS)	肠道易激综合征，一种慢性应激相关性疾病，特征是腹泻、便秘和伴随肠道节律性收缩的疼痛
megacolon [megəˈkəʊlən]	巨结肠，极度扩张的结肠。一般是先天性的，也可能发生在急性溃疡性结肠炎
melena [məˈliːnə]	黑便，因肠道出血所致的黑色柏油样粪便。常见于新生儿，也可能是胃肠道出血的体征
obstipation [ˌɒbstiˈpeiʃən]	顽固性便秘，极度便秘
pernicious anemia [pəˈniʃəd]	恶性贫血，用于为不能分泌内因子所致的一种贫血，内因子是吸收维生素 B_{12} 所必须的物质
pilonidal cyst [pailəˈnaidəl]	藏毛囊肿，一种骶区真皮囊肿，通常位于臀部间隙的顶部
thrush [θrʌʃ]	鹅口疮，由念珠菌引起的口或喉咙的真菌感染；表现为黏膜白斑或溃疡
Vincent disease	文森特病，重度牙龈炎与坏死；坏死性溃疡性牙龈炎（necrotizing ulcerative gingivitis）；战壕口腔牙龈炎（trench mouth）
诊断与治疗	
appendectomy [ˌæpenˈdektəmi]	阑尾切除术，手术切除阑尾
bariatrics [ˌbæriˈætriks]	肥胖病学，与预防和控制肥胖和与肥胖相关疾病的医学分支（源自于希腊语 baros，意为"重量"）
bariatric surgery	减肥手术，在治疗病态肥胖中用手术将胃缩小，并限制营养吸收。最常见的是胃分流术，将胃分区并将上半部与小肠（空肠）直接接合（图12-16）
Billroth operations	胃切除术与胃与十二指肠吻合（Billroth I）或胃与空肠吻合（Billroth II，图12-17）
gavage [gəˈvɑːʒ]	管饲，通过鼻胃管直接喂食到胃的过程
lavage [ˈlævidʒ]	灌洗，清洗体腔；冲洗（irrigation）
manometry [məˈnɒmitri]	测压法，测量压力；与胃肠道相关时，测量门静脉系的压力，这个压力是阻塞的体征
Murphy sign	墨菲体征，当用手指用力按压肋骨右弓（肝下）以下部位时，不能做深呼吸，预示胆囊疾病
nasogastric (NG) tube	鼻胃管，从鼻插入胃的管道（图12-18），可用于清空胃、用药、给液或胃容物采样
parenteral hyperalimentation	胃肠外高营养补液，为不能进食的人完全静脉喂食。又称为胃肠道外全面营养（total parenteral nutrition，TPN）
percutaneous endoscopic gastrostomy (PEG) tube	经皮内镜胃造瘘管，插入胃长期喂食的管道（图12-19）

Terminology	补充术语（续表）
vagotomy [və'gɒtəmi]	迷走神经切断术，在胃溃疡治疗中，切断迷走神经脉冲以减少胃酸的分泌。以前要通过手术，现在用药物即可
药物	
antacid [ænt'æsid]	抑酸剂，抑制酸性的药物，通常用于抑制胃酸
antidiarrheal ['æntidəri:l]	止泻剂，通过降低超蠕动或减少刺激物的吸收以及顺滑肠道内壁治疗或预防腹泻
antiemetic [æntimetik]	止吐剂，缓解或预防恶心和呕吐的药物
antiflatulent [æntaif'lætjʊlənt]	抗气胀药，预防或缓解胃肠气胀的药物
antispasmodic [æntispæz'mɑdik]	解痉药，缓解痉挛的药物，通常针对平滑肌
emetic [i'metik]	催吐剂，用于引起呕吐的药物
histamine H₂ antagonist	组胺 H₂ 受体拮抗药，通过干扰组胺 H₂ 受体减少胃酸分泌的药物。用于治疗溃疡和其他胃肠道疾病，也被称为 H₂ 受体阻断剂（H₂-receptorblocking agent）
laxative ['læksətiv]	轻泻药，促进大肠排泄的药物。包括兴奋剂、高渗物质、粪便柔软剂和成形剂
proton pump inhibitor (PPI)	质子泵抑制剂，通过阻止氢离子（质子）进入胃抑制胃酸分泌的药物

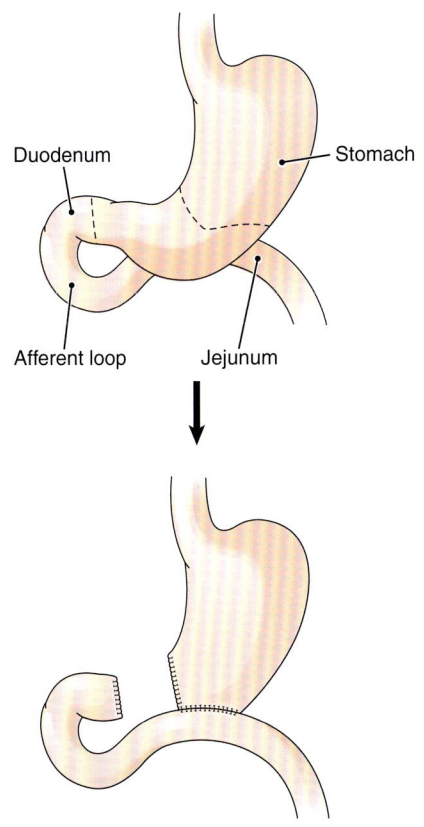

图 12-16 胃旁路。为了治疗病态肥胖，在胃中制造小囊以限制食物摄取。在胃空肠吻合术中，小囊绕过胃接到空肠以并减少营养物吸收

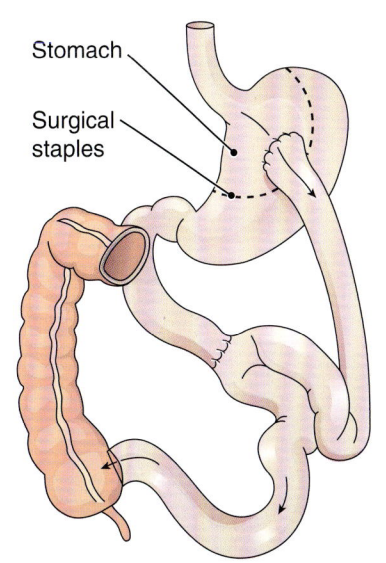

图 12-17 胃肠造口术（Billroth Ⅱ 手术）。虚线显示被切除的部分

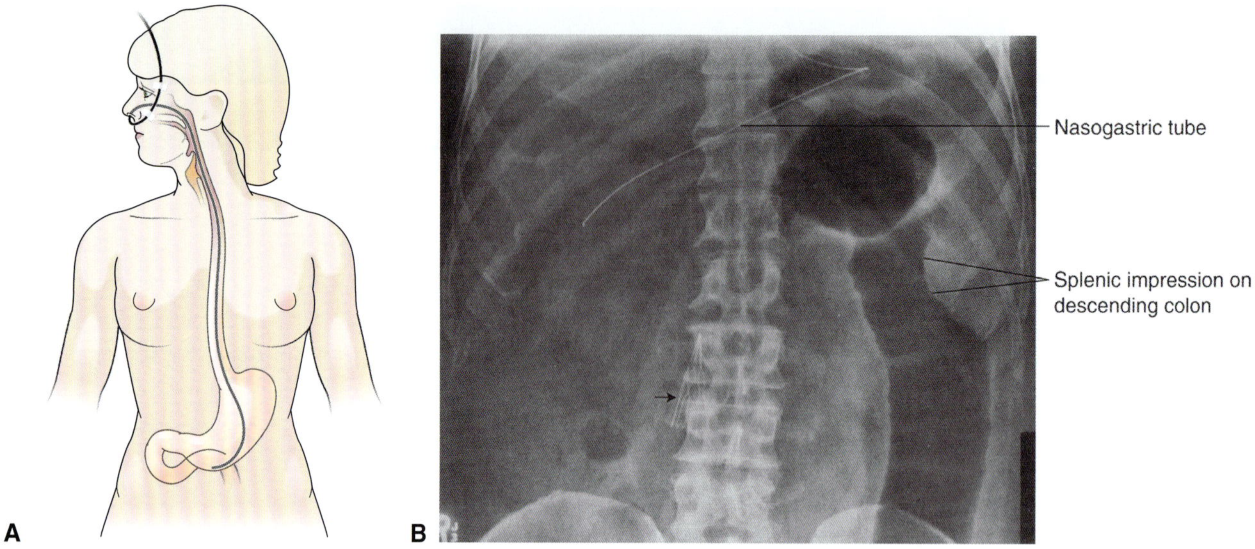

图 12-18 鼻胃（NG）管。A. 显示 NG 管在适当位置的图；B. 腹部 X 线片显示 NG 管。下腔静脉中显示出的过滤器（箭头）意在捕获可能起源于下肢和骨盆的栓塞

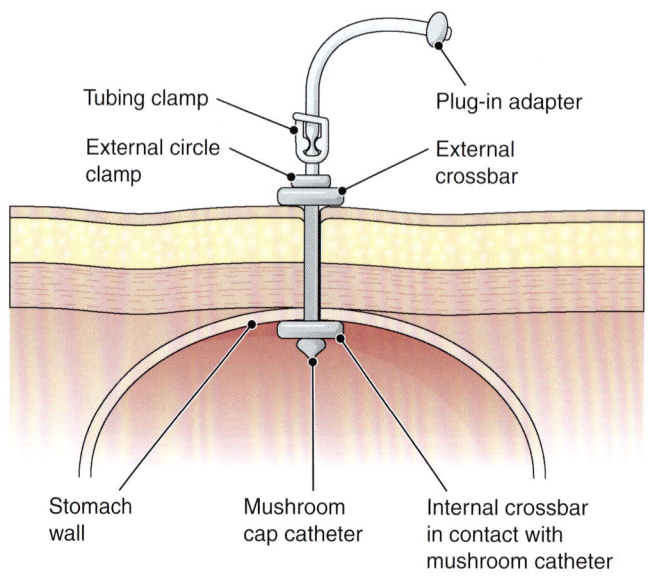

图 12-19 经皮内镜胃造瘘（PEG）管。显示管在胃中的适当位置

Terminology 缩略语

BE	Barium enema (for radiographic study of the colon)	钡灌肠（用于结肠X线造影检查）
BM	Bowel movement	肠道运动
CBD	Common bile duct	胆总管
EGD	Esophagogastroduodenoscopy	食管胃十二指肠镜检查
ERCP	Endoscopic retrograde cholangiopancreatography	内镜逆行胰胆管造影术
FAP	Familial adenomatous polyposis	家族性腺瘤性息肉病
GERD	Gastroesophageal reflux disease	胃食管反流病
GI	Gastrointestinal	胃肠的
HAV	Hepatitis A virus	甲型肝炎病毒
HBV	Hepatitis B virus	乙型肝炎病毒
HCV	Hepatitis C virus	丙型肝炎病毒
HDV	Hepatitis D virus	丁型肝炎病毒
HEV	Hepatitis E virus	戊型肝炎病毒
HCl	Hydrochloric acid	盐酸
IBD	Inflammatory bowel disease	炎症性肠病
IBS	Irritable bowel syndrome	肠道易激综合征
LES	Lower esophageal sphincter	食管下括约肌
NG	Nasogastric (tube)	鼻胃（管）
N&V	Nausea and vomiting	恶心和呕吐
N/V/D	Nausea, vomiting, and diarrhea	恶心、呕吐和腹泻
PONV	Postoperative nausea and vomiting	手术后恶心和呕吐
PPI	Proton pump inhibitor	质子泵抑制剂
TPN	Total parenteral nutrition	胃肠道外全面营养
UGI	Upper gastrointestinal	上消化道

Case Study Revisited
案例研究再访

B. F.'s Follow-Up Study

When B.F. returns after four weeks for his followup appointment in primary care, he explains that he started feeling better, so he stopped taking the medicine after three weeks. Now his symptoms have returned. They are waking him up at night, and he also now reports experiencing mild dysphagia. The physician explained that he must remain on his medication and emphasized the importance of going to his endoscopy appointment. Results from this study indicate that B. F. does indeed have moderate erosive esophagitis. There is a small hiatal hernia present as well.

B. F. is prescribed a PPI, 40 mg/day and encouraged to take it on a regular basis. He is counseled to decrease the fat in his meals, avoid lying down for at least two hours after meals, and limit alcohol intake. He returns six weeks later with marked improvement in compliance and total control of his symptoms. He is instructed to continue the PPI and to return in six months for reassessment.

B. F. 的研究随访

当 B. F. 在 4 个星期后回到初级保健进行随访，他说开始感觉好一些了，所以他在 3 周后停止服药。现在他的症状复发了，这些症状让他夜间无法入睡，并有轻度吞咽困难。医生解释说，他必须继续服药，并强调了内窥镜检查预约的重要性。内窥镜检查结果表明 B. F. 的确具有中度侵蚀性食管炎，还有一个小的食管裂孔疝。

医生又给 B. F. 开了 PPI，40mg /d，并鼓励他定期服用。还建议他减少膳食中的脂肪，避免在饭后至少 2 小时内躺下，并限制酒精摄入。6 个星期后回来，他遵医嘱良好，症状得到了很好的控制。他被指示继续服用 PPI，并在 6 个月内重新评估。

CHAPTER 12 复习

标记练习

消化系统

在对应的下划线上写出每个编号部分的名称。

Anus
Ascending colon
Cecum
Descending colon
Duodenum (of small intestine)
Esophagus
Gallbladder
Liver
Mouth
Pancreas

Parotid salivary gland
Pharynx
Rectum
Sigmoid colon
Small intestine
Stomach
Sublingual salivary gland
Submandibular salivary gland
Transverse colon

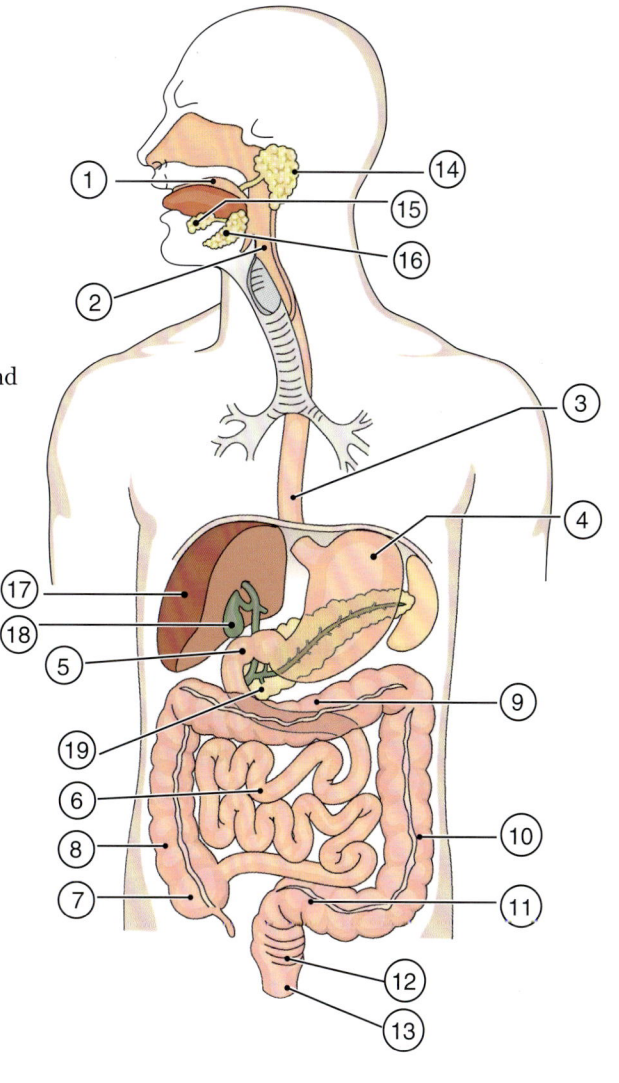

1. _____
2. _____
3. _____
4. _____
5. _____
6. _____
7. _____
8. _____
9. _____
10. _____
11. _____
12. _____
13. _____
14. _____
15. _____
16. _____
17. _____
18. _____
19. _____

消化附属器官

在对应的下划线上写出每个编号部分的名称。

Common bile duct   Gallbladder
Common hepatic duct   Liver
Cystic duct   Pancreas
Diaphragm   Pancreatic duct
Duodenum   Spleen

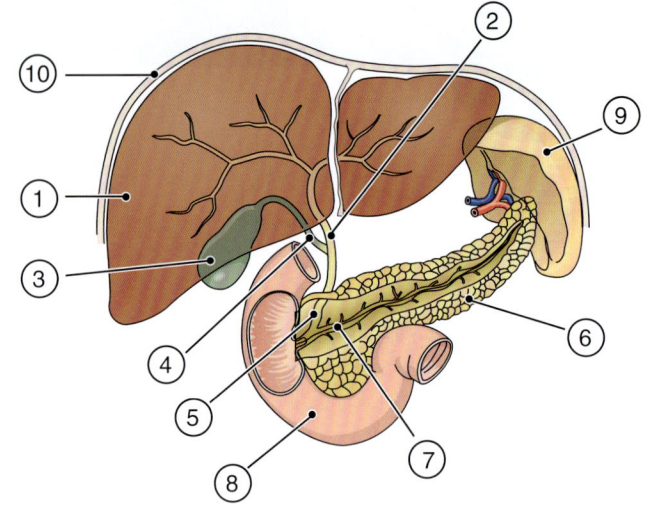

1. _____
2. _____
3. _____
4. _____
5. _____
6. _____
7. _____
8. _____
9. _____
10. _____

术语

匹配

匹配下列术语，在每个题号的左侧写上适当的字母。

____ 1. sublingual   a. pertaining to the cheek
____ 2. emetic   b. pertaining to the gum
____ 3. gingival   c. substance that induces vomiting
____ 4. agnathia   d. hypoglossal
____ 5. buccal   e. absence of the jaw

____ 6. enzyme   a. tooth decay
____ 7. caries   b. wave-like muscular contractions
____ 8. ileum   c. organic catalyst
____ 9. peristalsis   d. terminal portion of the small intestine
____ 10. icterus   e. jaundice

____ 11. choledochal   a. a type of liver disease
____ 12. cholelithotripsy b. pertaining to the common bile duct
____ 13. cholangiectasis c. crushing of a biliary calculus
____ 14. leukoplakia   d. dilatation of a bile duct
____ 15. cirrhosis   e. white patches on a mucous membrane

补充术语

____ 16. eructation   **a.** part of the stomach near the esophagus

____ 17. cardia   **b.** chewing

____ 18. achlorhydria   **c.** belching

____ 19. bolus   **d.** lack of hydrochloric acid in the stomach

____ 20. mastication   **e.** a mass, as of food

____ 21. gavage   **a.** swallowing

____ 22. bruxism   **b.** tooth grinding

____ 23. deglutition   **c.** malnutrition and wasting

____ 24. cachexia   **d.** feeding through a tube

____ 25. chyme   **e.** partially digested food

____ 26. antiflatulent   **a.** agent that controls loose watery stools

____ 27. antidiarrheal   **b.** agent that relieves heartburn, counteracts acidity

____ 28. antiemetic   **c.** agent that relieves or prevents gas

____ 29. antacid   **d.** agent that relieves spasm

____ 30. antispasmodic   **e.** agent that relieves or prevents nausea and vomiting

填空

31. Any surgical procedure to reduce the size of the stomach in the treatment of obesity is described as_____.

32. The blind pouch at the beginning of the colon is the_____.

33. The hepatic portal system carries blood to the_____.

34. The organ that stores bile is the_____.

35. The large serous membrane that lines the abdominal cavity and supports the abdominal organs is_____.

36. Glossorrhaphy is suture of the_____.

37. The palatine tonsils are located on either side of the_____.

38. Dentin is the main substance of a(n)_____.

39. From its name you might guess that the buccinator muscle is in the_____.

40. An enterovirus is a virus that infects the_____.

41. The anticoagulant heparin is found throughout the body, but it is named for its presence in the_____.

42. The substance cholesterol is named for its chemical composition (sterol) and for its presence in_____.

参见本章开头的 B.F. 案例研究。

43. Protrusion of the stomach through an opening in the diaphragm is termed a(n)_____.

44. Difficulty in swallowing is technically called_____.

45. The histamine-2 receptor antagonist used to treat B.F. reduces secretion of (see Chapter 8) _____.

定义

写出下列定义的单词。

46. liver enlargement_____

47. a dentist who specializes in treating the tissues around the teeth_____

48. surgical excision of the stomach _____
49. surgical repair of the palate _____
50. narrowing of the pylorus _____
51. inflammation of the pancreas _____
52. medical specialist who treats diseases of the stomach and intestine _____
53. surgical creation of an opening into the colon _____
54. surgical creation of a passage between the stomach and the duodenum _____
55. within (intra-) the liver _____

复数

写出下列单词的复数形式。

56. diverticulum _____
57. gingiva _____
58. calculus _____
59. anastomosis _____

拼写检查

写出下列术语的正确拼写。

60. hietal hernia _____
61. dyspepsia _____
62. inginal herna _____
63. icterus _____
64. pyeloric stenosis _____
65. diarryhea _____

真假判断

检查以下语句。如果语句为真，则在第一个空白处写入 T；如果语句为假，则在第一个空格中写入 F，并通过在第二个空格中替换带下划线的单词来更正语句。

	True or False	Correct Answer

66. In the opening case study, B.F. is experiencing his epigastric pain in the region <u>below</u> the stomach. _____ _____
67. The middle portion of the small intestine is the <u>duodenum</u>. _____ _____
68. Polysialia is the excess secretion of <u>bile</u>. _____ _____
69. The cystic duct carries bile to and from the <u>gallbladder</u>. _____ _____
70. The appendix is attached to the <u>cecum</u>. _____ _____
71. The common hepatic duct and the cystic duct merge to form the <u>common bile duct</u>. _____ _____
72. An emetic is an agent that promotes <u>diarrhea</u>. _____ _____
73. A <u>lavage</u> is an irrigation of a cavity. _____ _____

排除

在下列每组中，为与其余不相配的单词加下划线，并解释你选择的理由。

74. gingiva — villus — palate — uvula — incisor

75. spleen — cecum — colon — rectum — anus

76. pancreas — gallbladder — liver — pylorus — salivary glands

77. diarrhea — emesis — nausea — regurgitation — amylase

缩略语

写出下列缩略语的含义。

78. N&V
79. NG
80. TPN
81. GERD
82. EGD
83. GI
84. HCl
85. PPI
86. PEG (tube)
87. HAV

单词构建

使用给出的单词组成部分写出下列定义的单词。

-al   cec/o   r   -pexy   -cele   proct/o   -itis   -rhaphy   ile/o

88. inflammation of the cecum
89. suture of the rectum
90. fixation of the cecum
91. hernia of the rectum
92. pertaining to the ileum and cecum
93. fixation of the ileum
94. inflammation of the rectum
95. suture of the cecum
96. inflammation of the ileum

单词分析

定义下列单词，并给出每个单词组成部分的含义。如果需要，可以使用词典。

97. myenteric ［ˌmaiən'terik］ _____

    a. my/o _____

    b. enter/o _____

    c. -ic _____

98. cholescintigraphy ［'kəʊlsintigrəfi］ _____

    a. chole _____

    b. scinti _____

    c. -graphy _____

99. parenteral ［pə'rentərəl］ _____

    a. par(a) _____

    b. enter/o _____

    c. -al _____

100. nasogastric ［neizəʊ'gæstrik］ _____

    a. nas/o _____

    b. gastr/o _____

    c. -ic _____

101. xerostomia ［ˌziərə'stəʊmjə］ _____

    a. xero _____

    b. stoma _____

    c. –ia _____

Additional Case Studies
补充案例研究

Case Study 12-1: Cholecystectomy
案例研究 12-1：胆囊切除术

G. L., a 42-year-old obese Caucasian woman, entered the hospital with nausea and vomiting, flatulence and eructation, a fever of 100.5F, and continuous right upper quadrant (RUQ) and subscapular pain. Examination on admission showed rebound tenderness in the RUQ with a positive Murphy sign. Her skin, nails, and conjunctivae were yellowish, and she reported frequent clay-colored stools. Her leukocyte count was 16,000. An ERCP and ultrasound of the abdomen suggested many small stones in her gallbladder and possibly in the common bile duct. Her diagnosis was cholecystitis with cholelithiasis.

A laparoscopic cholecystectomy was attempted with an intraoperative cholangiogram and common bile duct exploration. Because of G. L.'s size and some unexpected bleeding, visualization was difficult, and the procedure was converted to an open approach. Small stones and granular sludge were irrigated from her common duct, and the gallbladder was removed. She had a T-tube inserted into the duct for bile drainage; this tube was removed on the second postoperative day. An NG tube in place before and during the surgery was also removed on Day 2. She was discharged on the fifth postoperative day with a prescription for prn pain medication.

G. L. 是一名 42 岁的白种人肥胖妇女，因恶心、呕吐、肠胃气胀和呕吐、发热 100.5 F、连续右上腹部（RUQ）和肩胛下疼痛进入医院。入院检查显示右上腹部反跳痛，墨菲征阳性。她的皮肤、指甲和结膜是淡黄色的，她主诉常常有土色的大便。她的白细胞计数是 16 000。内镜下逆行胰胆管造影术（ERCP）和腹部超声提示在胆囊中有许多小的结石，在胆总管中可能也有。诊断结果是有胆石症伴胆囊炎。

尝试为她做腹腔镜胆囊切除术和术中胆管造影和胆总管探查。由于 G. L. 的身材和一些意想不到的出血，难以做到可视化，该手术被改为开放式手术。小石子和颗粒泥被从她的胆总管中冲洗出来，胆囊被切除。有一个 T 管被插入她的胆管引流管道，手术后第 2 天被取出。在手术之前和手术期间的引流管也在第 2 天被移除。她在术后第 5 天出院，并给予在需要时处方药物镇痛。

Case Study 12-2: Colonoscopy with Biopsy
案例研究 12-2：结肠镜检查活检

S. M., a 24 YO man, had a recent history of lower abdominal pain with frequent loose mucoid stools. He described symptoms of occasional dysphagia, dyspepsia, nausea, and aphthous ulcers of his tongue and buccal mucosa. A previous barium enema examination showed some irregularities in the sigmoid and rectal segments of his large bowel. Stool samples for culture, ova, and parasites were negative. His tentative diagnosis was irritable bowel syndrome. He followed a lactose-free, low-residue diet and took Imodium to reduce intestinal motility. His gastroenterologist recommended a colonoscopy. After a two-day regimen of a soft to clear liquid diet, laxatives, and an enema, the morning of the procedure, he reported to the endoscopy unit. He was transported to the procedure room. ECG electrodes, a pulse oximeter sensor, and a blood pressure cuff were applied for monitoring, and an IV was inserted in S. M.'s right arm. An IV bolus of propofol was given, and S.M. was positioned on his left side. The colonoscope was gently inserted through the anal sphincter and advanced proximally.

The physician was able to advance past the ileocecal

S. M. 是一名 24 岁的男性，近期有下腹部疼痛、频繁松散的黏液样大便的病史。他描述了偶尔吞咽困难、消化不良、恶心与舌头和口腔黏膜口疮性溃疡的症状。以前的钡灌肠检查显示他的大肠的乙状结肠和直肠节段有一些异常。大便样本的培养物中卵清蛋白和寄生虫为阴性。他的暂时诊断是肠易激综合征。他一直保持无乳糖、低残留的饮食，并服用盐酸洛哌丁胺以降低肠蠕动。他的胃肠科医生建议进行结肠镜检查。在为期 2 天的软食到流食、通便和灌肠调整之后，在手术当天的早晨他来到了内窥镜检查病房。他被送到手术室，使用心电监护仪、脉搏血氧计传感器和血压袖带进行监测，并在右臂进行静脉输液（IV）。S. M. 被给予异丙酚的静脉推注，并置于左侧位，将结肠镜轻轻插入肛门括约肌并向近端推进。

医生能够将结肠镜推进通过回盲瓣，检查整个结肠。

valve, examining the entire length of the colon. Ulcerated granulomatous lesions were seen throughout the colon with a concentration in the sigmoid segment. Many biopsy specimens were taken. The mucosa of the distal ileum was normal. Pathology examination of the biopsy samples was expected to establish a diagnosis of IBD.

在整个结肠中观察到溃疡性肉芽肿性病变，在乙状结肠中比较集中，采集了许多活检标本。回肠末端的黏膜正常。活检样本的病理检查预期能够确定炎性肠炎诊断。

案例研究问题

多项选择。选择正确的答案，在每个题号的左侧写上你选择的字母。

____ 1. Flatulence and eructation represent
   a. regurgitation of chyme
   b. sounds heard only by abdominal auscultation
   c. passage of gas or air from the GI tract
   d. muscular movement of the alimentary tract

____ 2. Subscapular pain is experienced（图 5-7）
   a. above the navel
   b. below the shoulder blade
   c. below the sternum
   d. beside the shoulder blade

____ 3. Yellowish conjunctivae indicate
   a. emesis
   b. jaundice
   c. inflammation
   d. ptosis

____ 4. The common duct is more properly called the
   a. common bile duct
   b. common duodenal duct
   c. unified cystic duct
   d. joined bile duct

____ 5. The Murphy sign is a test for pain
   a. under the ribs on the left
   b. near the spleen
   c. in the lower right abdomen
   d. under the ribs on the right

____ 6. The NG tube is inserted through the _____ and terminates in the _____.
   a. nose, stomach
   b. nostril, gallbladder
   c. glottis, nephron
   d. anus, cecum

____ 7. Dysphagia and dyspepsia are difficulty or pain with
   a. chewing and intestinal motility
   b. swallowing and digestion
   c. breathing and absorption
   d. swallowing and nutrition

____ 8. The buccal mucosa is in the
   a. nostril, medial side
   b. mouth, inside of the cheek
   c. greater curvature of the stomach
   d. base of the tongue

____ 9. A gastroenterologist is a physician who specializes in study of
   a. mouth and teeth
   b. stomach, intestines, and related structures
   c. musculoskeletal system
   d. nutritional and weight loss diets

____ 10. The splenic and hepatic flexures are bends in the colon near the
   a. liver and splanchnic vein
   b. common bile duct and biliary tree
   c. spleen and appendix
   d. spleen and liver

____ 11. Intestinal motility refers to
   a. peristalsis
   b. chewing
   c. absorption
   d. ascites

____ **12.** A colonoscopy is

    a. a radiograph of the small intestine

    b. an endoscopic study of the esophagus

    c. an upper endoscopy with biopsy

    d. an endoscopic examination of the large bowel

____ **13.** The ileocecal valve is

    a. part of a colonoscope

    b. at the distal ileum

    c. in the pylorus

    d. at the proximal ileum

写出下列缩略语的含义。

14. ERCP_____

15. RUQ_____

16. NG_____

17. IBD_____

写出案例研究中下列含义的单词。

18. presence of stones in the gallbladder_____

19. endoscopic surgery of the gallbladder_____

20. inflammation of the gallbladder_____

21. radiographic study of the gallbladder and biliary system_____

22. ring of muscle that regulates the distal opening of the colon_____

23. surgical excision of tissue for pathology examination_____

CHAPTER 13

泌尿系统

预测试

多项选择。选择正确的答案，并在每个题号的左侧写上你选择的字母。

____1. The organ that forms urine is the
   a. cystic duct
   b. bladder
   c. gallbladder
   d. kidney

____2. The tube that carries urine out of the body is the
   a. ureter
   b. pylorus
   c. urethra
   d. peristalsis

____3. The hormone erythropoietin stimulates production of
   a. leukocytes
   b. saliva
   c. red blood cells
   d. platelets

____4. Micturition is the scientific term for
   a. urination
   b. digestion
   c. breathing
   d. retention

____5. With reference to the urinary system, the root cyst/o means
   a. ureter
   b. urinary stasis
   c. urinary bladder
   d. kidney

____6. Nephritis is inflammation of the
   a. liver
   b. intestine
   c. bladder
   d. kidney

____7. Separation of substances by passage through a membrane is termed
   a. absorption
   b. deglutition
   c. centrifugation
   d. dialysis

____8. A substance that promotes urinary output is a(n)
   a. hypertensive
   b. diuretic
   c. channel blocker
   d. enzyme

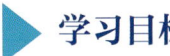

学习目标

学完本章后,应该能够:

1. ▶ 描述泌尿系统的功能。
2. ▶ 列举并描述泌尿道的器官,并给出它们的功能。
3. ▶ 识别肾元的组成部分。
4. ▶ 说明肾与血液循环之间的关系。
5. ▶ 描述尿液形成的过程。
6. ▶ 说明尿液如何传输并排出体外。
7. ▶ 识别并使用与泌尿系统相关的词根。
8. ▶ 描述泌尿系统的6种主要疾病。
9. ▶ 解释用于泌尿系统的缩略语。
10. ▶ 分析案例研究中与泌尿系统相关的医学术语。

Case Study: E. O.'s Stress Incontinence
案例研究:E. O. 的压力性尿失禁

Chief Complaint

E. O. is a 52-year-old Asian female with a history of stress incontinence. The condition has affected her quality of life, as she is not able to be active in athletics without worrying about urinary leakage under physical strain. E. O. has cut back on her sports participation and currently is involved in only two golf leagues. Although the incontinence continues to be a problem, she does not want to take medication or have corrective surgery. E. O. heard about a minimally invasive research protocol that could potentially address the incontinence. She decided to investigate to see if she would be a candidate for the study.

Examination

E. O. met with the research nurse who explained the study to her. She was told the study hoped to achieve around 75 percent improvement, which E. O. found acceptable. A urologic history was taken involving questions relating to urinary frequency, urgency, and nocturia (nighttime urination). A few procedures were required at the beginning of the study that would determine eligibility. E. O. was required to provide a clean-catch specimen and underwent a cystometrography (CMG) and a cystoscopy. The results indicated that she would be a good candidate for the research trial. She was required to maintain a urinary diary for two weeks and record when the stress incontinence and urgency occurred. E. O. proceeded with the study.

Clinical Course

The clinical study involved taking muscle cells from E.O.'s thigh, growing them in a laboratory, and then reinserting cultured stem cells (myoblasts) into the area surrounding the urethra. Theoretically, these actively growing cells would promote sphincter muscle development and provide greater control of urination. The urologist took a punch biopsy from E. O.'s thigh muscle to obtain the necessary cells. After laboratory processing, the active cells were injected into place. They were allowed to settle and grow for three months, at which time another CMG and cystoscopy were performed. A comparison was made with the original test results to see if there was any improvement in the stress incontinence. All procedures were conducted in the office with minimal discomfort.

主诉

E. O. 是一名52岁的亚洲女性,有压力性尿失禁病史。这种情况影响了她的生活质量,因为需要担心身体紧张下的尿泄漏,她不能活跃在各种运动之中。E. O. 已经减少了体育运动的参与,目前仅参与两个高尔夫球联赛。虽然尿失禁仍然是一个问题,她不想服药或进行矫正手术。E. O. 听说一种微创研究可能解决失禁问题,她决定试试看她是否能够成为该研究的候选人。

检查

E. O. 会见了向她解释该研究项目的研究护士。她被告知这项研究希望获得75%左右的改善,E. O. 认为可以接受。记录泌尿系统病史涉及与尿频、尿急和夜尿等有关问题。在研究开始时,需要一些程序来确定资格。E. O. 被要求提供清洁捕获标本并进行膀胱内压描记法(cystometrography,CMG)和膀胱镜检查。结果表明她将是研究试验的良好候选人。她需要在2周内保持每日尿的记录,并记录压力性尿失禁和尿急发生的时间。E. O. 开始了这项研究。

临床病程

临床研究涉及从E. O. 的大腿获取肌肉细胞,让它们在实验室中生长,然后将培养的干细胞(myoblasts,成肌细胞)重新插入到尿道周围的区域。理论上,这些活跃的生长细胞将促进括约肌肌肉发育并提供更有力的排尿控制。泌尿科医生从E. O. 的大腿肌肉进行穿刺活检以获得必要的细胞。实验室处理后,将活性细胞注射到位。这些细胞会定居并生长3个月,届时进行另一次CMG和膀胱镜检查。与原始测试结果进行比较,以查看压力性尿失禁是否有任何改善。所有步骤都在医生办公室进行,只有最小程度的不适。

简介

泌尿系统（urinary system）排泄新陈代谢的废物。在形成并排除尿液（urine）的过程中，泌尿系统还调节体液的成分、总量和酸碱平衡。肾（kidney）的活动以多种方式影响人体循环，泌尿系统对维持体内平衡（homeostasis）至关重要。如图 13-1 所示，泌尿系统由下列部分构成：

- 两个肾，是形成尿液的器官。
- 两根输尿管（ureter），将尿液从肾输送到膀胱。
- 膀胱（bladder），储存并排出尿液。
- 尿道（urethra），将尿液输送到体外。

肾

肾（kidney）是将从血液中过滤出来的物质形成尿液的器官。除了代谢废物以外，尿液还包含水和离子，所以它的形成对调节体液总量和成分非常重要。另外，肾还产生两种作用于循环系统的物质：

- 红细胞生成素（erythropoietin，EPO），一

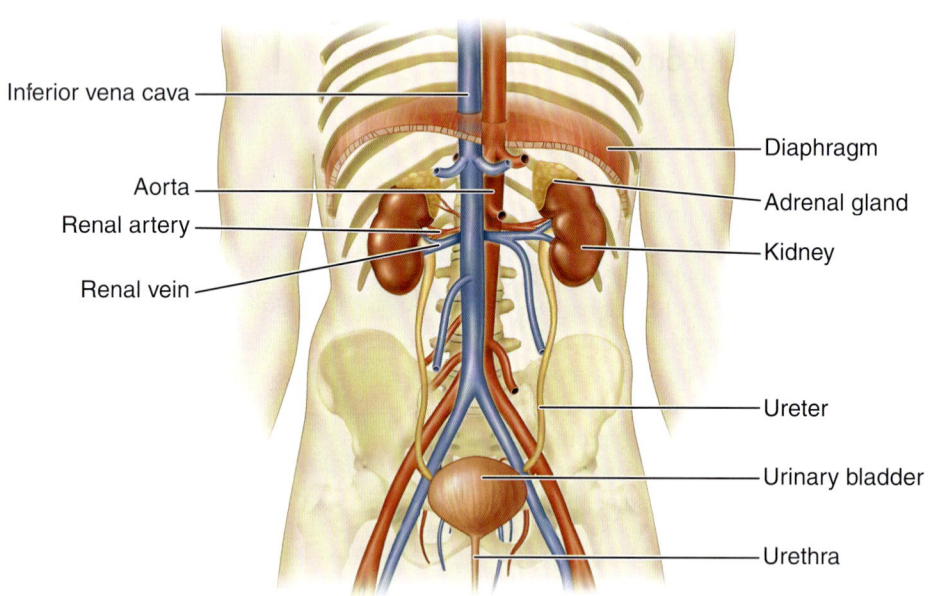

图 13-1　泌尿系统。该系统由肾（kidey）、输尿管（ureter）、膀胱（urinary bladder）和尿道（urethra）组成。这里还显示了隔膜、附近的血管和肾上腺（adrenal glard）

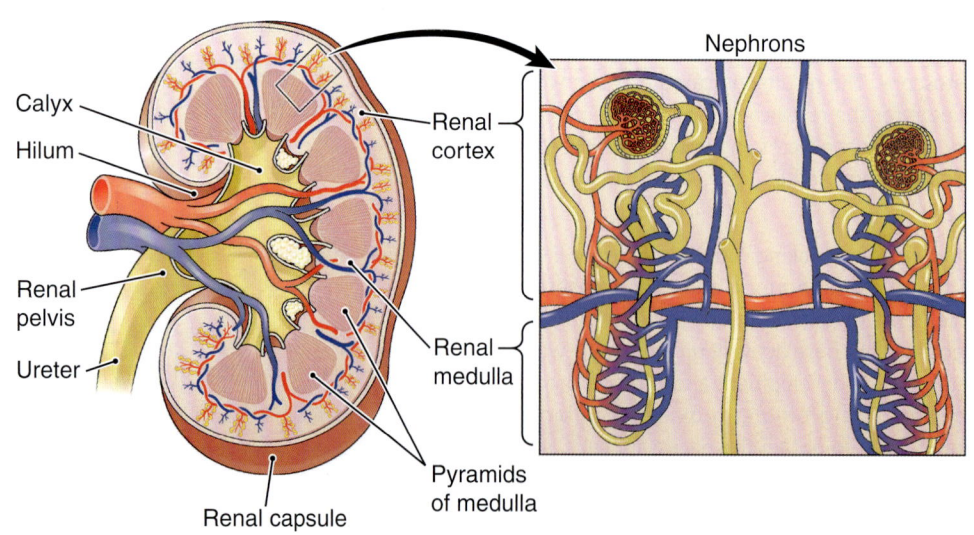

图 13-2　肾。通过肾的纵向截面（左）显示其内部结构，肾门是血管和导管与肾的连接点，肾元的放大图。每个肾含有超过 100 万个肾元（右）

框 13-1 聚焦单词

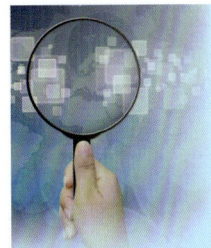

有双重意义的单词

有些单词出现在不只一个人体系统中，代表不同的结构。肾的髓质（medulla）是该器官的内部部分，像肾上腺、卵巢（ovary）、淋巴结等器官也可以分为中心髓质和外部皮质。但 medulla 意为"髓"，这个名词也指骨髓、脊髓和大脑脊髓的部分延髓（medulla oblongata）。

在心脏和大脑中都有室（ventricle）。单词 fundus 意为器官的后部或基底，子宫（uterus）的基底是远离子宫颈的上半圆的部分，与胃的情况相同。眼底则是眼睛最中心的一层，视网膜（retina）就位于那里。macula 是一个斑点，眼睛的 macula（黄斑）是视觉最敏锐的一点，耳朵的 macula（听斑）包含平衡感受器。

在解释医学词汇时，了解单词使用的上下文通常是很重要的。

种刺激骨髓中红细胞生产的激素。
- 肾素（renin），一种升高血压的酶。它会激活一种被称为血管紧张素（angiotensin）的血液成分，引起血管收缩。被称为 ACE 抑制剂（血管紧张素转化酶抑制剂，angiotensin-converting enzyme inhibitors）的药物通过干扰血管紧张素的生产来降低血压。

肾的位置和结构

肾位于腰部（lumbar region）腹膜之后。在每个肾的顶部，有一个肾上腺。肾包围在一个纤维结缔组织囊之中，外面覆盖着脂肪。最外层的结缔组织支撑着肾，并将其固定在身体壁上。

如果从内部观察（图 13-2），能看到肾有一个外层区域肾皮质（renal cortex）和一个内层区域肾髓质（renal medulla，框 13-1）。肾髓质被分为三角形的肾锥体（renal pyramid），这些锥体是由肾元（nephron）的袢和收集小管组成，肾元是肾的功能单元。每个收集小管将尿液排到被称为肾盏（calyx，源自于意为"杯子"的拉丁语单词）的尿液集中区。几个较小的肾小盏（minor calix）组成一个肾大盏（major calyx），然后主肾盏（major calix）联合构成肾盂（renal pelvis），肾盂是输尿管的上部漏斗形部分。

肾元

肾脏微小的工作单元是肾元（nephron，图 13-3），每一个这样的微小结构基本上是一根卷曲的小管，折叠成不同的形状。小管起始于一个杯形的肾小球囊（glomerular capsule），肾小球囊是肾元的血液过滤装置。然后，小管折叠成为近端小管（proximal tubule），伸直形成肾单位袢（nephron loop）（也被称为亨利氏环，loop of Henle），再次卷曲成为远端小管（distal tubule），最后伸直形成收集管。

图 13-3 肾元及其供血。肾元根据身体不断变化的需要调节尿液中的水、废物和其他物质的比例。肾元由肾小球囊、肾曲小管、肾元环（亨利氏套）和收集管组成。血液过滤在通过肾小球囊中的肾小球时发生。进入肾元的物质可以通过周围的管周毛细血管返回到血液中

肾的供血

血液通过肾动脉进入肾。肾动脉是腹部大动脉的一个短分支，进入肾组织后继续分支成为更小的血管，直至最终血液被带进肾小球囊在被称为肾小球（glomeruli）的一丛毛细血管中循环。血液通过一系列最终合并成为肾静脉的血管离开肾，肾静脉汇入下腔静脉（inferior vena cava）。

尿液形成

随着血液流过肾小球，血液压力迫使物质穿过肾小球壁和肾小球囊壁，进入到肾元。进入肾元的液体被称为肾小球滤液（glomerular filtrate），主要由水、电解质、可溶性废物、营养和毒素组成。主要的废物是尿素（urea），一种含氮的蛋白质代谢副产品。滤液中不应含有任何细胞或蛋白质，如白蛋白。

废物和毒素必须被排出，但大多数水、电解质和营养必须返回血液，否则人很快会饥饿并脱水。这一返回过程被称为肾小管重吸收（tubular reabsorption），发生在肾元周围的管周毛细血管网（peritubular capillaries）。

随着滤液流过肾元，其他过程会进一步调节其成分和 pH 值。滤液的浓度也受脑垂体激素（pituitary hormone）作用的调节。抗利尿激素（Antidiuretic hormone，ADH）会促进水的再吸收，进而使滤液浓度上升。最终的滤液被称为尿液，进入采集管后被排出。利尿剂（diuretic）是促进尿输出量增加的物质，被用于治疗高血压和心力衰竭，以减少体液总量和降低心脏负荷（参见第 9 章）。

尿液的输送和排出

尿液从肾盂中流出，通过左右输尿管进入膀胱储存（图 13-4）。随着膀胱充盈，它从其基底上的一个稳定的三角向上膨胀。这个膀胱三角区上面两个角是输尿管的开口，下面是尿道的开口（图 13-4）。三角区的稳定性能够防止尿液反流进入输尿管。

膀胱充满会刺激膀胱肌肉的反射收缩，并将尿液通过尿道排出。女性的尿道比较短（约 4cm），只输送尿液；男性的尿道比较长（约 20cm），输送尿液和精液。

排空尿液在技术上被称为排尿（micturition 或 urination），由尿道周围的两块括约肌调节。尿道内括约肌（internal urethral sphincter）在尿道进口周围，非自主地执行功能；尿道外括约肌由意识控制，不能留住尿液被称为尿失禁（urinary incontinence）。

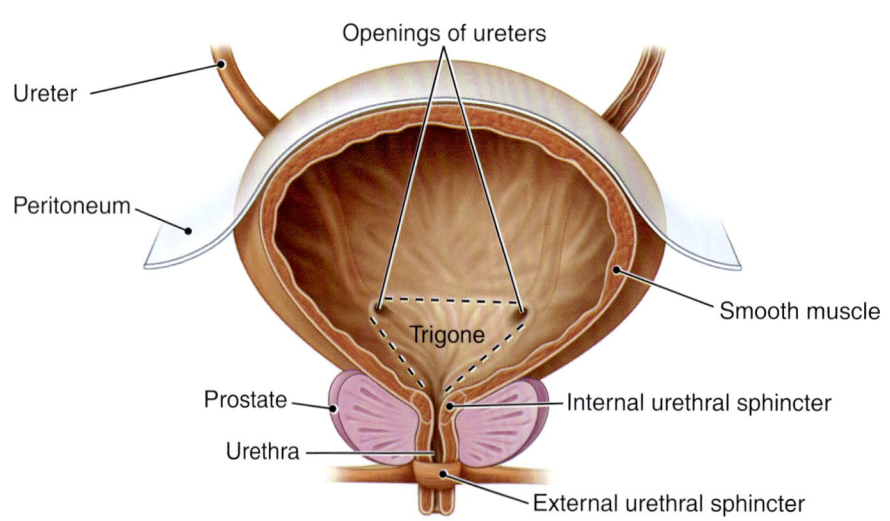

图 13-4 膀胱。图示为雄性膀胱的内部。膀胱底板中的膀胱三角区是由输尿管和尿道的开口标记的三角形区域。尿道穿过男性的前列腺

Terminology 关键术语

正常结构和功能

antidiuretic hormone (ADH) [ˌæntidɑijʊˈretik]	抗利尿激素，脑垂体腺释放的一种引起肾中水再吸收的激素
angiotensin [ˌændʒiəʊˈtensən]	血管紧张素，一种升高血压的物质，在血液中被肾素激活，肾素是肾生产的一种酶
calyx [ˈkeiliks]	肾盏，肾盂中的杯状腔体，也常用 calix（复数：calices，词根：cali, calic）
diuresis [ˌdaijʊəˈriːsis]	排尿，一般意指增加尿排泄
diuretic [ˌdaijuˈretik]	利尿剂，增加尿排泄量的物质；与排尿相关的
erythropoietin (EPO) [iriθrəˈpɔiətin]	红细胞生成素，一种由肾产生的刺激骨髓中红细胞生产的激素
glomerular capsule [gˈlɒmrjʊlə]	肾小球囊，起始于肾元的杯形结构，在肾小球周围，接收从血液中过滤出的物质；又称为鲍曼囊（Bowman capsule）
glomerular filtrate [ˈfiltreit]	肾小球滤液，液体和从血液中过滤出的可溶解物质，通过肾小球囊进入肾元
glomerulus [gləʊˈmeərjʊləs]	肾小球，肾小球囊中的毛细血管丛（复数：glomeruli，词根：glomerul/o）
kidney [ˈkidni]	肾，一个排泄器官（词根：ren/o, nephr/o）；两个肾过滤血液并形成尿液，尿液包含代谢废物和其他物质，以调节体液的水、电解质和酸碱平衡
micturition [ˌmiktjʊˈriʃn]	排尿，排空尿液；也常用 urination
nephron [ˈnefrɒn]	肾元，肾的微小功能单元；肾元与血管共同过滤血液，并平衡尿液的成分
renal cortex [ˈriːnəl ˈkɔː(r)teks]	肾皮质，肾的外层部分；包含肾元的
renal medulla [miˈdʌlə]	肾髓质，肾的内层部分，包含元和运输尿液到肾盂的导管
renal pelvis [ˈpelvis]	肾盂，输尿管扩展的上端，从肾接收尿液；希腊语词根 pyel/o 意为"盆"
renal pyramid [ˈpirəmid]	肾锥体，肾髓质中的三角形结构，由肾元袢和收集管组成
renin [ˈriːnin]	肾素，肾产生的一种酶，能够激活血液中的红细胞生成素
trigone [ˈtraigəʊn]	膀胱三角区，由输尿管的两个开口和尿道开口在膀胱基底构成的三角区（图 13-4）
tubular reabsorption [ˈtjuːbjələ(r)]	肾小管重吸收，肾小球滤液中的物质通过管周毛细血管网返回血液
urea [jʊˈriːə]	尿素，尿液中的含氮废物
ureter [jʊˈriːtə]	输尿管，将尿液从肾输送到膀胱的管道（词根：ureter/o）
urethra [jʊˈriːθrə]	尿道，将尿液从膀胱运输出体外的管道（词根：urethr/o）
urinary bladder [ˈblædə(r)]	膀胱，储存并排除肾排泄的尿液的器官（词根：cyst/o, vesic/o）
urination [ˌjʊəriˈneiʃn]	排尿，排空尿液，也常用 micturition
urine [ˈjʊərin]	尿，肾排泄的液体，由水、电解质、尿素、其他代谢和色素废物构成。生病时尿液中会出现多种其他物质（词根：ur/o）

与泌尿系统相关的词根

参见表 13-1 和表 13-2

表 13-1　与肾相关的词根

词根	含义	示例	示例定义
ren/o	肾	suprarenal [su:pə'ri:nəl]	肾上的
nephr/o	肾	nephrosis [ni'frəʊsis]	肾病
glomerul/o	肾小球	juxtaglomerular [dʒʌkstəglɒ'merʊlə]	肾小球旁
pyel/o	肾盂	pyelectasis [paie'lektəsis]	肾盂扩张
cali/o, calic/o	肾盏	caliceal [kæli'si:l]	肾盏的；也拼写为 calyceal

练习 13-1

使用词根 ren/o 写出下列单词。

1. before or in front of (pre-) the kidney
2. behind (post-) the kidney
3. above the kidneys
4. around the kidneys

使用词根 nephr/o 写出下列单词。

5. the medical specialist who studies the kidney
6. any disease of the kidney
7. poisonous or toxic to the kidney
8. softening of the kidney
9. enlargement of the kidney

使用适当的词根写出下列单词。

10. incision into the kidney
11. inflammation of the renal pelvis and kidney
12. plastic repair of the renal pelvis
13. radiograph of the renal pelvis
14. inflammation of a glomerulus
15. incision of a renal calyx
16. hardening of a glomerulus
17. dilatation of a renal calyx

表 13-2　与泌尿道相关的词根（肾除外）

词根	含义	示例	示例定义
ur/o	尿，泌尿系统	urosepsis [jʊ'rəʊsepsis]	尿脓毒病
urin/o	尿	nocturia [nɒk'tjʊəriə]	夜尿症（词根：noct/i）
ureter/o	输尿管	ureterostenosis [jʊəri:tərɒste'nəʊsis]	输尿管狭窄
cyst/o	膀胱	cystocele ['sistəsi:l]	膀胱膨出
vesic/o	膀胱	intravesical [intrei'vesikəl]	膀胱内的
urethr/o	尿道	urethrotome [jʊə'reθrəʊtəʊm]	尿道刀

练习 13-2

使用词根 ur/o 形成下列单词。

1. any disease of the urinary tract _____
2. radiography of the urinary tract _____
3. a urinary calculus (stone) _____
4. presence of urinary waste products in the blood _____

词根 ur/o 用于后缀 -uria，意为"尿液或排尿的状态"，请使用 -uria 形成下列单词。

5. lack of urine _____
6. presence of pus in the urine _____
7. urination at night _____
8. painful or difficult urination _____
9. presence of blood (hemat/o) in the urine _____

后缀 -uresis 意为"排尿"，请使用 -uresisi 写出下列单词。

10. increased excretion of urine _____
11. lack of urination _____
12. excretion of sodium (natri-) in the urine _____
13. excretion of potassium (kali-) in the urine _____

以上几个单词的形容词结尾是 -uretic，与 diuretic（多尿的）和 natriuretic（尿钠排泄的）的结尾一样。请使用适当的词根形成下列单词。

14. surgical fixation of the urethra _____
15. surgical creation of an opening in the ureter _____
16. suture of the urethra _____
17. endoscopic examination of the urethra _____
18. herniation of the ureter _____

练习 13-2 （续表）

使用词根 cyst/o 形成下列单词。

19. inflammation of the urinary bladder _____
20. radiography of the urinary bladder _____
21. an instrument for examining the interior of the bladder _____
22. incision of the bladder _____
23. discharge from the bladder _____

使用词根 vesic/o 形成下列单词。

24. above the urinary bladder _____
25. pertaining to the urethra and bladder _____

定义下列术语。

26. cystalgia ［sis'tældʒiə］ _____
27. ureterotomy ［juəri:tə'rɒtəmi］ _____
28. transurethral ［trænzjuə'ri:θrəl］ _____
29. uropoiesis ［uərə'pɔii:sis］ _____

泌尿系统的临床表现

感染

感染尿路的微生物一般是通过尿道进入，然后上升到膀胱，引起膀胱炎（cystitis）。如果不做治疗，感染可能进一步上升进入尿路。感染微生物通常是大便携带的结肠细菌，特别是大肠杆菌（Escherichia coli）。尽管泌尿路感染（urinary tract infection，UTI）也发生于男性，但更常见于女性，因为女性尿道比较短，而且其开口比男性更靠近肛门。不良的如厕习惯和尿潴留（urinary stasis）也是促进因素。在医院中，泌尿系统感染可能是由涉及泌尿系统的治疗所致，特别是导尿术（catheterization），将管道插入膀胱以抽出尿液（图 13-5）。不多见的情况中，尿路感染起始于血液，并下降进入泌尿系统。

涉及肾和肾盂的感染被称为肾盂肾炎（pyelone

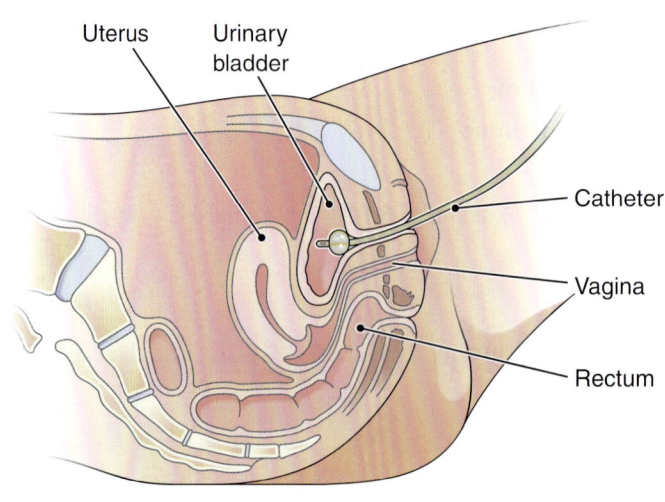

图13-5 内置导尿管。图示的导尿管被置于女性膀胱中

phritis）。如同膀胱炎一样，该病症的体征包括尿痛或排尿困难（dysuria）、尿液出现细菌和脓，分别称为细菌尿（bacteriuria）和脓尿（pyuria）。

尿道炎（urethritis）是尿道的炎症，通常与性传播感染相关，例如淋病（gonorrhea）和衣原体（chlamydial）感染（参见第 14 章）。

肾小球肾炎

尽管名称简单地意为肾小球和肾的炎症，肾小球肾炎（glomerulonephritis）是免疫反应后继发的一种特定病症。它通常是针对其他系统感染的反应，常见的是呼吸道的链球菌感染或皮肤感染，还可能伴随自身免疫疾病，如红斑狼疮。肾小球肾炎的症状有高血压、水肿和少尿（oliguria），而且尿的浓度很高。因为肾组织受损，血液和蛋白质进入肾元，导致血尿（hematuria）和蛋白尿（proteinuria）。血液细胞还可能形成肾小球的小模型，被称为管型（cast），在尿液中能够被发现。大多数肾小球肾炎患者能够完全康复，但有些病例，特别是老年患者，该疾病可能导致慢性肾衰竭（chronic renal failure，CRF）或终末期肾病（end-stage renal disease，ESRD）。在这种情况下，尿素和其他含氮化合物会在血液中积累，引起尿毒症（uremia），这些含氮化合物会影响中枢神经系统，引起易怒、食欲减退、麻痹和其他症状，还会有电解质失衡和酸中毒。

肾病综合征

肾小球肾炎是肾病综合征的起因之一，该疾病会使肾小球渗透性变强，导致蛋白质流失。肾病综合征其他可能的起因包括肾静脉血栓、糖尿病（diabetes）、全身红斑狼疮、毒素或肾小球受损的其他情况。

肾病综合征的特征是蛋白尿和低蛋白血症。低血清蛋白水平会影响毛细血管的交换，并导致水肿。由于肝要通过释放脂蛋白（lipoprotein）补偿蛋白质的流失，还可能会使血脂升高。

急性肾衰竭

受伤、休克、毒素、感染和其他肾脏疾病可能损伤肾元，导致急性肾衰竭（acute renal failure，ARF）。肾功能快速损失，造成少尿和血液中含氮废物的积累。肾不能排泄钾会引起血钾过高，伴随其他电解质失衡和酸中毒（框 13-2）。当肾小管坏死时，病症可能发展为急性肾小管坏死（acute tubular necrosis，ATN）。

肾衰竭可能导致需要肾透析（kidney dialysis）或最终进行肾移植。透析是指物质穿过半透膜的运动，在肾受损或被摘除的情况下，这种方法被用于将有害或不需要的物质从人体内排出（图 13-6）。有两种透析方式：

- 血液透析（hemodialysis），血液通过一个由透析液（dialysate）包围的膜，透析液将血液中有害物质滤出，达到清洁血液的目的。做血液透析的患者每周要到透析中心做 3 次长达 4 小时的治疗。一些患者可以使用比较简单的机器每天在家进行治疗。框 13-3 给出了透析治疗的职业信息。
- 腹膜透析（peritoneal），透析液被引入腹膜

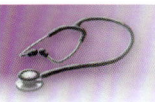

框 13-2

临床观点
钠和钾：不平衡的原因和后果

体液中的钠和钾浓度是水和电解质平衡的重要量度。体液中过量的钠称为高钠血症（hypernatremia），取自于钠的拉丁语名称 natrium。这种病症伴有脱水和严重呕吐，并可能引起高血压、水肿、抽搐和昏迷。低钠血症（hyponatremia），体液中的钠缺乏，可来自水中毒（过度水合）、心力衰竭、肾衰竭、肝硬化、pH 值不平衡或内分泌紊乱，它可以导致肌肉无力、低血压、意识混乱、休克、抽搐和昏迷。

术语高钾血症（hyperkalemia）取自拉丁语钾的名称 kalium，它是指体液中过量的钾，可能由肾衰竭、脱水和其他原因引起。其体征和症状包括恶心、呕吐、肌肉无力和严重的心律失常。低钾血症（hypokalemia）或体液低钾可能是由于服用利尿剂导致钾与水一起损失。这也可能是由于 pH 值不平衡或从肾上腺皮质分泌过多的醛固酮导致钾排泄。低钾血症会导致肌肉疲劳、麻痹、意识混乱、通气不足（hypoventilation）和心律失常。

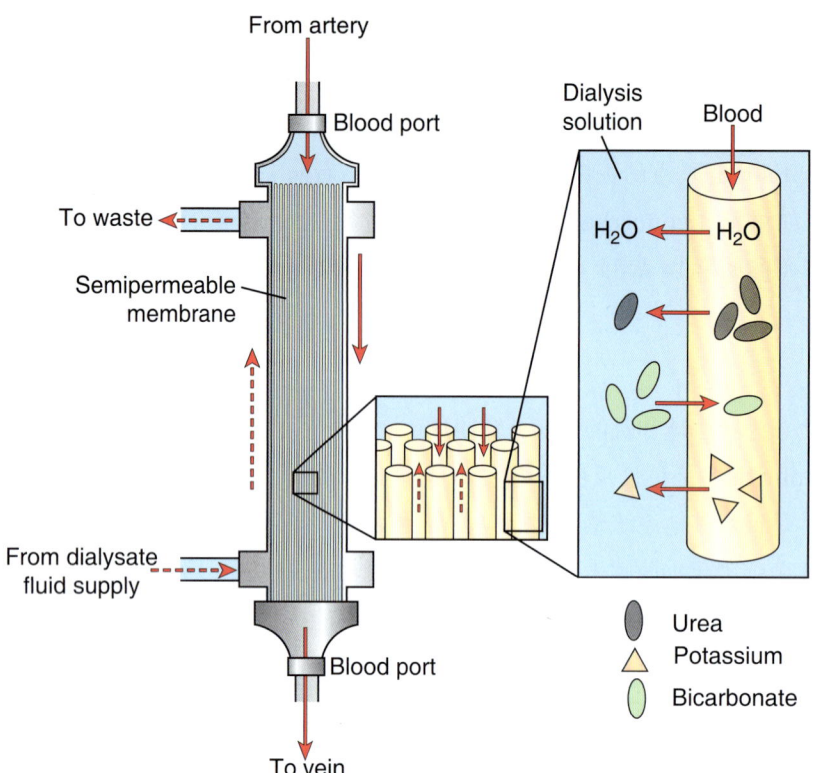

图 13-6 血液透析。半透膜将患者的血液与透析溶液分离。该膜允许除血浆蛋白和血细胞之外的所有血液成分在两个隔室之间扩散。水、电解质和其他溶解的物质从较高浓度移动到较低浓度,除去废物,并恢复血液的适当成分

腔（peritoneal cavity），透析液与废物一起被定期抽出并置换（图 13-7）。在持续不卧床腹膜透析（continuous ambulatory peritoneal dialysis，CAPD）中，液体在白天每隔一定的时间间隔进行交换；在持续循环性腹膜透析（continuous cyclic peritoneal dialysis，CCPD）中，液体在夜间交换。

尿路结石

尿路结石（urinary lithiasis）与导致血液中钙含量增加的感染、刺激、饮食或激素失衡有关。大多数尿路结石是由钙盐构成的，但也可能由其他物质组成。引起结石形成的原因包括脱水、感染、尿液 pH 值异常、尿潴留和新陈代谢紊乱。结石一般会在肾中形成，并可能移入膀胱（图 13-8）。这会导致剧痛，被

框 13-3

健康职业
血液透析技术员

血液透析技术员（hemodialysis technician），也称为肾技术员或肾脏技术员，专门向患有肾衰竭的患者提供安全和有效的肾透析治疗。在治疗开始之前，技术员准备透析溶液并确保透析机是清洁、无菌的并且处于适当的工作状态。技术员测量和记录患者的体重、体温和生命体征，将导管插入患者的手臂，并将透析机与导管连接。在透析期间，技术员监测患者的不良反应并防止任何设备故障。在治疗完成后，技术人员再次测量并记录患者的体重、温度和生命体征。为了执行这些职责，血液透析技术员需要完整的知识和临床培训。美国的大多数血液透析技术员接受来自大学或技术学校的培训，许多州要求技术员获得认证。

血液透析技术人员在各种环境中工作，例如医院、诊所和患者家中。随着人口老龄化，肾脏疾病的发病率预计上升，血液透析的需求量也会上升。有关这个职业的更多信息，请联系全国肾脏病学技术协会（National Association of Nephrology Technicians）www.dialysistech.net。

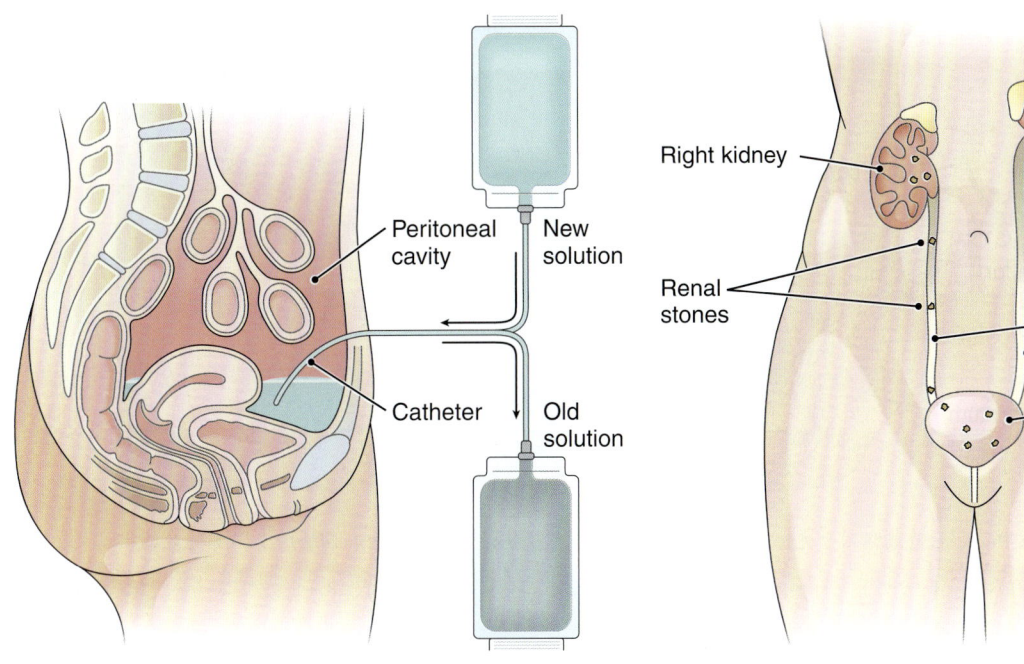

图 13-7　腹膜透析。腹膜内衬腹膜腔，是一种富含小血管的半透膜。废物从血管网络扩散到腹膜腔中的透析液中

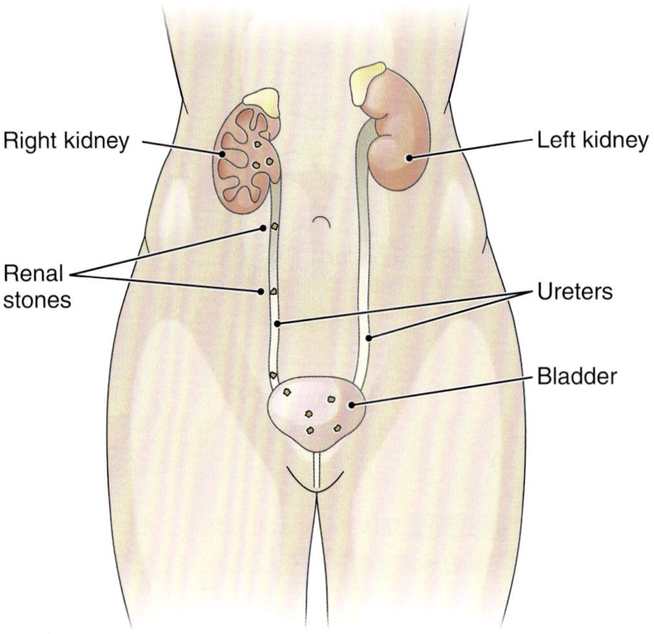

图 13-8　尿道中的结石形成。图中示出了各种可能的结石形成位置

称为肾绞痛（renal colic），所导致的阻塞会引发感染，并引起肾盂积水（hydronephrosis）。

由于 X 线不能透过，结石通常可以用简单的腹部 X 线透视检查出来。结石自己可能被溶解并排出体外，如果不能，则需要进行取石术（lithotomy）或通过内窥镜取出。在体外震波碎石术（extracorporeal shock-wave lithotripsy）中，外部的冲击波被用来粉碎结石（图 13-9）。

癌症

膀胱癌与职业性暴露于化学品、寄生虫感染和吸烟相关。一个关键症状是突然、无痛的血尿（hematuria）。通常，通过膀胱镜观察膀胱内壁能够看到肿瘤（图 13-10）。膀胱镜也可以用于活组织采样分析。

如果治疗不能有效地永久去除肿瘤，可能需要做膀胱切除术（cystectomy）。在这种情况下，输尿

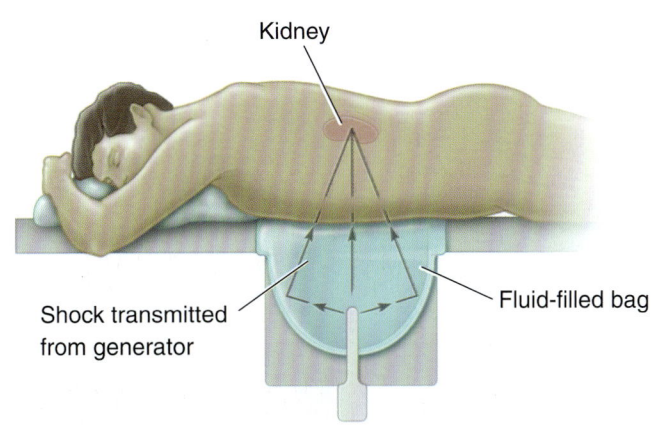

图 13-9　碎石术。冲击波用于打碎肾结石，并允许他们通过尿道排出。该过程称为体外冲击波碎石术

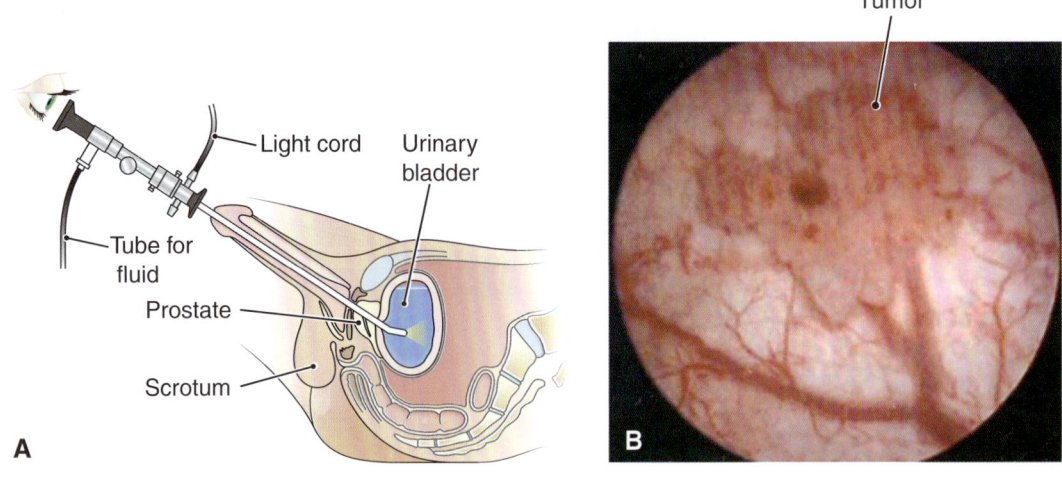

图 13-10 膀胱中。A.无菌流体用于充满膀胱。膀胱镜用于检查膀胱、取活检标本和切除肿瘤；B.膀胱癌，通过膀胱镜观察

管必须在其他地方排放，例如利用回肠通道术（ileal conduit）通过回肠（图 13-11）或肠道的其他部分直接排出身体表面。

癌症也可能涉及肾和肾盂。诊断膀胱癌和其他泌尿系统疾病的方法还有超声波、CT 扫描和 X 线造影研究，例如静脉尿路造影术（intravenous urography，IVU）（图 13-12），也被称为静脉肾盂造影术（intravenous pyelography，IVP）和逆行性肾盂造影术（retrograde pyelography）。

尿液分析

尿液分析（urinalysis，UA）是一种简单且广泛使用的泌尿道疾病诊断方法。当人体其他系统的副产品被排入尿液时，尿液分析也能显示这些系统的失调。在常规尿液分析中，要检查尿液的颜色和浑浊度（存在细菌的迹象），要记录尿比重（specific gravity，SG）和 pH 值，还要测试化学成分，例如葡萄糖、酮体（ketones）和血红蛋白等。尿液还要使用显微镜检查细胞、结晶和管型（cast）。在更细致的测试中，药物、酶、激素和其他代谢物都要做分析，还可能要做细菌培养。

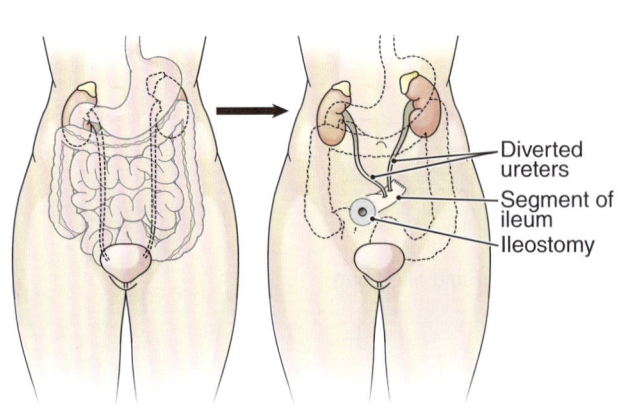

图 13-11 回肠膀胱术。在该手术中，当膀胱被切除或不起作用时，输尿管通过回肠排出身体表面

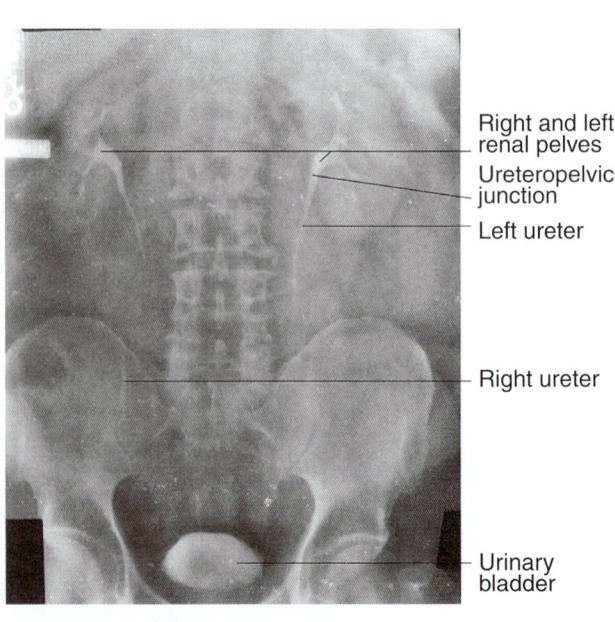

图 13-12 静脉尿路造影。图像显示了肾盂、输尿管和膀胱

Terminology 关键术语

病症

bacteriuria [bæk'tiəriəriə]	细菌尿，尿液中存在细菌
cast [kɑ:st]	管型，在尿液中出现的肾小管固体模型
cystitis [si'staitis]	膀胱炎，膀胱的炎症，一般是感染所致
dysuria [dis'juəriə]	排尿困难，排尿疼痛或困难
glomerulonephritis [gləʊmerjʊləʊnef'raitis]	肾小球肾炎，肾的炎症，主要涉及肾小球。急性肾小球肾炎一般发生于身体其他部位感染之后；慢性肾小球肾炎起因不一，通常会导致肾衰竭
hematuria [ˌhi:mə'tju:riə]	血尿，尿液中出现血液
hydronephrosis [ˌhaidrəni'frəʊsis]	肾盂积水，阻塞引起的肾盂尿液积累；会引起膨胀和肾萎缩
hypokalemia [haipəʊkə'li:mjə]	低钾血症，血液中缺钾
hyponatremia [haipɒnə'tremiə]	低钠血症，血液中缺钠
hypoproteinemia [haipɒprəʊti:'ni:miə]	低蛋白血症，血液中蛋白含量下降；可能是肾受损所致的蛋白质流失引起的
hyperkalemia [haipəkə'li:miə]	高钾血症，血液中钾含量过高
hypernatremia [haipənə'tri:miə]	高钠血症，血液中钠含量过高
nephrotic syndrome [ni'frəʊtik]	肾病综合征，肾小球受损导致蛋白质在尿液中流失所致的病症，包括低血浆蛋白（hypoproteinemia）、水肿、血脂升高，也被称为肾病（nephrosis）
oliguria [ɒli'gjʊəriə]	少尿，尿液排放量很少
proteinuria [prəʊti:n'jʊəriə]	蛋白尿，尿液中出现蛋白质，主要是白蛋白
pyelonephritis [paiələʊni'fraitis]	肾盂肾炎，肾盂和肾的炎症，一般是由感染引起的
pyuria [pai'jʊəriə]	脓尿，尿液中出现脓
renal colic ['ri:nəl 'kɔlik]	肾绞痛，与通道结石相关的肾区放射性疼痛
uremia [jʊ'ri:miə] 尿毒症	用于肾功能不全所致的血液中出现尿素和其他含氮物质等毒素
urethritis [ˌjʊərə'θraitis]	尿道炎，尿道的炎症，一般是由感染引起的
urinary stasis [ˈjʊərəˌneri: ˈsteisis]	尿潴留，尿液流动停滞；也称为尿停滞（urinary stagnation）

诊断与治疗

catheterization [kæθirai'zeiʃən]	导尿术，将导管插入尿道或膀胱，以抽出尿液（图13-5）
cystoscope ['sistəskəʊp]	膀胱镜，检查膀胱内部的仪器。也被用于取出外来异物、手术和其他治疗
dialysis [ˌdai'æləsis]	透析，通过半透膜进行物质分离。当肾受损或缺失时，透析被用来排除体内的有害物质。有两种透析方式，血液透析（hemodialysis）和腹膜透析（peritoneal dialysis）

Terminology 关键术语（续表）

术语	释义
hemodialysis [ˌhi:mədai'ælisis]	血液透析，通过半透膜去除血液中的有害物质（图 13-6）
intravenous pyelography (IVP) [paiə'lɒgrəfi]	静脉肾盂造影，参见：静脉尿路造影（图 13-12）
intravenous urography (IVU) [jʊə'rɒgrəfi]	静脉尿路造影，在静脉使用能够通过尿液排泄的造影剂后的 X 线造影；也被称为排泄性尿路造影（excretory urography）或静脉肾盂造影，不过后者不是很准确，因为这一方法不仅显示肾盂
lithotripsy ['laiθəʊtripsi]	碎石，使用外部冲击波粉碎结石（图 13-9）
peritoneal dialysis [peritə'ni:əl]	腹膜透析，通过在腹膜腔引入透析液，然后排出液体来去除体内的有害物质（图 13-7）
retrograde pyelography ['retrəgreid]	逆行肾盂造影，通过尿道将造影剂注入肾的肾盂造影
specific gravity (SG)	比重，物质重量与同体积水重量之比。正常尿液的比重为 1.015~1.025，患病时该数值会升高或下降
urinalysis (UA) [ˌjʊəri'nælisis]	尿液分析，尿液的实验室研究，包括物理性质、化学性质和显微镜图像
手术	
cystectomy [sis'tektəmi]	膀胱切除术，手术切除全部或部分膀胱
ileal conduit ['iliəl 'kɒndjuit]	回肠通道术，通过连接尿道和回肠的一个隔离分段使尿路改道。分段的一端是封闭的，另一端通过腹壁的开口排泄。当膀胱被切除或不起作用时，需要执行这种手术（图 13-11），也被称为回肠膀胱
lithotomy [li'θɒtəmi]	取石术，切开一个器官以去除结石
renal transplantation	肾移植，将捐献者的肾手术移植给患者

Terminology 补充术语

正常结构与功能

术语	释义
aldosterone [æl'dɒstərəʊn]	醛固酮，一种肾上腺分泌的激素，能够调节肾的电解质排泄
clearance ['kliərəns]	肾血浆清除率，肾每分钟能够清洁的血浆量，也常用 renal pasma clearance
creatinine [kri:'ætini:n]	肌酸酐，一种含氮的肌肉代谢副产品。血液肌酸酐含量升高时肾衰竭的迹象
detrusor muscle [di'tru:sə]	逼尿肌，膀胱壁上的肌肉
glomerular filtration rate (GFR)	肾小球滤过率，两个肾每分钟形成的滤液量
maximal transport capacity (Tm)	最大输送能力，给定物质通过肾小管的最大速率，也常用 tubular maximum
renal corpuscle ['kɔ:pʌsl]	肾小体，将肾小球囊和肾小球视为一个单元，是肾的过滤装置

Terminology 补充术语（续表）

症状与病症

anuresis [ˈənrisis]	无尿，缺少尿液
anuria [ənˈjʊəriə]	无尿，缺少尿液的形成
azotemia [æzəˈtiːmiə]	氮质血症，血液中含氮废物，特别是尿素含量升高
cystocele [ˈsistəsiːl]	膀胱膨出，膀胱疝入阴道（图 15-12）；也常用 vesicocele
dehydration [ˌdiːhaiˈdreiʃn]	脱水，体液过度流失
diabetes insipidus [ˌdaiəˈbiːtiːz inˈsipidəs]	尿崩症，抗利尿激素生产不足引起的病症，会导致稀释尿液过量排泄和极度口渴
enuresis [ˌenjʊəˈriːsis]	遗尿，不自主排尿，通常在夜间；又称为尿床（bed-wetting）
epispadias [epiˈspeidiəs]	尿道上裂，尿道在阴茎背表面上的一个凹槽或裂口开口的一种先天性疾病；也拼写为 anaspadias
glycosuria [ˌglaikəʊˈsjʊəriə]	糖尿，尿液中出现葡萄糖，如糖尿病病例
horseshoe kidney	马蹄肾，两个肾的下极点先天性结合，形成一个马蹄形器官（图 13-13）
hydroureter [haidrəjʊəˈriːtə]	输尿管积水，因阻塞产生的输尿管尿充盈
hypospadias [haipəˈspeidiəs]	尿道下裂，尿道在阴茎下表面或阴道内开口的先天性疾病（图 13-14）
hypovolemia [haipəʊvəˈliːmiə]	血容量不足，血容量降低
neurogenic bladder [njʊərəʊˈdʒenik ˈblædə]	神经性膀胱功能障碍，由中枢神经系统损伤所致的任何膀胱功能障碍
nocturia [nɒkˈtjʊəriə]	夜尿症，夜间过量排尿（词根：noct/o 意为"夜间"）
polycystic kidney disease [pɒliˈsistik]	多囊肾，肾脏扩张并含有许多囊的遗传疾病（图 13-15）
polydipsia [ˌpɒliˈdipsiə]	烦渴，极度口渴
polyuria [ˌpɒliˈjəriə]	多尿症，排泄大量尿液，如在糖尿病病例中
retention of urine [riˈtenʃn]	尿潴留，因为无法排尿所致的尿液在膀胱中积累
staghorn calculus [ˈstæghɔːn ˈkælkjələs]	鹿角状结石，充满肾盂和肾盏的肾结石，形状像"鹿角"（图 13-16）
ureterocele [jʊəriːtərəʊˈseliː]	输尿管囊肿，输尿管进入膀胱开口附近囊样扩张，通常是先天性输尿管开口狭窄所致（图 13-17）
urinary frequency	尿频，不增加平均输出量的排尿需要
urinary incontinence [inˈkɔntinəns]	尿失禁，不能留住尿液，可能起源于神经系统疾病、脊髓外伤、骨盆肌肉无力、尿潴留或膀胱功能受损。在急迫性尿失禁（urgency incontinence）中，一个迫切的要求会引起突然排尿，患者根本来不及进入卫生间。在压力性尿失禁（stress incontinence）中，在例如咳嗽、打喷嚏或锻炼这样的用力活动期间，尿液会流出来

Terminology 补充术语（续表）

urinary urgency [ˈɜːdʒənsi]	尿急，突然需要排尿
water intoxication [ɪnˌtɒksɪˈkeɪʃən]	水中毒，过量摄入或保留水，钠浓度降低。可能是过量饮水、过量的抗利尿激素或用纯水替代大量的体液所致。会引起细胞环境失衡，造成水肿和其他失调
Wilms tumor	肾母细胞瘤，恶性肾肿瘤，一般发生于5岁以下儿童
诊断	
anion gap [ˈænaɪən gæp]	阴离子间隙，电解质失衡的一种度量
blood urea nitrogen(BUN)	血尿素氮，氮在血液中以尿素的形式存在，血尿素氮含量升高显示血液中含氮废物增加和肾衰竭
clean-catch specimen	清洁采样，在彻底清洁尿道开口后采集的中段尿样，以将污染概率降到最小
cystometrography [sɪstəˈmetrəʊgrəfi]	膀胱内压描记法，一种研究膀胱功能的方法，将膀胱充满液体或空气，测量在不同充满程度下膀胱肌肉所承受的压力
protein electrophoresis (PEP) [iˌlektrəʊfəˈriːsɪs]	蛋白电泳，尿蛋白实验室研究，用于诊断多发性骨髓炎（multiple myeloma）、全身性红斑狼疮和淋巴肿瘤
urinometer [jʊəriˈnɒmɪtə]	尿比重计，测量尿液比重的仪器
治疗	
indwelling Foley catheter [ˈɪnˈdwelɪŋ]	留置气囊导尿管，一端带有气囊的导尿管，气囊能够防止导管离开膀胱（图13-5）
lithotrite [ˈlɪθətraɪt]	碎石器，粉碎膀胱结石的仪器

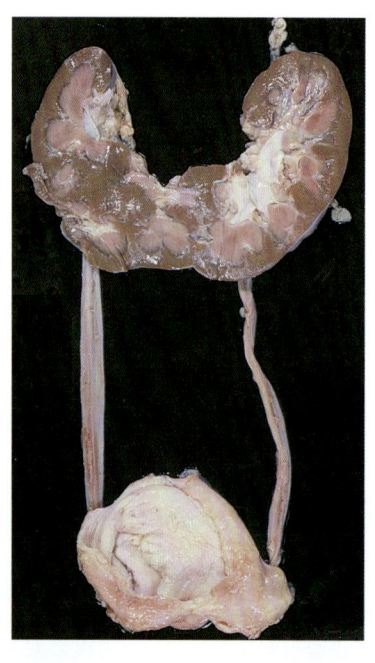

图13-13 马蹄肾。照片显示肾脏在两端融合

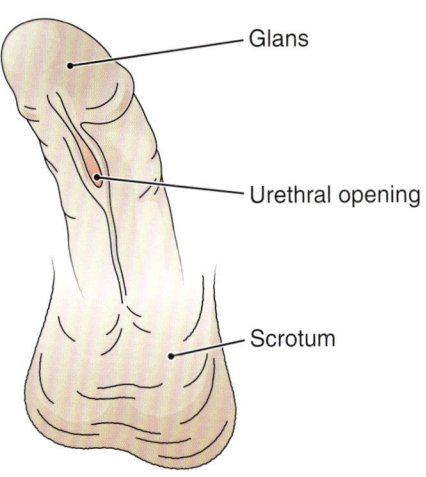

图 13-14 **尿道下裂**。图中显示尿道在阴茎侧表面上的开口

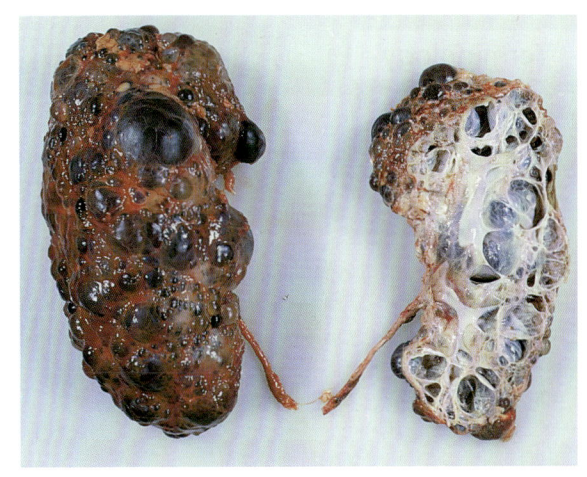

图 13-15 **成人多囊性疾病**。肾脏扩大，活组织几乎完全被不同大小的囊肿替代。（左）表面视图；（右）纵截面

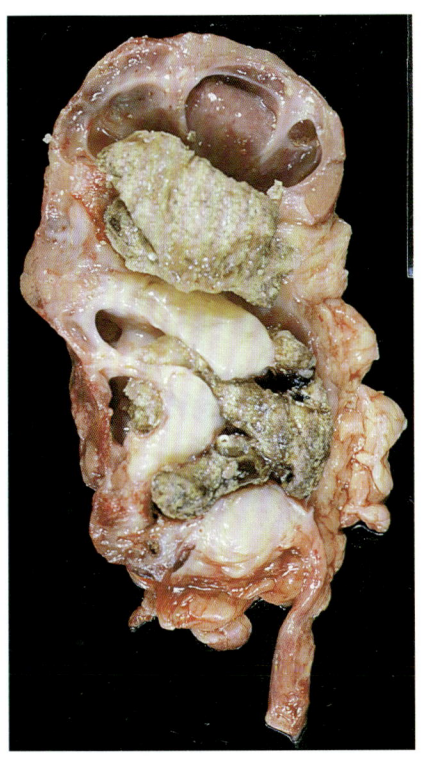

图 13-16 **鹿角结石**。肾显现出肾积水和插入扩张的肾盏的结石

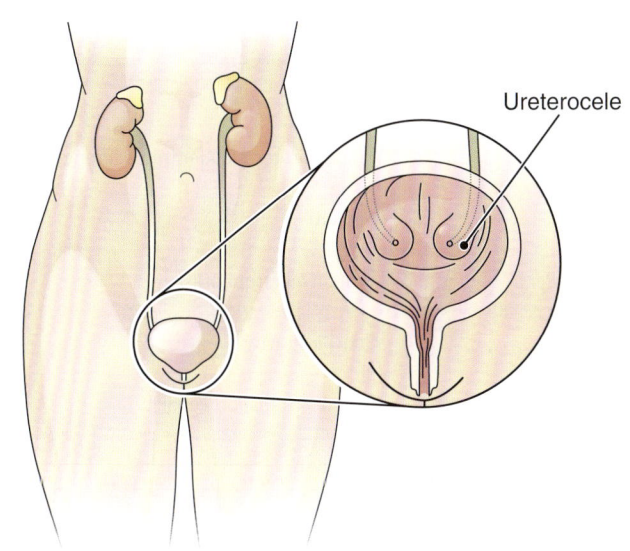

图 13-17 **输尿管疝**。输尿管突出到膀胱，所产生的阻塞导致尿液回流到输尿管（输尿管积水）和肾盂（肾积水）

Terminology	缩略语	
ACE	Angiotensin-converting enzyme	血管紧张素转化酶
ADH	Antidiuretic hormone	抗利尿激素
ARF	Acute renal failure	急性肾衰竭
ATN	Acute tubular necrosis	急性肾小管坏死

Terminology 关键术语（续表）

BUN	Blood urea nitrogen	血尿素氮
CAPD	Continuous ambulatory peritoneal dialysis	持续不卧床腹膜透析
CCPD	Continuous cyclic peritoneal dialysis	持续循环性腹膜透折
CMG	Cystometrography; cystometrogram	膀胱内压描记法；膀胱内压图
CRF	Chronic renal failure	慢性肾衰竭
EPO	Erythropoietin	红细胞生成素
ESRD	End-stage renal disease	终末期肾病
ESWL	Extracorporeal shock wave lithotripsy	体外冲击波碎石术
GFR	Glomerular filtration rate	肾小球滤过率
GU	Genitourinary	泌尿生殖器官的
IVP	Intravenous pyelography	静脉肾盂造影
IVU	Intravenous urography	静脉尿路造影
K	Potassium	钾
KUB	Kidney-ureter-bladder (radiography)	肾尿道膀胱（X线造影）
Na	Sodium	钠
PEP	Protein electrophoresis	蛋白电泳
SG	Specific gravity	比重
Tm	Maximal transport capacity	最大输送能力
UA	Urinalysis	尿液分析
UTI	Urinary tract infection	泌尿系统感染

Case Study Revisited 案例研究再访

E. O.'s Follow-Up Study

E. O. had excellent results from the implanted autograft of muscle cells. There was no retention of urine, and the incontinence and urgency had all but disappeared. After a year, E. O. continued to experience about a 95 percent success rate from her stress incontinence and had a much improved quality of life score.

E. O. 的随访研究

E. O. 的自体肌肉细胞移植的效果极好。没有尿潴留，并且尿失禁和尿急症状全部消失。1年后，E. O. 95%的压力性尿失禁得到了成功的控制，并且生活质量大大提高。

复习

标记练习

泌尿系统

在相应的行上写入每个编号部分的名称。

Adrenal gland　　　　Renal artery
Aorta　　　　　　　　Renal vein
Diaphragm　　　　　　Ureter
Inferior vena cava　　Urethra
Kidney　　　　　　　　Urinary bladder

1. _____
2. _____
3. _____
4. _____
5. _____
6. _____
7. _____
8. _____
9. _____
10. _____

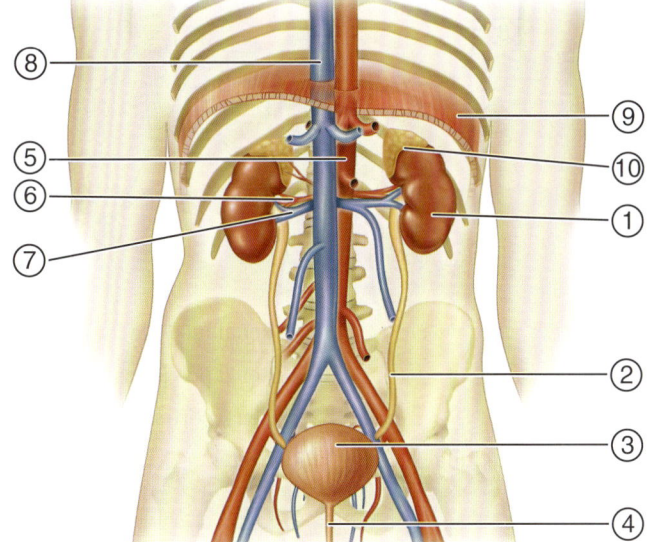

肾

在相应的行上写入每个编号部分的名称。

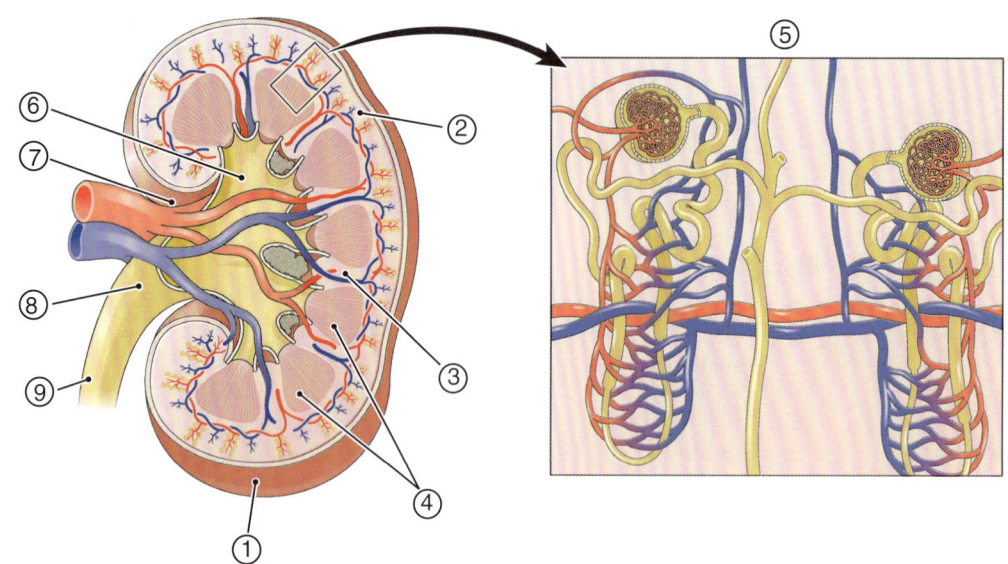

Calyx
Hilum
Nephrons
Pyramids of medulla
Renal capsule

Renal medulla
Renal pelvis
Renal cortex
Ureter

1. _____
2. _____
3. _____
4. _____
5. _____
6. _____
7. _____
8. _____
9. _____

膀胱

在相应的行上写入每个编号部分的名称。

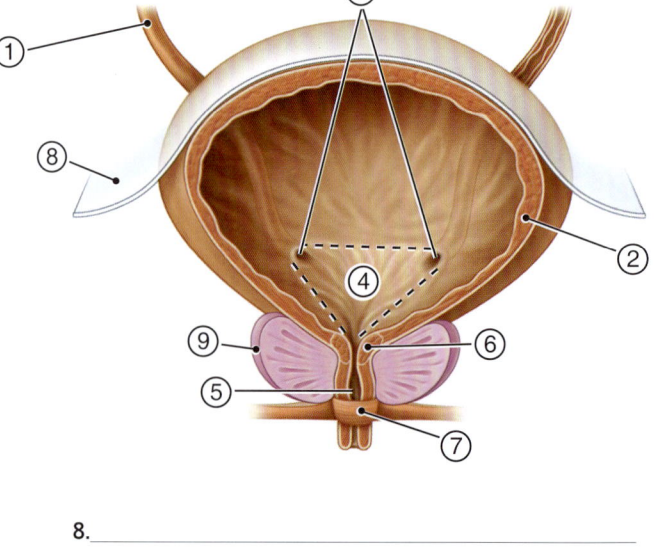

External urethral sphincter
Internal urethral sphincter
Openings of ureters
Peritoneum
Prostate

Smooth muscle
Trigone
Ureter
Urethra

1. _____
2. _____
3. _____
4. _____
5. _____
6. _____
7. _____
8. _____
9. _____

匹配

匹配以下术语，在每个数字左侧写出适当的字母。

____ 1. hematuria   a. blood in the urine

____ 2. oliguria   b. proteinuria

____ 3. chromaturia   c. elimination of small amounts of urine

____ 4. albuminuria   d. abnormal color of urine

____ 5. pyuria   e. pus in the urine

____ 6. renal cortex   a. absence of a bladder

____ 7. nephron   b. stagnation, as of urine

____ 8. stasis   c. deficiency of urine

____ 9. acystia   d. kidney's outer portion

____ 10. uropenia   e. microscopic functional unit of the kidney

补充术语

____ 11. aldosterone   a. amount of filtrate formed per minute by the kidney

____ 12. diabetes insipidus   b. condition caused by lack of ADH

____ 13. incontinence   c. nitrogenous metabolic waste

____ 14. glomerular filtration rate   d. hormone that regulates electrolytes

____ 15. creatinine   e. inability to retain urine

____ 16. polydipsia   a. excessive thirst

____ 17. enuresis   b. bed-wetting

____ 18. azoturia   c. presence of excess nitrogenous waste in the urine

____ 19. anuresis   d. congenital misplacement of the ureteral opening

____ 20. hypospadias   e. lack of urination

填空

21. Collection of urine in the renal pelvis is a result of obstruction _____.

22. The cluster of capillaries within the glomerular capsule is the _____.

23. An enzyme released by the kidneys that acts to increase blood pressure is _____.

24. Micturition is the scientific term for _____.

25. Laboratory study of the urine is a(n) _____.

26. The main nitrogenous waste product in urine is _____.

参照本章开头的 E.O. 案例研究。

27. E.O.'s inability to retain urine is termed urinary _____.

28. A midstream urine sample collected after thorough cleansing of the urethral opening is called a(n) _____.

29. Endoscopic examination of the urinary bladder is termed _____.

拼写检查

在术语右侧的线上写出正确的拼写。

30. catheter _____
31. uretha _____
32. dysurea _____
33. calysx _____
34. cystoceal _____
35. hypercalemia _____
36. intravesicle _____

真假判断

检查以下语句。如果语句为真，则在第一个空白处写入 T。如果语句为假，则在第一个空格中写入 F，并通过在第二个空格中替换带下划线的单词来更正语句。

	True or False	Correct Answer
37. A reniform structure is shaped like the <u>bladder</u>.	_____	_____
38. Pyelitis is inflammation of the <u>renal pelvis</u>.	_____	_____
39. A nephrotropic substance acts on the <u>kidney</u>.	_____	_____
40. The inner portion of the kidney is the <u>cortex</u>.	_____	_____
41. The tube that carries urine out of the body is the <u>ureter</u>.	_____	_____
42. EPO stimulates the production of <u>red blood cells</u>.	_____	_____
43. A lithotomy is an incision to remove a <u>calculus</u>.	_____	_____
44. Natriuresis refers to the excretion of <u>potassium</u> in the urine.	_____	_____

定义

定义下列单词。

45. urethrostenosis ［jʊəri:θrəsti'nəʊsis］ _____
46. polyuria ［ˈpɒliˈjəriə］ _____
47. nephrotoxic ［nefrəˈtɒksik］ _____
48. juxtaglomerular ［dʒʌkstəgloˈmerʊlə］ _____
49. calicectomy ［kæliˈkəʊtəmi］ _____
50. pararenal ［pɑ:rəˈri:nəl］ _____

写出下列定义的单词。

51. Physician who specializes in the kidney (nephr/o) _____
52. Dilatation of the renal pelvis and calices _____
53. Softening of a kidney (nephr/o) _____
54. Incision of the bladder (cyst/o) _____
55. Any disease of the kidney (nephr/o) _____
56. Radiograph of the bladder (cyst/o) and urethra _____
57. Plastic repair of a ureter and renal pelvis _____
58. Inflammation of the renal pelvis and the kidney _____

59. Surgical creation of an opening between a ureter and the sigmoid colon_____

排除

在下列每组中，给与其余内容不相配的单词加下划线，并解释你的选择理由。

60. capsule — cast — pyramid — nephron — cortex
_____

61. nephron loop — distal convoluted tubule — glomerular capsule — calyx — proximal convoluted tubule
_____

62. ileal conduit — specific gravity — dialysis — cystoscopy — lithotripsy
_____

反义词

写出下列单词的反义词。

63. dehydration _____

64. hypovolemia _____

65. diuretic _____

66. hyponatremia _____

67. uresis _____

形容词

写出下列单词的形容词形式。

68. ureter _____

69. nephrology _____

70. uremia _____

71. diuresis _____

72. nephrosis _____

73. calyx _____

74. urethra _____

复数

写出下列单词的复数形式。

75. pelvis _____

76. calyx _____

77. glomerulus _____

跟随流程

描述尿液流动的路径，通过在每个题号前的下划线填上字母 A 到 G，使下列每个步骤按正确次序排列。

____ **78.** Fluid or glomerular filtrate enters the nephron

____ **79.** Urine flows into the collecting ducts to be eliminated

____ 80. Urine flows from the ureters to the bladder

____ 81. Tubular reabsorption, or return process of nutrients, water, and electrolytes, occurs

____ 82. Blood flows through the glomerulus

____ 83. Urine is drained from the renal pelvis to the ureters

____ 84. Urine flows from the bladder to the urethra

单词构建

使用给出的单词组成部分写出下列定义的单词。

> graph-　　ren/o　　-al　　intra-　　vesic/o　　-y　　ur/o　　inter-　　lith　　log　　supra-

85. radiographic study of the urinary tract ____

86. pertaining to the kidney ____

87. within the kidney ____

88. radiographic study of the kidney ____

89. within the bladder ____

90. above the kidney ____

91. study of the urinary tract ____

92. between the kidneys ____

93. pertaining to the bladder ____

94. a urinary tract stone ____

缩略语

写出下列缩略语的含义。

95. SG ____

96. ADH ____

97. EPO ____

98. IVP ____

99. Na ____

100. GFR ____

101. UA ____

单词分析

定义下列单词，并给出每个单词组成部分的含义。如果需要，可以使用词典。

102. hemodialysis ［ˌhi:mədai'ælisis］ ____

　　a. hem/o ____

　　b. dia ____

　　c. lysis ____

103. cystometrography ［sistə'metrəugrəfi］ ____

　　a. cyst/o ____

　　b. metr/o ____

　　c. -graphy ____

104. ureteroneocystostomy ［jʊəriːtəwʌniːəʊsisˈtəʊstəmi］ _____

    a. ureter/o _____

    b. neo _____

    c. cyst/o _____

    d. –stomy _____

Additional Case Studies
补充案例研究

Case Study 13-1: Renal Calculi
案例研究 13-1：肾结石

A. A., a 48-year-old woman, was admitted to the inpatient unit from the ER with severe right flank pain unresponsive to analgesics. Her pain did not decrease with administration of 100 mg of IV meperidine. She had a three-month history of chronic UTI. Six months ago, she had been prescribed calcium supplements for low bone density. Her gynecologist warned her that calcium could be a problem for people who are "stone formers." A. A. was unaware that she might be at risk. An IV urogram showed a right staghorn calculus. The diagnosis was further confirmed by a renal ultrasound. A renal flow scan showed normal perfusion and no obstruction. Kidney function was 37 percent on the right and 63 percent on the left. The pain became intermittent, and A.A. had no hematuria, dysuria, frequency, urgency, or nocturia. Urinalysis revealed no albumin, glucose, bacteria, or blood; there was evidence of cells, crystals, and casts.

A. A. was transferred to surgery for a cystoscopic ureteral laser lithotripsy, insertion of a right retrograde ureteral catheter, and right percutaneous nephrolithotomy. A ureteral calculus was fragmented with a pulsed-dye laser. Most of the staghorn was removed from the renal pelvis with no remaining stone in the renal calices. She was discharged two days later and ordered to strain her urine for the next week for evidence of stones.

A. A. 是一名 48 岁的女性，从急诊室进入院，严重的右侧腹痛对镇痛药无反应，给予 100mg 哌替啶，疼痛没有减轻。她有 3 个月的慢性尿路感染史。6 个月前，因为低骨密度，医生给她开了钙补充剂。她的妇科医生警告她，钙对"结石患者"可能造成问题。A. A. 不知道她可能会面临风险。静脉尿路造影（IV urogram）显示有右侧鹿角状结石。肾脏超声检查进一步证实了诊断。肾血流扫描显示正常灌注且无阻塞。右侧肾功能是 37%，左侧是 63%。疼痛变得间歇性，并且 A.A. 没有血尿、排尿困难、尿频、尿急或夜尿。尿分析显示没有白蛋白、葡萄糖、细菌或血液；有细胞、晶体和管型的证据。

A. A. 被转到外科做膀胱镜输尿管激光碎石术（cystoscopic ureteral laser lithotripsy），插入右侧倒置输尿管导管，并做右侧经皮肾穿刺术。输尿管结石被脉冲染料激光（pulsed-dye laser）破碎，大多数鹿角状结石被从肾盂取出，肾中没有残余的结石。她 2 天后出院，并被嘱咐下周过滤尿液以证明结石的存在。

Case Study 13-2: End-Stage Renal Disease
案例研究 13-2：晚期肾病

M. C., a 20 YO part-time college student, has had chronic glomerulonephritis since age 7. He has been treated at home with CAPD for the past 16 months as he awaits kidney transplantation. His doctor advised him to go immediately to the ER when he reported chest pain, shortness of breath, and oliguria. On admission, M. C. was placed on oxygen and given a panel of blood tests and an ECG to rule out an acute cardiac episode. His hemoglobin was 8.2, and his hematocrit was 26 percent. He had bilateral lung rales. ABGs were: pH, 7.0; $Paco_2$, 28; Pao_2, 50; HCO_3, 21. His BUN, serum creatinine, and BUN/creatinine ratio were abnormally high. His ECG and liver enzyme studies were normal. His admission diagnosis was ESRD, fluid overload, and metabolic acidosis. He was typed and crossed for blood; tested for HIV, hepatitis B antigen, and sexually transmitted disease; and sent to hemodialysis. A bed was reserved for him on the transplant unit.

M. C. 是一名 20 岁的兼职大学生，自 7 岁起就患有慢性肾小球肾炎。在他等待肾移植的过去 16 个月里，他在家接受连续性可动式腹膜透析治疗。他的医生在他报告胸痛、呼吸短促和少尿时建议立即去急诊室。入院时，M. C. 被输氧，并做了一组血液测试和心电图以排除急性心脏病发作。他的血红蛋白是 8.2，血细胞比容是 26%。他有双侧肺啰音。动脉血气（ABG）测试结果为：pH7.0；$PaCO_2$28；$PaO_2$50；$HCO_3$21。他的血尿素氮（blood urea nitrogen, BUN）、血清肌酐和 BUN/肌酐比异常高，心电图和肝酶分析正常。他的入院诊断是晚期肾病（end-stage renal disease, ESRD）、体液超负荷和代谢性酸中毒。他被测定血型（typed），还做了交叉配血试验，测试 HIV、乙型肝炎抗原和性传播疾病；并被送去做血液透析。在移植部门为他安排了一张病床。

案例研究问题

多项选择，选择正确的答案，在每个题号的左侧写出你选择的字母。

____ 1. The term perfusion means

    a. metabolism

    b. size

    c. passage of fluid

    d. surrounding tissue

____ 2. The term percutaneous means

    a. under the skin

    b. on the surface

    c. with a catheter

    d. through the skin

____ 3. M.C.'s chronic glomerulonephritis means that he has had

    a. long-term kidney stones

    b. an acute bout of kidney infection

    c. short-term bladder inflammation

    d. a long-term kidney infection

____ 4. Renal dialysis can be performed by shunting venous blood through a dialysis machine and returning the blood to the patient's arterial system. This procedure is called

    a. hemodialysis

    b. arteriovenous transplant

    c. CAPD

    d. glomerular filtration rate

写出案例研究中下列含义的术语。

5. Intravenous injection of contrast dye and radiographic study of the urinary tract _____

6. Presence of blood in the urine _____

7. Referring to endoscopy of the urinary bladder _____

8. Surgical incision for removal of a kidney stone _____

9. Production of a reduced amount of urine _____

10. Getting up to go to the bathroom at night _____

11. Crushing a stone _____

12. Kidney replacement _____

缩略语，定义下列缩略语。

13. UTI _____

14. CAPD _____

15. BUN _____

16. ESRD _____

17. HIV _____

CHAPTER 14

男性生殖系统

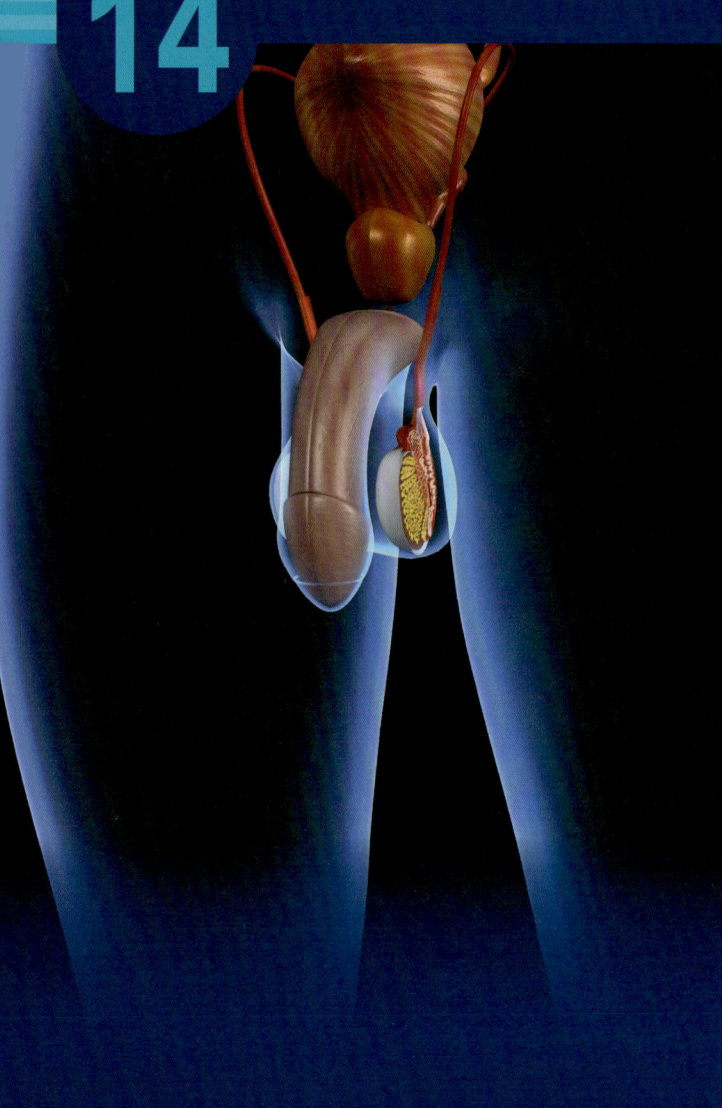

预测试

多项选择，选择正确的答案，并在每个题号左侧写出你选择的字母。

____1. The male germ cell, or gamete, is the
   a. ovum
   b. testis
   c. spermatozoon
   d. semen

____2. Gametes develop in a gonad, which in males is called the
   a. vas deferens
   b. seminal vesicle
   c. penis
   d. testis

____3. The main male sex hormone is
   a. testosterone
   b. renin
   c. estrogen
   d. amylase

____4. The secretion that transports gametes in males is
   a. bile
   b. semen
   c. urine
   d. pepsin

____5. The gland below the bladder in males is the
   a. scrotum
   b. prostate
   c. adrenal
   d. parotid

____6. Orchitis is inflammation of the
   a. bladder
   b. kidney
   c. penis
   d. testis

学习目标

学完本章后，应该能够：

1 ▶ 描述男性生殖系统的器官，并指出各个器官的功能。
2 ▶ 了解精子从其在睾丸中发育直至被释放的过程。
3 ▶ 描述精液的成分及功能。
4 ▶ 识别并使用与男性生殖系统相关的词根。
5 ▶ 描述男性生殖系统的6种主要的疾病。
6 ▶ 解释用于男性生殖系统的缩略语。
7 ▶ 分析几个案例研究中关于男性生殖系统的医学术语。

Case Study: C. S.'s Benign Prostatic Hyperplasia and TURP
案例研究：C. S. 的良性前列腺增生和经尿道前列腺电切术（TURP）

Chief Complaint

C. S., a 60-year-old teacher, was having a decreased force of his urine stream and ejaculation, hesitancy, and sensation of incomplete bladder emptying. He had tried using prostate-health herbal supplements without any real benefit for two years. He decided to make an appointment with a urologist.

Examination

The urologist took a history and examined the patient. C. S. reported no dysuria, hematuria, or flank pain. He had no history of UTI, epididymitis, prostatitis, renal disease, or renal calculi. His medical history was otherwise not significant to his urologic complaint.

Rectal examination revealed a 50-g prostate with slight firmness in the right prostatic lobe. The physician ordered a bladder ultrasound, which was performed later that week. The results indicated no intravesical lesions or prostate protrusion into the bladder base.

A transabdominal ultrasound was ordered and showed a residual urine volume of 120 mL. A urinalysis revealed normal values except for the following: WBC = 8; RBC = 10; bacteria = trace.

C. S. was diagnosed with benign prostatic hyperplasia (BPH) with bladder neck obstruction and was scheduled for a transurethral resection of the prostate (TURP). His urologist explained the procedure and what to expect pre- and postoperatively. The office staff notified the hospital to schedule the surgery. The next day, the hospital admissions department called C.S., went through normal admissions procedures, and scheduled a surgery date.

Clinical Course

C. S. was NPO the night before the surgery. He was taken to the operating room and was given a spinal anesthetic for the procedure. It had already been explained to him that the surgery would take about an hour and that he would be awake during the procedure but would not feel any pain. A resectoscope was used to trim the enlarged prostatic tissue. At the end of the surgery, a Foley catheter was inserted into the bladder and left in place to drain the urine and permit irrigation of the bladder to remove any clots. C. S. tolerated the procedure well and was transferred to the recovery room and later to his hospital room. He was encouraged to drink plenty of fluids postoperatively.

主诉

C. S. 是一名60岁的教师，排尿和射精无力，怀疑并感觉不能完全排空膀胱。他试着使用前列腺（prostate）健康草药补充剂，2年没有任何实际效果。他决定预约泌尿科医生（urologist）。

检查

泌尿科医生记录了病历，并检查了患者。C. S. 报告没有排尿困难、血尿或侧腹疼痛。他没有尿路感染（UTI）、附睾炎（epididymitis）、前列腺炎（prostatitis）、肾脏疾病或肾结石（renal calculi）的病史。他的病史在其他方面对他的泌尿系统疾病并不重要。

直肠检查显示前列腺50g，前列腺右叶轻微变硬。医生安排在1周后做膀胱超声（bladder ultrasound）检查，结果表明没有膀胱内病变（intravesical lesion）或前列腺突出进入膀胱基底。

又做了经腹超声（transabdominal ultrasound）检查，结果显示尿残余量为120mL。除了WBC = 8、RBC = 10、细菌 = 微量，尿分析结果显示正常。

C. S. 被诊断为伴有膀胱颈阻塞的良性前列腺增生（benign prostatic hyperplasia，BPH），并被安排做经尿道前列腺切除术（transurethral resection of the prostate，TURP）。他的泌尿科医生解释了手术过程和术前及术后的预期，办公室工作人员通知医院安排手术。第2天，医院住院部门通知C. S. 办理正常的入院程序，并安排了手术日期。

临床病程

C. S. 在手术前一天晚上被禁食。他被带到手术室，并为手术做了脊髓麻醉（spinal anesthetic）。他已经被告知手术将需要大约1小时，并且他在手术期间将保持清醒，但不会感到任何疼痛。使用前列腺切除器（resectoscope）对扩张的前列腺组织做了修整。手术结束时，将导尿管（Foley catheter）插入并保留在膀胱中以排出尿液，并允许灌注膀胱以清除所有凝块。C. S. 对整个手术程序耐受良好，并被转移到恢复室，随后进入病房。他被鼓励在术后喝大量液体。

简介

男性和女性的性腺（gonad）都生产生殖细胞（reproductive cell），又称为配子（gamete），和激素。配子是由减数分裂（meiosis）产生的，在减数分裂中，细胞分裂会使染色体（chromosome）数量从46减到32。当男性和女性配子在受精（fertilization）结合时，原始染色体数量就恢复了。

性激素协助配子的产生，在怀孕（pregnancy）和哺乳（lactation）期发挥功能，并产生第二性征（secondary sex characteristics），例如与男女性别（gender）相关的身材大小、体型、体毛和嗓音等。

生殖道的发育与泌尿道紧密相关，在女性，这两个系统完全分离，而男性的生殖系统和泌尿系统共用一个通道——尿道。因此，这两个系统一起被称为生殖泌尿系统（genitourinary，GU）或泌尿生殖系统（urogenital），在治疗男性生殖系统疾病和泌尿系统疾病时，要咨询泌尿科医生。

睾丸

男性生殖细胞、精子细胞或精子（spermatozoon，复数形式为 spermatozoa）是由一对睾丸（testis，复数形式为 testes）产生的，睾丸悬挂在体外的阴囊（scrotum）之中（图14-1）。尽管睾丸是在腹腔中发育的，它们会在出生前或出生后很短时间内通过腹股沟管（inguinal canal）下降到阴囊中（图14-2）。

从性成熟（sexual maturation）或青春期（puberty）开始，精子便在睾丸中卷曲的生精小管（seminiferous tubule）中持续形成（图14-3）。精子的发育需要特殊的滋养细胞（sertoli cells）和男性激素，或称为雄性激素（androgen）——主要是睾丸素的协助。这些激素在位于生精小管之间的间质细胞（interstitial cell）中产生。男性和女性性腺都由脑下垂体前叶释放的促卵泡激素（follicle-stimulating hormone，FSH）和黄体生成素（luteinizing hormone，LH）产生刺激。男性和女性的激素的化学成分是相同的，不过它们是根据其在女性生殖中的作用命名的。在男性，促卵泡激素刺激滋养细胞并促进精子的形成，黄体生成素刺激间质细胞产生睾丸素。

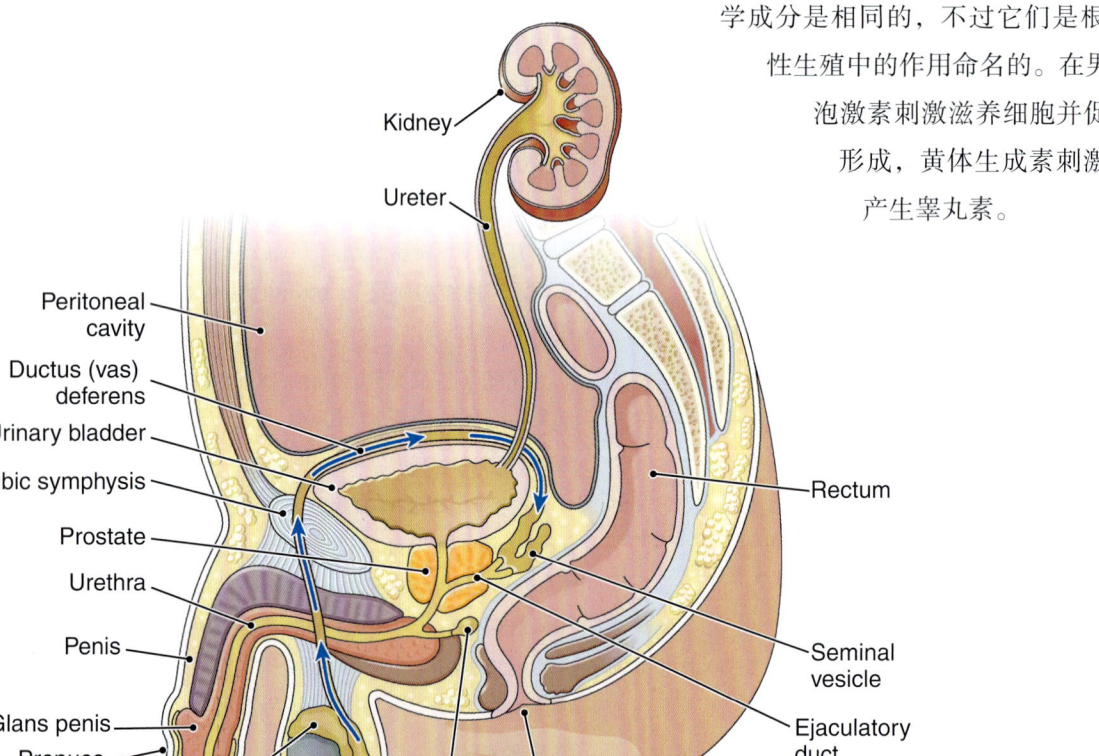

图14-1 **男性生殖系统**。图中也显示了部分泌尿系统和消化系统

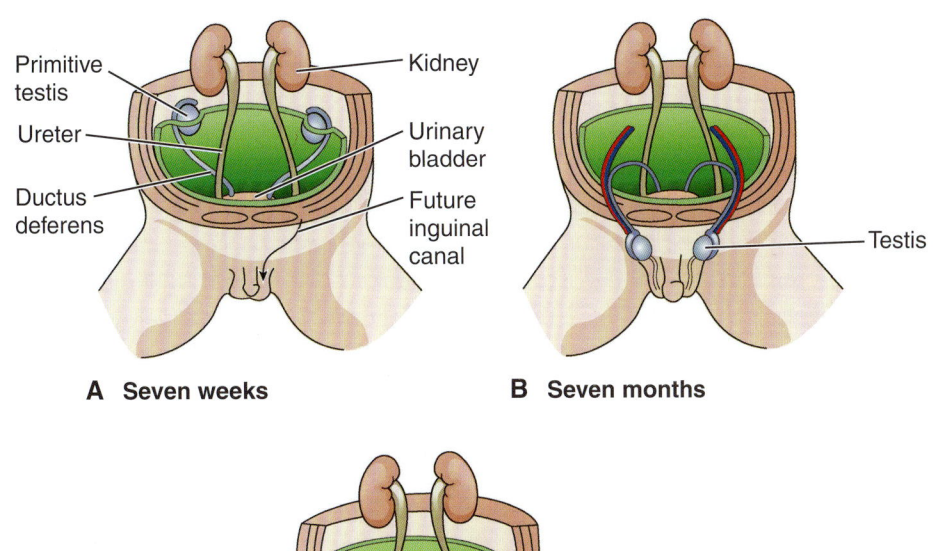
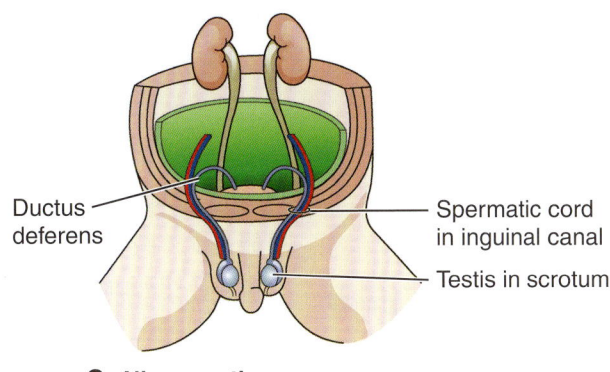

图 14-2　睾丸下降。图中显示了在胎儿发育期间的三个不同时间的腹股沟的形成和睾丸的下降。A. 在 7 周时，睾丸在背腹壁；B. 在 7 个月时，睾丸通过腹股沟管；C. 在 9 个月时，睾丸在阴囊中通过精索悬吊

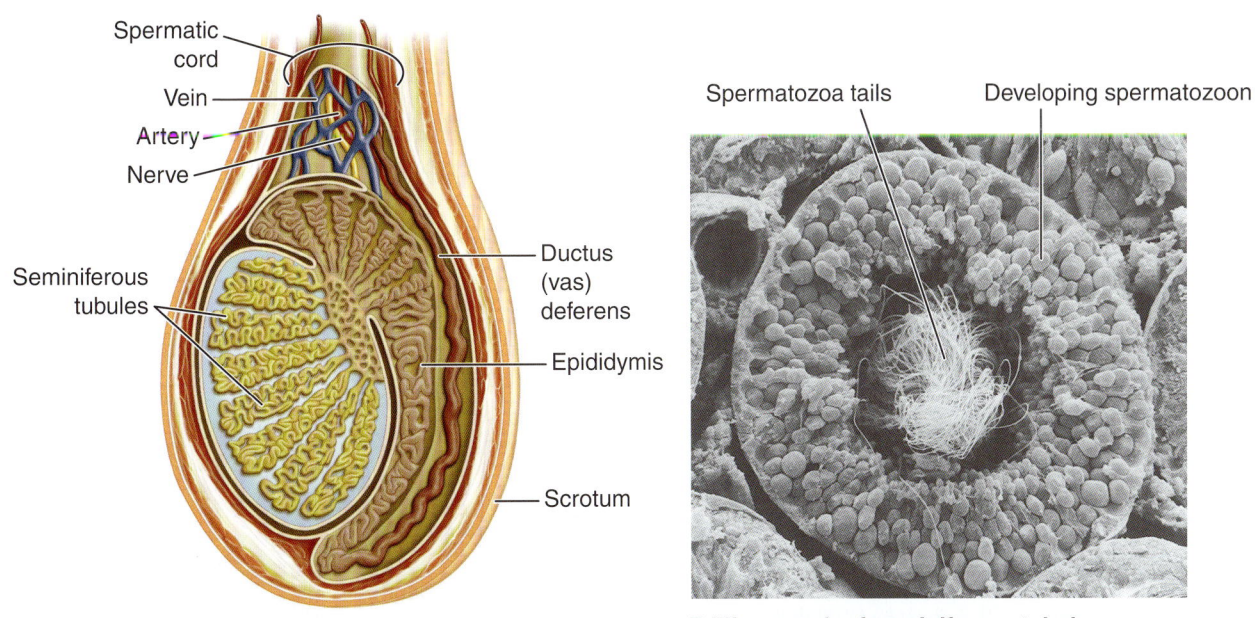

图 14-3　睾丸。A. 阴囊中的睾丸位置显示生精小管的结构，还显示了附睾和精索；B. 精子在睾丸中生精小管内发育

框 14-1

聚焦单词
到底是哪个？

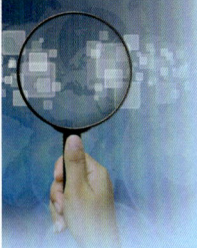

许多人体结构和治疗方法会有两个或多个名称，这一情况使学习医学术语变得更加困难。这种一物多名的情况的发生可能是因为不同的命名发生在不同的时间或地点，或者是因为处于一个名称向另一个名称转换的状态，而新的名称尚未被广泛采用。

从睾丸通向尿道的管道原来被称为输精管（vas deferens），vas 是管道（vessel）通用名词。为了区别于血管（blood vessel），将输精管命名为 ductus deferens。不过，原来的名称还在使用，因为男性绝育手术输精管切除术仍然被称为 vasectomy，而不是"ductusectomy"。

类似的不一致也出现在其他系统。dorsal 和 posterior 的含义都是背面，ventral 和 anterior 的含义都是前面。人类生长激素（human growth hormone）也被称为 somatotropin，升高血压的激素抗利尿激素又被称为血管加压素（vasopressin）。

在神经系统，包含神经传导物质的轴突（axon）末端的小肿胀——突触小结被不同地称为 endfeet、end-bulb、terminal knob、terminal feet 和其他更多的名称。在女性中，将卵细胞（ovary）从卵巢（ovary）输送到子宫（uterus）的输卵管被称为 uterine tube、或者 Fallopian tube、或者 oviduct、或者……

精子的输送

精子在产生之后被储存在每个睾丸表面卷曲的管道——附睾（epididymis，图 14-1 和 14-3）之中，直至射精（ejaculation）将它们推入一系列通向体外的通道。首先是输精管（ductus deferens 或 vas deferens），包含在精索（spermatic cord）之中，与神经和为睾丸供血的血管在一起（图 14-2 和 14-3）。精索通过腹股沟管上升进入腹腔，输精管在那里离开精索进入膀胱（框 14-1 讨论通用交叉名称对学习医学术语的挑战）。

输精管的一个短的延续是射精通道，穿过膀胱下的前列腺（prostate gland）将精子送入尿道。最终，精子与其他分泌物混合穿过尿道，通过阴茎（penis）释放（图 14-1）。

阴茎

尿道海绵体部（penile urethra）输送尿液和精液（semen）。阴茎是男性的性交（sexual intercourse 或 coitus）器官，由三段海绵状组织组成。海绵状组织充血就会产生勃起（erection）——阴茎变硬。如图 14-4 所示，两个阴茎海绵主体（corpora cavernosa）在两侧，尿道海绵体（corpus spongiosum）在中间，尿道穿过尿道海绵体。尿道海绵体在顶部扩张成为龟头（glans penis），阴茎头由松软的皮肤——包皮（prepuce 或 foreskin）覆盖。

手术切除包皮被称为包皮环切术（circumcision），可能是出于医学原因所做，但更常见的出于卫生、文化偏好或宗教原因所做。

精液的形成

精液是输送精子的浓稠的微白色液体，其中包含精子细胞、来自于三种附属腺体的分泌物（图 14-1）。附属腺体分别是：

- 成对的精囊（seminal vesicle），分别向射精管释放它们的分泌物。
- 前列腺，分泌进入膀胱下尿道的初段。
- 两个尿道球腺（bulbourethral gland，cowper gland），分泌进入前列腺之后的尿道。

这些腺体共同产生微碱性混合分泌物，能够滋养并输送精子，并通过中和女性阴道的酸性保护精子。

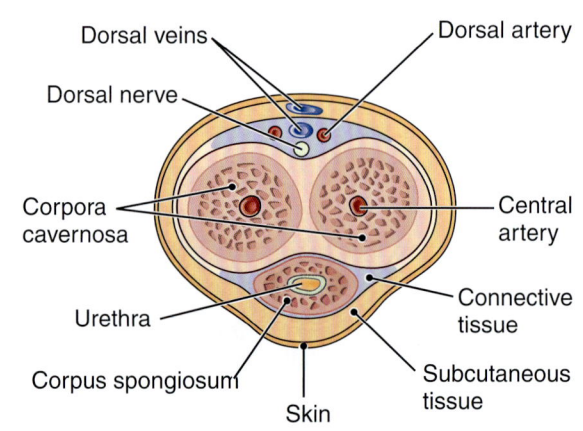

图 14-4　阴茎。这个横截面显示勃起的阴茎（海绵主体和尿道海绵体），尿道、血管和神经位于中心

Terminology 关键术语

正常结构与功能

androgen [ˈændrədʒən]	雄性激素，任何有雄性特征的激素；词根 andr/o 意为"雄性"
bulbourethral gland [bʌlbəreˈθrəl]	尿道球腺，前列腺后尿道侧的小腺体，分泌部分精液，也被称为库珀氏腺（Cowper gland）
circumcision [ˌsɜːkəmˈsiʒn]	包皮环切术，手术切除包皮前端
coitus [ˈkɔitəs]	性交，同 sexual intercourse
ductus deferens [ˈdʌktəs ˈdefərənz]	输精管，将精子从附睾输送到射精管的管道，也拼写为 vas deferens
ejaculation [iˌdʒækjuˈleiʃn]	射精，精液从男性尿道射出
ejaculatory duct	射精管，输精管和精囊合并形成的管道，携带精子和精液进入尿道
epididymis [ˌepiˈdidimis]	附睾，睾丸表面卷曲的管道，储存精子直至射精
erection [iˈrekʃn]	勃起，阴茎或阴蒂的坚挺或硬化，通常是因为性兴奋
follicle-stimulating hormone (FSH)	促卵泡激素，垂体前叶分泌的作用于性腺的激素。在男性，促卵泡激素刺激间质细胞，并促进精子发育
gamete [ˈgæmiːt]	配子，成熟的生殖细胞，男性是精子，女性是卵子
glans penis	龟头，阴茎的球状前端
gonad [ˈgəʊnæd]	性腺，睾丸或卵巢
inguinal canal [ˈiŋgwinl kəˈnæl]	腹股沟管，男性睾丸降入精囊的管道
interstitial cell [ˌintəˈstiʃl]	间质细胞，位于睾丸的生精小管中的细胞，主要产生睾丸素
luteinizing hormone (LH) [ˈluːtiːəˌnaiziŋ]	促黄体生成素，垂体前叶分泌的作用于性腺的激素。在男性，促黄体生成素刺激间质细胞产生睾丸素
meiosis [maiˈəʊsis]	减数分裂，一种形成配子的细胞分裂方式，导致细胞中有 23 条染色体，是其他人体细胞染色体数量的一半（源自于希腊语 meiosis 意为"减少"）
penis [ˈpiːnis]	阴茎，男性性交和排尿器官（形容词 penile）
pituitary gland [piˈtuːiˌteriː]	脑垂体，位于大脑底部的内分泌腺
prepuce [ˈpriːpjuːs]	包皮，阴茎龟头的皮肤褶层，也常用 foreskin
prostate gland [ˈprɒsteit]	前列腺，男性膀胱下尿道周围的腺体，对精液分泌有贡献（词根：prostat/o）
puberty [ˈpjuːbəti]	青春期，获得性生殖能力并开始发育第二性征的时期
scrotum [ˈskrəʊtəm]	阴囊，包含睾丸的双囊（词根：osche/o）
semen [ˈsiːmen]	精液，输送精子的浓稠的分泌物（词根：semin, sperm/i, spermat/o）
seminal vesicle [ˈsemənəl ˈvesikl]	精囊，膀胱后面一个囊样腺体，对精液分泌有贡献（词根：vesicul/o）

Terminology 关键术语

Sertoli cell	滋养细胞，生精小管中协助精子发育的细胞；也被称为支持细胞（sustentacular cell）
spermatic cord ［spɜː'mætɪk］	精索，附着在睾丸上的索状结构，包含输精管、血管和神经，包围在一个纤维鞘中（图14-3）
spermatozoon ［ˌspɜːmətəˈzəʊən］	精子，成熟的男性生殖细胞（复数 spermatozoa，词根：sperm/i, spermat/o）
testis ［ˈtestɪs］	睾丸，男性生殖腺（词根：test/o, orchi/o, orchid/o）；复数形式为 testes；也拼写为 testicle
testosterone ［teˈstɒstərəʊn］	睾丸素，主要的雄性激素
vas deferens	输精管，同 ductus deferens

与男性生殖系统相关的词根

参见表14-1

表14-1 男性生殖系统的词根

词根	含义	示例	示例定义
test/o	睾丸	testosterone ［teˈstɒstərəʊn］	睾丸素
orchi/o, orchid/o	睾丸	anorchism ［ænɔːrˈkɪzəm］	无睾症
osche/o	阴囊	oscheal ［ˈɒstʃəl］	阴囊的
semin	精液	inseminate ［ɪnˈsemɪneɪt］	授精
sperm/i, spermat/o	精液，精子	polyspermia ［ˌpɒlɪˈspɜːmjə］	精液过多
epididym/o	附睾	epididymitis ［ˌepɪˌdɪdɪˈmaɪtɪs］	附睾炎
vas/o	输精管，血管	vasostomy ［ˈvæsɒstəmɪ］	输精管复通
vesicul/o	精囊	vesiculogram ［vəˈsɪkjʊləgræm］	精囊造影片
prostat/o	前列腺	prostatometer ［ˌprɒsteɪˈtɒmɪtə］	前列腺测量仪

练习14-1

定义下列单词。

1. spermatogenesis ［ˌspɜːmətəʊˈdʒenɪsɪs］ _____
2. prostatodynia ［ˌprɒstətəʊˈdɪnjə］ _____

练习 14-1

3. oscheoplasty [ɔustʃi:əup'læsti] _____
4. epididymectomy [epidaidi'mektəmi] _____
5. orchialgia [ɔ:ki'ældʒiə] _____
6. testopathy ['testəpəθi] _____
7. orchiepididymitis [ɔ:kiepididi'maitis] _____

使用词根 orchi/o 写出下列定义的单词，还要用词根 orchid/o 写出每个单词。

8. surgical fixation of a testis _____
9. plastic repair of a testis _____
10. surgical removal of a testis _____

使用词根 spermat/o 写出下列定义的单词。

11. Condition of having sperm in the urine (-uria) _____
12. Destruction (-lysis) of sperm _____
13. Excessive discharge (-rhea) of semen _____
14. Subnormal concentration of sperm in semen _____
15. A sperm-forming cell _____

单词结尾 –spermia 意为"精子或精液的状态"。为 –spermia 加一个前缀构成下列定义的单词。

16. presence of blood in the semen _____
17. lack of semen _____
18. secretion of excess (poly/o) semen _____
19. presence of pus in the semen _____

写出下列定义的单词。

20. excision of the ductus deferens _____
21. tumor of the scrotum _____
22. suture of the vas deferens _____
23. excision of the prostate gland _____
24. radiographic study of a seminal vesicle _____
25. inflammation of a seminal vesicle _____
26. incision of the epididymis _____

男性生殖系统的临床表现

感染

男性生殖道的大多数感染是性传播感染（sexually transmitted infection，STI）（框 14–2）。美国最常见的性传播感染是沙眼衣原体（Chlamydia trachomatis）引起的，主要会引起男性尿道炎（urethritis）。沙眼衣原体还会引起性病淋巴肉芽肿（lymphogranuloma venereum），这是一种与淋巴结病相关的性传播感染，在热带区域最常见。这两种形式的衣原体感染都可以用抗生素治疗。

淋病（gonorrhea）是由淋球菌（gonococcus，

GC）引起的。感染通常以尿道为中心，引起带有灼痛的尿道炎、有脓性分泌物和排尿困难。如果不治疗，疾病会扩散到生殖系统。淋病可以用抗生素治疗，但淋球菌会很快发展为耐药性。

另一种性传播感染是由病毒引起的疱疹（herpes）感染。其他性传播感染将在第 15 章讨论。

流行性腮腺炎（mumps）是非性传播病毒疾病，能够感染睾丸并导致不育（sterility）。其他微生物也会感染生殖道，引起尿道炎、前列腺炎（prostatitis）、睾丸炎（orchitis）或附睾炎。

良性前列腺增生

随着男性年龄增大，前列腺通常会增大，被称为良性前列腺增生（benign prostatic hyperplasia，BPH）。尽管不是癌症，这种增生组织会挤压膀胱附近的尿道，干扰排尿。如果阻塞得不到纠正，可能继发尿潴留（urinary retention）、感染和其他并发症。

用药放松前列腺和膀胱颈附近的肌肉被用于治

框 14-2 供你参考
性传播感染

疾病	微生物	说明
细菌的		
chlamydial infection 衣原体感染	D 至 K 型沙眼衣原体	生殖泌尿道上行感染，可能扩散到女性的骨盆，引起盆腔炎（pelvic inflammatory disease, PID）
lymphogranuloma venereum 性病淋巴肉芽肿	L 型沙眼衣原体	带有腹股沟淋巴结肿胀的一般性感染；生殖系统组织瘢痕化
gonorrhea 淋病	淋球菌	生殖泌尿路感染。在男性表现为尿道炎，在女性为阴道分泌物和宫颈炎（cervicitis），会导致盆腔炎。可能为全身感染，可能传染给新生儿。抗生素治疗
bacterial vaginosis 细菌性阴道炎	Gardnerella vaginalis 阴道加德菌	带有恶臭分泌物的阴道感染
syphilis 梅毒	Treponema pallidum 梅毒螺旋体	一期：下疳（chancre）；二期：全身感染和梅毒性疣（syphilitic warts）；三期：其他系统退化。引起自发性流产、死产和致命的畸形，用抗生素治疗
病毒的		
AIDS 艾滋病（获得性免疫缺陷综合征）	HIV（人类免疫缺陷病毒）	影响免疫系统 T 细胞的通常会致命的疾病，会使患者虚弱，并导致其他疾病
genital herpes 生殖器疱疹	herpes simplex virus (HSV) 单纯性疱疹病毒	痛苦的生殖系统损伤。在女性可能是宫颈癌的风险因素之一；新生儿感染通常会致命，目前无法治愈
hepatitis B 乙型肝炎	HBV 乙型肝炎病毒	引起肝脏发炎，可能是急性的，或可发展成慢性病毒携带状态。与肝癌有关
condyloma acuminatum 尖锐湿疣	HPV 人乳头瘤病毒	良性生殖器疣。在女性，易患宫颈非典型增生（cervical dysplasia）和宫颈癌。有针对流行株的疫苗
原虫的		
Trichomoniasis 滴虫病	Trichomonas vaginalis 阴道毛滴虫	阴道炎。绿色、多泡分泌物，瘙痒；性交疼痛（dyspareunia）、排尿疼痛（dysuria）

疗良性前列腺增生的症状。α肾上腺素能受体阻滞剂（Alphaadrenergic blocking agent），例如坦索罗辛（tamsulosin）与这些区域的交感神经刺激相互冲突，能够改善尿液流动速。因为睾丸素会刺激前列腺增大，干扰前列腺睾丸素活动的药物可能延缓疾病的进展，例如非那雄胺（finasteride）。锯棕榈（saw palmetto）是一种矮生棕榈树，其浆果提取物能够以同样的方式发生作用。锯棕榈被发现能够推迟某些良性前列腺增生病例的手术需要。

在深度良性前列腺增生病例中，可能需要前列腺切除术（prostatectomy）。当手术通过尿道执行时，这一方法被称为经尿道前列腺切除术（transurethral resection of the prostate，TURP，图14–5A）。也可以通过经尿道前列腺切开术（transurethral incision of the prostate，TUIP）降低尿道的压力（图14–5B）。外科医生还会使用激光束或热量破坏前列腺组织。良性前列腺增生可以通过直肠指检（digital rectal examination，DRE）或造影研究进行诊断。

癌症

前列腺癌

前列腺癌（prostatic cancer）是男性最常见的恶性肿瘤，中年以上男性与癌症相关的死亡中，只有肺癌和结肠癌的致死病例超过前列腺癌。医生通常能够通过直肠指诊发现前列腺癌。前列腺特异性抗原（prostate-specific antigen，PSA）血液测试也有助于早期检查。在有前列腺癌的情况下，这种蛋白质的产生会增加，不过其他前列腺疾病也会使它的生产量升高。

前列腺癌的TNM分期系统包括以下几类：
- T1：肿瘤不能通过直肠检查触及，需要活组织或异常PAS检查。
- T2：肿瘤可触及，并局限于前列腺。
- T3：肿瘤在前列腺以外局部扩散。
- M：远处转移。

治疗方法包括手术（前列腺切除术，prostatectomy）、放射性治疗（放疗）、雄性激素抑制（雄性激素会刺激前列腺的生长）和化学治疗（化疗）。放疗通常通过植入放射性粒子进行，另一种被称为"观察等待"或递延治疗的方法主要是监测，而不做治疗。选择这种方法是基于患者的年龄、肿瘤的侵入度和不治疗肿瘤对患者有生之年造成伤害的可能性。

睾丸癌

成年男性的睾丸癌发生率低于1%。睾丸癌通常发生在25~45岁，没有显示出基因遗传的迹象。这

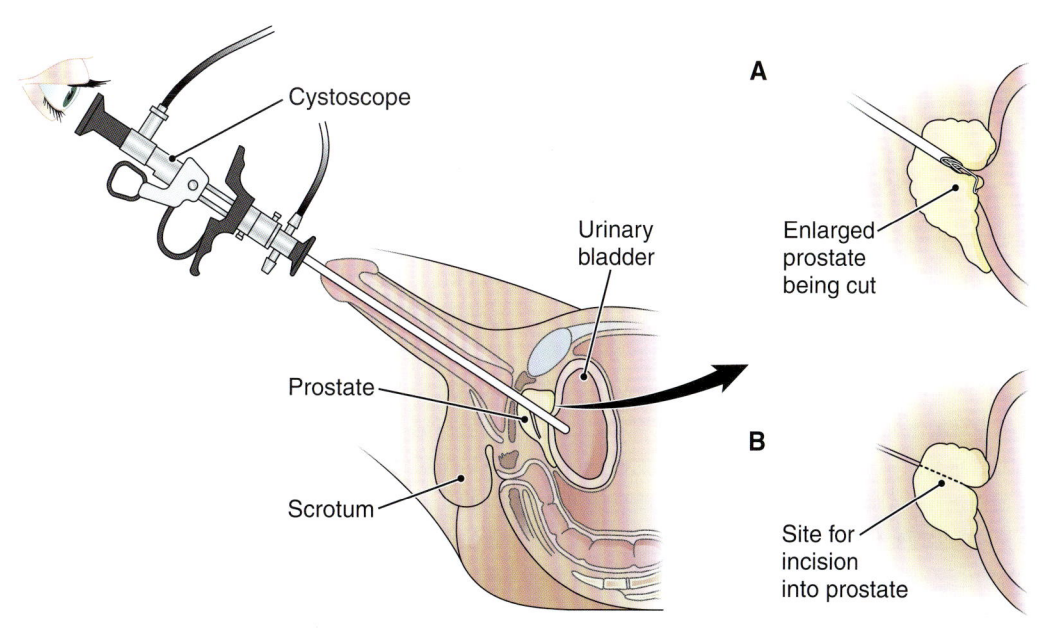

图14-5　前列腺手术程序。A. 经尿道前列腺切除术（TURP），在膀胱开口处除去部分前列腺。B. 经尿道前列腺切开术（TUIP），在前列腺中进行一个或两个切口以减小尿道的压力

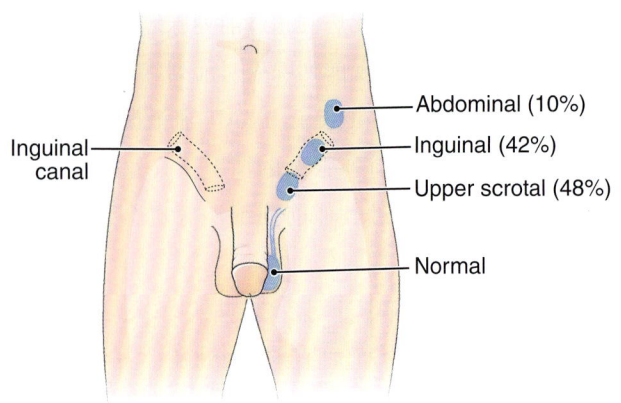

图 14-6 隐睾症。睾丸不能下降到阴囊。在大多数情况下，睾丸保留在阴囊的上部或腹股沟管中。图中显示了不同位置的百分比

种癌症典型地始发于生殖细胞，并可能扩散到腹部淋巴结。一半以上的睾丸肿瘤会释放能够在血液中检测出来的标志物。治疗包括睾丸切除术（orchiectomy）、放疗和化疗。

隐睾症

在出生时一个或两个睾丸没有降入阴囊是比较常见的（图14-6），这被称为隐睾症（cryptorchidism），字母意为隐藏（crypt/o）睾丸（orchid/o）。这种情况一般会在1岁以内自我矫正，如果没有，则必须通过手术矫正，以避免不育和癌症风险上升。

不育症

不能生育或生育能力降低被称为不育症（infertility）。不育症的起因可能是遗传性的、激素引起的、疾病相关的或暴露于化学或物理制剂所致，最常见的起因是性传播感染。完全不能生育后代可被称为绝育（sterility）。男性可以通过切除并封闭两侧输精管（vasectomy）自愿绝育（图15–5）。

勃起功能障碍

勃起功能障碍（erectile dysfunction，ED），也被称为阳痿（impotence），是指男性因为无法启动或保持勃起直至射精而不能完成性交。这种病例的10%~20%为心理性的，即情感因素引起的，例如压力、情绪低落或心理创伤。更常见的是生理因素引起的，包括：

- 血管疾病，例如动脉硬化、静脉曲张或糖尿病引起的损伤。
- 神经系统问题，由肿瘤、外伤、糖尿病影响以及放射性或手术引起的伤害所致。
- 药物的不良反应，例如降压药、抗溃疡药或食欲抑制剂。

治疗勃起功能障碍的药物通过扩张阴茎中的动脉来增加进入阴茎的血流。非药物治疗包括矫形手术、真空泵吸取血液进入阴茎、阴茎注射扩张血管和人工

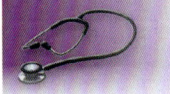

框 14-3

临床观点
勃起功能障碍

全世界有不少男性及其伙伴受到勃起功能障碍的影响，不能获得并保持勃起。尽管更常见于65岁以上的男性，但勃起功能障碍可能发生于任何年龄，而且可能有许多原因。

勃起是自主神经系统和阴茎血管相互作用的结果。性唤起刺激阴茎中的副交感神经（parasympathetic nerve），释放一种被称为一氧化氮（nitric oxide，NO）的化合物。这种物质激活血管平滑肌中一种能够促进血管扩张的酶，增加流入阴茎的血流，并引起勃起。引起勃起功能障碍的身体因素会阻止这些生理变化。

以勃起的生理机制为目标的药物能够帮助那些勃起功能障碍的男性，包括西地那非（sildenafil，商品名称为伟哥，Viagra）、伐地那非（vardenafil）和他达拉非（tadalafil）。这些药物能够防止血管扩张的中断，因而延长一氧化氮的作用。尽管对80%的勃起功能障碍有效，这些可能引起一些相对较小的不良反应，包括头痛、鼻塞、肠胃不适和淡蓝色视觉。使用硝酸盐药物治疗心绞痛的男性一定不要使用这些药物，因为硝酸盐会提升一氧化氮的水平，与治疗勃起功能障碍和延长一氧化氮作用的药物一起可能导致威胁生命的血压过低。低血压和心力衰竭的男性也禁用这些药物。

阴茎（penile prosthesis）。框 14-3 有关于勃起功能障碍的更多信息。

医生助手协助泌尿科和许多其他医学领域的患者检查和护理。框 14-4 描述了这一专业的职业。

腹股沟疝

腹股沟管会构成腹壁上的弱点，可能导致疝。在最常见的腹股沟疝（inguinal hernia）（图 14-7），一个腹部器官，通常是肠道，进入腹股沟管，并可能延伸到阴囊之中。这是一种间接的、或外部的腹股沟疝。在直接的或内部的腹股沟疝中，器官通过腹壁突出进入阴囊。如果对该器官的供血被切断，疝被称为是绞窄的（strangulated）。手术矫正疝被称为疝修补术（herniorrhaphy）。

框 14-4

健康职业
医生助理

医生助理（physician assistant, PA）在内科医生和外科医生的监督下进行医疗工作。他们接受过诊断、治疗和预防保健方面的培训。他们还获得治疗轻伤的许可。在美国几乎所有的州，他们都可以开处方药。根据工作环境，他们还可以管理医疗业务并监督其他医务人员。

在医疗服务不足的地区，他们可以在自己的专业方向独立工作，并根据需要与医生进行协商。许多医生助理在普通外科或内科、儿科或家庭医学诊所工作。如果他们的专业是外科，他们可以在手术之前和之后为患者提供护理，或者协助手术。

医生助理必须完成正式的 6 年教育计划，4 年的本科工作和 2 年硕士学位。大多数医生助理项目要求候选人具有学士学位，核心科学课程，以及在军事或一些其他联合健康领域的临床经验。成功完成一个教学年和一年的临床轮换之后，医生助理必须通过全国考试的认证。他们也可以通过国家医生助理认证委员会（National Commission on Certification of Physician Assistants, NCCPA）获得认证（PA-C），并通过继续教育维持认证。工作前景非常好，特别是医院需要通过增加人员配置来弥补医疗人员的变化。更多相关信息，请联系美国医生助理协会（American Academy of Physician Assistants），网址：www.aapa.org。

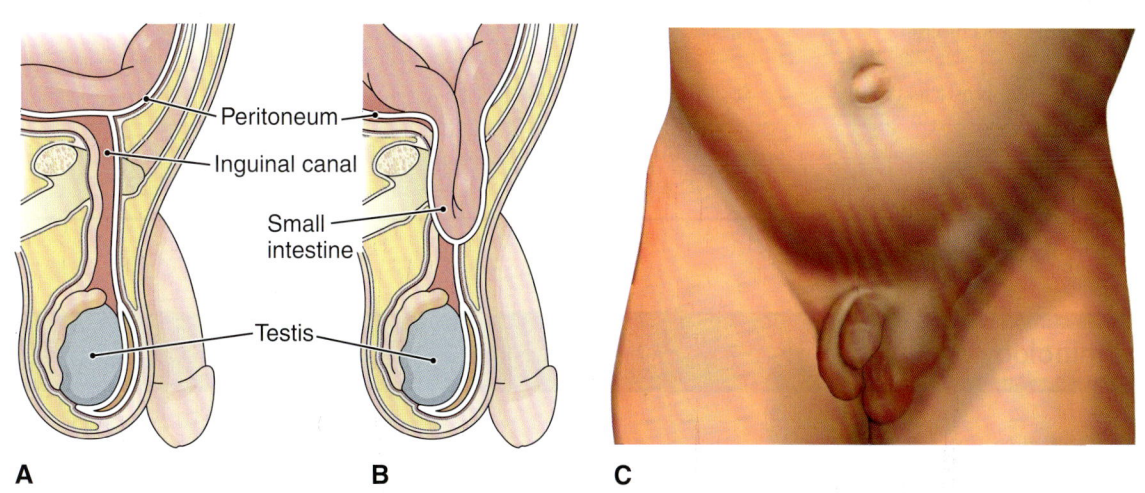

图 14-7 腹股沟疝。A. 正常；B. 腹壁中的弱点允许肠或其他腹部内容物突出到腹股沟管内，疝囊是腹膜的延伸；C. 腹股沟疝可在腹股沟区域和阴囊中引起可见的隆起

Terminology 关键术语

病症

benign prostatic hyperplasia (BPH)	良性前列腺增生，非恶性的前列腺扩大，通常随年龄增加而发生。也被称为良性前列腺肥大（benign prostatic hypertrophy）
cryptorchidism [krip'tɔ:kidizəm]	隐睾症，睾丸未能降入阴囊（图 14-6）
epididymitis [ˌepiˌdidi'maitis]	附睾炎，附睾的炎症，通常是泌尿系统感染或性传播感染所致
erectile dysfunction [iˈrektail]	勃起功能障碍，男性因为无法启动或保持勃起直至射精而不能完成性交；又称为阳痿（impotence）
impotence ['impətəns]	阳痿，勃起功能障碍
infertility [ˌinfɜ:'tiləti]	不育，产生后代的能力下降
inguinal hernia ['ingwinl 'hə:njə]	腹股沟疝，肠道或其他腹部器官通过腹股沟管或腹壁突出进入阴囊
orchitis [ɔ:'kaitis]	睾丸炎，睾丸的炎症；可能是受伤、腮腺炎病毒或其他感染所致
prostatitis [ˌprɒstə'taitis]	前列腺炎，前列腺的炎症；常与泌尿系统感染和性传播感染一起出现
sexually transmitted infection (STI)	性传播感染，通过性活动传播的感染（框 14-2），也被称为性传播疾病（sexually transmitted disease, STD），曾被成为性病（venereal disease, VD，源自于爱神维纳斯 Venus）
sterility [stə'riləti]	绝育，完全不能生产后代
urethritis [ˌjʊərə'θraitis]	尿道炎，尿道的炎症，通常是淋病和衣原体感染所致

手术

herniorrhaphy [hɜ:ni'ɔ:rəfi]	疝修补术，手术修补疝
prostatectomy [ˌprɒstə'tektəmi]	前列腺切除术，手术切除前列腺
vasectomy [və'sektəmi]	输精管切除术，切除输精管，通常切除两侧的输精管，以实现绝育（图 15-5），可能通过尿道完成手术（经尿道切除术 transurethral resection）

Terminology 补充术语

正常结构与功能

emission [i'miʃn]	泌精，排出精液
genitalia [ˌdʒeni'teiliə]	生殖器，与生殖相关的器官，分为内、外两部分
insemination [inˌsemi'neiʃn]	授精，向女性阴道导入精液
orgasm ['ɔ:gæzəm]	性高潮，一种身体和情感的兴奋状态，特别是在性交顶峰时发生的

Terminology 关键术语

phallus ['fæləs]	阴茎，男性生殖器（形容词：phallic）
病症	
balanitis [bælə'nitis]	龟头炎，龟头及其黏膜的炎症（词根：balan/o 意为"龟头"）
bladder neck obstruction (BNO)	膀胱颈梗阻，膀胱出口尿液流动堵塞；常见起因是良性前列腺增生
hydrocele ['haidrəsi:l]	鞘膜积液，囊样腔体液体积累，特别是覆盖睾丸或精索的包囊
phimosis [fai'məusis]	包茎，包皮开口狭窄，以致于包皮不能被推到龟头之后
penis priapism ['praiəpizəm]	阴茎勃起异常，阴茎异常、疼痛、持续的勃起，可能是药物或精索的特定损伤所致
seminoma [semi'nəumə]	精原细胞瘤，一种睾丸肿瘤
spermatocele ['spɜ:mətəusi:l]	精子囊肿，一种包含精子的附睾囊肿（图 14-8）
varicocele ['værikəusi:l]	精索静脉曲张，精索静脉扩张（图 14-8）
诊断与治疗	
brachytherapy [b'rækiθerəpi]	短距离放射治疗，将封装于胶囊中的放射源，例如放射性粒子直接放置于肿瘤之中或附近组织的放射疗法（源自于希腊语 brachy- 意为"短"）
castration [kæ'streiʃn]	阉割，手术切除睾丸或卵巢。能够抑制性腺的激素和药物能够产生功能性阉割
Gleason tumor grade	格里森肿瘤分级，前列腺中癌症严重性变化的评估系统，评估结果为格里森评分（Gleason score）
resectoscope [ri'sektəskəup]	电切镜，经尿道从膀胱、前列腺、子宫或尿道切除组织的内窥镜仪器

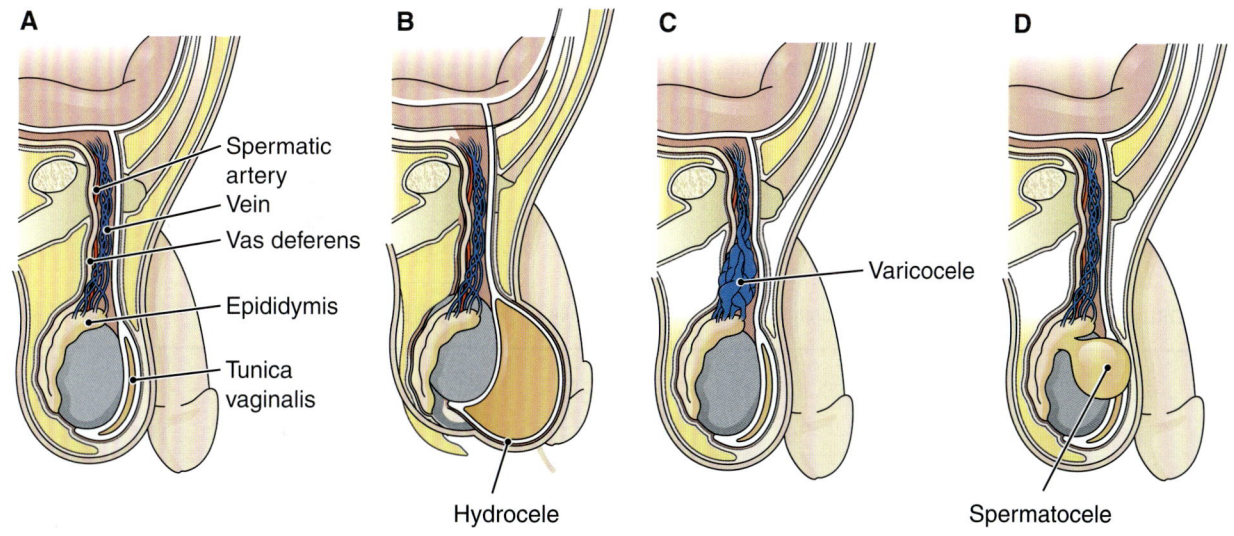

图 14-8 阴囊异常。A. 正常；B. 水肿；C. 精索静脉曲张；D. 精子囊肿

Terminology 缩略语

AIDS	Acquired immunodeficiency syndrome	艾滋病（获得性免疫缺陷综合征）
BNO	Bladder neck obstruction	膀胱颈梗阻
BPH	Benign prostatic hyperplasia (hypertrophy)	良性前列腺增生（肥大）
DRE	Digital rectal examination	直肠指检
ED	Erectile dysfunction	勃起功能障碍
FSH	Follicle-stimulating hormone	促卵泡激素
GC	Gonococcus	淋球菌
GU	Genitourinary	泌尿生殖的
HBV	Hepatitis B virus	乙型肝炎病毒
HIV	Human immunodeficiency virus	人类免疫缺陷病毒
HSV	Herpes simplex virus	单纯性疱疹病毒
LH	Luteinizing hormone	促黄体生成素
NGU	Nongonococcal urethritis	非淋病性尿道炎
PSA	Prostate-specific antigen	前列腺特异性抗体
STD	Sexually transmitted disease	性传播疾病
STI	Sexually transmitted infection	性传播感染
TPUR	Transperineal urethral resection	经会阴尿道切除术
TSE	Testicular self-examination	睾丸自检
TUIP	Transurethral incision of prostate	经尿道前列腺切开术
TURP	Transurethral resection of prostate	经尿道前列腺切除术
UG	Urogenital	泌尿生殖的
UTI	Urinary tract infection	尿路感染
VD	Venereal disease (sexually transmitted infection)	性病（性传播感染）
VDRL	Venereal Disease Research Laboratory (test for syphilis)	性病研究实验室（梅毒测试）

Case Study Revisited
案例研究再访

C. S.'s Follow-Up

On the morning of the second postoperative day, the Foley catheter was removed, and C. S. was able to void on his own. He experienced dysuria and some burning when urinating, but otherwise did not have any postoperative complications.

He was aware that the painful urination might persist for a few weeks. He remained in the hospital through the second day and then was discharged home with specific instructions. He was to follow up with his urologist in a week.

C. S. 的随访

在术后第 2 天早晨，导尿管被移除，C. S. 能够自己排尿。排尿时他经历了排尿困难和一些灼热，但除此之外没有任何术后并发症。

他被告知排尿疼痛可能会持续几个星期。术后第 2 天留他在医院，然后带着具体的医嘱出院回家。1 周后他的泌尿科医生会对他进行随访。

CHAPTER 14 复习

标记练习

男性生殖系统

在对应的下划线上写出每个编号部分的名称。

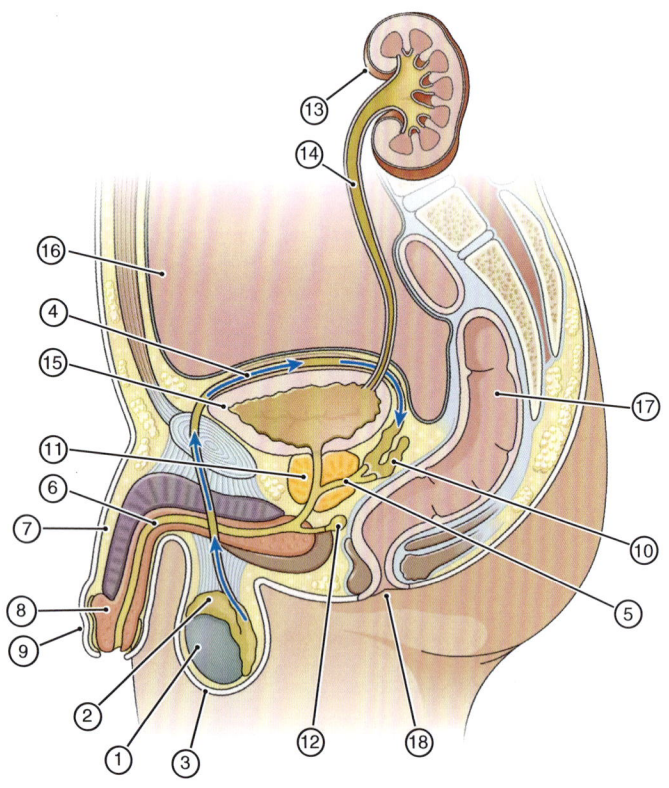

Anus
Bulbourethral (Cowper) gland
Ductus (vas) deferens
Ejaculatory duct
Epididymis
Glans penis

Kidney
Penis
Peritoneal cavity
Prepuce (foreskin)
Prostate
Rectum

Scrotum
Seminal vesicle
Testis
Ureter
Urethra
Urinary bladder

1. _____
2. _____
3. _____
4. _____
5. _____
6. _____
7. _____
8. _____
9. _____
10. _____
11. _____
12. _____
13. _____
14. _____
15. _____
16. _____
17. _____
18. _____

匹配

匹配下列术语，在每个题号的左侧写上适当的字母。

___ 1. gamete　　　　　　a. reproductive cell
___ 2. androgen　　　　　b. start of sexual maturity
___ 3. gonad　　　　　　c. hormone that produces male characteristics
___ 4. puberty　　　　　d. cell division that forms the gametes
___ 5. meiosis　　　　　e. sex gland

___ 6. vasectomy　　　　a. excision of the ductus deferens
___ 7. circumcision　　　b. erectile dysfunction
___ 8. impotence　　　　c. surgical removal of the foreskin
___ 9. glans　　　　　　d. end of the penis
___ 10. coitus　　　　　e. sexual intercourse

补充术语

___ 11. priapism　　　　a. narrowing of the foreskin opening
___ 12. phallic　　　　　b. prolonged erection of the penis
___ 13. genitalia　　　　c. tumor of the testis
___ 14. phimosis　　　　d. reproductive organs
___ 15. seminoma　　　　e. pertaining to the penis

___ 16. spermatocele　　a. inflammation of the glans penis
___ 17. balanitis　　　　b. a form of radiation treatment
___ 18. castration　　　c. discharge of semen
___ 19. emission　　　　d. removal of the testes
___ 20. brachytherapy　e. epididymal cyst

填空

21. The main male sex hormone is _____.
22. The two glands that secrete into the urethra just below the prostate gland are the _____.
23. The thick fluid that transports spermatozoa is _____.
24. The male gonad is the _____.
25. The channel through which the testis descends is the _____.
26. The sac that holds the testis is the _____.

定义

定义下列术语。

27. vasorrhaphy ［veiˈsɒrəphi］ _____
28. anorchism ［ænɔːrˈkizəm］ _____
29. oscheoma ［ˈɒstʃiːəʊmə］ _____
30. vesiculography ［vəˈsikjʊləgrəphi］ _____

31. prostatometer ［prɒsteiˈtəmitə］_____
32. hemospermia ［ˈheməzpəmiə］_____

写出下列定义的单词。

33. surgical fixation of the testis_____
34. stone in the scrotum_____
35. surgical incision of the epididymis_____
36. plastic repair of the scrotum_____
37. surgical creation of an opening between two parts of a cut ductus deferens (done to reverse a vasectomy)_____

在本章开头的 C.S. 案例研究中找出下列每个定义的单词（参见第 13 章）。

38. blood in the urine_____
39. painful urination_____
40. within the urinary bladder_____
41. overdevelopment of tissue_____
42. instrument for excising tissue_____

拼写检查

在下列术语右侧的下划线上写出正确的拼写。

43. testostirone_____
44. semin_____
45. prostrate_____
46. epididimis_____
47. hyospadias_____

真假判断

检查以下语句。如果语句为真，则在第一个空格处写上 T；如果语句为假，则在第一个空格中写上 F，并通过在第二个空格中替换带下划线的单词来更正语句。

	True or False	Correct Answer
48. Any male sex hormone is an androgen.	_____	_____
49. The adjective seminal refers to the seminal vesicle.	_____	_____
50. The spirochete Treponema pallidum causes syphilis.	_____	_____
51. Herpes simplex is a virus.	_____	_____
52. The ureter carries both urine and semen in males.	_____	_____
53. FSH and LH are produced by the pituitary gland.	_____	_____
54. Spermatogenesis begins at puberty.	_____	_____

排除

在下列每组中，为与其余不相配的单词加下划线，并解释你选择的理由。

55. bulbourethral gland — prostate — testis — spermatic cord — seminal vesicle
_____

56. FSH — semen — testosterone — androgen — LH

57. condyloma acuminatum — gonorrhea — hernia — AIDS — herpes

形容词

写出下列单词的形容词形式。

58. semen_____

59. prostate_____

60. penis_____

61. urethra_____

62. scrotum_____

缩略语

写出下列缩略语的含义。

63. BPH_____

64. STI_____

65. ED_____

66. GC_____

67. PSA_____

68. GU_____

69. TURP_____

跟随流程

描述精液流动的路径，通过在每个题号前的下划线填上字母 A 到 F，使下列每个步骤按正确次序排列。

____ **70.** ejaculatory duct delivers sperm to the urethra

____ **71.** sperm cells, mixed with other secretions, travel through the prostate gland

____ **72.** sperm cells mix with secretions from the seminal vesicle

____ **73.** sperm is propelled through ductus deferens

____ **74.** sperm cells are manufactured and stored in the epididymis

____ **75.** cells travel in the urethra through the penis to be released

单词构建

使用给出了单词组成部分写出下列定义的单词。

| -ar | -tomy | -graphy | -genesis | spermat/o | vas/o | -plasty | -itis | -ic | -cyte | -lysis | vesicul/o |

76. plastic repair of the ductus deferens _____

77. destruction of sperm cells _____

78. pertaining to the seminal vesicle _____

79. x-ray study of the vas deferens _____

80. inflammation of the seminal vesicle _____
81. pertaining to spermatozoa _____
82. cell that develops into a sperm cell _____
83. incision of the ductus deferens _____
84. formation of spermatozoa _____
85. radiographic study of the seminal vesicle _____

单词分析

定义下列单词，并给出每个单词组成部分的含义。如果需要，可以使用词典。

86. hydrocelectomy ［haidrəuse'lektəmi］ _____
    a. hydr/o_____
    b. -cele_____
    c. ecto_____
    d. tom/o_____
    e. -y_____

87. spermicidal ［ˌspɜ:mi'saidl］ _____
    a. sperm/i_____
    b. -cide_____
    c. -al_____

88. cryptorchidism ［krip'tɔ:kidizəm］ _____
    a. crypt_____
    b. orchid/o_____
    c. -ism_____

89. vasovesiculitis ［veisəuvesik'jʊlaitiz］ _____
    a. vas/o_____
    b. vesicul/o_____
    c. -itis_____

90. polyspermia ［pɒli'spɜ:mjə］ _____
    a. poly_____
    b. sperm/o_____
    c. –ia_____

Additional Case Studies
补充案例研究

Case Study 14-1: Herniorrhaphy and Vasectomy
案例研究 14-1：疝修补术和输精管结扎术

L. D., a 48-year-old married dock worker with three children, had inguinal bulging and pain on exertion when he lifted heavy objects. An occupational health service advised a surgical referral. The surgeon diagnosed L. D. with bilateral direct inguinal hernias and suggested that he not delay surgery, although he was not at high risk for a strangulated hernia. L. D. asked the surgeon if he could also be sterilized at the same time. He was scheduled for bilateral inguinal herniorrhaphy and elective vasectomy.

During the herniorrhaphy procedure, an oblique incision was made in each groin. The incision continued through the muscle layers by either resecting or splitting the muscle fibers. The spermatic vessels and vas deferens were identified, separated, and gently retracted. The spermatic cord was examined for an indirect hernia. Repair began with suturing the defect in the rectus abdominis muscles, transverse fascia, cremaster muscle, external oblique aponeurosis, and Scarpa fascia with heavy-gauge synthetic nonabsorbable suture material.

The vasectomy began with the identification of the vas deferens through the scrotal skin. An incision was made, and the vas was gently dissected and retracted through the opening. Each vas was clamped with a small hemostat, and a 1-cm length was resected. Both cut ends were coagulated with electrosurgery and tied independently with a fine-gauge absorbable suture material. The testicles were examined, and the scrotal incision was closed with an absorbable suture material.

L. D. 是一名 48 岁的已婚船坞工人，有 3 名子女。当他举重物时，腹股沟肿胀，劳累时疼痛。职业卫生服务机构建议外科转诊。外科医生诊断 L. D. 为双侧直接腹股沟疝（direct inguinal hernias），并建议他不要延迟手术，虽然他不是高风险的窒息性疝。L. D. 问外科医生是否也可以同时做绝育。他被安排进行双侧腹股沟疝修补术（herniorrhaphy）和选择性输精管切除术（vasectomy）。

在疝修补手术过程中，在每个腹股沟中做一个斜切口，切口通过切除或分裂肌肉纤维连续通过肌肉层。精索血管和输精管被识别、分离并轻轻地缩回。检查精索是否存在间接疝。修复开始于用大口径合成不可吸收缝合材料缝合腹直肌（rectus abdominis muscle）、腹横筋膜（transverse fascia）、提睾肌（cremaster muscle）、腹外斜肌腱膜（external oblique aponeurosis）和斯卡帕筋膜（Scarpa fascia）的损伤。

输精管切除术开始于通过阴囊皮肤鉴别输精管。切开一个切口，轻轻地切开输精管并通过开口缩回。用小止血钳夹住每个输精管，切除长度为 1cm。两个切割端用电外科手术凝固，并用细口径可吸收缝合材料独立扎结。检查睾丸，用可吸收缝合材料封闭阴囊切口。

Case Study 14-2: Erectile Dysfunction
案例研究 14-2：勃起功能障碍

R.G., a 67-year-old attorney, was at his annual appointment with his internist when he decided to discuss what he considered an embarrassing subject, erectile dysfunction (ED). R.G. was happily married with four grown children and had continued to enjoy an active sexual relationship with his wife, until recently. He was having difficulty sustaining an erection. He had seen so much media publicity on this subject that he decided to bring it up with his physician. At the conclusion of the appointment, the internist ruled out any psychogenic causes or adverse effects of medications, such as an antidepressant or an antihypertensive, that could predispose to ED. He recommended that R.G. schedule a follow-up visit to his urologist to make certain there were no underlying physical factors that would contribute to his impotence.

R.G. 是一名 67 岁的律师，当他决定讨论他认为令人尴尬的勃起功能障碍（erectile dysfunction，ED）时，他约见了他的内科医生。R.G. 婚姻幸福，有 4 个已成年的孩子，并与他的妻子一直享受积极的性生活，直到最近他难以维持勃起。他看到很多媒体宣传这个问题，他决定带着这个问题找他的医生。在约见结束时，内科医生排除了可能易患勃起功能障碍的任何心理原因或药物不良反应，例如抗抑郁药或抗高血压药。他建议 R.G. 安排随后约见他的泌尿科医生，以确定没有引起阳痿的潜在身体因素。

R. G. made an appointment with the urologist whom he had seen about 10 years ago when he was diagnosed with BPH. At that time, the physician had reviewed various therapies with R. G., so R.G. felt comfortable discussing his present concerns.

The urologist's examination ruled out trauma, vascular disorders, or tumors. It was decided to have R.G. try an ED medication. The physician explained that the impotence agents work by targeting the physiologic mechanisms of erection. They promote vasodilation to increase blood flow to the penis. Side effects of the medications were also discussed. R. G was relieved that he had no tumor or other disease condition. He understood the therapy plan and left with follow-up instructions.

R. G. 预约了在 10 年前为他诊断出良性前列腺增生的泌尿科医生。当时，那位医生已经为 R. G. 评估了各种疗法，所以与他讨论目前关注的问题，R. G. 感到很舒服。

泌尿科医生的检查排除了创伤、血管疾病或肿瘤。他决定让 R. G. 尝试使用治疗勃起功能障碍的药物。医生解释了阳痿药物针对勃起的生理机制的作用原理，这些药物能够促进血管舒张，增加血液流向阴茎，还讨论了药物的不良反应。由于没有肿瘤或其他疾病状况，R.G 放松了许多。他了解了治疗计划，带着后续的指导信息离开了。

案例研究问题

多项选择。选择正确的答案，在每个题号的左侧写出你选择的字母。

_____ 1. The term for male sterilization surgery is

    a. herniorrhaphy

    b. circumcision

    c. vagotomy

    d. vasectomy

_____ 2. An oblique surgical incision follows which direction?

    a. slanted or angled

    b. superior to inferior

    c. lateral

    d. circumferential

_____ 3. When the ends of the vas were coagulated with electrosurgery, they were

    a. dilated

    b. sealed

    c. sutured

    d. clamped

_____ 4. A urologist is a physician who treats health and disease conditions of the

    a. male reproductive system

    b. urinary system

    c. digestive system

    d. a and b

_____ 5. Impotence is a condition that

    a. precedes a vasectomy

    b. is synonymous with ED

    c. refers to the inability to maintain penile erection

    d. b and c

_____ 6. BPH is a condition of the prostate gland that

    a. is cancerous

    b. causes impotence

    c. requires vasodilation agents as treatment

    d. may cause urinary retention and infection

_____ 7. The ED drugs Viagra and Cialis target the physiologic mechanisms of erection by

    a. increasing urinary and semen flow

    b. dilating arteries in the penis to increase blood flow

    c. increasing neurotransmitters to treat underlying psychogenic causes

    d. b and c

写出案例研究中下列含义的术语。

8. surgical repair of a weak abdominal muscle in the groin area on both sides_____

9. entrapment of a bowel loop in a hernia_____

10. inflammation of the glans penis_____

11. narrowing of the distal opening of the foreskin_____

12. originating in the mind_____

13. widening of blood vessels_____

14. drug for treatment of high blood pressure_____

CHAPTER 15

女性生殖系统、妊娠与分娩

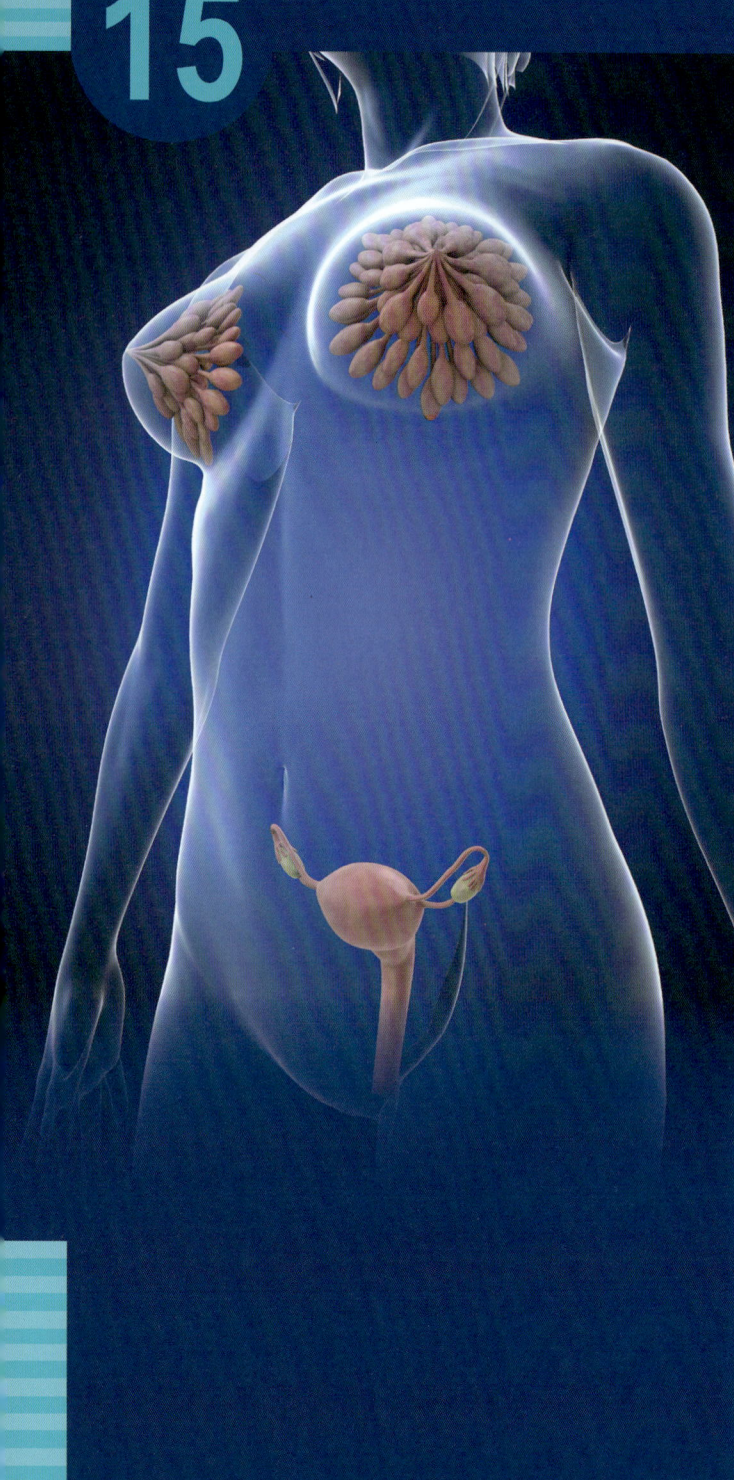

▶ 预测试

多项选择，选择正确的答案，并在每个题号左侧写出你选择的字母。

_____ 1. The female gonad is the
   a. uterus
   b. cervix
   c. ovary
   d. testis

_____ 2. The two ovarian hormones are
   a. testosterone and estrogen
   b. estrogen and progesterone
   c. thyroxine and progesterone
   d. progesterone and testosterone

_____ 3. Use of artificial methods to prevent fertilization is termed
   a. antiception
   b. coitus
   c. contraception
   d. gestation

_____ 4. During the first two months of growth, the developing offspring is called a(n)
   a. neonate
   b. embryo
   c. zygote
   d. fetus

_____ 5. The structure that nourishes the developing fetus is the
   a. mammary gland
   b. cervix
   c. placenta
   d. follicle

_____ 6. Production of milk is technically called
   a. ovulation
   b. lactation
   c. corpus luteum
   d. parturition

_____ 7. The roots metr/o and hyster/o mean
   a. uterus
   b. vagina
   c. follicle
   d. ovary

_____ 8. Any disorder present at birth is described as
   a. hereditary
   b. genetic
   c. congenital
   d. familial

学习目标

学完本章后，应该能够：

1 ▶ 描述女性生殖道，并给出每个部位的功能。
2 ▶ 描述乳腺的构造和功能。
3 ▶ 概述月经周期中的各项事件。
4 ▶ 列出四种避孕方法，并给出示例。
5 ▶ 描述女性生殖系统的 7 种疾病。
6 ▶ 概述在受孕后前 2 个月中发生的事件。
7 ▶ 描述胎盘的结构和功能。
8 ▶ 描述胎儿循环的两种适应性改变，并给出它们的目的。
9 ▶ 描述分娩的 3 个阶段。
10 ▶ 列出乳汁分泌的激素和神经控制。
11 ▶ 识别并使用与女性生殖系统、妊娠和分娩相关的词根。
12 ▶ 描述妊娠与分娩的 6 种疾病。
13 ▶ 定义两类先天性疾病，并给出示例。
14 ▶ 解释女性生殖系统相关的缩略语。
15 ▶ 分析几个案例研究中与女性生殖系统、妊娠和分娩相关的医学术语。

Case Study: A. Y.'s Cesarean Section
案例研究：A. Y. 的剖腹产

Chief Complaint

A. Y. is a 29-year-old gravida 2, para 1, at 39 weeks of gestation. Her first pregnancy resulted in a cesarean section. She had had an uneventful pregnancy with good health, moderate weight gain, good fetal heart sounds, and no signs or symptoms of pregnancy-induced hypertension. A.Y. went to the hospital when she realized she was going into labor.

Examination

A. Y. had been in active labor for several hours, fully effaced and dilated, yet unable to progress. Her obstetrician ordered an x-ray pelvimetry test that revealed CPD (cephalopelvic disproportion) with the fetus in the right occiput posterior position. Changes in fetal heart rate indicated fetal distress. A.Y. was transported to the OR for an emergency C-section under spinal anesthesia.

Clinical Course

After being placed in the supine position, A. Y. had a urethral catheter inserted, and her abdomen was prepped with antimicrobial solution. After draping, a transverse suprapubic incision was made. Dissection was continued through the muscle layers to the uterus, with care not to nick the bladder. The uterus was incised through the lower segment, 2 cm from the bladder. The fetal head was gently elevated through the incision while the assistant put gentle pressure on the fundus. The baby's mouth and nose were suctioned with a bulb syringe, and the umbilical cord was clamped and cut. The baby was handed off to an attending pediatrician and OB nurse and placed in a radiant neonate warmer bed. The Apgar score was 9/9. The placenta was gently delivered from the uterus, and the scrub nurse checked for three vessels and filled two sterile test tubes with cord blood for laboratory analysis. A. Y. was given an injection of Pitocin to stimulate uterine contraction. The uterus and abdomen were closed, and A. Y. was transported to the PACU (postanesthesia care unit).

主诉

A.Y. 是一名 29 岁的第 2 次怀孕的孕妇，已经分娩 1 次，现在是妊娠的 39 周。她的第一次怀孕是剖腹产。她健康状况良好，体重适度增加，胎音良好，没有妊娠期高血压综合征的体征或症状，孕期平静。当 A.Y. 意识到要分娩时，她去了医院。

检查

A. Y. 已经努力分娩了几个小时，子宫口已充分扩张，但依然没有进展。她的产科医生指示进行 X 线透光率检查，显示 CPD（头盆不称）和胎儿右枕骨后位，胎儿心率的变化表明胎儿窘迫。A.Y. 在脊髓麻醉下运送到手术室的 C 段。

临床病程

置于仰卧位后，A. Y. 被插入尿管，腹部用抗微生物溶液准备。在覆盖后，行横向的耻骨上切口，通过肌肉层到子宫继续切开，并小心地避免切破膀胱。子宫通过下段被切开，距膀胱 2cm。胎儿头部被通过切口轻轻地升高，助手对子宫底施加轻微的压力。婴儿的口和鼻用球形注射器抽吸，夹紧并切割脐带。婴儿被转交给一名儿科主治医生和手术室护士，并放置在一个发热的新生儿暖床上，Apgar 评分为 9/9。胎盘从子宫轻轻取出，手术助理护士检查 3 个血管，并用脐带血填充两个无菌试管用于实验室分析。A. Y. 被给予催产素注射以刺激子宫收缩。子宫和腹部关闭，A. Y. 被运送到 PACU（麻醉后护理病房）。

简介

与男性一样，女性的生殖系统也由内部器官和外生殖器构成。尽管乳房（breast），或乳腺（mammary gland）不是生殖系统的组成部分，但也在该系统中进行讨论，因为其功能是为婴儿提供营养。

与男性连续产生配子不同，女性配子的形成是周期性的，每个月经周期（menstrual cycle）释放一个卵子。每个月，子宫（uterus）都准备好接受一个受精卵（fertilized egg）。如果发生受精，发育中的后代将由胎盘（placenta）提供营养和保护，并由液体包围，直至出生。如果释放的卵子没有受精，子宫内壁会在月经（menstruation）期间脱落。

女性生殖系统

卵巢

雌性性腺是一对卵巢（ovary），由盆腔内的韧带固定在子宫的两侧（图15-1）。女性的配子，卵子（egg）或卵细胞（ovum，复数形式为ova）在卵巢中发育。

每个月会有几个卵细胞成熟，每个卵细胞都处于一个被称为卵泡（ovarian follicle）的细胞簇中。在排卵（ovulation）时，通常只有一个卵细胞被从卵巢释放，其余的成熟卵细胞则会退化。卵泡会留下来继续执行其功能，如果卵子未受精，卵泡会保留大约2周；如果受精，则保留大约2个月。

输卵管、子宫和阴道

排卵后，卵子进入输卵管（uterine tube，也常用fallopian tube或oviduct），输卵管附着于子宫的上侧部（图15-1）。输卵管在子宫之上呈拱形，有被称为伞毛（fimbriae）的手指状突起，将从卵巢中释放出的卵子扫入输卵管。

子宫是为发育中的后代提供营养的器官。子宫呈梨形，上部是圆的基底，中间是一个三角形的腔体，下面是狭窄的子宫颈（cervix），子宫颈突入阴道（vagina）。在上阴道子宫颈周围的凹处是穹隆（fornix）。在宫颈后壁，腹膜向下倾斜形成一个盲袋，

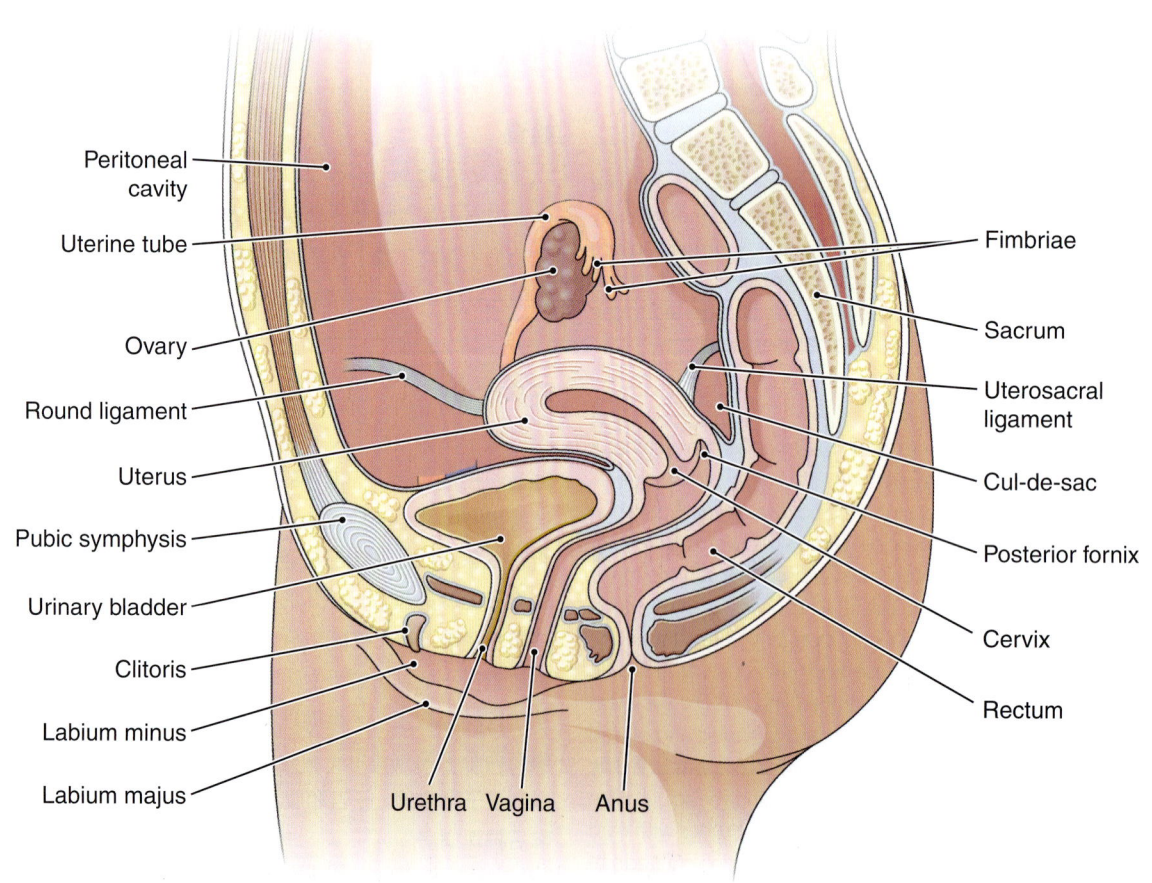

图15-1 **女性生殖系统。** 图中所示为生殖系统和一些相邻结构在一起的矢状截面

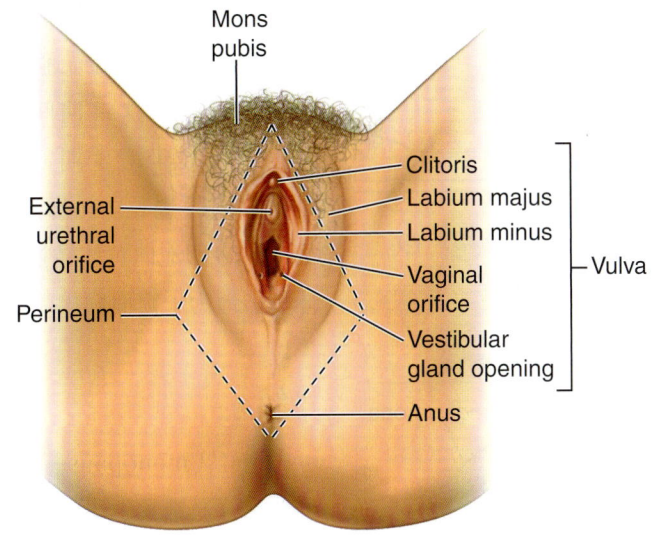

图 15-2 女性外生殖器。外阴与附近的结构和会阴的轮廓一起示出，会阴从阴道延伸至肛门

是腹腔的最低点。

子宫壁的最内层子宫内膜（endometrium）供血丰富，在怀孕期间，它接受受精卵并成为胎盘的一部分。如果没有发生受精，子宫内膜会在月经期脱落。子宫壁的肌肉层是子宫肌层（myometrium）。

阴道是一个肌肉管道，在性交期间接受阴茎，还用作产道，并输送月经流出体外（图15-1）。

外生殖器官

女性所有外生殖器官统称为外阴（vulva）（图15-2），包括外部的大阴唇（labium majus）和包围阴道和尿道开口的内部小阴唇（labium minus）。尿道开口前面的阴蒂（clitoris）起源上类似于阴茎，并对性刺激有反应。

男性和女性大腿之间从外生殖器官到肛门之间的区域被称为会阴（perineum）。在分娩时，可能会在阴道和肛门之间做一个切口，以便于生产并避免组织撕裂，这一方法被称为外阴切开术（episiotomy）。这一方法实际上是会阴切开术（perineotomy），因为词根 episi/o 意为"外阴"。

乳腺

乳腺，或乳房主要由腺体组织和脂肪构成（图15-3），它们的功能是为新生儿提供营养。乳腺分泌的人奶通过导管输送到乳头（nipple）。

月经周期

女性的生殖活动开始于青春期初潮（menarche），也就是第一次月经。每个月的月经周期由来自于脑垂体前叶的激素控制，男性的生殖活动也受该激素的控制。

促卵泡激素（follicle-stimulating hormone，FSH）通过引起粒细胞成熟进入卵泡（图15-4）开始月经周期。卵泡分泌雌性激素，雌性激素启动子宫内膜发育准备接受受精卵。

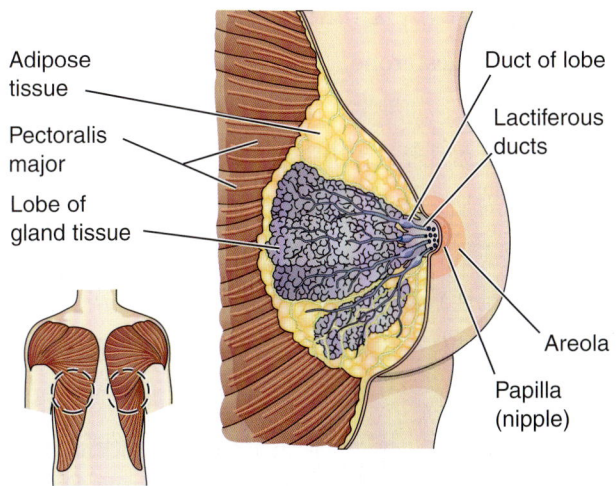

图 15-3 乳房截面

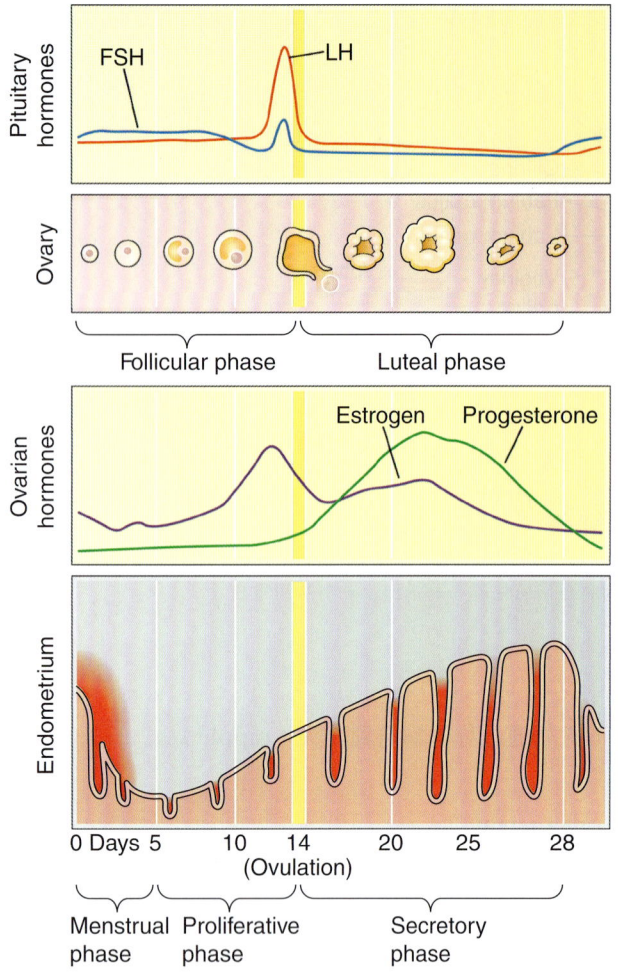

一个月经周期进程中卵巢和子宫发生的同步变化。排卵之前的时间被描述为卵巢的卵泡期（follicular phase），因为这一期间包含卵泡的发育。这一期间的子宫处于增生期（proliferative phase），标志是子宫内膜生长。排卵后，卵巢处于黄体期（luteal phase），卵泡向黄体转换。子宫则处于分泌期，其腺体积极地为子宫内膜接受可能的受精卵植入做准备。

绝经

绝经（menopause）就是每个月的月经周期不再继续，这通常发生于 45~55 岁。生殖激素水平下降，卵巢逐渐退化。一些女性会经历不愉快的综合征，例如潮热（hot flash）、头痛、失眠（insomnia）、情绪波动和泌尿系统问题，还有些人生殖道萎缩，阴道干燥。最重要的是，雌性激素水平的下降会伴随骨质疏松（osteoporosis）。

医生可能采用激素替代疗法（hormone replacement therapy，HRT）来减轻绝经综合征。这种治疗通常要服用雌性激素和黄体酮（progestin），以尽量降低子宫内膜癌症的风险。雌性激素替代能够减轻随年龄增长出现的骨质疏松。不过，对激素替代疗法安全性的关注，已经引起在绝经早期使用该疗法的重新考虑。对最广泛使用的激素替代疗法的研究显示，延长使用该疗法会增加子宫内膜癌、乳腺癌、心脏病和血栓的风险。对激素替代疗法安全性以及为没有子宫的女性单独使用雌性激素的研究还在继续。

除激素替代疗法以外，抗抑郁药物和维生素 E 也能够帮助减轻绝经综合征，局部使用雌性激素和湿润剂能够减轻阴道干燥。如果需要，还可以使用非激素的增加骨密度的药物。锻炼和有足够钙含量的平衡饮食对保持健康非常重要。

图 15-4 乳房截面。月经周期。图中显示了在平均 28 天的月经周期内垂体和卵巢激素、卵巢以及子宫的变化，在第 14 天有排卵。卵巢中的不同阶段被命名为卵泡发育阶段和黄体形成阶段。子宫中的阶段是根据子宫内膜的变化命名的

第二垂体激素是促黄体生成素（luteinizing hormone，LH），触发排卵和卵泡向黄体（corpus luteum）的转变。这个结构位于卵巢的左后侧，分泌孕激素（progesterone）和雌性激素，进一步促进子宫内膜的生长。如果没有发生受精，激素水平会下降，子宫内膜会在月经过程中脱落。

月经周期平均是 28 天，月经的第 1 天作为月经周期的第 1 天，排卵大约发生在第 14 天。在整个月经周期，雌性激素和孕激素向脑垂体反馈以调节促卵泡激素和促黄体生成素的产生。激素避孕法通过提供雌性激素和孕激素，抑制脑垂体释放促卵泡激素和促黄体生成素，阻止排卵，但不干扰月经。撤销激素之后的月经周期是无卵的，即没有月经之前的排卵。

图 15-4 显示了在脑垂体和排卵激素影响下的

避孕

避孕（contraception）是使用人工手段防止卵子受精或受精卵在子宫着床。临时性避孕方法的功能为：

- 阻止精子进入子宫（例如避孕套和隔膜）。
- 防止受精卵着床（例如子宫内避孕器）。
- 防止排卵（例如激素）。激素的使用方法在剂量和给药途径上有所不同，例如口服、注射、

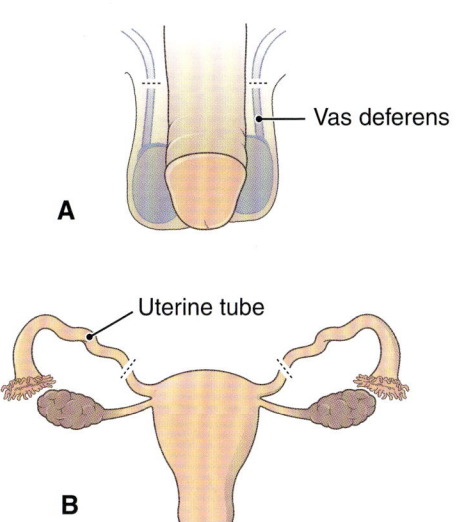

图 15-5 绝育。A. 输精管切除术。B. 输卵管结扎术

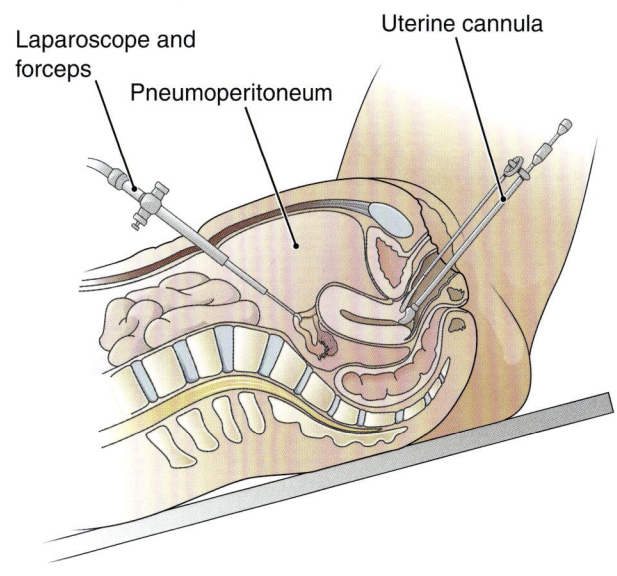

图 15-6 腹腔镜绝育。腹膜腔充气（气腹），并通过小切口用腹腔镜切开输卵管

皮贴和阴道环。

所谓的事后避孕药（morning-after pill）旨在用于紧急避孕，在无保护性交 72 小时内服用能够大大降低怀孕（pregnancy）的机率。一种名为"B 计划"的产品包含 2 剂隔 12 小时服用的黄体酮。

手术绝育能够提供最有效，而且通常是永久的避孕。在男性，就是输精管切除术；在女性，就是输卵管结扎术（tubal ligation），两侧的输卵管被切开并结扎（图 15-5）。执行输卵管结扎术的优选方法是通过腹壁的腹腔镜手术（图 15-6）。

除美国以外的其他国家，RU486（米非司酮，mifepristone）被更多地用于避孕。它通过阻断孕激素，引起子宫内膜分解来终止早期怀孕。从技术上讲，RU486 是引发流产的药物（abortifacient），而不是避孕药物。框 15-1 给出了当前使用的主要避孕方法。每种方法都有优点和缺点，根据有效性排序。请注意，只有男性和女性避孕套能够预防性传播疾病的扩散。

框 15-1 供你参考：目前使用的主要避孕方法

方法	说明
手术	
vasectomy/tubal ligation 输精管切除术/输卵管结扎术	切开并结扎输送配子的管道
激素	
birth control pills 避孕药	雌性激素和黄体酮或者单独口服黄体酮以避免排卵
birth control shot 避孕针	每 3 周注射一次人工合成孕激素，以避免排卵
birth control patch 避孕贴	贴在身体上通过皮肤使用雌性激素和黄体酮的粘贴；贴 3 周，第 4 周取下

框 15-1

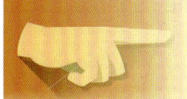

供你参考

目前使用的主要避孕方法

birth control ring 避孕环	插入阴道从内部释放激素的柔韧的环；放置 3 周，第 4 周取出
阻隔	
condom 避孕套	阻止精子接触卵子的套。男性避孕套套在勃起的阴茎上，女性避孕套放入阴道并盖住子宫颈
diaphragm (with spermicide) 隔膜（带杀精剂）	盖住子宫颈的橡胶帽，防止精子进入
contraceptive sponge(with spermicide) 避孕海绵（带杀精剂）	柔软的、包含杀精剂的一次性发泡盘，用水湿润后插入阴道
intrauterine device (IUD) 宫内避孕器	通过阴道插入子宫的金属或塑料装置；通过释放铜或避孕激素防止受精和着床
其他	
spermicide 杀精剂	用于杀死精子的化学物质，最好与阻隔方法一起使用
fertility awareness 安全期避孕	根据月经史、基础体温或宫颈黏液的性质确定月经周期中可能受孕的时间段，在此期间禁欲

Terminology 关键术语

女性生殖系统

正常结构与功能

cervix ［'sɜːviks］	子宫颈，通常指子宫下部狭窄的部分（词根：cervic/o）；也常用 cervix uteri
clitoris ［'klɪtərɪs］	阴蒂，尿道开口前的小的可勃起的组织体，起源上类似于阴茎（词根：clitor/o, clitorid/o）
contraception ［ˌkɒntrə'sepʃn］	避孕，防止怀孕
corpus luteum ［'luːtiːəm］	黄体，卵泡在排卵后发育成的小的黄色结构，能够分泌孕激素和雌性激素
culdesac ［'kʌl də sæk］	陷凹，盲袋，例如直肠与子宫直接的陷凹；直肠子宫陷凹（rectouterine pouch，图 15-1）
endometrium ［ˌendəʊ'miːtriəm］	子宫内膜，子宫内壁
estrogen ［'iːstrədʒən］	雌性激素，产生女性特征并为子宫接受受精卵做准备的一组激素。最活跃的是雌二醇（estradiol）
fallopian tube ［fə'lɒpeən］	输卵管，参见 uterine tube
fimbria ［'fɪmbrɪə］	伞毛，输卵管的手指形扩展，其波动能够捕获被释放的卵子（图 15-1）（复数形式为 fimbriae）

Terminology 关键术语（续表）

follicle-stimulating hormone (FSH)	促卵泡生成素，脑垂体前叶分泌的一种作用于性腺的激素。在女性，它刺激卵子在卵巢中成熟
fornix ['fɔːniks]	穹隆，一个拱形空间，例如阴道的最上壁与子宫颈直接的空间（图 15-1）；源自于拉丁语意为"拱"
labium majus ['leibiəm mə'dʒəs]	大阴唇，形成外阴两侧的大的皮肤褶皱（词根：labi/o 意为"唇"，复数形式为 labia majora）
labium minus ['leibiəm 'mainəs]	小阴唇，大阴唇内侧的小皮肤褶皱（复数形式为 labia minora）
luteinizing hormone (LH) ['luːtiːəˌnaiziŋ]	促黄体生成素，脑垂体前叶分泌的一种作用于性腺的激素。在女性，它刺激排卵和黄体的形成
mammary gland ['mæməri]	乳腺，女性能够分泌乳汁的特殊腺体（词根：mamm/o, mast/o）；也常用 breast
menarche [mə'nɑːkiː]	初潮，第一个月经期，通常发生于青春期
menopause ['menəpɔːz]	绝经，女性月经周期停止
menstruation [ˌmenstru'eiʃn]	月经，周期性排泄血液和未怀孕子宫内壁的黏膜组织（词根：men/o, mens）；也常用 menstrual period 和 menses
myometrium [maiə'metriəm]	子宫肌层，子宫的肌肉壁
ovarian follicle [əʊˈveəriːən ˈfɔlikəl]	卵泡，卵子在其中成熟的一簇细胞
ovary ['əʊvəri]	卵巢，女性性腺（词根：ovari/o, oophor/o）
ovulation [ˌɒvjʊ'leiʃn]	排卵，从卵巢释放成熟的卵子（源自于 ovule，意为"小蛋"）
ovum ['əʊvəm]	卵子、卵细胞，女性配子或生殖细胞（词根：oo, ov/o，复数形式为 ova）
perineum [ˌperi'niːəm]	会阴，人腿之间从外生殖器到肛门的区域（词根：perine/o）
progesterone [prə'dʒestərəʊn]	黄体酮，黄体和胎盘分泌的一种激素，在怀孕期供养子宫内膜
tubal ligation ['tjuːbl lai'geiʃən]	输卵管结扎术，手术堵塞输卵管以到达绝育（图 15-5 和 15-6）
uterine tube ['juːtərain]	输卵管，从子宫上侧部延伸出来的管道，将卵子输送到子宫（词根：salping/o）。也被称为 fallopian tube 或 oviduct
uterus ['juːtərəs]	子宫，接受受精卵并在怀孕期间维持后代发育的器官（词根：uter/o, metr, hyster/o，框 15-2）
vagina [və'dʒainə]	阴道，子宫颈至外阴直接的肌肉管道（词根：vagin/o, colp/o）
vulva ['vʌlvə]	外阴，女性外生殖器官（词根：vulv/o, episi/o）

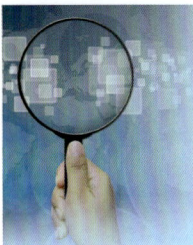

框 15-2 聚焦单词
疯狂的想法

在了解子宫词根 hyster/o 的起源时，大多数女性都会感到震惊。它源自于单词 hysterical（癔病的）和 hysterics（歇斯底里），词根相同，而且是基于一个非常古老的信念——女性的精神障碍源自于子宫。

疑病症患者是那些怀疑自己有想象中的疾病的人，单词 hypochondriac（疑病症患者）的起源也是有与上面类似的历史。hypochondriac 起源于腹部的上部，古人相信那里是精神障碍的所在地。

与女性生殖系统相关的单词组成部分

参见表 15-1 至 15-3。

表 15-1　女性生殖系统和卵巢的词根

词根	含义	示例	示例定义
gyn/o, gynec/o	女性	gynecology [ˌgaini'kɒlədʒi]	妇科学
men/o, mens	月亮、月经	premenstrual [ˌpriːˈmenstruəl]	经前期
oo	卵子	oocyte ['əʊəsait]	卵母细胞
ov/o, ovul/o	卵子	anovulatory [ænɒvjʊ'lətəri]	无排卵
ovari/o	卵巢	ovariopexy [əʊværiːəʊ'peksi]	卵巢固定术
oophor/o	卵巢	oophorectomy [ˌəʊəfə'rektəmi]	卵巢切除术

练习 15-1

定义下列单词。

1. gynecopathy [ˌdʒinə'kɒpəθi] _____
2. intermenstrual [intə(ː)'menstruəl] _____
3. oogenesis [ˌəʊə'dʒenisis] _____
4. ovulation [ˌɒvjʊ'leiʃn] _____
5. ovarian [əʊ'veəriən] _____
6. oophoritis [ˌəʊəfə'raitis] _____

练习 15-1 （续表）

写出下列定义的单词。

7. rupture (-rhexis) of an ovary _____
8. pertaining to ovulation _____
9. profuse bleeding (-hagia) at the time of menstruation _____

单词 menorrhea 意为"月经"。在 menorrhea 上加一个前缀构成下列定义的单词。

10. scanty menstrual flow _____
11. absence of menstruation _____
12. painful or difficult menstruation _____

使用词根 ovari/o 写出下列单词。

13. incision into an ovary _____
14. surgical puncture of an ovary _____
15. hernia of an ovary _____

使用词根 oophor/o 写出下列单词。

16. surgical repair of an ovary _____
17. malignant tumor of the ovary _____

表 15-2　输卵管、子宫和阴道的词根

词根	含义	示例	示例定义
salping/o	输卵管	salpingoplasty ［sælpingəʊpˈlæsti］	输卵管成形术
uter/o	子宫	intrauterine ［ˌɪntrəˈjuːtəraɪn］	宫内
metr/o, metr/i	子宫	metrorrhea ［metrɒˈriə］	子宫漏
hyster/o	子宫	hysterotomy ［ˈhɪstəˈrɒtəmi］	子宫切开术
cervic/o	子宫颈	endocervical ［endəʊˈsɜːvaɪkl］	子宫颈内的
vagin/o	阴道	vaginometer ［ˈvædʒɪnəmɪtə］	阴道测量器
colp/o	阴道	colpostenosis ［kɒlpɒsteˈnəʊsɪs］	阴道狭窄

练习 15-2

定义下列单词。

1. hysterography
   [histə'rɒgrəfi] _____

2. metromalacia
   [metrəumə'leiʃə] _____

3. vaginoplasty
   [vædʒinɒp'læsti] _____

4. colpodynia
   ['kɒlpədiniə] _____

5. salpingectomy
   [ˌsælpin'dʒektəmi] _____

6. uterovesical
   [juːtəəʊ'vesikəl] _____

7. intracervical
   [intrei'sɜːvaikl] _____

写出下列单词。

8. surgical fixation of a uterine tube _____
9. radiographic study of the uterine tube _____

词根 salping/o 来自于意为"管"的单词 salpinx。在 salpinx 上加一个前缀写出下列单词。

10. collection of fluid in a uterine tube _____
11. presence of pus in a uterine tube _____

请注意词根 salping/o 和 oophor/o 是如何组成 salpingo-oophoritis（输卵管和卵巢炎）的。写出下列单词。

12. surgical removal of a uterine tube and ovary _____

使用给出的词根写出下列单词。

13. surgical fixation of the uterus (hyster/o) _____
14. pertaining to the uterus (uter/o) _____
15. narrowing of the uterus (metr/o) _____
16. radiograph of the uterus (hyster/o) and uterine tubes _____
17. through the cervix _____
18. prolapse of the uterus (metr/o) _____
19. hernia of the vagina (colp/o) _____
20. inflammation of the vagina (vagin/o) _____

表 15-3　女性附属结构的词根

词根	含义	示例	示例定义
vulv/o	外阴	vulvar ['vʌlvə]	外阴的
episi/o	外阴	episiotomy [iˌpi:si'ɒtəmi]	外阴切开术
perine/o	会阴	perineal [peri'ni:əl]	会阴的
clitor/o, clitorid/o	阴蒂	clitorectomy [klitɔ':ektəmi]	阴蒂切除术
mamm/o	乳房、乳腺	mammoplasty ['mæməplæsti]	乳房成形术
mast/o	乳房、乳腺	amastia [ə'mɑ:stiə]	无乳房

练习 15-3

写出下列单词。

1. excision of the vulva (vulv/o)
2. suture of the vulva (episi/o)
3. pertaining to the vagina (vagin/o) and perineum
4. enlargement of the clitoris
5. radiographic record of the breast (mamm/o)
6. inflammation of the breast (mast/o)
7. excision of the breast

女性生殖系统的临床表现

感染

框 14-2 给出了引起男性和女性性传播感染的主要微生物。

生殖器疱疹（genital herpes）影响了超过 25% 的美国成年人，目前无法治愈。一旦发生感染，病毒将在神经系统中生存，引起断断续续的发病，包括生殖器疼痛、瘙痒、灼痛和排尿问题。病毒很容易在性伴侣之间扩散，即使他们没有疾病的活动体征。怀孕的妇女会在分娩期间将病毒传染给婴儿，可能导致残疾，甚至死亡。基本的卫生习惯和使用安全套能够减少病毒的扩散。

能够感染外阴和阴道的真菌是白色念珠菌（candida albicans），会引起念珠菌病（candidiasis）。所致的阴道炎（vaginitis）会引起瘙痒，并排出浓稠、白色、乳酪样的分泌物。怀孕、糖尿病和服用抗生素、类固醇或避孕药都易患此感染。如果感染反复发作，患者的伴侣应接受治疗，以预防再感染。治疗需要使用抗真菌药物（mycostatics）。

盆腔炎（pelvic inflammatory disease，PID）是从生殖器官扩散到盆腔的感染，最常见的是由淋病衣原体（chlamydia）所致，但在条件适当时，生存在生殖道的细菌也可能引起感染。盆腔炎是一种很严重的疾病，可能导致败血症（septicemia）或休克。输卵管炎（salpingitis）会封闭输卵管，并引起不育（infertility）。

子宫肌瘤

子宫肌瘤（fibroid）是良性的平滑肌肿瘤，通常发生于子宫肌层（myometrium，图 15-7）。这种肿

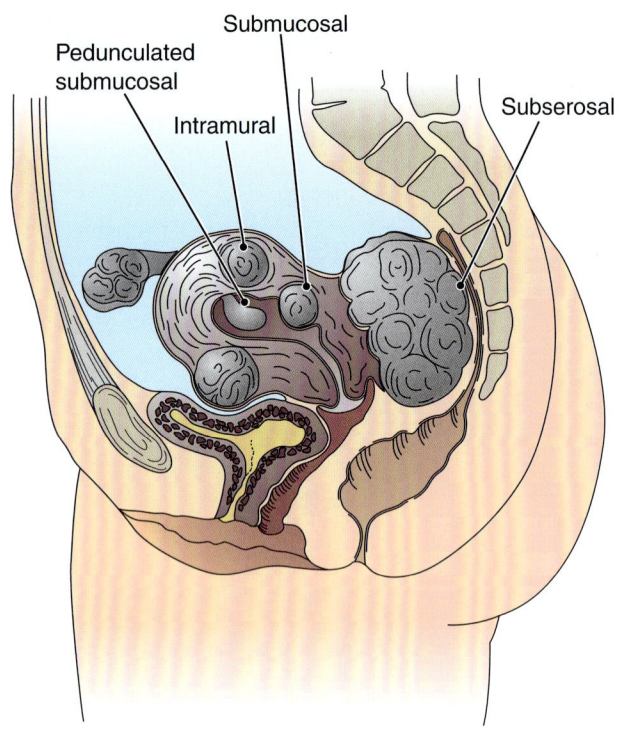

图 15-7 子宫平滑肌瘤（子宫肌瘤）。图中示出了各种可能的位置。它们可以在子宫壁内（intramural）、黏膜下（submucosal）、在茎上（pedunculated）或外部浆膜下（subserosal）。图中显示一个肿瘤压迫膀胱，另一个肿瘤压迫直肠

瘤在技术上被称为平滑肌瘤（leiomyoma），是最常见的子宫病症之一，通常没有症状，也不需要治疗。不过，子宫肌瘤可能引起月经大出血（menorrhagia）和直肠或膀胱压力。治疗包括：

- 抑制刺激子宫肌瘤生长的激素。
- 手术切除子宫肌瘤（myomectomy）。
- 手术切除子宫（hysterectomy）。
- 子宫肌瘤栓塞术（uterine fibroid embolization，UFE），减少子宫切除术的使用。经过特殊训练的放射科医生使用一个插管或在子宫动脉注射少量合成颗粒。这些颗粒会阻止对子宫肌瘤的供血，使其收缩。

子宫内膜异位症

子宫内膜组织在子宫外生长被称为子宫内膜异位症。通常会涉及卵巢、输卵管、腹膜和其他盆腔器官（图 15-8）。受正常激素的刺激，子宫内膜组织会引起炎症、子宫肌瘤和周围区域的粘连，导致疼痛、痛经（dysmenorrhea）和不育。腹腔镜检查（laparoscopy）被用于诊断子宫内膜异位，也被用于切除异常组织。

月经失调

月经异常包括月经流量太少（oligomenorrhea）或太多（menorrhagia）和闭经（amenorrhea）。痛经（dysmenorrhea）通常发生在月经的开始，并持续 1~2 天。这些病症被统称为功能失调性子宫出血（dysfunctional uterine bleeding，DUB）。这些病症可能是激素失衡、全身性疾病或子宫疾病引起的，

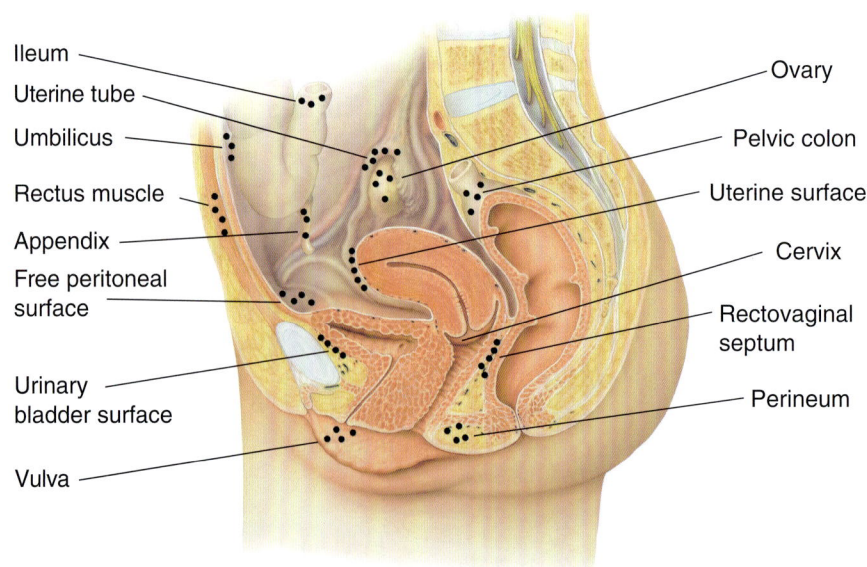

图 15-8 子宫内膜异位症。子宫内膜组织几乎可以在子宫外腹膜腔内的任何地方生长，引起炎症和其他并发症

最常见于青春期或接近更年期。在其他时间段，则通常与生活变化和情绪紧张相关。

经前期综合征（premenstrual syndrome，PMS）是在月经周期后半段出现的症状，包括情绪变化、疲劳、腹胀、头痛和食欲变化。经前期综合征的起因尚在研究之中，通过激素治疗、抗抑郁药物或抗焦虑药物可以缓解症状，锻炼、饮食控制、休息和放松也有帮助。避免接触咖啡因，服用维生素 E 可能减轻乳房疼痛，还应该喝足够的水，并限制盐的摄入。

多囊卵巢综合征

在这里讨论多囊卵巢综合征（polycystic ovarian syndrome，PCOS）是因为这种病症最先被描述的症状是卵巢增大，并有多个囊肿。尽管卵巢会显示出异常，但这些体征并不一定出现于多囊卵巢综合征。多囊卵巢综合征是一种内分泌疾病，涉及雄性激素和雌性激素升高感染脑垂体促卵泡激素和促黄体生成素的正常分泌。其影响包括：

- 停止排卵和不育。
- 月经流量太少或闭经。
- 多毛症（hirsutism），过量雄性激素所致。
- 胰岛素抵抗，导致糖尿病。
- 肥胖。

多囊卵巢综合征治疗需要使用激素调节激素失衡，用药物提高对胰岛素的响应，降低体重（雌性激素在脂肪组织中产生），有时需要切除部分卵巢。

女性生殖道的癌症

子宫内膜癌

子宫内膜癌是女性生殖道最常见的癌症。有风险的女性应当定期做活组织检查，因为子宫内膜癌并不总是能够通过简单的组织测试巴氏涂片（papanicolaou smear）检测出来。治疗包括子宫切除术（hysterectomy，图 15-9）和放疗。

小部分病例发生在子宫内膜增生（hyperplasia）之后。增生的组织可以通过刮宫术（dilation and curettage，D&C）切除，在刮宫术过程中，子宫颈被扩张，子宫内壁被用刮匙刮削。

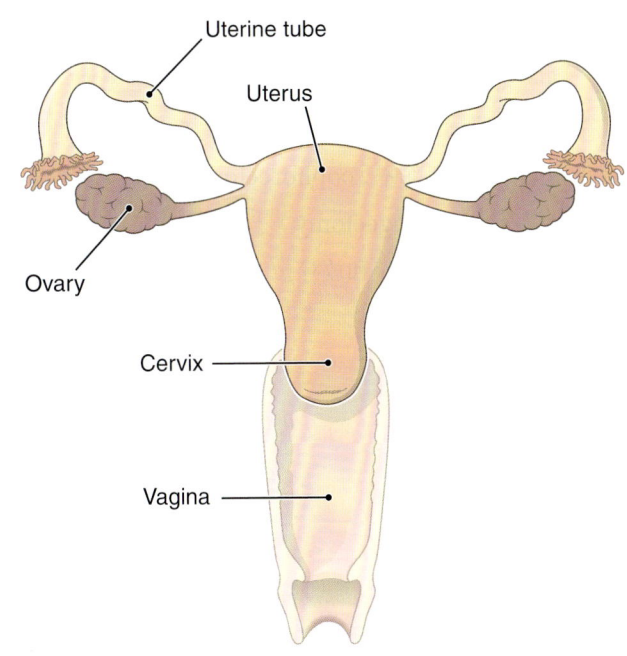

图 15-9 子宫切除术。子宫切除术（hysterectomy）是手术切除子宫。切除卵巢（oophorectomy）和子宫管（salpingectomy）可以是单侧或双侧

宫颈癌

几乎所有宫颈癌的患者都被人乳头瘤病毒（human papillomavirus，HPV）感染，这种病毒会引起生殖器疣（genital wart）。发病还与性活动频繁和其他性传播病毒感染有关，例如疱疹。

在 1940 和 1950 年代，合成类固醇己烯雌酚（diethylstilbestrol，DES，被用于避免流产）。接受这种药物治疗的女性所生的女儿显示出患子宫颈和阴道癌症的风险升高。这些女性需要做定期检查。

宫颈癌发生之前通常有子宫颈内壁上皮细胞的异常生长（dysplasia）。基于涉及的组织深度，这种增生被分级为 CIN I、II 或 III。CIN 代表宫颈上皮内瘤样病变（cervical intraepithelial neoplasia）。宫颈癌可以通过巴氏涂片（pap smear）、阴道镜（colposcope）和活组织检查诊断。在锥形活组织检查中（图 15-10），要从子宫颈内壁上切下一块锥形的组织进行研究。通常在这一过程中，所有其他异常组织细胞也都会被切除。

卵巢癌

卵巢癌死亡率很高，因为它没有明显的早期症状，至今也没有准确的常规筛查测试。女性可能会忽略卵

巢癌可能的模糊症状，例如腹胀、排便习惯改变、背痛、排尿变化、异常出血、体重减轻和疲乏无力。通常在诊断出癌症时，肿瘤已经侵入骨盆和腹部。可能需要卵巢（卵巢切除术，oophorectomy）和输卵管（输卵管切除术，salpingectomy）与子宫一起切除（图15-9），同时进行化疗和放疗。

乳腺癌

在美国与癌症相关的女性死亡病例中，乳腺癌（breast cancer）仅次于肺癌。乳腺癌通过淋巴结核血液迅速转移到其他部位，如肺、肝、骨骼和卵巢。

诊断

乳腺癌诊断的第一步是简单的触诊。定期的乳房自检（breast self-examination，BSE）极其重要，因为许多乳腺癌都是女性自己发现的。

乳腺造影（mammography）会提供乳房的二维X线图像，是乳腺癌的标准诊断方法（图15-11）。一些健康组织建议40岁以上的女性应每年做一次乳腺造影检查，另一些医疗专业人士建议等到50岁以上，除非属于高风险人群，例如有乳腺癌家族史的女性。在数字乳腺造影中，图像被储存在计算机中，而不是胶片上。这些图像可以被电子处理，以便于解释说明，也便于储存和检索，或传送给其他医疗机构。

超声和核磁共振是乳腺造影的辅助手段，超声能够显示乳腺造影可见的团块是否属于良性囊肿，使用造影剂的核磁共振能够显示象征肿瘤的异常血管形成。

任何有疑问的乳房组织都必须通过针头吸出或手术切除做活组织检查。在立体性向活检中，医生使用计算机导向的成像系统定位有疑问的组织，并使用针头采样。这一方法比手术活检侵入性更小。

乳腺导管原位癌（ductal carcinoma in situ，DCIS）是一种源于乳导管内壁增生的乳腺癌。这种癌起初只局限于乳导管，并不侵入附件的组织或扩散，

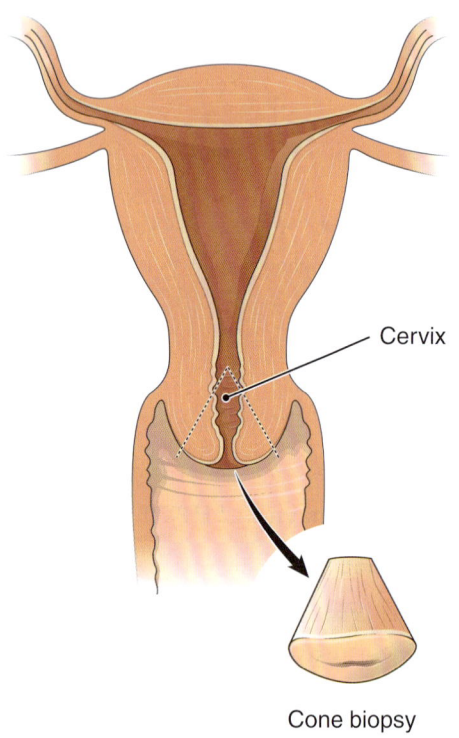

图 15-10　子宫颈锥体活检

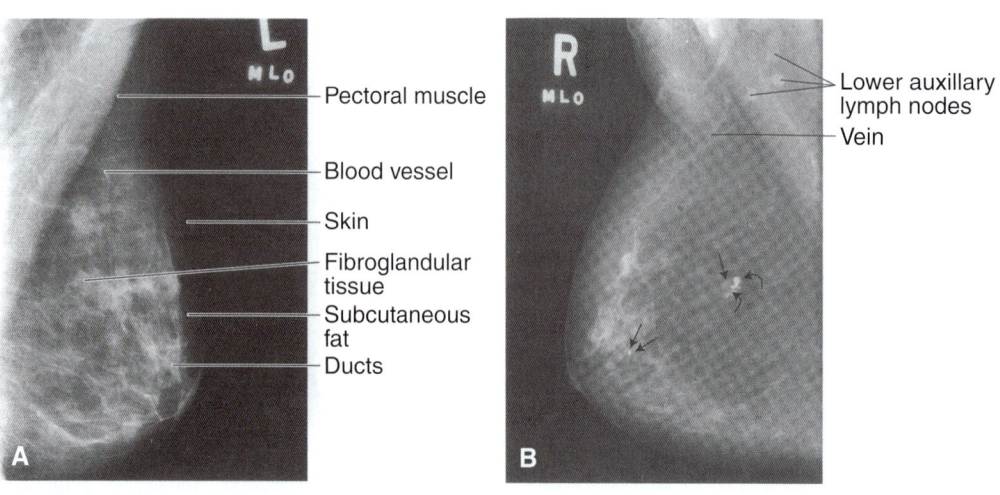

图 15-11　乳房 X 线片。A. 正常乳房 X 线片，左乳房；B. 右乳房乳房 X 线片显示病变（箭头）。在乳房 X 线片中，脂肪组织显示为灰色，乳腺组织、钙沉积和良性或癌性肿瘤显示为白色

通常能够被早期检查出来。

治疗

乳腺癌的治疗一般是某种形式的乳房切除术（mastectomy），或切除部分乳房组织：

在根治性乳房切除术（radical mastectomy）中，这个乳房都被切除，乳房下的肌肉和腋下淋巴结也会被切除。

在乳房改良根治术（modified radical mastectomy）中，乳房和淋巴结被切除，保留肌肉。

在乳房区段切除术（segmental mastectomy）或乳房肿瘤切除术（lumpectomy）中，只切除肿瘤。如果肿瘤比较小，而且手术后有追加治疗，这种方法与根治性手术治疗的生存率同样高。

手术能够评估肿瘤的扩散程度，并使用前哨淋巴结活检（sentinel node biopsy）保留淋巴组织。一种染色剂或放射性示踪剂能够确认最先从肿瘤接受淋巴液的淋巴结。针对这些"前哨淋巴结"进行的肿瘤扩散可能性的研究可以指导进一步的治疗。

通常在乳房手术后，患者要接受化疗和/或放疗。目前，在某些病例中能够只对肿瘤区域传送放射线（短距离放射治疗，brachytherapy），取代向整个乳房的照射。通过在乳房组织中短时间插管或植入提供放射源。

乳腺癌治疗的发展涉及到基因研究和肿瘤分析，使得治疗能够对每个特定的病例更有针对性。大约8%的乳腺癌与在家庭中传播的基因缺陷（BRCA1或BRCA2）有关，具有这些遗传倾向的女性能够被认真地排查或预防性地治疗。

一些特定的药物能够治疗乳腺癌，包括：
- 阻止雌性激素产生或抑制乳房组织中雌性激素受体的药物，如果肿瘤对该激素有响应的话。
- 抑制肿瘤生长因子的药物。
- 抑制为肿瘤供血的血管生长的药物（血管生成抑制剂，antiangiogenesis agents）。

这些药物和其他抗癌药在补充术语中有详细列表。

Terminology 关键术语

女性生殖系统

病症

candidiasis	[ˌkændəˈdaɪəsəs]	念珠菌病，念珠菌真菌感染，是阴道炎常见起因
dysmenorrhea	[ˌdɪsmenəʊˈriːə]	痛经，月经疼痛或困难。一种由感染、使用宫内避孕器、子宫内膜异位、前列腺素产生更多或其他原因所致的病症
endometriosis	[ˌendəʊˌmiːtriˈəʊsɪs]	子宫内膜异位症，子宫内膜组织生长到子宫之外，通常是在盆腔（图15-8）
fibroid	[ˈfaɪbrɔɪd]	子宫肌瘤，子宫平滑肌良性肿瘤（参见leiomyoma）
leiomyoma	[laɪəʊmaɪˈəʊmə]	平滑肌瘤，平滑肌良性肿瘤，通常在子宫壁（子宫肌层）。在子宫的平滑肌瘤能够引起出血和膀胱或直肠压力（图15-7）
pelvic inflammatory disease (PID)		盆腔炎，生殖道感染扩散到盆腔的情况，通常是由性传播的淋病或衣原体感染
salpingitis	[ˌsælpɪnˈdʒaɪtɪs]	输卵管炎，输卵管的炎症，通常是尿路感染或性传播感染所致。慢性输卵管炎可能导致不育或宫外孕（ectopic pregnancy）
vaginitis	[ˌvædʒəˈnaɪtɪs]	阴道炎，阴道的炎症

诊断与治疗

colposcope	[ˈkɒlpəskəʊp]	阴道镜，检查阴道和子宫颈的装置

Terminology	关键术语（续表）

女性生殖系统

cone biopsy	锥形活检，从子宫颈内壁切下一块锥形组织进行细胞学检查；也被称为宫颈锥切术（conization）
dilation and curettage (D&C) [kjʊəˈretidʒ]	刮宫术，扩张子宫颈，用刮匙刮削子宫内壁的治疗方法
hysterectomy [ˌhistəˈrektəmi]	子宫切除术，手术切除子宫，做这一手术的最常见原因是肿瘤；通常输卵管和卵巢也会被切除（图 15-9）
mammography [mæˈmɒgrəfi]	乳腺造影，为检测乳腺癌所进行的乳房 X 线检查，所获得的图像为乳腺 X 线片（mammogram，图 15-11）
mastectomy [mæˈstektəmi]	乳房切除术，切除乳房组织以消除恶性肿瘤
oophorectomy [ˌəʊəfəˈrektəmi]	卵巢切除术，手术切除卵巢（图 15-9）
Pap smear	巴氏涂片，子宫颈或阴道所采集的细胞的研究，用于癌症的早期检测；也被称为 Papanicolaou smear 或 Pap test
salpingectomy [ˌsælpinˈdʒektəmi]	输卵管切除术，手术切除输卵管（图 15-9）
sentinel node biopsy [ˈsentinl]	前哨淋巴结活检，最先从肿瘤接受淋巴液的淋巴结的活组织检查，用于确定癌症的扩散程度
stereotactic biopsy	立体定向活检，使用计算机导向成像系统定位怀疑组织并切除样本进行研究的穿刺活检

Terminology	补充术语

女性生殖系统

正常结构与功能

adnexa [ædˈneksə]	附件，附属器官，例如子宫附件——卵巢、输卵管和子宫韧带
areola [əˈriːələ]	色晕，一个色素环，例如乳头周围的深色区域
graafian follicle	赫拉夫卵泡，成熟的卵巢卵泡
greater vestibular gland [vesˈtibjʊlə]	前庭大腺，阴道开口附近前庭一侧的分泌黏液的小腺体；也被称为巴托兰腺（Bartholin gland）
hymen [ˈhaimən]	处女膜，部分覆盖阴道开口的黏膜褶皱
mons pubis [ˌmɒnzˈpjuːbis]	阴阜，青春期后形成的在耻骨联合前部的有毛发的圆形肉隆起
oocyte [ˈəʊəsait]	卵母细胞，未成熟的卵细胞
perimenopause [ˈpiərimɪnəpɔːz]	围绝经期，绝经之前一段时间；开始于月经周期不规律的时候，结束于最后一次月经后 1 年，平均 3~4 年

Terminology 补充术语（续表）

女性生殖系统

vestibule ['vestibju:l]	前庭，小阴唇之间的空间，包括尿道口、阴道和前庭大腺导管

病症

cystocele ['sistəsi:l]	膀胱膨出，进入阴道壁的膀胱疝（图 15-12）
dyspareunia [dispə'ru:niə]	性交困难，性交时疼痛
fibrocystic disease of the breast [faibrəʊ'sistik]	乳房纤维囊肿，乳房中有可触知的肿块，通常伴随疼痛和增生。必须通过诊断将这些在月经周期中的肿块变化与恶性肿瘤区别开来
hirsutism ['hɜ:sju:tizəm]	多毛症，毛发生长过多
leucorrhea [ˌlju:kə'ri:ə]	白带，白色或微黄的阴道排泄物。感染和其他病症会改变白带的量、颜色或气味
microcalcification	微钙化，小的钙沉积，在乳腺 X 线片上显示为白点。大多数微钙化是无害的，但有些可能表明有乳腺癌
prolapse of the uterus ['prəʊlæps]	子宫脱垂，子宫向下移位，有时子宫颈会突出阴道
rectocele ['rektəsi:l]	脱肛，进入阴道壁的直肠疝，也被称为直肠膨出（proctocele，图 15-12）

诊断与治疗

culdocentesis [kʌldəsen'ti:sis]	后穹窿穿刺术，从直肠子宫陷凹空间穿刺阴道壁为诊断采集液体
episiorrhaphy ['ipiziərəfi]	外阴缝合术，缝合外阴或外阴切开术（切开以便于分娩）的会阴切口
laparoscopy [ˌlæpə'rɒskəpi]	腹腔镜检查，腹部内窥镜检查；可能包括手术过程，例如输卵管结扎（图 15-6）
myomectomy [maiə'mektəmi]	子宫肌瘤切除术，手术切除子宫肌瘤
speculum ['spekjələm]	窥器，用于扩张通道或腔体开口以便检查的装置（图 7-13）
teletherapy [ˌteli'θerəpi]	远距放射疗法，通过外部射线源向肿瘤进行放射，相当于植入放射性物质（近距放射疗法 brachytherapy）或放射性核素全身给药（systemic administration of radionuclide）

药物

aromatase inhibitor (AI) [ərəʊ'mɑ:teis]	芳香酶抑制剂，抑制雌性激素产生的药物；用于对雌性激素有响应的绝经后乳腺癌的治疗。例如依西美坦（exemestane）、阿那曲唑（anastrozole）和来曲唑（letrozole）
bisphosphonate [bis'fɒsfəʊneit]	二磷酸盐，预防和治疗骨质疏松的药物；通过减少骨转换提高骨密度、例如阿仑膦酸钠（alendronate）和利塞膦酸钠（risedronate）
HER_2 inhibitor	HER_2 抑制剂，用于治疗显示对人表皮生长因子有过量受体（HER_2）的乳腺癌，例如曲妥单抗（trastuzumab）
paclitaxel [ˌpækli'tæksəl]	紫杉醇，从紫杉树中提取的抗肿瘤药，主要用于治疗乳腺癌和卵巢癌
selective estrogen receptor modulator (SERM)	选择性雌激素受体调节剂，作用于雌性激素受体的药物，例如他莫昔芬（tamoxifen）和雷洛昔芬（raloxifene），也被用于预防绝经后骨质疏松

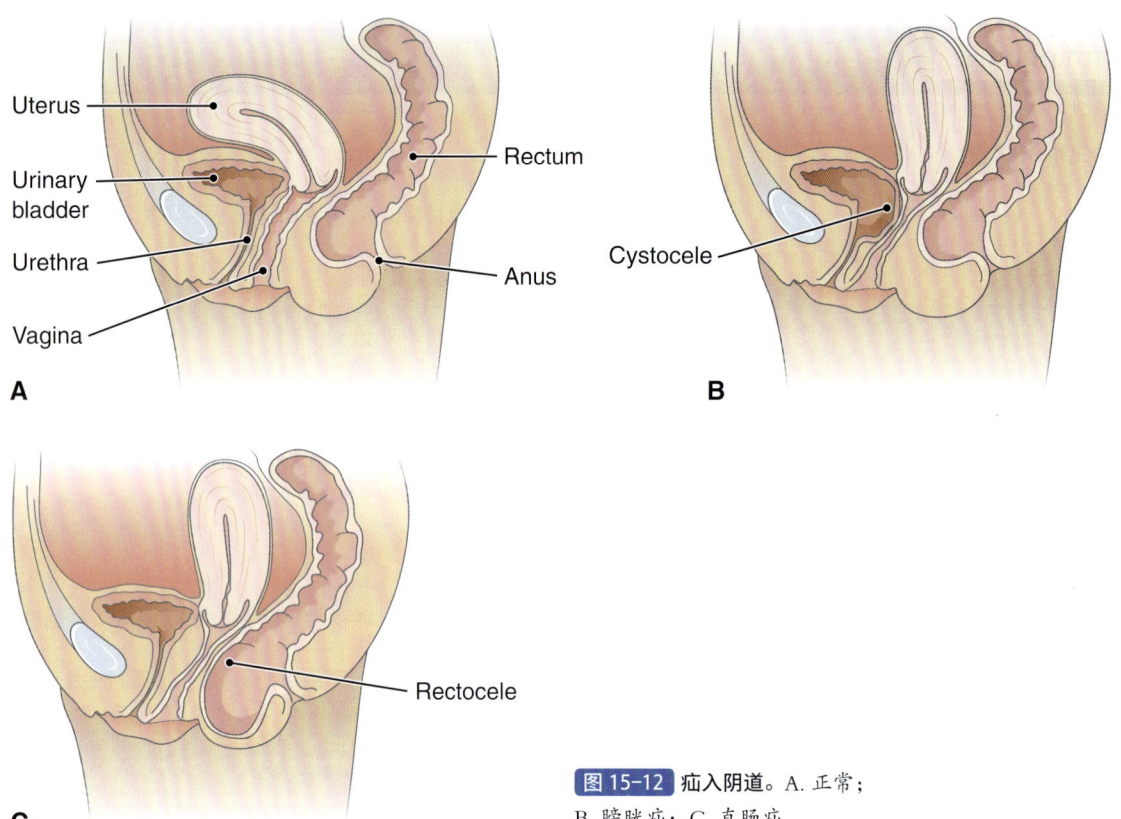

图 15-12 疝入阴道。A. 正常；B. 膀胱疝；C. 直肠疝

Terminology 缩略语

AI	Aromatase inhibitor	芳香酶抑制剂
BRCA1	Breast cancer gene 1	乳腺癌基因 1
BRCA2	Breast cancer gene 2	乳腺癌基因 2
BSE	Breast self-examination	乳房自检
BSO	Bilateral salpingo-oophorectomy	双侧输卵管卵巢切除术
BV	Bacterial vaginosis	细菌性阴道炎
CIN	Cervical intraepithelial neoplasia	宫颈上皮内瘤样病变
D&C	Dilation and curettage	刮宫术
DCIS	Ductal carcinoma in situ	乳腺导管原位癌
DES	Diethylstilbestrol	己烯雌酚
DUB	Dysfunctional uterine bleeding	功能失调性子宫出血
FSH	Follicle-stimulating hormone	促卵泡激素
GC	Gonococcus (cause of gonorrhea)	淋球菌（淋病的起因）
GYN	Gynecology	妇科学

Terminology	缩略语（续表）	
HPV	Human papillomavirus	人乳头瘤病毒
HRT	Hormone replacement therapy	激素替代疗法
IUD	Intrauterine device	宫内避孕器
LH	Luteinizing hormone	促黄体生成素
NGU	Nongonococcal urethritis	非淋病性尿道炎
PCOS	Polycystic ovarian syndrome	多囊卵巢综合征
PID	Pelvic inflammatory disease	盆腔炎
PMS	Premenstrual syndrome	经前期综合征
SERM	Selective estrogen receptor modulator	选择性雌激素受体调节剂
STD	Sexually transmitted disease	性传播疾病
STI	Sexually transmitted infection	性传播感染
TAH	Total abdominal hysterectomy	经腹全子宫切除术
TSS	Toxic shock syndrome	中毒性休克综合征
UFE	Uterine fibroid embolization	子宫肌瘤栓塞术
VD	Venereal disease (sexually transmitted disease)	性病（性传播疾病）

妊娠与分娩

受精和早期发育

精子穿透一个排出的卵细胞的结果是受精（图15-13）。在正常情况下，这一结合发生在输卵管。精子的核与卵细胞融合，染色体数量恢复为46，并形成一个合子（zygote）。随着合子通过输卵管向子宫运动，它迅速分裂。在6~7天内，受精卵到达子宫，并在子宫内膜上着床，胚胎（embryo）开始发育。

在胚胎最初8周的生长期间，所有主要的人体系统都已建立。胚胎组织产生人体绒毛膜促性腺激素（human chorionic gonadotropin，hCG），其作用是保持黄体对卵巢的功能，维护子宫内膜（尿液中出现hCG是最常见的怀孕测试的基础）。2个月后，胎盘激素接替这一功能，黄体退化。这时，胚胎已成为胎儿（fetus，图15-14）。

胎盘

在发育期间，胎儿由胎盘（placenta）提供营养。胎盘是由胚胎的最外层浆膜（chorion）和子宫的最内层子宫内膜形成的（图15-15）。在这里，母亲和胎儿的血流通过胎儿毛细血管发生交换。

脐带（umbilical cord）包含连接胎儿和胎盘的血管，胎儿的血液通过两根脐动脉进入胎盘。随着血液通过胎盘，血液带走营养和氧气，并排出二氧化碳和代谢废物。补充的血液通过一根脐静脉从胎盘输送给胎儿。

尽管母亲和胎儿的血流并不混合，所有的交换都通过毛细血管发生，一些物质还是能够双向通过胎盘。例如，一些病毒，如HIV和风疹病毒，以及一些药物、酒精和其他有害物质能够通过母亲传送给胎儿；胎儿的蛋白质能够进入母亲的血液，并引起免疫反应。

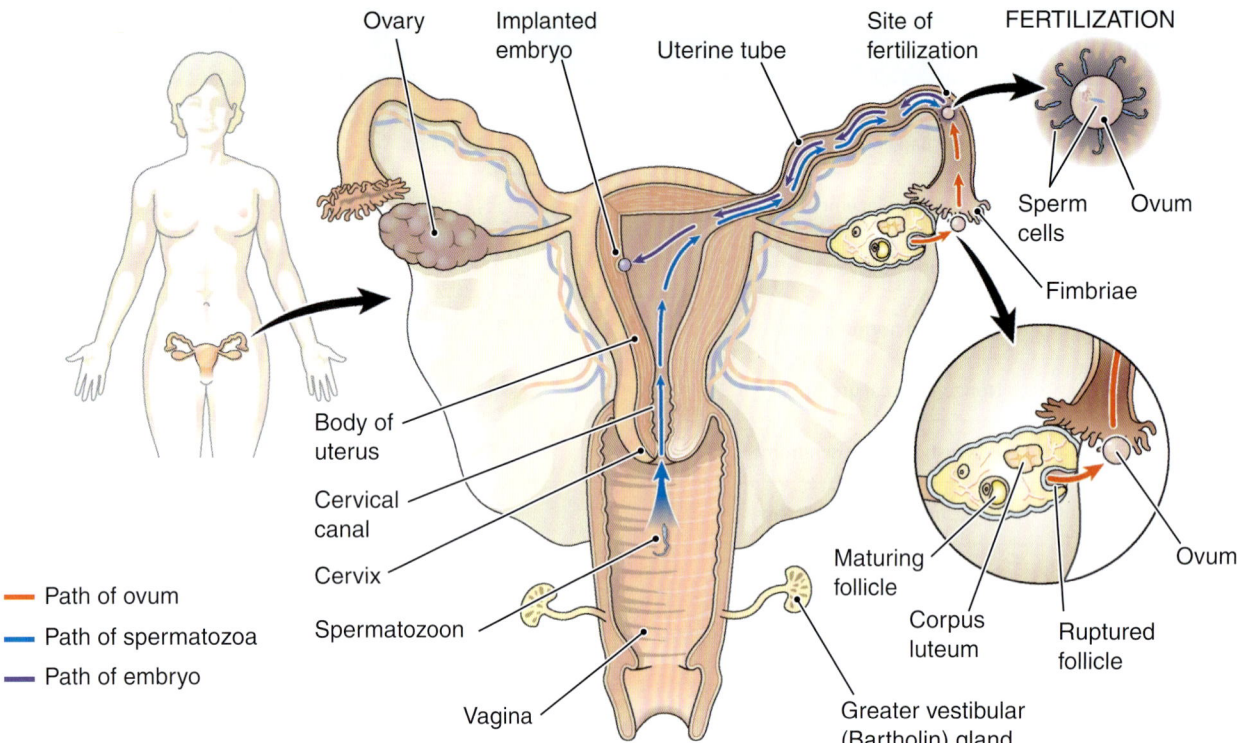

图 15-13 排卵和受精。箭头显示精子和卵子的通路。受精发生在子宫管中，之后受精卵在子宫壁上着床

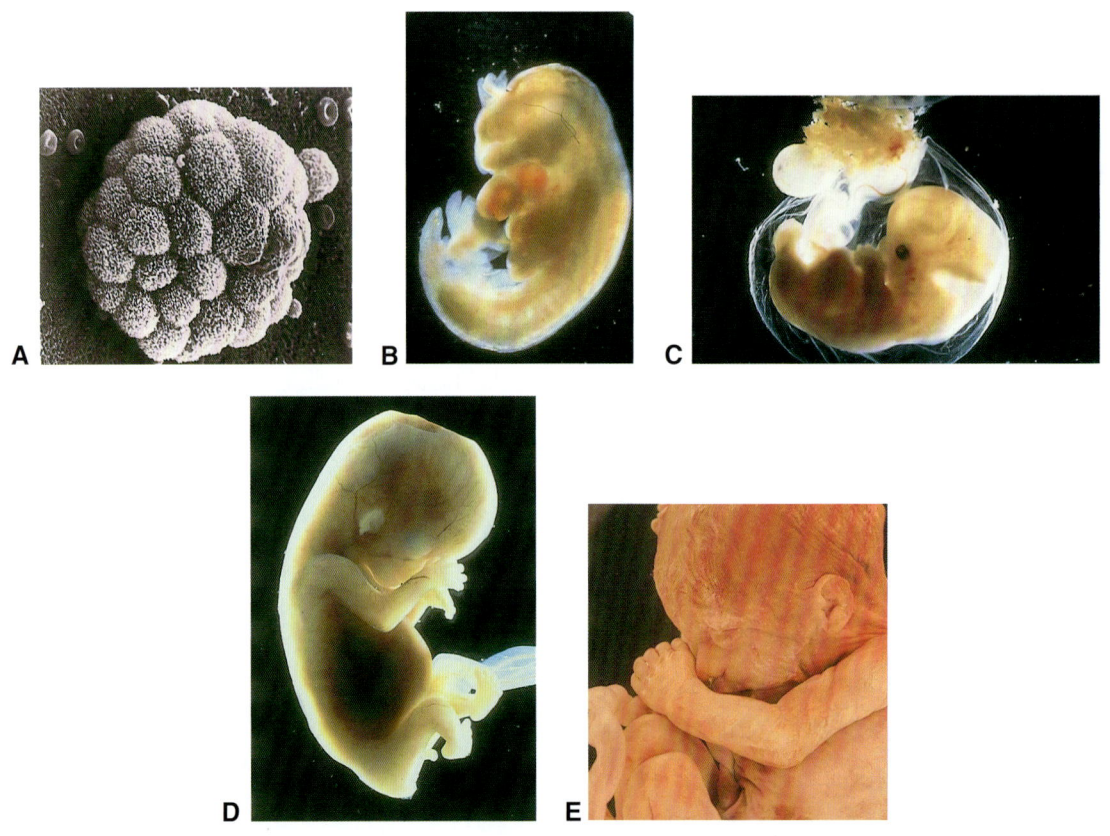

图 15-14 人的发育。图中显示了人类胚胎和早期胎儿。A. 受孕后 7~8 天在子宫中着床；B. 胚胎在第 32 天；C. 在第 37 天；D. 在第 41 天；E. 胎儿 12~15 周

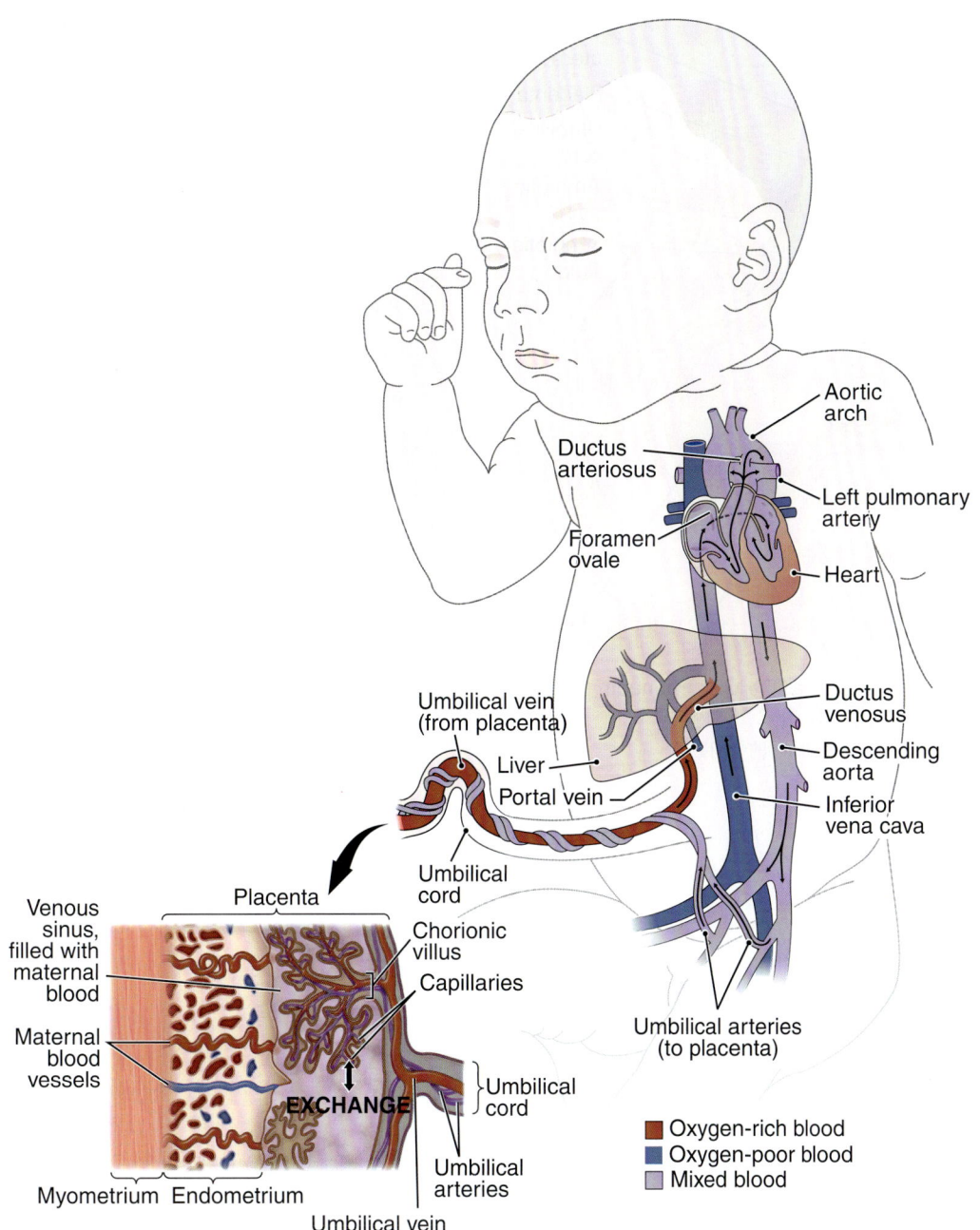

图 15-15 胎儿循环。颜色显示各种血管中血液的相对氧含量。气体、废物和营养物质通过胎盘中的毛细血管在胎儿和母亲之间交换

在妊娠（gestation）期间，胎儿被羊膜囊（amniotic sac）中的液体缓冲和保护（图 15-16），羊膜囊通常被称为羊水囊（bag of waters）。羊膜囊在分娩时会破裂。

胎儿循环

胎儿有几个适应性改变，其功能是绕过肺，不必为血液充氧。当血液从胎盘来到右心房，心房隔膜上的卵圆孔（foramen ovale）允许部分血液直接进入左心房，因而绕过了肺动脉。下一步，泵出右心室的血液通过连接肺动脉和降主动脉的动脉导管（descending aorta）直接分流到主动脉（图 15-15）。这两个通道在胎儿出生肺循环建立后都会关闭，如果没有关闭，将会给心脏增加负担，可能需要进行治疗。

分娩

怀孕的时间，从受精到分娩大约是 38 周或 266

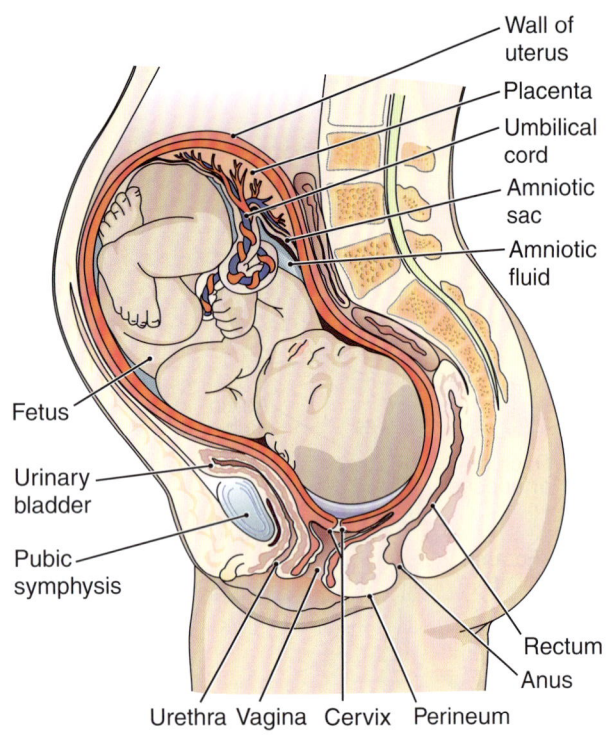

图 15-16 怀孕的子宫与完整的胎儿的中间截面

天。在实践中，从孕前最后一次月经周期（last menstrual period，LMP）第 1 天开始计算大约为 280 天或 40 周。为研究方便，怀孕期每三个月分为一期（三个月期 trimesters），每一期能够观察到确定的胎儿变化。

分娩（childbirth 或 parturition）分为三个阶段：

- 开始规律性的子宫收缩和子宫颈扩张。
- 胎儿的娩出。
- 排出胎盘和胎膜。

紧随分娩第三阶段之后的是子宫收缩和控制出血。这一情况的起因尚不完全了解，但肯定与来自于脑垂体后叶（posterior pituitary）的后叶催产素（oxytocin）和被称为前列腺素（prostaglandin）的其他激素有关。框 15-3 给出了关于助产士（midwife）和其他分娩助手的职业信息。

医院应用阿普加评分（Apgar score）来评估新生儿的健康状况。有五项特征：心率、呼吸、肌张力、对鼻插管的反应和皮肤颜色，在出生后 1min 和

框 15-3

健康职业

护理助产士和助产师

有各种与术语 midwife（助产士）相关的职称，每个职称都有不同的学术准备和认证。助产士（midwife）的字面意思是"与女人在一起"，这种执业被称为助产（midwifery [ˌmidˈwifəri]）。在美国，助产士的作用因教育程度、资格和执照而异。

一名认证护理助产士（certified nurse-midwife，CNM）要接受护理和助产学科的教育。认证助产士（certified midwife，CM）只接受助产士学科的教育。为了参加美国助产士认证委员会（American Midwifery Certification Board，AMCB）的考试，两个职称都需要硕士学位。每 5 年需要重新认证。认证护理助产士和认证助产士是从青少年到更年期的妇女提供初级保健。这包括常规妇科和生殖保健、妊娠、分娩和产后护理，以及围绝经期和绝经期管理。认证护理助产士在美国所有 50 个州、华盛顿特区和美国领土获得许可，并且在所有美国司法管辖区都有处方权。认证助产士在纽约、新泽西和罗德岛获得执照，他们可以在特拉华州和密苏里州执业，在纽约有处方权。大多数私人保险和医疗补助计划为认证护理助产士/认证助产士服务报销。大多数认证护理助产士/认证助产士在医院参与分娩，但他们也参与在家分娩，在分娩中心、诊所和健康部门工作。美国护士助产士学院（American College of Nurse-Midwives）在 www.acnm.org 有关于这些职业的信息。

认证专业助产士（Certified Professional Midwife，CPM）是一个独立的助产服务提供者，符合由北美助产士注册处（North American Registry of Midwives，NARM）制定的认证标准。这个专业不需要大学学历。认证专业助产士在美国 26 个州受到监管，其认证、许可和注册要求各不相同。认证专业助产士没有规定的权限，在一些州的私人保险和 10 个州的医疗补助计划报销在家庭和分娩中心的认证专业助产士服务。认证专业助产士在妊娠期、分娩和产后为妇女提供护理，并提供新生儿护理。认证专业助产士的专业协会是北美洲助产士联盟（Midwives Alliance of North America，MANA）和全国认证专业助产士协会（National）

助产师（doula 分娩助手）是在妊娠、分娩和分娩后与家庭合作的人。助产师提供情感和身体支持和教育。他们可以帮助产前准备和早期家庭分娩，并在整个住院期间继续提供支持。一些助产师被训练在产后提供护理，并且可以在分娩后为家庭提供支持。助产师名称 doula 来自希腊语，指的是家庭中最重要的女性仆人，可以协助女主人生孩子。助产师有一个专业协会为培训和认证制定标准。更多信息请访问 www.dona.org。

5min 时分别从 0~2 分打分。测试的最高分为 10 分，低分的婴儿需要医疗护理。

术语孕妇（gravida）是指怀孕的女性，术语产妇（para）是指已经分娩的女性。这意味着生产了一个能成活的婴儿（500g 以上的体重或 20 周以上的妊娠），无论婴儿在分娩时是否成活，也无论是单胞胎还是多胞胎。加在这两个术语上的前缀提示怀孕或分娩的次数，例如：

- nulli- 没有。
- primi-1 次。
- secondi-2 次。
- tri- 或 terti-3 次。
- quadri-4 次。
- multi- 多次。

也可以在术语后加一个数字，表示发生的次数，例如 gravida 1、para 3 等。

乳汁分泌

来自于脑垂体前叶的催乳激素（prolactin）和来自于胎盘的激素使乳腺开始分泌乳汁，被称为乳汁分泌（lactation）。婴儿的吸吮会刺激乳汁的释放，后叶催产素对乳汁的释放也是必须的。在分娩后最初几天，只产生初乳（colostrum）。初乳的成分与乳汁有些差异，含有保护性的抗体。

Terminology 关键术语

怀孕与分娩

正常结构与功能

amniotic sac [ˌæmniˈəʊtik]		羊膜囊，充满容纳着胎儿的液体的膜囊，也被称为羊膜（amnion）（词根：amnio）
Apgar score		阿普加评分，在出生后立即评价婴儿身体状况的评分系统。在分娩后 1 分钟和 5 分钟，有时在此之后为五项特征在 0~2 分之间评分。最高评分为 10 分，低分的婴儿需要医疗护理
chorion [ˈkɔːriɒn]		浆膜，胚胎的最外层，与子宫内膜一起形成胎盘（形容词为 chorionic）
colostrum [kəˈlɒstrəm]		初乳，分娩后最初几天产生乳汁前分泌的乳液
ductus arteriosus [ˈdʌktəs ɑːˈtɪəriəlsəs]		动脉导管，连接肺动脉和降大动脉的胎儿血管，允许血液绕过肺
embryo [ˈembriəʊ]		胚胎，合子至胎儿之间的发育期，从进入子宫的第 2~8 周（词根：embry/o）；形容词为 embryonic
fertilization [ˌfɜːtəlaiˈzeiʃn]		受精，卵子与精子的结合
fetus [ˈfiːtəs]		胎儿，从受精后第 3 个月至出生前在子宫发育中的孩子（词根：fet/o）；形容词为 fetal
foramen ovale [fəʊˈreimən əʊˈvæliː]		卵圆孔，胎儿心脏房间隔上的小孔，允许血液从心脏右侧直接流到左侧
gestation [dʒeˈsteiʃn]		妊娠期，从受孕至分娩的发育期
gravida [ˈgrævidə]		孕妇，怀孕的女性
human chorionic gonadotropin (hCG) [ˌkəʊriˈɒnik ˌɡɒnədəʊˈtrɒpin]		人绒毛膜促性腺激素，怀孕早期胚胎分泌的一种维持黄体的激素，以便黄体继续分泌激素

Terminology	关键术语（续表）
lactation [læk'teiʃn]	乳汁分泌，乳腺分泌乳汁
oxytocin [ˌɒksi'təʊsin]	催产素，刺激子宫收缩的一种脑垂体激素。它也刺激乳汁从乳房中释放
para ['pærə]	产妇，已生产可成活婴儿的女性。多胞胎被认为是单次妊娠
parturition [ˌpɑːtjʊ'riʃn]	分娩，生孩子（词根：nat/i）；也称为 labor（词根：toc/o）
placenta [plə'sentə]	胎盘，胎儿和母体组织构成的器官，能够为胎儿提供营养并维护胎儿的发育
prostaglandin [ˌprɒstə'glændin]	前列腺素，一组有不同作用的激素，其作用包括刺激子宫收缩
umbilical cord [ʌmˌbilikl 'kɔːd]	脐带，连接胎儿和胎盘的结构，包含在母亲与胎儿之间输送血液的血管
zygote ['zaigəʊt]	合子，受精卵

与妊娠和分娩相关的词根

参见表 15-4

表 15-4　妊娠和分娩的词根

词根	含义	示例	示例定义
amnio	羊膜、羊膜囊	diamniotic [diəmna'iəʊtik]	双羊膜腔的
embry/o	胚胎	embryonic [ˌembri'ɒnik]	胚胎的
fet/o	胎儿	fetometry [fe'tɒmitri]	胎儿测量法
toc/o	分娩	dystocia [dis'təʊʃiə]	难产
nat/i	分娩	neonate ['niːəʊneit]	新生儿
lact/o	乳汁	lactose ['læktəʊs]	乳糖
galact/o	乳汁	galactogogue [gə'læktəgɒg]	催乳剂
gravida	孕妇	nulligravida [nʌli'grævidə]	未孕妇
para	产妇	multipara [mʌl'tipərə]	多产妇

练习 15-4

定义下列单词。

1. prenatal
   [ˌpriːˈneitl] _____
2. embryogenesis
   [ˌembriəʊˈdʒenəsis] _____
3. neonatal
   [ˌniːəʊˈneitl] _____
4. fetoscopy
   [fiːˈtɒskəpi] _____
5. monoamniotic
   [mɒnəʊmnaˈiəʊtik] _____
6. agalactia
   [æˈɡælæktiə] _____
7. hypolactation
   [haipəʊlækˈteiʃn] _____

使用适当的词根写出下列单词。

8. study of an embryo _____
9. after birth _____
10. incision of the amnion (to induce labor) _____
11. cell (-cyte) found in amniotic fluid _____
12. any disease of an embryo _____
13. instrument for endoscopic examination of the fetus _____
14. rupture of the amniotic sac _____
15. study of the newborn _____
16. woman who is pregnant for the first time _____
17. woman who has been pregnant two or more times _____
18. woman who has never given birth _____
19. woman who has given birth to one child _____

使用意为"分娩状态"的后缀 –tocia 写出下列单词。

20. dry labor _____
21. slow labor _____

使用词根 galact/o 写出下列单词。

22. discharge of milk _____
23. cystic enlargement (-cele) of a milk duct _____

妊娠与分娩的临床表现

不孕

有 10%~15% 的夫妇想要孩子，但不能怀孕或不能维持怀孕。第 14 章和本节要讨论不育的一些起因。对男性而言，起因包括精子太少、精子活动力（sperm motility）低、输精管阻塞和勃起功能障碍。对女性而言，起因包括：

- 缺少排卵。
- 输卵管阻塞，感染或组织生长过多所致。
- 子宫问题，例如肿瘤或子宫内膜组织异常生长。
- 子宫颈瘢痕或感染。
- 阴道酸性过高伤害精子或有精子细胞抗体。
- 药物，包括停服避孕药之后暂时或永久的不孕。

框 15-4 介绍了一些在其他所有诊断和治疗方法都无效的情况下帮助不育夫妇的临床方法。

宫外孕

受精卵在子宫腔正常位置之外发育被称为宫外孕（ectopic pregnancy，图 15-17）。尽管可能发生在腹腔的其他任何地方，宫外孕通常发生在输卵管，导致输卵管妊娠。输卵管炎、子宫内膜异位和盆腔炎可能会阻塞卵子进入子宫的通道而导致宫外孕。输卵管妊娠的持续生长会使输卵管破裂，引起危险的大出血。宫外孕的症状有疼痛、压痛、肿胀和休克。通过测量

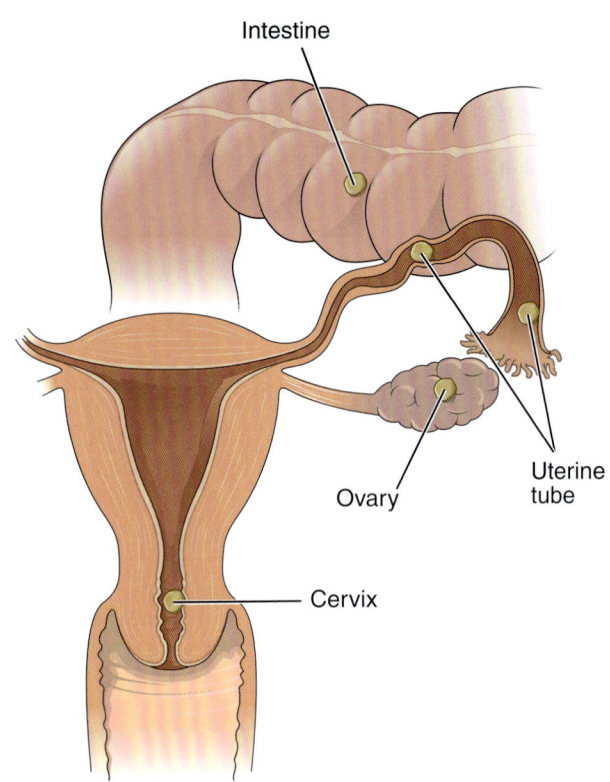

图 15-17 宫外孕。受精卵在子宫外发育的可能位置

人绒毛膜促性腺激素和超声造影可以诊断宫外孕，并可以通过腹腔镜检查确认。宫外孕需要立即手术，有时还要切除输卵管。

妊娠高血压综合征

妊娠高血压综合征（pregnancy-induced hypertens

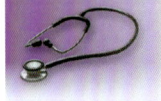

框 15-3

临床观点
辅助生殖技术：受孕的"艺术"

至少十分之一的美国夫妇受到不育的影响。辅助生殖技术，例如体外受精（in vitro fertilization，IVF）、配子输卵管内移植（gamete intrafallopian transfer，GIFT）和合子输卵管内移植（zygote intrafallopian transfer，ZIFT），能够帮助这些夫妇受孕。

体外受精（In vitro fertilization）是指卵子在母体之外的一个实验室器皿中受精，通常用于女性的输卵管阻塞或男性精子数量低的情况。参与体外受精的女性要服用激素，以排出几个卵子。然后，这些卵子被用针头抽出，并与其丈夫的精子结合。在几次分裂之后，一些受精卵被置于子宫，绕过了被阻塞的输卵管。其余的受精卵被冷冻储存，用于受孕失败情况下重复这一过程，或用于以后的怀孕。

配子输卵管内移植被用于女性至少有一侧输卵管正常，且男性精子数量足够的情况。如体外受精一样，女性要服用激素以排出几个卵子，卵子被采集后与丈夫的精子一起用插管植入输卵管。因此，在配子输卵管内移植中，受精发生于女性体内，而不是实验室的器皿中。

合子输卵管内移植是体外受精和配子输卵管内移植的组合。受精发生于实验室器皿，然后合子被植入输卵管。

在美国，辅助生殖技术因为缺少指导和限制，出现了一些问题。问题与储存胚胎和配子的使用、未经同意使用胚胎和捐献者不适当的疾病排查相关。另外，植入不只一个受精卵会导致多胞胎的发生，在一次怀孕中生产 7 或 8 个孩子，这种情况危害婴儿的生存和健康。

ion，PIH）也被称为子痫前期（preeclampsia）或妊娠毒血症（toxemia of pregnancy），是一种妊娠期间高血压伴随尿少（oliguria）、蛋白尿和水肿的状态。起因是激素失衡导致的血管收缩。如果不治疗，妊娠高血压综合征可能导致子痫（eclampsia），伴随癫痫和昏迷，还可能死亡。

流产

出于各种不同的原因，妊娠可能在胎儿能够在子宫外生存之前终止。流产是在怀孕 20 周或重量到达 500g 之前损失胚胎或胎儿。如果是自发的，这通常被称为早产（miscarriage）。大多数自发流产发生在怀孕的前 3 个月。原因包括目前身体健康状况差、激素失衡、宫颈机能不全、免疫反应、肿瘤和最常见的胎儿异常。如果所有妊娠组织没有完全除去，被描述为不完全流产，医生必须移除遗留组织。

人工流产（induced abortion）是有意识地终止妊娠。人工流产的常用方法是刮宫术（dilatation and evacuation，D&E）。

Rh 因子不相配

在特定的妊娠中，母亲与胎儿的血液不相配。如果母亲缺乏 Rh 血液抗原（参见第 10 章），而胎儿的 Rh 因子为阳性（从父亲获得），随着妊娠期间胎儿的血液穿过胎盘或分娩时进入母亲的血流，母亲的身体可能产生 Rh 抗体。如果此后的妊娠怀有一个 Rh 阳性的胎儿，抗体可能进入胎儿体内并破坏胎儿的红细胞。通过在怀孕期间和分娩后短时间内给予母亲预制的 Rh 抗体以消除其血液中的这些蛋白质，可以预防新生儿溶血症（hemolytic disease of the newborn，HDN）。

胎盘异常

如果胎盘附着接近或在子宫颈以上，而不是子宫的顶部，这种情况被称为胎盘前置（placenta previa）。这种异常可能在妊娠后期引起出血。如果出血严重，可能需要终止妊娠。

胎盘早剥（placental abruption 或 abruptio placentae）是指胎盘从其附着点过早分离。分离会引起出血，如果出血过多，可能导致胎儿或母亲死亡，或需要终止妊娠。起因包括受伤、母亲高血压和高龄妊娠。

乳腺炎

乳腺炎（mastitis）可能在任何时候发生，但一般发生于哺乳期的前几周。通常是金黄色葡萄球菌或链球菌通过乳头裂纹感染所致。乳房变得红肿、疼痛，患者可能会发冷、发热和全身不适。

先天性疾病

先天性疾病是在出生时就有的，包括两类：
- 发生在胎儿生长期间的发育性疾病。
- 父母通过生殖细胞传给孩子的遗传性（家族性 familial）疾病。

遗传性疾病是由基因或染色体细胞突变（mutation）引起的。突变可能涉及染色体数量或结构的变化，或者单一或多个基因的变化。遗传性疾病的出现和严重性还可能涉及异常基因与环境因素的相互作用。例如家族遗传的疾病，如糖尿病、心脏病、高血压和特定形态的癌症。框 15-5 介绍了一些最常见的遗传性疾病。

遗传疾病携带者是指带有不显现的基因缺陷，但可能会遗传给后代的人。实验室测试能够鉴别某些遗传疾病。畸形因素（teratogen）是因其胎儿发育畸形的主要原因，包括风疹（rubella）、单纯性疱疹（herpes simplex）和梅毒（syphilis）感染、酒精、药物、化学品和放射性等。在怀孕的前 3 个月，胎儿最容易受致畸因素的影响。

发育障碍包括闭锁（atresia）、无脑（anencephaly）、唇裂（cleft lip）、腭裂（cleft palate）和先天性心脏病等。脊柱裂（spina bifida）是脊柱闭合不完全，脊髓及其隔膜可能通过裂缝突出（图 15-19），这通常发生在腰部。如果没有组织突出，则被称为隐性脊柱裂（spina bifida occulta）。脊膜（meninges）通过裂口突出被称为脑脊髓膜突出（meningocele），在脊髓脊膜突出（myelomeningocele）病例中，脊髓及其隔膜都通过缺陷开口突出，如图 15-19D 和图 15-20 所示。请注意，叶酸，一种维生素 B，能够预防胚胎脊髓畸形，通常被称为神经管缺陷。这种维生

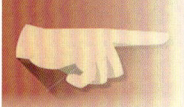

供你参考
遗传性疾病*

框 15-4

疾病	起因	说明
albinism [ˈælbinizəm] 白化病	隐性基因突变	缺少色素沉着
cystic fibrosis [ˌsistik faiˈbrəʊsis] 囊性纤维化	隐性基因突变	影响呼吸系统、胰腺和汗腺；白人最常见的遗传性疾病（参见第 11 章）
Down syndrome 唐氏综合征	多余的 21 号染色体	倾斜的眼睛、身材矮小、智力低下和其他疾病（图 15-18）；发病率随着母亲年龄的增加而上升；三体综合征
fragile X chromosome 脆性 X 染色体综合征	X 染色体（决定性别）缺陷	智力下降、自闭症（autism）、多动症（hyperactivity）；大头大耳；通过 X 染色体由母亲遗传给儿子（伴性的 sex-linked）
hemophilia [ˌhiːməˈfiliə] 血友病	X 染色体隐性突变	X 染色体遗传出血病，通常由母亲遗传给儿子
Huntington disease 亨廷顿病	显性基因突变	代谢改变破坏特定的神经细胞；出现在成年，约在 10 年内致命；引起运动与精神障碍
Klinefelter syndrome 克兰费尔特综合征	多余的 X 染色体	性发育不足，智力低下
Marfan syndrome 马方综合征	显性基因突变	结缔组织疾病，主动脉无力
neurofibromatosis [njʊəˈrəʊfaibrəʊmətəʊsis] 多发性神经纤维瘤	显性基因突变	多皮肤肿瘤，包含神经组织
phenylketonuria [fenəlkiːtəˈnjʊəriə] 苯丙酮尿症	隐性基因突变	缺乏代谢氨基酸的酶（苯丙氨酸，phenylalanine）；神经系统症状、精神发育迟滞、缺少色素；出生时测试；特殊饮食能够预防发育迟缓
sickle cell anemia 镰状细胞性贫血	隐性基因突变	形状异常的红细胞阻塞血管；主要影响黑人
Tay-Sachs disease 泰 - 萨克斯病	隐性基因突变	缺乏一种酶，引起脂肪在神经细胞和其他组织的积累；引起儿童早期死亡；影响东欧犹太人
Turner syndrome 特纳综合征	单 X 染色体	性不成熟、身材矮小、可能有智力低下

* 显性基因是特性始终出现的基因，即使只从父母一方遗传，也会影响后代。隐性基因是只有从父母双方遗传其特性才能影响后代的基因

素存在于蔬菜、肝脏、豆类（legumes）和种子中，现在被添加到包括麦片和面包等食品之中，以为年轻怀孕的女性尽早提供该维生素。

先天性疾病的诊断

许多先天性疾病能够在出生前被检测出来。超声扫描图（图 15-21）除了被用于妊娠监测和确定胎儿性别外，还能够揭示特定的胎儿畸形。在羊膜穿刺术（amniocentesis，图 15-22），用针头在羊膜腔中采集样本，用于分析化学异常。在实验室中培养的细胞被用于测试生化障碍。染色体组型（karyotype）被用于研究遗传物质（图 4-10）。

在绒毛采样（chorionic villus sampling，CVS）中，通过子宫颈获取包围胎儿薄膜的少量组织以进行分析。这种取样可以在怀孕的第 8~10 周进行，羊膜穿刺要在第 14~16 周才能进行。

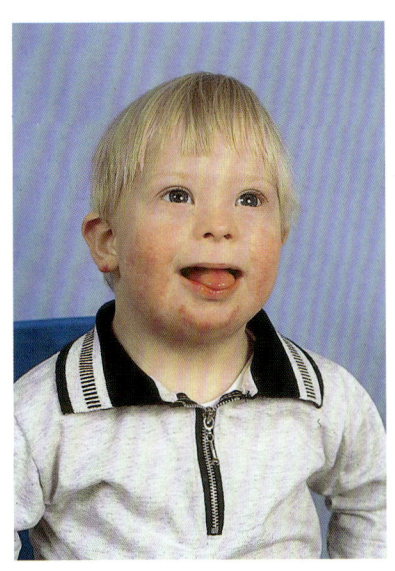

图 15-18 儿童唐氏综合征（21-三体综合征）。典型的面部特征在这张照片中可见

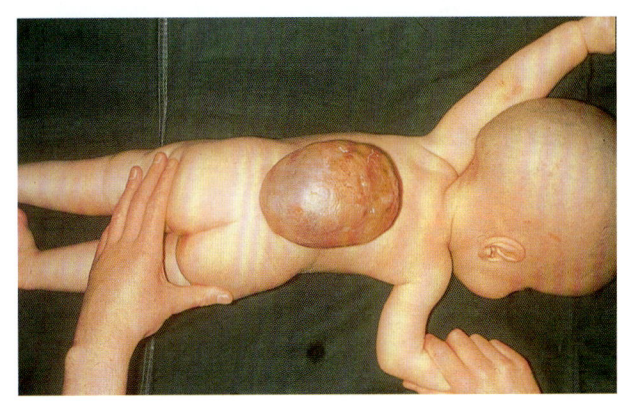

图 15-20 脊髓脊膜突出

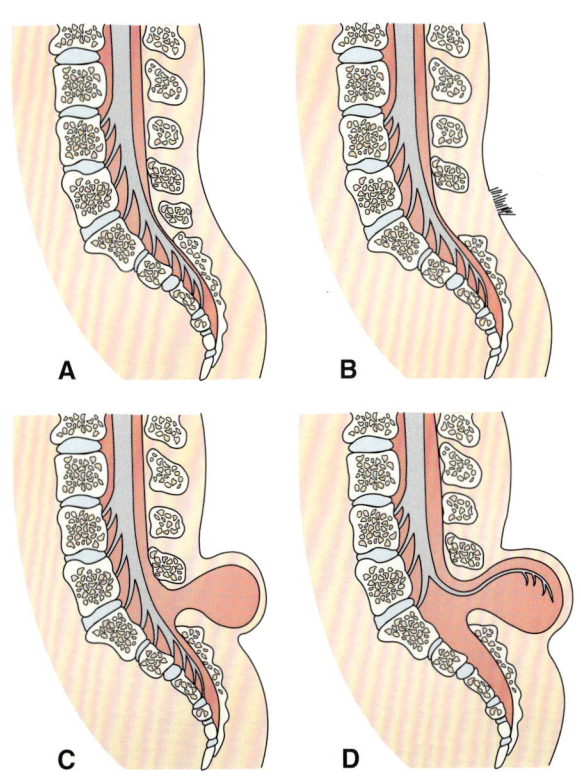

图 15-19 脊柱缺陷。A. 正常脊髓；B. 隐性脊柱裂；C. 脑脊膜突出；D. 脊髓脊膜突出

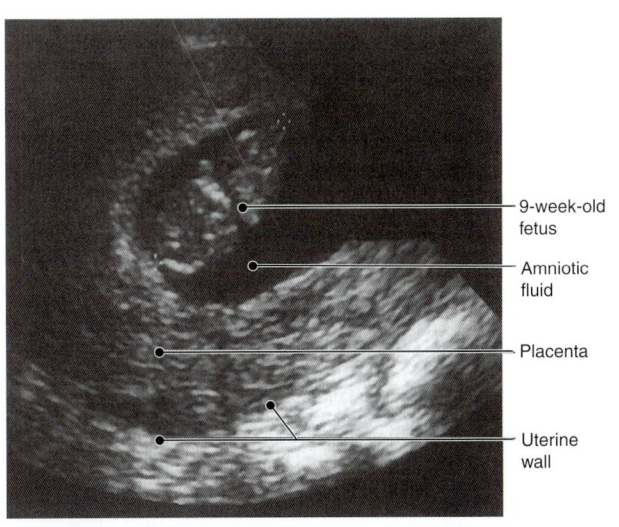

图 15-21 超声扫描图。这个经阴道超声扫描图检查显示一个 9 周龄的胎儿

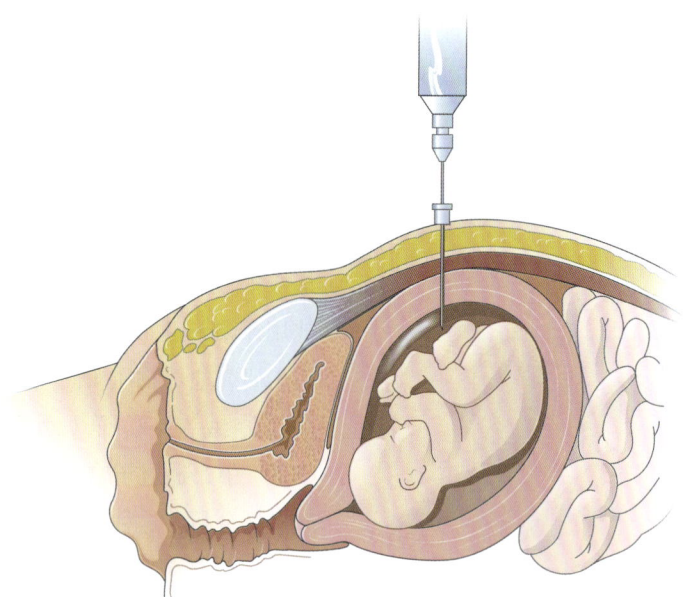

图15-22 羊膜腔穿刺术。从羊膜囊中取出样本，通过细胞和液体测试胎儿异常

Terminology　关键术语

妊娠与分娩

病症

abortion [ə'bɔːʃn]	流产，在胎儿能够在子宫外生存之前终止妊娠，通常在第20周或胎儿体重达到500g之前。可以是自发的，也可以是人工的。自发的流产通常被称为miscarriage
anencephaly [ænən'sefəli]	无脑，先天缺失大脑
atresia [eit'riːziə]	闭锁，正常身体开口先天性缺失或关闭
carrier ['kæriə(r)]	携带者，带有能够传播给下一代的未表达的基因缺陷的个人
cleft lip [kleft]	唇裂，上唇先天性开裂
cleft palate	腭裂，上颚先天性开裂
congenital disorder [kən'dʒenitl]	先天性疾病，出生时即出现的疾病。可以是发育性的或遗传性的（familial 家族性的）
eclampsia [i'klæmpsiə]	子痫，妊娠期间或分娩后发生的惊厥，与妊娠高血压综合征相关；形容词为eclamptic
ectopic pregnancy [ek'tɒpik]	异位妊娠，受精卵在子宫体外发育。通常发生于输卵管（tubal pregnancy，输卵管妊娠），但也可能发生于生殖道的其他部分或腹腔（图15-17）
hemolytic disease of the newborn (HDN) [hiː'mɒlitik]	新生儿溶血病，因母亲和胎儿血液之间Rh因子不兼容所致的疾病。Rh阴性目前对进入其体内的Rh阳性的胎儿红细胞会产生抗体，这些抗体会在妊娠后期破坏Rh阳性的胎儿的红细胞，除非用抗体消除母亲体内的Rh抗原。正式的名称为胎儿成红细胞增多病（erythroblastosis fetalis）

Terminology 关键术语（续表）

病症

术语	释义
mastitis [mæˈstaitis]	乳腺炎，乳腺的炎症，通常发生于哺乳的早期
mutation [mjuːˈteiʃn]	突变，细胞的基因发生变化。大多数突变是无害的，如果突变出现在性细胞中，会传播给后代
placental abruption [pləˈsentl]	胎盘早剥，胎盘过早分离；也常用 abruptio placentae
placenta previa [priˈvaiə]	前置胎盘，胎盘附着在子宫的下部，而不是正常的子宫上部。在妊娠晚期可能导致大出血
pregnancy-induced hypertension (PIH)	妊娠高血压综合征，妊娠晚期的中毒性状况，与高血压、水肿和蛋白尿相关，如果不治疗可能导致子痫。也被称为子痫前期（preeclampsia）和妊娠毒血症（toxemia of pregnancy）
spina bifida [ˌspainə ˈbifidə]	脊柱裂，脊柱闭合先天性缺陷，脊髓和脊髓膜可能通过裂口突出（图15-19和图15-20）
teratogen [təˈrætədʒən]	致畸原，引起胎儿发育畸形的因素（词根：terat/o 意为"畸形胎儿"）；形容词为 teratogenic

诊断与治疗

术语	释义
amniocentesis [ˌæmniəʊsenˈtiːsis]	羊膜穿刺术，经腹腔穿刺羊膜囊采集羊水进行测试。对细胞和羊水的测试能够揭示先天性畸形、血液不相配和胎儿的性别（图15-22）
chorionic villus sampling (CVS) [kəʊriˈɒnik]	绒毛采样，通过子宫颈采集绒毛细胞进行胎儿测试。可以在妊娠早期在羊膜穿刺术之前进行
dilatation and evacuation (D&E)	刮宫术，扩张子宫颈，并用刮匙刮除受孕产物
karyotype [ˈkæriəˌtaip]	染色体组型，根据大小降序排列的细胞染色体图片；能够揭示染色体自身和数量或排列次序的畸形（词根：kary/o 意为"细胞核"；图4-10）
ultrasonography [ˌʌltrəsəˈnɒɡrəfi]	超声波造影，使用高频声波产生器官或组织的影像（图15-21）。在产科被用于诊断怀孕、多胞胎和畸形，也用于研究和测量胎儿。获得的图像被称为超声图像（ultrasonogram）

Terminology 补充术语

妊娠与分娩

正常结构与功能

术语	释义
afterbirth [ˈɑːftəbɜːθ]	胞衣，分娩后的胎盘和羊膜
antepartum [ˌæntiˈpɑːtəm]	产前，分娩之前
Braxton Hicks contractions	布雷希氏收缩，妊娠期中的子宫无痛性收缩，在第3个3月期收缩频率和强度都会上升。这种收缩是在为分娩而加强子宫

Terminology 补充术语（续表）

正常结构与功能

chloasma [kləʊˈæzmə]	黄褐斑，妊娠期间脸上出现的褐色色素沉着，也常用 melasma
fontanel [ˌfɒntəˈnel]	囟门，胎儿颅骨之间由薄膜覆盖的空间，出生后会逐渐骨化。也可拼写为 fontanelle
intrapartum [ɪntrəˈpɑːtəm]	分娩期的，在分娩期间发生的
linea nigra [ˈlɪniə ˈnɪɡrə]	黑中线，妊娠晚期在肚脐和阴阜之间的腹部可能出现的黑色条纹
lochia [ˈləʊkɪə]	恶露，分娩后子宫排出的血液、黏液和组织混合物
meconium [məˈkəʊnɪəm]	胎粪，新生儿的第一次粪便
peripartum [periˈpɑːtəm]	围产期，妊娠末期和分娩后前几个月
postpartum [ˌpəʊstˈpɑːtəm]	产后的，分娩之后
premature [ˈpremətʃə(r)]	早产的，婴儿在器官完全发育之前出生；也常用 immature
preterm [ˌpriːˈtɜːm]	早产的，早产儿，在怀孕37周以内出生的婴儿
puerperium [ˌpjuːəˈpɪərɪəm]	产褥期，分娩后前42天，在此期间，母亲的生殖器官通常会恢复正常（词根：puer 意为"儿童"）
striae atrophicae [stˈraɪiː æˈtrɒfɪkɪ]	萎缩纹，皮肤被长时间拉伸之后收缩出现的粉色或灰色的条纹；妊娠纹（stretch marks, striae gravidarum）
umbilicus [ʌmˈbɪlɪkəs]	脐，腹部的瘢痕，标志着胎儿脐带的附着点；也常用 navel
vernix caseosa [ˌkeɪsiːˈəʊsə]	胎脂，覆盖并保护胎儿的奶酪样沉着

病症

cephalopelvic disproportion [sefəˈləʊpelvɪk]	头盆不称，胎儿的头比母亲骨盆出口大的情况，也被称为胎盆不称（fetopelvic disproportion）
choriocarcinoma [kɔːrɪəʊkɑːsɪˈnəʊmə]	绒毛膜癌，一种由胎盘组织构成的罕见的恶性肿瘤
galactorrhea [ɡæˈlæktɒrɪə]	乳溢症，乳汁分泌过多或哺乳停止后继续产生乳汁。通常是催乳激素分泌过多所致，可能预示有垂体肿瘤
hydatidiform mole [haɪˈdeɪtɪdɪfɔːm]	葡萄胎，胎盘组织良性增生。胎盘扩张成葡萄样的囊，肿瘤可能会侵入子宫壁，引起破裂。也被称为胞状畸胎（hydatid mole）
hydramnios [haɪdˈræmnɪːəʊz]	羊水过多，也常用 polyhydramnios
oligohydramnios [ˌɒlɪɡəʊhaɪdˈræmnɪːəʊz]	羊水过少，缺乏羊水
patent ductus arteriosus (PDA)	动脉导管未闭，出生后动脉导管的存留，血液继续绕过肺动脉进入大动脉
puerperal infection [pjʊ(ː)ˈəːpərəl]	产褥感染，分娩后生殖道感染

Terminology 补充术语（续表）

诊断与治疗

abortifacient [əˌbɔːtəˈfeɪʃənt]	堕胎药，诱发流产的药物
alpha-fetoprotein (AFP) [ˈælfəfetˈɒprəʊtiːn]	甲胎蛋白，在特定的胎儿疾病情况下，羊水和母亲血清中含量会上升的一种胎儿蛋白质
artificial insemination (AI) [ɪnˌsemɪˈneɪʃn]	人工授精，为受孕将活的精子置入阴道或子宫颈。精液可以来自其丈夫、伴侣或捐献者
cesarean section [sɪˈzeərɪən]	剖宫产术，为分娩胎儿切开腹壁和子宫
endometrial ablation [əˈbleɪʃn]	子宫内膜切除术，为治疗目的选择性地破坏子宫内膜；用于减轻月经过多
extracorporeal membrane oxygenation (ECMO) [ˌekstrəkɔːˈpɔːrɪəl]	体外膜式氧合，一种肺旁路技术，脱氧的血液通过一个环路为血液充氧，然后返回人体。被用于预后良好的呼吸衰竭的新生儿和儿科患者
in vitro fertilization (IVF)	体外受精，一种在无法自然受精情况下达成受精的临床方法。取出卵子，在实验室使其受精，再将合子置入子宫或输卵管（zygote intrafallopian transfer，ZIFT，合子输卵管移植）。另一种方法是取出卵子，并将卵子和精子细胞一起置入输卵管（gamete intrafallopian transfer，GIFT，配子输卵管移植，框15-4）
obstetrics [əbˈstetrɪks]	产科学，治疗妊娠、分娩和产后期女性的医学分支。通常与妇科学在一起
pediatrics [ˌpiːdɪˈætrɪks]	儿科学，治疗儿童与儿童疾病的医学分支（词根：ped/o 意为"儿童"）
pelvimetry [pelˈvɪmɪtrɪ]	骨盆测量，通过人工检查和X线片研究测量骨盆，以确定是否可以通过阴道分娩胎儿
presentation [ˌpreznˈteɪʃn]	先露、胎位，描述通过阴道或直肠检查能够感觉到的胎儿的部分身体。正常情况下头最先露出（颅顶胎位，vertex presentation），但有时是臀部（臀位）、脸或其他部位先露

Terminology 缩略语

妊娠与分娩

AB	Abortion	流产
AFP	Alpha-fetoprotein	甲胎蛋白
AGA	Appropriate for gestational age	适于胎龄儿
AI	Artificial insemination	人工授精
ART	Assisted reproductive technology	辅助生殖技术
C-section	Cesarean section	剖宫产术

Terminology 缩略语（续表）

妊娠与分娩

CPD	Cephalopelvic disproportion	头盆不称
CVS	Chorionic villus sampling	绒毛采样
D&E	Dilatation and evacuation	刮宫术
ECMO	Extracorporeal membrane oxygenation	体外膜式氧合
EDC	Estimated date of confinement	预产期
FHR	Fetal heart rate	胎儿心率
FHT	Fetal heart tone	胎儿心音
FTND	Full-term normal delivery	足月顺产
FTP	Full-term pregnancy	足月妊娠
GA	Gestational age	胎龄
GIFT	Gamete intrafallopian transfer	配子输卵管移植
hCG	Human chorionic gonadotropin	人绒毛膜促性腺激素
HDN	Hemolytic disease of the newborn	新生儿溶血病
IVF	In vitro fertilization	体外受精
LMP	Last menstrual period	末次月经日期
NB	Newborn	新生儿
NICU	Neonatal intensive care unit	新生儿重症监护室
OB	Obstetrics, obstetrician	产科学、产科医生
PDA	Patent ductus arteriosus	动脉导管未闭
PIH	Pregnancy-induced hypertension	妊娠高血压综合征
PKU	Phenylketonuria	苯丙酮尿症
SVD	Spontaneous vaginal delivery	正常分娩
UC	Uterine contractions	子宫收缩
UTP	Uterine term pregnancy	子宫妊娠
VBAC	Vaginal birth after cesarean section	剖宫产术后阴道分娩
ZIFT	Zygote intrafallopian transfer	合子输卵管移植

Case Study Revisited
案例研究再访

A.Y.'s Follow-Up Study

A.Y. was encouraged to get up and walk the next day. Her incision was healing well, and there were no signs of infection. She was able to tolerate a regular diet and required minimal medication for pain. A.Y. experienced minor discomfort with breast-feeding initially, but she and the baby began to get into a routine, and the feeding progressed well. A.Y.'s husband offered needed support and encouragement and was very helpful with their 3-year-old son, who missed his mom. Both baby and mom were doing well and were discharged home. A.Y.'s mother was stopping by every day to take care of the "big brother," help with meals, and do some light housekeeping so A.Y. could get some important rest.

A.Y. 的检查随访

A.Y. 被鼓励第 2 天起床行走。她的切口愈合良好，没有感染的迹象。她能够耐受正常饮食，并需要最少量的药物镇痛。A.Y. 经历了最初母乳喂养的轻微不适，但她和婴儿已经开始正常，喂养进展状况良好。A.Y. 的丈夫提供了所需的支持和鼓励，并照顾他们 3 岁的思念妈妈的儿子。婴儿和妈妈都做得很好，并被送回家。A.Y. 的母亲每天都来照顾"大哥"，帮助他吃饭，做一些清洁家务，这样 A.Y. 就可以有时间休息。

CHAPTER 15 复习

标记练习

女性生殖系统

在对应的下划线上写出每个编号部分的名称。

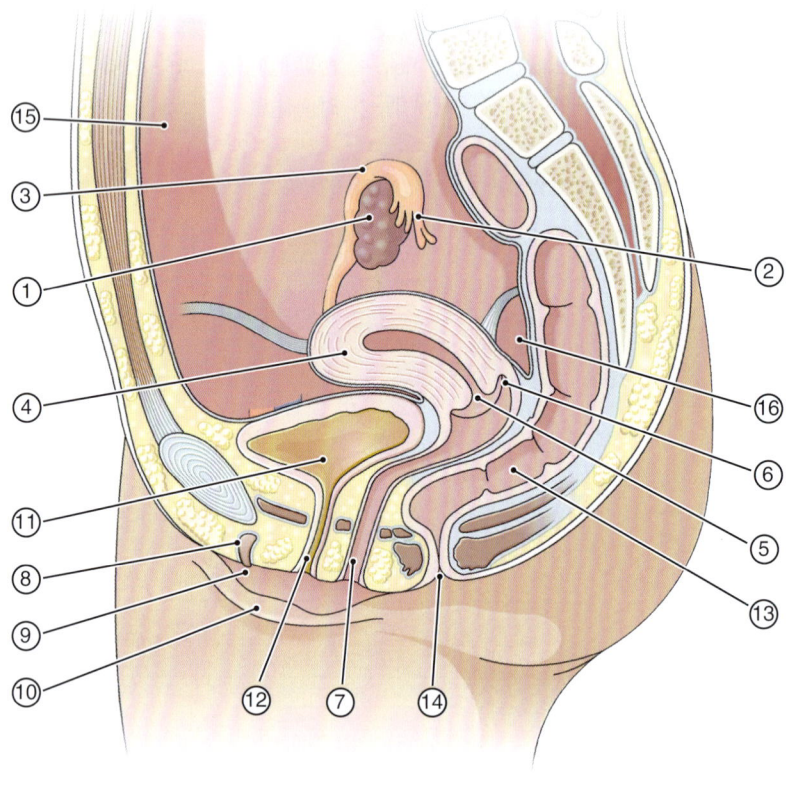

Anus   Uterine tube   Cervix
Peritoneal cavity   Clitoris   Posterior fornix
Cul-de-sac   Rectum   Fimbriae
Urethra   Labium majus   Urinary bladder
Labium minus   Uterus   Ovary
Vagina

1. _____
2. _____
3. _____
4. _____
5. _____
6. _____
7. _____
8. _____
9. _____
10. _____
11. _____
12. _____
13. _____
14. _____
15. _____
16. _____

排卵和受精

在对应的下划线上写出每个编号部分的名称。

Cervix
Body of uterus
Fimbriae
Greater vestibular (Bartholin) gland
Implanted embryo
Ovary
Ovum
Sperm cells (spermatozoa)
Uterine tube
Vagina

1. _____
2. _____
3. _____
4. _____
5. _____
6. _____
7. _____
8. _____
9. _____
10. _____

术语

匹配

匹配下列术语，在每个题号的左侧写上适当的字母。

____ 1. vulva   a. fertilized egg
____ 2. gestation   b. female erectile tissue
____ 3. oxytocin   c. external female genitalia
____ 4. zygote   d. period of development in the uterus
____ 5. clitoris   e. hormone that stimulates labor

____ 6. menostasis   a. first menstrual period
____ 7. metrorrhagia   b. excess uterine bleeding
____ 8. menarche   c. suppression of menstruation
____ 9. gynecogenic   d. wasting of uterine tissue
____ 10. metratrophia   e. producing female characteristics

____ 11. eclampsia   a. fibroid
____ 12. mutation   b. absence of a normal body opening
____ 13. teratogen   c. genetic change
____ 14. atresia   d. convulsions and coma occurring during pregnancy
____ 15. leiomyoma   e. cause of fetal abnormality

补充术语

____ **16.** puerperium   **a.** uterine discharge after childbirth

____ **17.** linea nigra   **b.** period after childbirth

____ **18.** meconium   **c.** first feces of the newborn

____ **19.** hymen   **d.** membrane that covers the vaginal opening

____ **20.** lochia   **e.** dark line on the abdomen from umbilicus to pubic region

____ **21.** hirsutism   **a.** excess of amniotic fluid

____ **22.** dyspareunia   **b.** pain during intercourse

____ **23.** vernix caseosa   **c.** whitish vaginal discharge

____ **24.** leukorrhea   **d.** excess hair growth

____ **25.** polyhydramnios   **e.** fetal protective covering

填空

26. The instrument for examining the vagina and cervix is the _____.

27. The female gonad is the _____.

28. The herniation of the rectum into the vaginal wall is called _____.

29. The ovarian follicle encloses a developing _____.

30. The organ that nourishes and maintains the developing fetus is the _____.

31. The secretion of milk from the mammary glands is called _____.

32. Loss of an embryo or fetus before 20 weeks or 500 g is termed a(n) _____.

33. Parametritis ［ˌpærəmi'traitis］ means inflammation of the tissue near the _____.

34. Polymastia ［ˌpɔli'mæstiə］ means the presence of more than one pair of _____.

拼写检查

在下列术语右侧的下划线上写出正确的拼写。

35. oophorectomy _____

36. premenstrual _____

37. salpinjectomy _____

38. dysmennarrhea _____

39. clef palate _____

真假判断

判断下列语句。如果语句为真，在第一个空格上写上 T；如果语句为加，在第一个空格上写上 F，并在第二个空格上通过替换带下划线的单词更重语句。

	True or False	Correct Answer
40. Agalactia is the lack of <u>milk</u> production.		
41. For the first two months, the developing offspring is called a <u>fetus</u>.		
42. The muscular wall of the uterus is the <u>endometrium</u>.		
43. After ovulation, the ovarian follicle becomes a <u>fimbriae</u>.		
44. Fertilization of an ovum occurs in the <u>uterus</u>.		

45. The Pap smear is a test for <u>cervical</u> cancer. _____ _____
46. Parturition is <u>childbirth</u>. _____ _____
47. The fallopian tube is the <u>uterine tube</u>. _____ _____
48. A fontanel is the soft spot between the cranial bones. _____ _____

定义

定义下列术语。

49. retrouterine ['rətrəʊtərain] _____
50. hysteropathy [his'terəpəθi] _____
51. metromalacia [metrəʊmə'leiʃə] _____
52. pyosalpinx [paiəʊ'sælpiŋks] _____
53. colpostenosis [kɒlpɒste'nəʊsis] _____
54. vulvodynia [vʌlvə'dainiə] _____
55. postnatal ['pəʊst'neitl] _____
56. inframammary [infrɑ:'mæmeəri] _____
57. extraembryonic ['ekstrə,embrai'ɒnik] _____
58. tripara [trai'pærə] _____
59. teratogenic [,terətə'dʒenik] _____

写出下列单词。

60. hernia of a uterine tube _____
61. suture of the vulva (episi/o) _____
62. narrowing of the uterus (metr/o) _____
63. surgical removal of the uterus (hyster/o) and uterine tubes _____
64. radiograph of the breast (mamm/o) _____
65. abnormal or difficult labor _____
66. rupture of the amniotic sac _____
67. study of the embryo _____
68. measurement of a fetus _____

在本章开头 A.Y. 的案例研究中，找出下列术语。

69. term that refers to a pregnant woman _____
70. upper rounded portion of the uterus _____
71. measurement of the pelvis _____
72. above the pubic bone _____
73. test to measure the health of a newborn _____
74. newborn _____

反义词

写出下列单词的反义词。

75. oligohydramnios _____
76. postnatal _____

77. dystocia
78. ovulatory
79. extrauterine

形容词

写出下列单词的形容词形式。

80. cervix
81. uterus
82. perineum
83. vagina
84. embryo
85. amnion

复数

写出下列单词的复数形式。

86. ovum
87. cervix
88. fimbria
89. labium

排除

在下列每组中，为与其他不相配的单词加上下划线，并解释你选择的理由。

90. amniocentesis — chorionic villus sampling — karyotype — ultrasonography — candidiasis

91. hemophilia — albinism — measles — PKU — cystic fibrosis

92. colostrum — progesterone — LH — estrogen — FSH

93. umbilical cord — labia majora — amniotic fluid — chorion — placenta

94. placental abruption — spina bifida — pregnancy-induced hypertension — placenta previa — eclampsia

跟随流程

描述卵子从产生到受精的路径，通过在每个题号前的下划线填上字母 A 到 D，使下列每个步骤按正确次序排列。

____ 95. uterine tube
____ 96. fimbriae
____ 97. ovary
____ 98. uterus

单词构建

用给出的单词组成部分写出下列定义的单词。

| -graphy | episi/o | -plasty | intra- | cervic/o | mamm/o | -itis | -al | -tomy | trans- |

99. plastic repair of the vulva _____

100. inflammation of the cervix _____

101. radiographic study of the breast _____

102. plastic repair of the breast _____

103. radiographic study of the cervix _____

104. incision of the vulva _____

105. within the cervix _____

106. plastic repair of the cervix _____

107. incision of the cervix _____

108. through the cervix _____

缩略语

写出下列缩略语的含义。

109. hCG _____
110. DUB _____
111. LMP _____
112. FHR _____
113. GA _____
114. VBAC _____

单词分析

定义下列单词，并给出每个单词组成部分的含义。如果需要，可以使用词典。

115. antiangiogenesis ［ænti:əngi':əʊdʒenəsis］ _____
    a. anti _____
    b. angi/o _____
    c. gen _____
    d. e/sis _____

116. gynecomastia ［gainikəʊ'mæstiə］ _____
    a. gynec/o _____
    b. mast/o _____
    c. -ia _____

117. oxytocia ［ˌɒksi'təʊʃə］ _____
    a. oxy _____
    b. toc _____
    c. -ia _____

118. oligohydramnios ［ˌɒligəʊhaid'ræmni:əʊz］ _____
    a. oligo _____
    b. hydr/o _____

c. amnio(s) _____

119. galactorrhea [gæ'læktɒriə] _____

  a. galact/o_____

  b. (r)rhea_____

120. anencephaly [ænən'sefəli] _____

  a. an _____

  b. encephal/o_____

  c. -y_____

Additional Case Studies
补充案例研究

Case Study 15-1: Total Abdominal Hysterectomy with Bilateral Salpingo-oophorectomy
案例研究 15-1：附带双侧输卵管卵巢切除术的经腹全子宫切除术

M.T., a 60-year-old gravida 2, para 2, had spent three months under the care of her gynecologist for treatment of postmenopausal bleeding and cervical dysplasia. She had had several vaginal examinations with Pap smears, a uterine ultrasound, colposcopy with endocervical biopsies, and a D&C with cone biopsy. She wanted to take hormone replacement therapy, but her doctor thought she was at too much risk with the abnormal cells on her cervix and the excessive bleeding.

She had a TAH and BSO under general anesthesia with no complications and an uneventful recovery. Her uterus had been prolapsed on abdominal examination, but there was no sign of malignancy or PID. The pathology report revealed several uterine leiomyomas and stenosis of the right uterine tube. She was discharged on the second postoperative day with few activity restrictions.

M.T. 是一名 60 岁的 2 次怀孕、2 次分娩的女性，因绝经后出血和宫颈非典型增生接受妇产科医生 3 个月的治疗。她曾经进行过多次阴道检查、子宫超声、子宫颈活检阴道镜检查和 D & C 锥切活检。她想采取激素替代疗法，但她的医生认为因子宫颈异常细胞和过多的出血，风险过高。

她在全身麻醉下做了经腹全子宫切除术（total abdominal hysterectomy，TAH）和双侧输卵管卵巢切除术（bilateral salpingo-oophorectomy，BSO），没有并发症，顺利恢复。腹部检查显示她的子宫脱垂，但没有恶性或盆腔炎（pelvic inflammatory disease，PID）的迹象。病理报告显示几个子宫平滑肌瘤和右输卵管狭窄。她在术后第 2 天出院，几乎没有活动限制。

Case Study 15-2: In Vitro Fertilization
案例研究 15-2：体外受精

C. A. had worked as a technologist in the IVF laboratory at University Medical Center for four years. Her department was the advanced reproductive technology program. Although her work was primarily in the laboratory, she followed each patient through all five phases of the IVF and embryo transfer treatment cycle: follicular development, aspiration of the preovulatory follicles, sperm preparation, IVF, and embryo transfer. Her department does both GIFT and ZIFT.

While the female patient is in surgery having an ultrasound-guided transvaginal oocyte retrieval, C. A. examines the recently donated sperm for motility and quantity. She prepares to inoculate the sample into the cytoplasm of the ova as soon as she receives the cells from the OR. After inoculation, she places the sterile petri dish with the fertilized oocytes into an incubator until they are ready to be introduced into the female patient.

C. A. 曾在大学医学中心的 IVF 实验室担任技术专家 4 年，她的部门执行了一个先进的生殖技术项目。尽管她的工作主要是在实验室，她跟随了每个患者所有五个阶段的体外受精（in vitro fertilization ,IVF）和胚胎转移治疗周期：卵泡发育、排卵前的卵泡、精子准备、IVF 和胚胎移植。她的部门既做配子卵管内移植，也做合子卵管内移植。

在女性患者做超声引导的经阴道卵母细胞摘取手术时，C. A. 检查最近捐赠的精子的运动性和数量。一旦接收到来自手术室的细胞，她就将样本接种到卵细胞的细胞质中。接种后，她将无菌培养皿中的受精的卵母细胞放入培养箱中，直至它们能够被植入女性患者身体中。

案例研究问题

多项选择。选择正确的答案，在每个题号的左侧写出你选择的字母。

____ 1. M.T. is a gravida 2, para 2. This means
   a. she has four children from two pregnancies
   b. she has had two pregnancies and two births
   c. she has had four pregnancies and two births
   d. she has one set of twins

____ 2. An endocervical biopsy is
   a. a cone-shaped tissue sample from the uterine fundus
   b. a tissue sample from within the neck
   c. a tissue sample from the lining of the cervix
   d. a scraping of tissue cells from the vaginal wall

____ 3. A curettage is a(n)
   a. suturing
   b. scraping
   c. incision
   d. examination

____ 4. A colposcopy is an endoscopic examination of the
   a. vagina
   b. fundus
   c. intraperitoneal pelvic floor
   d. uterus and uterine tubes

____ 5. Another name for a leiomyoma is a(n)
   a. ectopic pregnancy
   b. uterine fibroid
   c. myoma
   d. b and c

____ 6. Pregnancy-induced hypertension is also called
   a. placenta previa
   b. congenital mutation
   c. ectopic pregnancy
   d. preeclampsia

写出案例研究中下列含义的术语。

7. displaced downward _____
8. cell produced by fertilization _____
9. an immature egg cell _____
10. pertaining to the structure in which an egg ripens _____

定义下列缩略语。

11. D&C _____
12. BSO _____
13. HRT _____
14. TAH _____
15. IVF _____
16. GYN _____
17. ZIFT _____

CHAPTER 16

内分泌系统

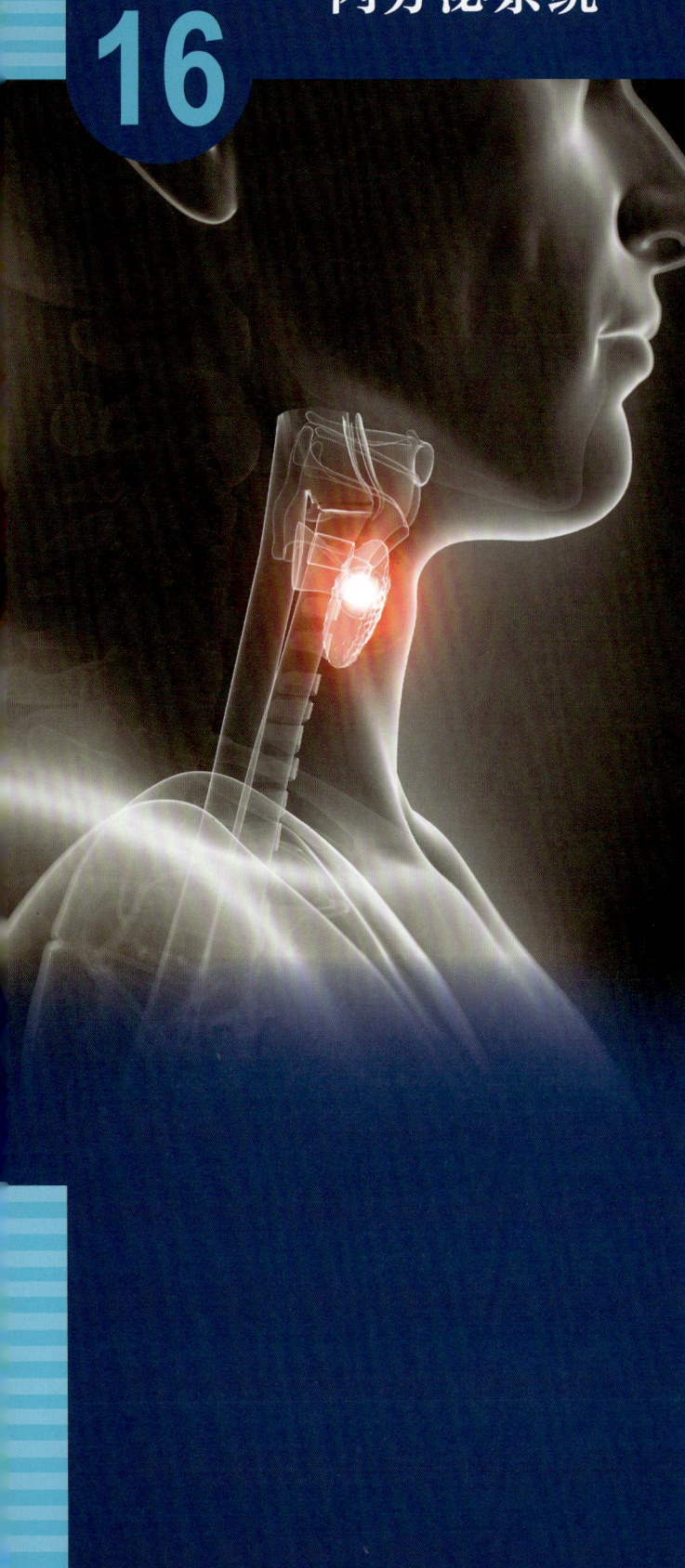

预测试

多项选择。选择正确的答案，在每个题号的左侧写出你选择的字母。

____ 1. The secretions of the endocrine glands are called
   a. enzymes
   b. sera
   c. lymph
   d. hormones

____ 2. The small gland in the brain that controls other glands is the
   a. thymus
   b. pituitary
   c. appendix
   d. corpus luteum

____ 3. The glands that are located above the kidneys are the
   a. adrenals
   b. thyroid
   c. follicles
   d. fimbriae

____ 4. Gigantism results from overproduction of
   a. erythropoietin
   b. oxytocin
   c. growth hormone
   d. prolactin

____ 5. Diabetes mellitus involves the hormone insulin, which is made in the
   a. kidney
   b. seminal vesicle
   c. thymus
   d. pancreas

____ 6. A goiter involves the
   a. zygote
   b. calyx
   c. adrenal
   d. thyroid

学习目标

学完本章后,应该能够:

1 ▶ 定义激素。
2 ▶ 比较类固醇和氨基酸激素。
3 ▶ 给出内分泌腺的位置和结构。
4 ▶ 例举内分泌腺产生的激素,简单描述每个腺体的功能。
5 ▶ 识别并使用与内分泌系统相关的词根。
6 ▶ 描述内分泌系统的主要疾病。
7 ▶ 解释内分泌学使用的缩略语。
8 ▶ 分析几个案例研究中与内分泌系统相关的医学术语。

Case Study: J. D.'s Graves Disease
案例研究:J. D. 的格雷夫斯病

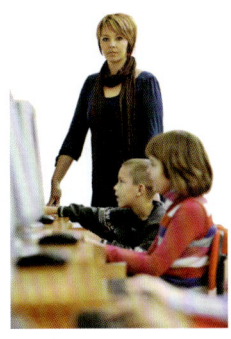

Chief Complaint

J. D. is a 35-year-old second grade teacher. Her husband has been noticing that she has been very energetic over the past few months, more so than usual. She is constantly working or cleaning, and she is up during the night, unable to sleep. J. D. says that she has felt nervous and jittery for the past few months. Her husband encouraged her to make an appointment with her physician.

Examination

J. D.'s internist, Dr. Gilbert, was able to make a few observations when he walked into the examination room. J. D. had lost weight since her last appointment, and her eyes were protruding. Normally a quiet and happy person, she appeared irritable and abrupt. She complained about her edginess, dry eyes, and inability to sleep. She also mentioned that she can't tolerate the heat and frequently perspires. She said she just hasn't been "feeling herself" as of late. Dr. Gilbert examined her, and when palpating her neck, he noted an enlarged thyroid. He also noted a dermopathy on her shins where the skin had thickened and had red patches. Her vital signs were pretty consistent with previous examinations, except that she was a bit tachycardic. Dr. Gilbert suspected hyperthyroidism. He ordered some blood work to check her thyroid levels and confirm his diagnosis.

Clinical Course

Results of the laboratory work verified Dr. Gilbert's suspicion. He discussed the diagnosis of the autoimmune disorder of hyperthyroidism, also known as Graves disease or diffuse toxic goiter, with J. D. and her husband. He provided them the results of the T3 and T4 laboratory work and explained that the high levels meant her thyroid was overactive. He explained the treatment options, including antithyroid medication, partial or total thyroidectomy, or radiation therapy. Dr. Gilbert felt that a medical regimen would be appropriate for J. D. and ordered the antithyroid drug Tapazole. He also ordered eye drops for the exophthalmos.

主诉

J. D. 是一名 35 岁的二年级教师。她的丈夫注意到她在过去几个月里精力非常充沛,远超过平时。她不断地工作或做清洁,在夜间无法入睡。J. D. 说她在过去几个月感到紧张和不安。她的丈夫督促她约见医生。

检查

J. D. 的内科医生是 Gilbert 博士,当他走进检查室时做了一些观察。自上次约见以来,J. D. 的体重减轻,眼睛突出。她通常是一个安静和快乐的人,现在却出现了急躁和粗暴。她主诉精神紧张、眼睛干燥并无法入睡。她还提到不能忍受热并经常出汗,说最近一直感觉"没有着落"。Gilbert 博士为她做了检查,当触摸她的脖子时,他注意到甲状腺肿大,还注意到她的皮肤病,皮肤增厚,有红色斑块。除了有点心动过速,她的生命体征与以前的检查非常一致。Gilbert 博士怀疑她有甲状腺功能亢进症。他安排了血液甲状腺水平检查,确认了他的诊断。

临床病程

实验室研究结果证实了 Gilbert 博士的怀疑。他与 J. D. 和她的丈夫讨论了甲状腺功能亢进症的自身免疫疾病的诊断,这种病也称被为格雷夫斯病或弥漫性毒性甲状腺肿。他向他们提供了 T_3 和 T_4 的实验室检查结果,并解释高水平意味着她的甲状腺过度活动。他解释了治疗选择,包括抗甲状腺药物、部分或全部甲状腺切除术或放射治疗。Gilbert 博士认为医疗方案适用于 J. D.,并开了抗甲状腺药物塔巴唑和用于治疗眼球突出的眼药水。

简介

人体的主要控制系统是内分泌（endocrine）和神经系统（在第 17 和 18 章讨论）。内分泌系统由广泛分布的腺体组成，这些腺体分泌被称为激素的调节性物质。因为激素被释放到血液之中，内分泌腺又被称为无管腺（ductless gland），而外分泌腺（exocrine gland），例如汗腺和消化腺，其分泌物通过导管到达体外。尽管在血液中循环的激素能够到达身体的各个部分，但只有特定的组织会对特定的激素产生反应。被特定激素影响的组织被称为靶组织（target tissue），靶组织细胞膜或细胞内有特定的受体，能够使特定的激素发生作用。

激素

激素的产生量极小，但作用极强。通过对不同的靶组织的作用，它们影响人体的生长、新陈代谢、生殖活动和行为（框 16-1 介绍了一些关于血液中循环的物质对人体影响的传统的看法。）从化学上讲，激素可以分为两类：

- 类固醇激素（steroid hormone）由脂肪制成。类固醇是由性腺和肾上腺皮层（cortex）产生的。
- 由氨基酸构成的激素，包括蛋白质和类似蛋白质的化合物。除性腺和肾上腺皮层外，所有的内分泌腺都产生氨基酸激素。

激素的产生主要由负反馈控制，即激素本身或激素作用的某种产物作为激素下一步生产的控制，是一种自我调节系统。激素的产生也受神经系统或其他激素的控制。

内分泌腺

请参照图 16-1 确定下面介绍的各内分泌腺的位置。框 16-2 列出了各个

图 16-1 内分泌腺

框 16-1

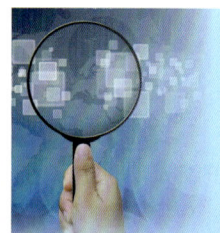

聚焦单词
你的体液良好吗？

在古代，人们接受这样一种理论，即人的健康状态取决于四种体液的平衡。这些被称为"humor"的体液是黄胆汁、黑胆汁、黏液（phlegm）和血液。这四种体液中的任何一种的优势地位能够决定一个人的情绪或气质。黄胆汁引起愤怒、黑胆汁引起压抑、黏液使人迟钝、血液则决定快乐和乐观。

尽管我们已经不再相信体液学说，但我们的词汇表之中还有一些形容词反应出这些早期的信念。胆汁质（choleric）形容一个人受黄胆汁的影响，神经胶质（melancholic）形容受黑胆汁的影响（melano- 意为"黑或暗"），多血质（sanguine）的人"随大流儿"。

体液（humor）一词还存留在现在的形容词体液的（humoral）之中，表示由血液或其他体液输送的物质。这一名词被应用于激素和其他影响身体反应的循环物质。体液免疫（humoral immunity）是基于血流中所携带抗体的免疫。

框 16-2

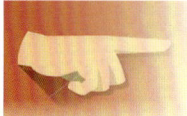

供你参考
内分泌腺及其分泌的激素

腺体	激素	主要功能
anterior pituitary 垂体前叶	growth hormone (GH)（somatotropin）生长激素	促进身体组织生长
	thyroid-stimulating hormone (TSH) 促甲状腺激素	刺激甲状腺产生甲状腺素
	adrenocorticotropic hormone (ACTH) 促肾上腺皮质激素	刺激肾上腺皮层产生皮质激素，在压力情况下（受伤、疼痛）协助保护身体
	follicle-stimulating hormone (FSH) 促卵泡激素	刺激卵泡的生长和激素活性；刺激睾丸的生长，促进精子细胞的发育
	luteinizing hormone (LH) 促黄体生成素	引起女性在卵泡破裂处发育黄体；刺激男性睾丸素的分泌
	prolactin（PRH）催乳素	刺激乳腺分泌乳汁
posterior pituitary 垂体后叶	antidiuretic hormone（ADH）抗利尿激素	促进水在肾小管的再吸收；引起血管收缩
	oxytocin 后叶催产素	引起子宫收缩；引起乳汁从乳腺中排出
thyroid 甲状腺	thyroxine（T_4）甲状腺素和 triiodothyronine（T_3）三碘甲状腺氨酸	提高代谢速率和热量的产生，影响身体和心理活动；是正常生长所必需的
parathyroid 甲状旁腺	parathyroid hormone（PTH）甲状旁腺素	调节血液与骨骼之间钙的交换，提高骨密度
adrenal cortex 肾上腺皮质	cortisol (hydrocortisone) 皮质醇	协助碳水化合物、蛋白质和脂肪的代谢；应激时生效
	aldosterone 醛固酮	协助调节电解质和水的平衡
	sex hormones 性激素	可能影响第二性征
adrenal medulla 肾上腺髓质	epinephrine 肾上腺素	应激反应，提高呼吸、血压和心率
Pancreatic 胰腺	islet insulin 胰岛素	协助葡萄糖进入细胞，是细胞营养代谢所必需的；降低血糖水平
	glucagon 胰高血糖素	刺激肝释放葡萄糖，因而提高血糖水平
pineal 松果腺	melatonin 褪黑素	调节情绪、性发育和应对环境光线的每日周期性变化
testis 睾丸	testosterone 睾酮	刺激性器官的生长和发育以及第二性征的发育；刺激精子细胞的成熟
ovary 卵巢	estrogen 雌激素	刺激主要性器官的生长和第二性征的发育
	progesterone 黄体酮	为受精卵着床准备子宫内壁；协助维护妊娠；刺激乳腺分泌组织的发育

>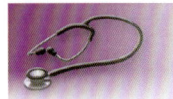
>
> ## 临床观点
> ### 生长激素：临床应用正在增长
>
> 框 16-3
>
> 生长激素是垂体前叶产生的。它主要是在深度睡眠的开始阶段释放，所以认为你在睡眠时长高的古老信念实际上是有其成立基础的。尽管生长激素在早期生长中主要影响骨骼和肌肉的发育，其实它在人的整个生命期间对大多数其他组织都有一定的刺激作用。它的另一个名称是 somatotropin，源自于意为"身体"的 soma 和意为"作用于"的 tropin。在应激时释放的生长激素能够在血糖水平下降时促进肝脏输出富有能量的脂肪酸。童年时期缺乏生长激素会导致侏儒症，该激素最初只为生长激素缺乏的儿童处方使用。现在，生长激素已经被批准给那些处于最低年龄身高百分比的儿童使用。如果儿童仍处于生长期，生长激素的使用会导致身高极度提高。因为生长激素会提高肌肉量，它也会被吹捧为健美和抗衰老良药。不过，生长激素可能有一些不良反应，其长期作用尚不明确。临床使用的生长激素最初是从尸体的脑垂体获得的，现在可以通过基因工程生产。

内分泌腺和它们所分泌的激素及其作用。

脑垂体

垂体腺，或脑垂体（hypophysis），是大脑下面的一个小腺体，分为前叶（adenohypophysis）和后叶（neurohypophysis）。下丘脑（hypothalamus）是大脑的一部分，连接并控制脑垂体的两个叶。

脑垂体前叶产生六种激素，其中之一是生长激素（somatotropin），它刺激骨骼的生长并作用于其他组织（框 16-3）。其余的垂体激素调节其他腺体，包括甲状腺、肾上腺、性腺和乳腺（框 16-2）。后缀 -tropin 表示激素作用于其他腺体，如促性腺激素（gonadotropin）。形容词性的后缀是 -tropic，例如促肾上腺皮质的（adrenocorticotropic）。

垂体后叶释放两种实际上由下丘脑产生的激素，它们被存储在垂体后叶，直至被需要：

- 抗利尿激素（antidiuretic hormone，ADH）作用于肾，以保留水和促进血管收缩。这两种作用都会提升血压。
- 后叶催产素（oxytocin）刺激子宫收缩，并促进哺乳期乳房的乳汁分泌。

甲状腺和甲状旁腺

甲状腺由喉和上段气管两侧的两个叶组成。两个叶由一个狭窄的带（峡，isthmus）连接（图 16-2）。甲状腺分泌一种激素混合物，主要是甲状腺素（thyroxine，T_4）和三碘甲状腺氨酸（triiodothyronine，T_3）。因为甲状腺激素包含碘，实验室能够通过跟踪碘的水平测量这些激素，并研究甲状腺的活动。血液中大多数甲状腺激素都与蛋白质结合，主要是甲状腺结合球蛋白（thyroxinebinding globulin，TBG）。

甲状腺后叶的表面上有 4~6 个很小的影响钙代谢的甲状旁腺（parathyroid）（图 16-2）。甲状旁腺激素（parathyroid hormone，PTH）调节血液与骨骼之间的钙交换，在需要时提高血液中钙的水平。

肾上腺

肾上腺（adrenal gland）位于肾的顶部，分为两个不同的区域：外皮层（cortex）和内髓质（medulla）（图 16-4）。肾上腺生产的激素参与人体对压力的反应。皮层分泌类固醇激素：

- 皮质醇（cortisol、hydrocortisone）调动脂肪和碳水化合物储备增加血液中的营养。它还能够减少炎症，并以此为目的在临床使用。
- 醛固酮（aldosterone）使肾在排泄钾的同时保留钠和水。
- 性激素，主要是睾酮（testosterone），产生量很少，但其重要性尚不明了。一些运动员非法且危险地使用类似睾酮的类固醇来提高肌肉的大小、强度和耐力（框 20-1）。

肾上腺的内髓质产生肾上腺素（adrenaline）以应对压力。肾上腺素与神经系统共同协助人体应对物理和情绪的挑战。

胰腺

胰腺的内分泌部分是胰岛（pancreatic islet），

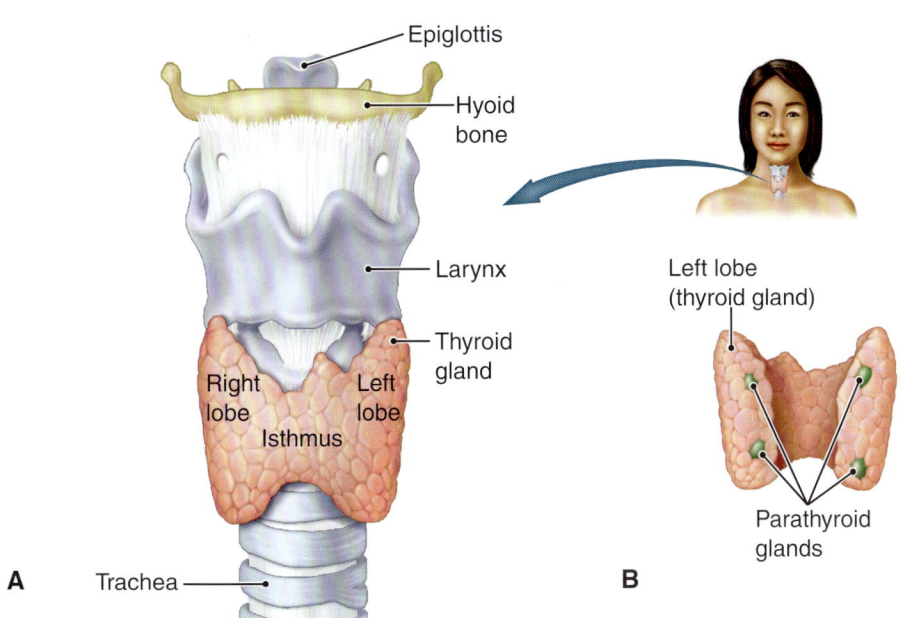

图 16-2 甲状腺和甲状旁腺。A. 甲状腺有两个叶,由峡部连接。这个前视图示出了与喉部中的其他结构相关的腺体;B. 甲状旁腺嵌入甲状腺的后部

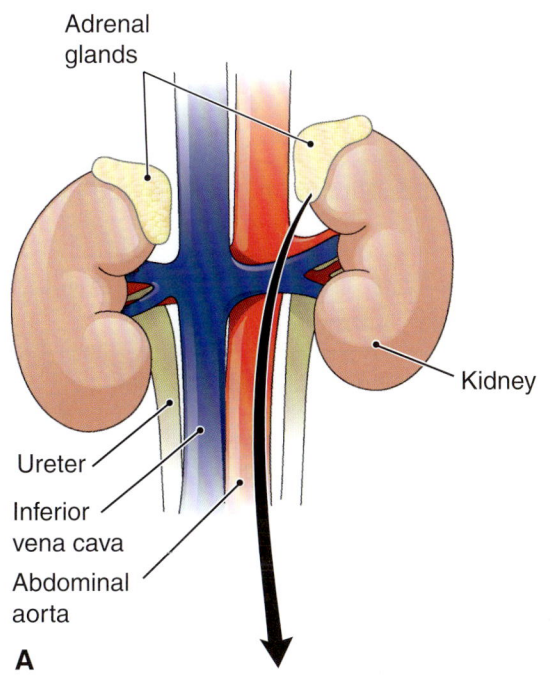

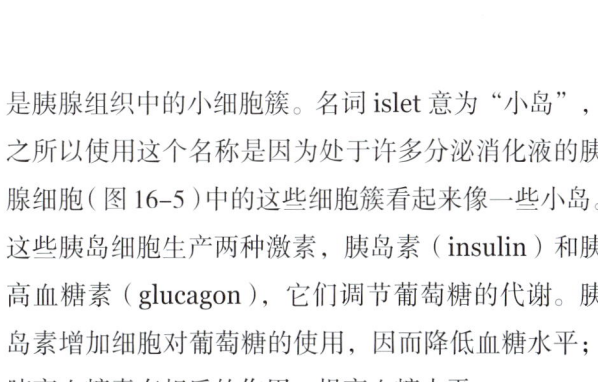

图 16-4 胰腺细胞显微图。在产生消化液的细胞簇中可见到光染色的胰岛细胞

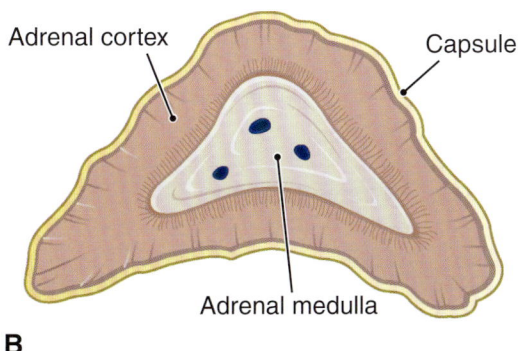

图 16-3 肾上腺。A. 肾顶部的肾上腺;B. 肾上腺分为髓质和皮层,各分泌不同的激素

是胰腺组织中的小细胞簇。名词 islet 意为"小岛",之所以使用这个名称是因为处于许多分泌消化液的胰腺细胞(图 16-5)中的这些细胞簇看起来像一些小岛。这些胰岛细胞生产两种激素,胰岛素(insulin)和胰高血糖素(glucagon),它们调节葡萄糖的代谢。胰岛素增加细胞对葡萄糖的使用,因而降低血糖水平;胰高血糖素有相反的作用,提高血糖水平。

其他内分泌组织

其他三类分泌激素的腺体:
- 松果体(pineal gland)是大脑中的一个小腺

体（图16-1）。它针对环境光线的变化调节情绪、日常节律和性发育。它分泌的激素是褪黑素（melatonin），一些人在跨时区旅行时服用它协助调节睡眠 - 清醒周期。
- 胸腺（thymus）在第9章中讨论过，分泌激素胸腺素（thymosin），协助免疫系统中T细胞的发育。胸腺位于胸上部心脏之上，在生命早期非常重要，但在成年或萎缩并变得无关紧要。
- 性腺（gonad），第14和15章讨论了睾丸和卵巢，因为它们除了产生性细胞之外还分泌激素，所有也是内分泌腺。

其他器官，包括胃、肾、心脏和小肠，也都分泌激素。不过，它们都有其他的主要功能，因此在它们各自所属的系统进行说明。

最后，前列腺素（prostaglandin）是一组由许多细胞产生的激素，它们有不同的作用，包括刺激子宫收缩、促进炎症和血管收缩。因为它们最初是在前列腺被发现的，所以被称为前列腺素。

Terminology 关键术语

正常结构与功能

术语	释义
adrenal gland [əˈdriːnl glænd]	肾上腺，在肾表面上的腺体。外皮质层分泌类固醇激素，内髓质分泌应激反应的肾上腺素（词根：adren/o）
endocrine [ˈendəʊkrɪn]	内分泌的，与分泌激素进入血液的内分泌腺相关的
hormone [ˈhɔːməʊn]	激素，内分泌腺的分泌物，是一种在血液中循环，并对组织、器官或腺体有调节作用的物质
hypophysis [haɪˈpɒfəsɪs]	脑垂体，垂体腺，名称源自于意为"之下"的hypo和意为"生长"的physis，因为该腺体在下丘脑之下发育（词根：hypophysi/o）
hypothalamus [ˌhaɪpəˈθæləməs]	下丘脑，大脑的一部分，控制垂体腺，并在维持自我平衡方面起作用
pancreatic islet [ˌpæŋkriˈætɪk ˈaɪlət]	胰岛，胰腺中的内分泌细胞簇，分泌激素调节葡萄糖的代谢；也被称为朗格汉斯岛（islet of Langerhans）或胰岛细胞（islet cells，词根：insul/o意为"岛"）
parathyroid gland [ˌpærəˈθaɪrɔɪd]	甲状旁腺，甲状腺后面的小内分泌腺，其作用是提高血钙的水平；通常有4~6个甲状旁腺（词根：parathyr/o, parathyroid/o），字面意为"甲状腺附近"
pineal gland [paɪˈniːəl]	松果体，大脑中的小腺体（图16-1），针对环境光线的变化调节情绪、日常节律和性发育。分泌褪黑素
pituitary gland [pɪˈtjuːɪtəri]	垂体腺，大脑底部的小内分泌腺。前叶分泌生长激素和刺激其他腺体的激素，后叶释放有下丘脑生产的抗利尿激素和后叶催产素（词根：pituitar/i）
prostaglandin [ˌprɒstəˈglændɪŋ]	前列腺素，一组身体各处产生的激素，有不同的作用，包括刺激子宫收缩和调节血压、血液凝结和炎症
receptor [rɪˈseptə(r)]	受体，细胞膜或细胞内的一个位置，激素能够附着于其上
steroid hormone [ˈstɪərɔɪd]	类固醇激素，由脂肪制成的激素，包括性激素和肾上腺皮质激素
target tissue	靶组织，激素对其发生作用的特定组织，也可以称为靶器官
thyroid gland [ˈθaɪrɔɪd]	甲状腺，喉与上端气管两侧的内分泌腺，其分泌的激素影响代谢和生长（词根：thyr/o, thyroid/o）

与内分泌系统相关的词根

参见表 16-1

表 16-1　与内分泌系统相关的词根

词根	含义	示例	示例定义
endocrin/o	内分泌腺或系统	endocrinopathy [ˌendəʊkraiˈnɒpəθi]	内分泌失调
pituitar/i	垂体腺	pituitarism [piˈtjuːitərizəm]	垂体功能障碍
hypophysi/o	垂体腺、脑垂体	hypophysial [haipəʊˈfiziəl]	垂体的
thyr/o, thyroid/o	甲状腺	thyrolytic [θirəˈlitik]	破坏甲状腺的
parathyr/o, parathyroid/o	甲状旁腺	hyperparathyroidism [haipəpærəˈθairɔidizəm]	甲状旁腺功能亢进
adren/o, adrenal/o	肾上腺，肾上腺素	adrenergic [ædrəˈnɜːdʒik]	肾上腺素的
adrenocortic/o	肾上腺皮质	adrenocorticotropic [əˈdriːnəʊˌkɔːtikəʊˈtrɒpik]	促肾上腺皮质的
insul/o	胰岛	insular [ˈinsjələ(r)]	胰岛的

练习 16-1

定义下列单词。

1. hypoadrenalism
   [haipəʊəˈdriːnəlizm] _____
2. thyrotropic
   [θaiˈrɒtrəpik] _____
3. hypophysectomy
   [haiˌpɒfiˈsektəmi] _____
4. endocrinology
   [ˌendəʊkriˈnɒlədʒi] _____
5. insuloma
   [insjuːˈləʊmə] _____

通过将后缀 -ism 添加到腺体名称或其词根上，再加上前缀 hyper- 或 hypo- 表示该腺体的活性过高或过低，从而形成由内分泌功能障碍引起的病症的名称。使用腺体的全名构成下列定义的词语。

6. condition of overactivity of the thyroid gland, as seen in J.D.'s opening case study_____
7. condition of underactivity of the parathyroid gland_____
8. condition of overactivity of the adrenal gland_____

练习 16-1

使用腺体的词根构成下列定义的单词。

9. condition of overactivity of the adrenal cortex _____
10. condition of underactivity of the pituitary gland (use pituitar/i) _____

写出下列定义的单词。

11. enlargement of the adrenal gland _____
12. excision of the thyroid gland, as mentioned in J.D.'s opening case study _____
13. any disease of the adrenal gland _____
14. physician who specializes in study of the endocrine system _____
15. inflammation of the pancreatic islets _____

内分泌系统的临床表现

内分泌疾病通常是激素生产过多（分泌过多，hypersecretion）或生产不足（分泌不足，hyposecretion）所致，也可能是在错误地时间分泌或靶组织反应不够所致。分泌异常的原因可能起源于腺体自身，或者是下丘脑或垂体未能释放适当数量的刺激激素所致。下面介绍了一些常见的内分泌疾病，因激素分泌过多或分泌不足所致的病症在框 16-4 中给出。

脑垂体

垂体腺瘤（pituitary adenoma，glandular tumor）通常会增加生长激素或促肾上腺皮质激素（adrenocort

---

框 16-4

供你参考
与内分泌失调相关的疾病*

激素	分泌过多	分泌不足
growth hormone 生长激素	gigantism 巨人症（儿童） acromegaly 肢端肥大症（成人）	dwarfism 侏儒症（儿童）
antidiuretic hormone	syndrome of inappropriate ADH (SIADH) 抗利尿激素失调综合征	diabetes insipidus 尿崩症
aldosterone 醛固酮	aldosteronism 醛固酮增多症	Addison disease 艾迪森病
cortisol 皮质醇	Cushing syndrome 库欣综合征	Addison disease 艾迪森病
thyroid hormone 甲状腺激素	Graves disease 格雷夫斯病，thyrotoxicosis 甲状腺功能亢进	infantile and adult hypothyroidism 婴幼儿和成人甲状腺功能减退症
insulin 胰岛素	hypoglycemia 低血糖	diabetes mellitus 糖尿病
parathyroid hormone 甲状旁腺激素	bone degeneration 骨骼退化	tetany 强直

* 发音和说明请参见关键术语

icotropic hormone，ACTH）的分泌。比较少见的是肿瘤影响催乳激素的分泌。儿童生长激素过量会引起巨人症（gigantism），对成年人会引起肢端肥大症（acromegaly），特征是手、足、颌与五官肥大。治疗方法是手术或药物切除肿瘤（垂体瘤切除术 adenomectomy），以降低血液中的生长激素水平。过量的促肾上腺皮质激素会过度刺激肾上腺皮质，导致库欣病（Cushing disease）。催乳激素增加会引起男性和女性分泌乳汁（乳溢症 galactorrhea）。垂体腺瘤的放射线研究通常会显示包含垂体的骨窝（蝶鞍 sella turcica）肿大。

由肿瘤或供血中断所致的垂体功能低下可能只涉及一种激素，但通常会影响所有功能，被称为全垂体功能减退症（panhypopituitarism）。这种状况的广泛影响包括侏儒症（dwarfism）（缺乏生长激素所致）、缺乏性发育和性功能、疲劳和虚弱。

缺乏来自于垂体后叶的抗利尿激素会导致尿崩症（diabetes insipidus），肾的保水功能降低。其症状是多尿（polyuria）和烦渴（polydipsia）。

不应将尿崩症与糖尿病（diabetes mellitus，DM）混淆，糖尿病是葡萄糖代谢疾病（后面将讨论）。这两种疾病有相同的多尿和烦渴症状，但有完全不同的起因。糖尿病是一种更为常见的疾病，当单独使用名词 diabetes 时，一般是指糖尿病。Diabetes 源自于希腊语意为"虹吸"的单词。

甲状腺

因为甲状腺激素影响许多组织的生长和功能，婴儿期缺乏这种激素会引起身体和心理发育迟缓（retardation）和其他一些症状，共同构成婴幼儿甲状腺功能减退症（infantile hypothyroidism）。如果不能在出生时得到诊断和治疗，会在 6 个月内导致心理发育迟缓。在美国和其他发达国家，所有新生儿都要进行甲状腺功能减退症测试。

成年人缺乏甲状腺激素会引起体重上升、嗜睡症（lethargy）、皮肤干粗、头发脱落和面部肿胀。还可能有生殖系统问题和肌肉无力、疼痛和僵硬。成年甲状腺功能减退症的常见起因是甲状腺自免疫破坏。儿童和成年甲状腺功能减退症都可以用甲状腺激素进行治疗。

甲状腺功能亢进（hyperthyroidism）的最常见形式是格雷夫斯病（Graves disease），也被称为弥漫性毒性甲状腺肿（diffuse toxic goiter）。这是一种自身免疫病，有抗体刺激增加甲状腺激素的生产。症状有体重减轻、易激动、手震颤和心率过快。最独特的体征是眼球突出，被称为眼球突出症

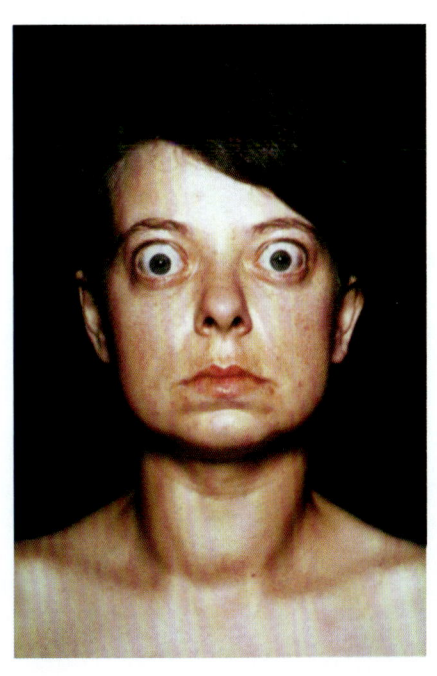

图 16-5 **格雷夫斯病**。一个甲状腺功能亢进症的年轻女子在脖子显现出一个团块和眼球突出

（exophthalmos），是由眼睛后面的组织肿胀所致（图16-5）。格雷夫斯病的治疗包括抗甲状腺药物、手术切除全部或部分甲状腺或放射性碘放疗。

甲状腺疾病的一个常见体征是甲状腺肿大（goiter）。但是，甲状腺肿大并不一定伴随甲状腺功能异常。饮食缺碘会引起简单的或无毒的甲状腺肿大，这种情况在发达国家很少见，因为在盐和其他零售食品中已经添加了碘。

甲状腺功能检查的常用方法是测量甲状腺的放射性碘的摄入（radioactive iodine uptake，RAIU）。实验室使用放射免疫检定法测量垂体促甲状腺激素（thyroid-stimulating hormone，TSH）的血液水平，该水平随甲状腺激素水平的变化而改变。总的和游离的甲状腺素（thyroxine，T_4）和三碘甲状腺氨酸（triiodothyronine，T_3）也可以测量，还有与甲状腺激素结合的甲状腺结合球蛋白TBG。服用放射性碘后的甲状腺扫描也被用于研究甲状腺的活动。

甲状旁腺

甲状旁腺过度活跃通常是肿瘤所致，会引起血液中钙水平升高。因为这些钙是从骨骼中获得的，所以会引起骨骼退化和骨痛。常见的不良反应是高水平钙循环所致的肾结石。

甲状旁腺的损害或甲状腺手术中常做的手术切除会导致血液钙水平下降，引起四肢和口周（perioral）的麻木（numbness）和刺痛（tingling），以及肌肉痉挛。服用钙可以治疗。

肾上腺

肾上腺皮质功能低下，也被称为艾迪森病（Addison disease），通常是肾上腺被自身免疫损伤所致，也可能是垂体促肾上腺皮质激素缺乏所致。缺乏肾上腺素会导致失水、低血压和电解质失衡，还会有虚弱、恶心和棕色色素沉着增加。棕色色素沉着增加是由垂体激素释放刺激皮肤色素细胞（melanocyte）引起的。一旦被诊断，艾迪森病需要通过替换皮质激素进行治疗。

肾上腺皮质激素过量会引起库欣综合征（Cushing syndrome）。该综合征的患者会有满月脸、躯干肥胖、虚弱、多毛（hirsutism）和液体潴留（图16-6）。库欣综合征最常见的起因是治疗时服用类固醇激素，肾上腺肿瘤是另一个可能的起因。如果疾病是由垂体肿瘤增加促肾上腺皮质激素的生产所致，就被称为库欣综合征。

胰腺与糖尿病

糖尿病（diabetes mellitus，DM）是最常见的内分泌疾病，也是严重的公共健康问题，身体细胞无法有效地利用葡萄糖。血液中积累了过量的葡萄糖，引起高血糖症（hyperglycemia）。多尿（polyuria）标志着要努力通过尿液排出多余的葡萄糖，被称为糖尿（glycosuria），其结果是脱水和烦渴（polydipsia），还有虚弱、体重减轻和多食（polyphagia）。不能利用碳水化合物，身体要燃烧更多的脂肪，这导致血液中酮体的积累，并转为酸中毒，被称为酮症酸中毒

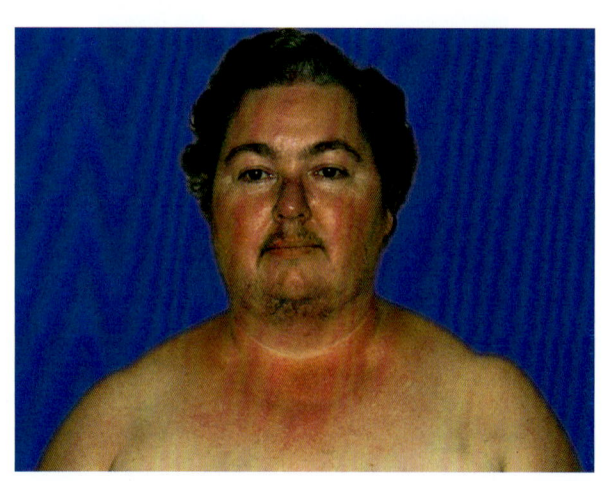

图16-6 **库欣综合征**。一个有满月脸、水牛背、面部毛发增多和头发稀疏的女性

（ketoacidosis）。如果不治疗，糖尿病会导致中枢神经系统饥饿和昏迷。糖尿病患者易患心血管、神经系统和视觉系统疾病、感染和肾衰竭。

糖尿病的类别

糖尿病分为两类：

- I 型糖尿病（type 1 diabetes mellitus，T1DM）是由自身免疫破坏胰岛细胞和胰腺不能产生胰岛素所致。I 型糖尿病会突然发病，通常发生于儿童和青少年。因为胰岛素水平很低或缺失，患者需认真监护并定期服用胰岛素。
- II 型糖尿病（type 2 diabetes mellitus，T2DM）占糖尿病病例的 90%。相比于 I 型糖尿病，遗传在 II 型糖尿病中有着更重要的作用。II 型糖尿病起始于细胞对胰岛素的抵抗，反馈刺激胰岛导致胰岛素过量生产，继而超负荷工作的胰岛细胞不能产生足够的胰岛素。大多数 II 型糖尿病患者与肥胖有关，特别是上半身肥胖。尽管常见于老年人，II 型糖尿病在年轻一代中的发病率正在上升，可能是因为肥胖、饮食不良和久坐不动的生活习惯的增加。

代谢综合征（metabolic syndrome），也被称为 X 综合征或胰岛素抵抗综合征，与 II 型糖尿病有关，被描述为由胰岛素抵抗引起的高血糖状态，伴随一些代谢疾病，包括高水平血浆甘油三酯、低水平高密度脂蛋白、高血压和冠状动脉粥样硬化性心脏病（冠心病）。

妊娠期糖尿病（gestational diabetes mellitus，GDM）是指妊娠期间的葡萄糖耐受不良（glucose intolerance）。这种失衡通常发生于有家族糖尿病史和肥胖的女性。有发病诱因的女性在妊娠期必须监测糖尿病体征，因为这种状况会引起母亲和胎儿的并发症。妊娠期糖尿病通常在分娩后消失，但也可能是后期发展糖尿病的迹象。像其他形式的糖尿病一样，首先要有合理的饮食，必要时进行胰岛素治疗。糖尿病可能继发其他内分泌疾病或需要皮质类固醇进行治疗，也可能是胰岛的遗传疾病所致。

诊断

通过测量禁食或不禁食的血浆葡萄糖水平可以诊断糖尿病。糖尿病的诊断标准是随机测试高于 200mg/dL 和空腹血糖（fasting plasma glucose，FPG）高于 126mg/dL。口服葡萄糖之后测量血糖水平被称为口服葡萄糖耐量测试（oral glucose tolerance test，OGTT）。空腹血糖受损（impaired fasting blood glucose，IFG）和糖耐量降低（impaired glucose tolerance，IGT）是葡萄糖正常反应和确认糖尿病之间的中间阶段。

治疗

I 型糖尿病的治疗必须每天 4~8 次监测血糖水平。传统上要针刺手指获得血液进行测试，但现在有新的方法通过皮肤监测血糖。还有连续监测系统，能够向患者警示高血糖和低血糖水平。胰岛素可以分次注射或通过胰岛素泵进行持续皮下胰岛素输注（continuous subcutaneous insulin infusion，CSII）。更新的计算机辅助泵能够监测血糖水平，并自动调节胰岛素的剂量。饮食必须认真控制，以保持血糖水平稳定。

在控制糖尿病的同时，患者每天都要监测自己的血糖水平。每几个月，医生能够通过糖化血红蛋白（glycated hemoglobin，HbA1c）测试获得长期血糖水平控制的更为精确的指征。该测试基于红细胞摄入的葡萄糖，能够反映测试前 2~3 个月的平均血糖水平。

锻炼和减轻体重是肥胖的 II 型糖尿病患者治疗的第一步，这些方法通常能够控制疾病的发展。可能需要使用增加胰岛素生产或改善细胞对胰岛素的反应的药物，必要时需要给予胰岛素治疗。

目前，胰岛素可以通过基因工程制造。不同的品种有不同的作用时间，能够交替使用以实现血糖水平调节。过量的胰岛素可能是胰腺肿瘤所致，但更多地发生于糖尿病患者服用了太多的胰岛素。产生的低血糖会导致胰岛素休克，要通过服用葡萄糖进行治疗。

片剂或胶囊、喷雾吸入和皮肤贴剂等使用胰岛素的方法仍处于研究之中。研究者还在研究移植健康胰岛细胞以补偿失效细胞的可能性。研究的另一个领域是应用免疫抑制反应治疗 I 型糖尿病。

用于诊断内分泌疾病的方法还有成像技术、血浆和尿液中激素或其代谢物的其他测量方法，以及涉及激素刺激与抑制的研究。

框 16-5 是关于营养师和营养学家的信息。这些健康职业的从业者为包括糖尿病和其他代谢疾病的患者提供健康饮食计划。

健康职业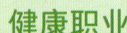

营养师和营养学家

框 16-5

营养师（dietitian）和营养学家（nutritionist）专门为诸如医院、学校和护理机构以及具有特定疾病的个人（例如糖尿病、肾脏疾病或心脏病）规划和监督饮食计划。他们评估客户的营养需求并设计个性化膳食计划。营养师和营养学家也在社区中工作，通过健康饮食教育公众预防疾病。公众对食品和营养认识的提高也为食品制造业带来了新的机会。为了履行其职责，营养师和营养学家需要完整的科学和临床背景。美国的大多数营养师和营养学家都接受来自大学或大学机构的培训，完成实习，并参加认证或注册考试。

营养师和营养学家的工作前景良好。随着美国人口继续老龄化，在医院和护理机构中对营养规划的需求预计将增加。此外，许多人现在重视健康饮食，会私下咨询营养学家。营养与饮食学院（The Academy of Nutrition and Dietetics）在 www.eatright.org 有关于这些职业的信息。

Terminology 关键术语

疾病

术语	释义
acromegaly [ˌækrə'megəli]	肢端肥大症，骨骼和软组织增生，特别是手、脚颌面部，成年人生长激素更多所致。该名称源自于意为"末端"的 acro 和意为"肿大"的 megal/o
Addison disease	艾迪森病，肾上腺皮质激素缺乏所致的疾病。特征是皮肤变暗、虚弱和水盐平衡失调
adenoma [ˌædə'nəʊmə]	腺瘤，腺体的肿瘤
adult hypothyroidism [ˌhaipəʊ'θairɔidizəm]	成年甲状腺功能减退症，成年人甲状腺机能减退的状况，患者面部干燥和蜡样肿胀；以前被称为黏液水肿 myxedema
Cushing disease	库欣病，因垂体生产过量的促肾上腺皮质激素所致的肾上腺皮质过度活跃
Cushing syndrome	库欣综合征，肾上腺皮质激素过多所致的状况，会引起肥胖、虚弱、高血糖、高血压和多毛症
diabetes insipidus [ˌdaiə'biːtiːz in'sipidəs]	尿崩症，用于来自垂体前叶的抗利尿激素不足引起的疾病，会导致极度干渴和产生大量稀释的尿液。单词 insipidus 意为"无味"，指尿液的稀释
diabetes mellitus (DM) ['melitəs]	糖尿病，用于胰岛素生产缺乏或对胰岛素响应的组织不足引起的葡萄糖代谢疾病。Ⅰ型糖尿病是胰岛细胞自免疫破坏所致，通常发生于儿童，需要使用胰岛素治疗。Ⅱ型糖尿病通常发生于肥胖的成年人，需要饮食、锻炼和提高胰岛素生产或活性的药物治疗，有时需要胰岛素。单词 mellitus 源自于拉丁语蜂蜜的词根，指尿液中糖的成分
exophthalmos [ˌeksɒf'θælməs]	眼球突出症，眼球突出，常见于格雷夫斯病
gigantism [dʒai'gæntizəm]	巨人症，儿童期间垂体生长激素过多引起的过度生长
glycated hemoglobin (HbA1c) test	糖化血红蛋白测试，一种测量红细胞生命周期内葡萄糖与血红蛋白的结合力的测试。测试结果反映 2~3 个月中的平均血糖水平，有助于评估糖尿病的长期疗效。也被称为 A1c 测试
glycosuria [ˌglaikəʊ'sjʊəriə]	糖尿，尿液含糖过量
goiter ['gɔitə]	甲状腺肿，甲状腺肿大，可能是毒性的或无毒的。单纯的（无毒）甲状腺肿是缺碘引起的

Terminology 关键术语

Graves disease	格雷夫斯病，由甲状腺功能亢进引起的自身免疫病，突出症状是眼球突出，也被称为弥漫性毒性甲状腺肿（diffuse toxic goiter）
hyperglycemia [ˌhaipəglaiˈsiːmiə]	高血糖症，血液中葡萄糖含量过高
hypoglycemia [ˌhaipəʊglaiˈsiːmiə]	低血糖症，血糖水平异常低
hypothyroidism [ˌhaipəʊˈθairɔidizəm]	甲状腺功能减退症，先天性缺乏甲状腺分泌引起的状况，特征是身体和心理发育迟缓。也被称为先天性甲状腺功能低下
insulin shock	胰岛素休克，过量使用胰岛素，引起甲状腺功能亢进症的状况
ketoacidosis [kiːtəʊæsiˈdəʊsis]	酮症酸中毒，过量酮体引起的酸中毒，如在糖尿病中；又称为糖尿病酸中毒
metabolic syndrome	代谢综合征，因细胞拒绝胰岛素引起的高血糖状态，如在Ⅱ型糖尿病中，同时伴有其他代谢失调；也被称为X综合征或胰岛素抵抗综合征
panhypopituitarism [pænhaipəʊpiˈtjuːitərizm]	全垂体功能衰减症，整个垂体腺功能低下
tetany [ˈtetəni]	强直，肌肉兴奋与痉挛，可能是低血钙和其他因素引起的

Terminology 补充术语

正常结构与功能

sella turcica [ˈselə ˈtəːsikə]	蝶鞍，包含垂体腺的蝶骨的鞍形凹陷（字面意为"土耳其鞍"）
sphenoid bone [ˈsfiːnɔid]	蝶骨，在颅底的一块包含垂体腺的骨骼

症状与病症

adrenogenital syndrome	肾上腺性征综合征，来自于肾上腺皮质的雄性激素生产过剩所致的病症，会导致男性化；可能是先天性或获得性的，通常是肾上腺肿瘤的结果
Conn syndrome	康恩综合征，肾上腺肿瘤引起的醛固酮增多症
craniopharyngioma [ˈkreiniəʊfəˌrindʒiəʊmə]	颅咽管瘤，垂体腺良性肿瘤
Hashimoto disease	桥本病，自身免疫起源的慢性甲状腺肿
impaired glucose tolerance (IGT)	糖耐量受损，葡萄糖摄入后的高血糖水平，可能预示边缘糖尿病
ketosis [kiːˈtəʊsis]	酮症，酮体，例如丙酮，在体内的积累。通常是由碳水化合物代谢缺乏或不完善所致，例如糖尿病和饥饿的情况下
multiple endocrine neoplasia (MEN)	多发性内分泌腺瘤，一种会引起多个内分泌腺肿瘤的遗传性疾病；根据涉及的腺体组合分类
pheochromocytoma [fiːəkrəʊməsaiˈtəʊmə]	嗜铬细胞瘤，肾上腺髓质或其他包含嗜铬细胞组织结构的良性肿瘤；phe/o意为"棕色"或"暗黑的"。肾上腺肿瘤会引起肾上腺素产量的增加

Terminology 补充术语

pituitary apoplexy [ˈæpəpleksi]	垂体卒中，与垂体肿瘤相关的垂体腺突然大出血和变性。常见症状包括头痛、视觉问题和意识损失
seasonal affective disorder (SAD)	季节性情绪失调，一种懒散、抑郁、极度嗜睡和暴食的情绪失调，通常发生在冬季。被认为与受外界光线影响的褪黑素水平有关（框 16-6）
Simmonds disease	西蒙兹病，垂体前叶功能低下（全垂体功能减退症，panhypopituitarism），通常是因为梗死；也被称为垂体恶质病（pituitary cachexia [kəˈkeksiə]）
thyroid storm	甲状腺危象，未治疗的或治疗不佳的甲状腺功能亢进患者发生的甲状腺功能亢进症状突然发作。可能是疾病或外伤带来的。也被称为 thyroid crisis（甲状腺危机）
thyrotoxicosis [ˌθairəʊˌtɒksiˈkəʊsis]	甲状腺功能亢进，甲状腺过于活跃导致的病症。症状包括焦虑、易怒、体重减轻和出汗。甲状腺功能亢进的主要例证的格雷夫斯病
von Recklinghausen disease	雷克林霍曾病，甲状旁腺激素生产过多引起的骨质疏松症
诊断与治疗	
fasting plasma glucose (FPG)	空腹血糖，禁食至少 8 小时后测量的血糖水平。结果等于或高于 126 mg/dL 的表明有糖尿病。也被称为 fasting blood glucose (FBG) 或 fasting blood sugar (FBS)
free thyroxine index（FTI, T7）	游离甲状腺素指数，基于 T_4 的出现量和 T_3 的吸收量的计算结果，被用于诊断甲状腺机能障碍
oral glucose tolerance test (OGTT)	口服葡萄糖耐量测试，在禁食的患者服用挑战性剂量的葡萄糖后测量血糖水平。被用于测量患者代谢葡萄糖的能力。2 小时样本测量结果等于或高于 200 mg/dL 表明有糖尿病
radioactive iodine uptake test (RAIU)	放射性碘吸收测试，测量甲状腺对放射性碘吸收的测试，被用于评估甲状腺的功能
radioimmunoassay [ˌreidiəʊˌimjuːnəʊˈæsei]（RIA）	放射性免疫分析，一种使用放射性标记的激素和特定抗体测量血浆中微量物质（特别是激素）的方法
thyroid scan	甲状腺扫描，服用放射性碘后的甲状腺成像
thyroxine-binding globulin (TBG) test	甲状腺结合球蛋白测试，测量血液中与 T_4 结合的主要蛋白质的测试
transsphenoidal adenomectomy	经蝶（骨）腺瘤切除术，通过蝶窦（蝶骨中的空间）切除垂体瘤

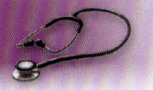

临床观点
季节性情绪失调

框 16-6

漫长黑暗的日子会让我们情绪低落，削弱我们前进的动力。这是据悉响应，还是存在物理基础？研究表明，环境中的光线量对人的行为的确有影响。有证据显示光线会改变那些受冬季黑暗日子严重影响的人们的情绪，这些人蒙患了季节性情绪失调症（seasonal affective disorder，SAD）。当白天变短时，这些人感觉昏昏欲睡、抑郁和焦虑。他们往往会暴食，特别是碳水化合物。

当光线照射眼睛的视网膜时，会启动神经脉冲减少大脑松果腺褪黑素的生产量。因为褪黑素会压抑情绪，光线的最终作用是提升情绪。早晨起床后光线照射 15 分钟通常就足够了，但有些人在早晚都需要更长的光照时间。其他的帮助包括有氧锻炼、压力管理技巧和抗抑郁药物。

Terminology 缩略语

A1c	Glycated hemoglobin (test)	糖化血红蛋白（测试）
ACTH	Adrenocorticotropic hormone	促肾上腺皮质激素
ADH	Antidiuretic hormone	抗利尿激素
BS	Blood sugar	血糖
CSII	Continuous subcutaneous insulin infusion	持续皮下胰岛素输注
DM	Diabetes mellitus	糖尿病
FBG	Fasting blood glucose	空腹血糖
FBS	Fasting blood sugar	空腹血糖
FPG	Fasting plasma glucose	空腹血糖
FSH	Follicle-stimulating hormone	促卵泡激素
FTI	Free thyroxine index	游离甲状腺素指数
GDM	Gestational diabetes mellitus	妊娠糖尿病
GH	Growth hormone	生长激素
HbA1c	Hemoglobin A1c; glycated hemoglobin	血红蛋白 A1c；糖化血红蛋白
I^{131}	Iodine-131 (radioactive iodine)	I^{131}（放射性碘）
IFG	Impaired fasting blood glucose	空腹血糖受损
IGT	Impaired glucose tolerance	糖耐量受损
LH	Luteinizing hormone	促黄体激素
MEN	Multiple endocrine neoplasia	多发性内分泌腺瘤
NPH	Neutral protamine Hagedorn (insulin)	中性鱼精蛋白锌胰岛素
OGTT	Oral glucose tolerance test	口服葡萄糖耐量试验
PRL	Prolactin	催乳激素
PTH	Parathyroid hormone	甲状旁腺激素
RAIU	Radioactive iodine uptake	放射性碘吸收
RIA	Radioimmunoassay	放射性免疫分析
SIADH	Syndrome of inappropriate antidiuretic hormone (secretion)	抗利尿激素分泌异常综合征
T1DM	Type 1 diabetes mellitus	Ⅰ型糖尿病
T2DM	Type 2 diabetes mellitus	Ⅱ型糖尿病

Terminology 缩略语

T_3	Triiodothyronine	三碘甲腺原氨酸
T_4	Thyroxine; tetraiodothyronine	甲状腺素；四碘甲状腺原氨酸
T_7	Free thyroxine index	游离甲状腺素指数
TBG	Thyroxine-binding globulin	甲状腺素结合蛋白
TSH	Thyroid-stimulating hormone	促甲状腺激素

Case Study Revisited 案例研究再访

J. D.'s Follow-Up

J. D. began her antithyroid medication therapy and began to feel better. She was able to concentrate more at work and found she was not as irritable with the children in school. She was sleeping better and began to add a few of the pounds she had previously lost. Her husband also noted the difference and mentioned this to Dr. Gilbert at the follow-up appointment four weeks later.

J. D. 的随访

J. D. 开始她的抗甲状腺药物治疗，开始感觉好些了。她能够更多地集中在工作中，对学校的孩子也不那么急躁了。她睡得好了，体重也恢复了。她的丈夫也注意到这一变化，并在4个星期后的随访中向 Gilbert 博士提到了这些。

CHAPTER 16 复习

标记练习

内分泌系统的腺体

在对应的下划线上写出每个编号部分的名称。

Adrenals
Hypothalamus
Ovaries
Pancreatic islets
Parathyroids
Pineal
Pituitary (hypophysis)
Testes
Thyroid

1. _____
2. _____
3. _____
4. _____
5. _____
6. _____
7. _____
8. _____
9. _____

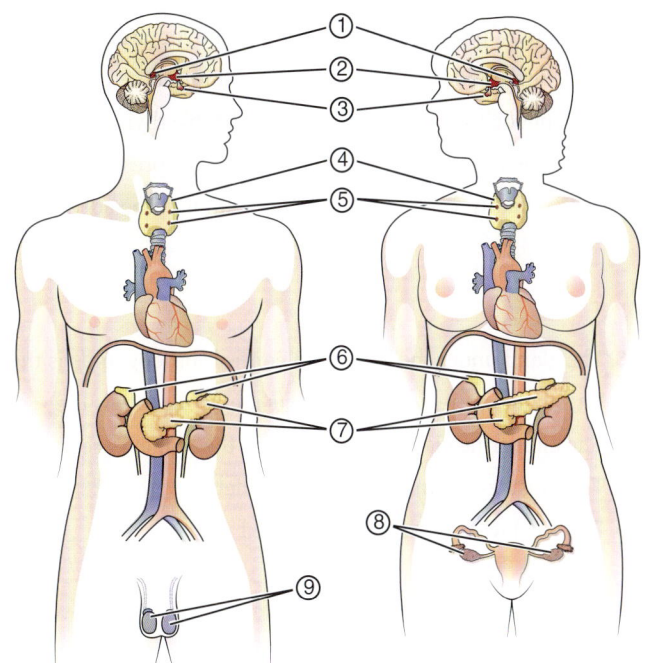

术语

匹配下列术语，在每个题号的左侧写上适当的字母。

____ 1. parathyroid   a. gland that is regulated by light
____ 2. posterior pituitary   b. small gland that acts to increase blood calcium levels
____ 3. hypothalamus   c. part of the brain that controls the pituitary
____ 4. anterior pituitary   d. gland that secretes ACTH
____ 5. pineal   e. gland that releases oxytocin

____ 6. epinephrine   a. hormone produced by the adrenal cortex
____ 7. growth hormone   b. somatotropin
____ 8. cortisol   c. pancreatic hormone that regulates glucose metabolism
____ 9. glucagon   d. hormone produced by the adrenal medulla
____ 10. melatonin   e. hormone from the pineal gland

____ 11. ADH   a. substance used to monitor blood glucose levels
____ 12. T_4 b. pituitary hormone that regulates water balance
____ 13. ACTH   c. a form of diabetes
____ 14. T2DM   d. thyroxine

____ 15. HbA1c   e. hormone that stimulates the adrenal cortex

____ 16. ketoacidosis   a. disorder that results from excess growth hormone
____ 17. adenoma   b. disorder caused by insufficient release of ADH
____ 18. Cushing syndrome   c. a result of uncontrolled diabetes
____ 19. acromegaly   d. disorder caused by overactivity of the adrenal cortex
____ 20. diabetes insipidus   e. neoplasm of a gland

补充术语

____ 21. craniopharyngioma   a. panhypopituitarism
____ 22. Simmonds disease   b. tumor of the pituitary gland
____ 23. pheochromocytoma   c. chronic thyroiditis
____ 24. Hashimoto disease   d. bony depression that holds the pituitary
____ 25. sella turcica   e. tumor of the adrenal medulla

填空

26. The gland under the brain that controls other glands is the_____.
27. The gland in the neck that affects metabolic rate is the_____.
28. The endocrine glands located above the kidneys are the_____.
29. The most common endocrine disorder is_____.
30. Excess glucose in the blood is called_____.

定义

定义下列单词。

31. thyrotomy [θaiˈrɒtəmi] _____
32. hypopituitarism [ˌhaipəʊpiˈtjuːitəˌrizəm] _____
33. hypophysiotropic [haipəʊfaiziːəʊˈtrɒpik] _____
34. adrenopathy [ˈædrinəpəθi] _____
35. adrenomegaly [ˈædrinəʊmegəli] _____
36. endocrinologist [ˌendəʊkriˈnɒlədʒist] _____

写出下列定义的单词。

37. tumor of the pancreatic islets   _____
38. destroying the thyroid gland   _____
39. pertaining to the adrenal cortex   _____

将腺体名称用作词根，写出下列定义的单词。

40. inflammation of the thyroid gland   _____
41. removal of one half (hemi-) of the thyroid gland _____
42. surgical removal of parathyroid gland   _____
43. overactivity of the adrenal gland   _____

使用词根 thyr/o 写出下列定义的单词。

44. acting on the thyroid gland　　　　＿＿＿＿＿＿＿＿＿＿＿＿＿＿

45. downward displacement of the thyroid gland　＿＿＿＿＿＿＿＿＿＿＿＿＿＿

46. any disease of the thyroid gland　＿＿＿＿＿＿＿＿＿＿＿＿＿＿

真假判断

检查下列语句，如果语句为真，在第一个空格上写上 T；如果语句为假，在第二个空格上写上 F，并通过在第二个空格上替换带下划线的单词更正语句。

	True or False	Correct Answer
47. Diabetes insipidus is caused by a lack of <u>thymosin</u>.	＿＿	＿＿＿＿＿
48. The hypophysis is the <u>pituitary</u> gland.	＿＿	＿＿＿＿＿
49. The outer region of an organ is the <u>medulla</u>.	＿＿	＿＿＿＿＿
50. The parathyroids regulate the element <u>sodium</u>.	＿＿	＿＿＿＿＿
51. Goiter is an enlargement of the <u>pineal</u> gland.	＿＿	＿＿＿＿＿
52. <u>Type 1</u> diabetes mellitus always requires insulin.	＿＿	＿＿＿＿＿
53. Thyroid hormones contain the element <u>iodine</u>.	＿＿	＿＿＿＿＿
54. The adrenal cortex produces <u>steroid</u> hormones.	＿＿	＿＿＿＿＿
55. Exophthalmos is protrusion of the <u>eyes</u>.	＿＿	＿＿＿＿＿
56. <u>Melatonin</u> regulates mood and daily cycles.	＿＿	＿＿＿＿＿

排除

在下列各组中，为与其余不相配的术语加下划线，并解释你选择的理由。

57. GH — TSH — FSH — PTH — ACTH

＿＿＿＿＿＿＿＿＿＿＿＿＿＿＿＿＿＿＿＿＿＿＿＿＿＿＿＿＿＿＿＿

58. Cushing syndrome — gigantism — dwarfism — acromegaly — thyrotoxicosis

＿＿＿＿＿＿＿＿＿＿＿＿＿＿＿＿＿＿＿＿＿＿＿＿＿＿＿＿＿＿＿＿

59. TBG — GDM — FPG — IGT — IFG

＿＿＿＿＿＿＿＿＿＿＿＿＿＿＿＿＿＿＿＿＿＿＿＿＿＿＿＿＿＿＿＿

60. testis — spleen — adrenals — parathyroids — pituitary

＿＿＿＿＿＿＿＿＿＿＿＿＿＿＿＿＿＿＿＿＿＿＿＿＿＿＿＿＿＿＿＿

单词构建

使用给出的单词组成部分形成下列定义的单词。

-ar　　adren/o　　-megal/o　　-oma　　thyr/o　　-ic　　-al　　trop　　-y　　insul/o　　path/o　　-lytic

61. any disease of the thyroid gland　　＿＿＿＿＿＿＿＿＿＿＿＿＿＿

62. acting on the adrenal gland　　＿＿＿＿＿＿＿＿＿＿＿＿＿＿

63. enlargement of the thyroid gland　　＿＿＿＿＿＿＿＿＿＿＿＿＿＿

64. pertaining to the gland above the kidney　　＿＿＿＿＿＿＿＿＿＿＿＿＿＿

65. enlargement of the adrenal gland　　＿＿＿＿＿＿＿＿＿＿＿＿＿＿

66. tumor of islet cells　　＿＿＿＿＿＿＿＿＿＿＿＿＿＿

67. destructive of thyroid tissue _____
68. any disease of the adrenal gland _____
69. acting on the thyroid gland _____
70. pertaining to pancreatic islet cells _____

单词分析

定义下列单词，并给出每个单词组成部分的含义。如果需要，可以使用词典。

71. craniopharyngioma (kra-ne-o-fah-rin-je-O-mah) _____
   a. crani/o _____
   b. pharyng/i _____
   c. -oma _____
72. panhypopituitarism (pan-hi-po-pih-TU-ih-tah-rism) _____
   a. pan _____
   b. hypo _____
   c. pituitar _____
   d. -ism _____
73. pheochromocytoma (fe-o-kro-mo-si-TO-mah) _____
   a. phe/o _____
   b. chrom/o _____
   c. cyt/o _____
   d. -oma _____
74. thyrotoxicosis (thi-ro-tok-sih-KO-sis) _____
   a. thyr/o _____
   b. toxic/o _____
   c. -sis _____
75. acromegaly _____
   a. acr/o _____
   b. megal/o _____
   c. y _____

给出腺体的名称

确定与下列病症相关的腺体。

76. diabetes mellitus _____
77. Addison disease _____
78. Graves disease _____
79. tetany _____
80. Simmonds disease _____

Additional Case Studies
补充案例研究

Case Study 16-1: Hyperparathyroidism
案例研究 16-1：甲状旁腺功能亢进

B. E., a 58 y/o woman with a history of hypertension, had a partial nephrectomy four years ago for renal calculi. During a routine physical examination, her total serum calcium level was 10.8 mg/dL. Her parathyroid hormone level was WNL; she was in no apparent distress, and the remainder of her physical examination and laboratory data were noncontributory.

B. E. underwent exploratory surgery for an enlarged right superior parathyroid gland. The remaining three glands appeared normal. The enlarged gland was excised, and a biopsy was performed on the remaining glands. The pathology report showed an adenoma of the abnormal gland. On her first postoperative day, she reported perioral numbness and tingling. She had no other symptoms, but her serum calcium level was subnormal. She was given one ampule of calcium gluconate. Within two days, her calcium level had improved, and she was discharged.

B. E. 是一名有高血压病史的 58 岁的女性，4 年前因肾结石做了部分肾切除术。在常规身体检查中，她的总血清钙水平为 10.8mg/dL。甲状旁腺激素水平在正常范围内；她没有明显的痛苦，她的身体检查和实验室数据的其他部分是无贡献的。

B. E. 为增大的右上甲状旁腺做了探查术。其余三个腺体看起来正常。增大的腺体被切除，并对剩余的腺体进行了活检。病理报告显示有异常的腺瘤。在术后第一天，她主诉口周麻木和刺痛，没有其他症状，但她的血清钙水平低于正常。给她用了一安瓿葡萄糖酸钙，2 天内钙水平有所改善，然后出院。

Case Study 16-2: Diabetes Treatment with an Insulin Pump
案例研究 16-2：胰岛素泵治疗糖尿病

M. G., a 32-year-old marketing executive, was diagnosed with type 1 diabetes at the age of 3. She vividly remembers her mother taking her to the doctor because she had an illness that caused her to feel extremely tired and very thirsty and hungry. She also had begun to wet her bed and had a cut on her knee that would not heal. Her mother had had gestational diabetes during her pregnancy with M. G., and at birth, M. G. was described as having "macrosomia" because she weighed 10 lb.

M. G. has managed her disease with meticulous attention to her diet, exercise, preventive healthcare, regular blood glucose monitoring, and twice-daily injections of regular and NPH insulin, which she rotates among her upper arms, thighs, and abdomen. She continues in a smoking cessation program supported by weekly acupuncture treatments. She maintains good control of her disease in spite of the inconvenience and time it consumes each day. She will be married next summer and would like to start a family. M.G.'s doctor suggested she try an insulin pump to give her more freedom and enhance her quality of life. After intensive training, she has received her pump. It is about the size of a deck of cards with a thin catheter that she introduces through a needle into her abdominal subcutaneous tissue. She can administer her insulin in a continuous subcutaneous insulin infusion (CSII) and in calculated meal bolus doses. She still has to test her blood for hyperglycemia and

M. G. 是一名 32 岁的营销主管，在 3 岁时被诊断患有 I 型糖尿病。她生动地记得她的母亲带她去看医生，因为她患了一种疾病，导致她感到极度疲倦、口渴和饥饿。她还开始尿床，在膝盖上有一个不会愈合的伤口。她的母亲在怀 M. G. 期间患有妊娠糖尿病。出生时，M.G. 被认为是一个"巨大儿"，因为她体重 10 磅。

M. G. 精心地控制她的疾病，精心关注饮食、运动、预防保健、定期血糖监测，在上臂、大腿或腹部上每日之次注射正常和中效胰岛素。她通过每周针灸治疗支持持续的戒烟计划。尽管每天都有不便且消耗时间，她仍然能够很好地控制疾病。她明年夏天会结婚，开始家庭生活。M. G. 的医生建议她尝试胰岛素泵给她更多的自由，提高她的生活质量。经过加强培训，她收到了她的胰岛素泵。它大概是一叠卡片大小，带有一根细导管，她将导管通过针头引入她的腹部皮下组织。她可以通过连续皮下胰岛素输注（CSII）和根据饮食计算的丸剂使用其胰岛素。当她的血糖过高时，她仍然需要测试血液的高血糖和低血糖，以及尿酮。她希望有一天能够做胰岛移植。

hypoglycemia and her urine for ketones when her blood glucose is too high. She hopes one day to have an islet transplantation.

案例研究问题

多项选择。选择正确答案，在每个题号的左侧写上你选择的字母。

____ 1. Renal calculi are

    a. kidney stones

    b. gallstones

    c. stomach ulcers

    d. bile obstructions

____ 2. B.E.'s serum calcium was 10.8 mg/dL, which is

    a. 5.4 mcg of calcium in her serous fluid

    b. 10.8 g of electrolytes in parathyroid hormone

    c. 10.8 mg of calcium in 100 mL of blood

    d. 21.6 L of calcium in 100 g of serum

____ 3. B.E. had perioral numbness and tingling. Perioral is

    a. peripheral to any orifice

    b. lateral to the eye

    c. within the buccal mucosa

    d. around the mouth

____ 4. Gestational diabetes occurs

    a. in a pregnant woman

    b. to any large fetus

    c. during menopause

    d. in a large baby with high blood glucose

____ 5. The term macrosomia describes

    a. excessive weight gain during pregnancy

    b. a large body

    c. an excessive amount of sleep

    d. inability to sleep during pregnancy

____ 6. M.G. injected the insulin into the subcutaneous tissue, which is

    a. present only in the abdomen, thighs, and upper arms

    b. a topical application

    c. below the skin

    d. above the pubic bone

____ 7. An islet transplantation refers to

    a. transfer of insulin-secreting cells into a pancreas

    b. transfer of parathyroid cells to the liver

    c. surgical insertion of an insulin pump into the abdomen

    d. a total pancreas and kidney transplantation

写出案例研究中下列含义的术语。

8. surgical excision of a kidney _____

9. tumor of a gland _____

10. single-use glass injectable medication container _____

11. high serum glucose _____

12. a large dose of a therapeutic agent _____

缩略语。定义下列缩略语。

13. WNL _____

14. NPH _____

15. CSII _____

CHAPTER 17

神经系统和行为障碍

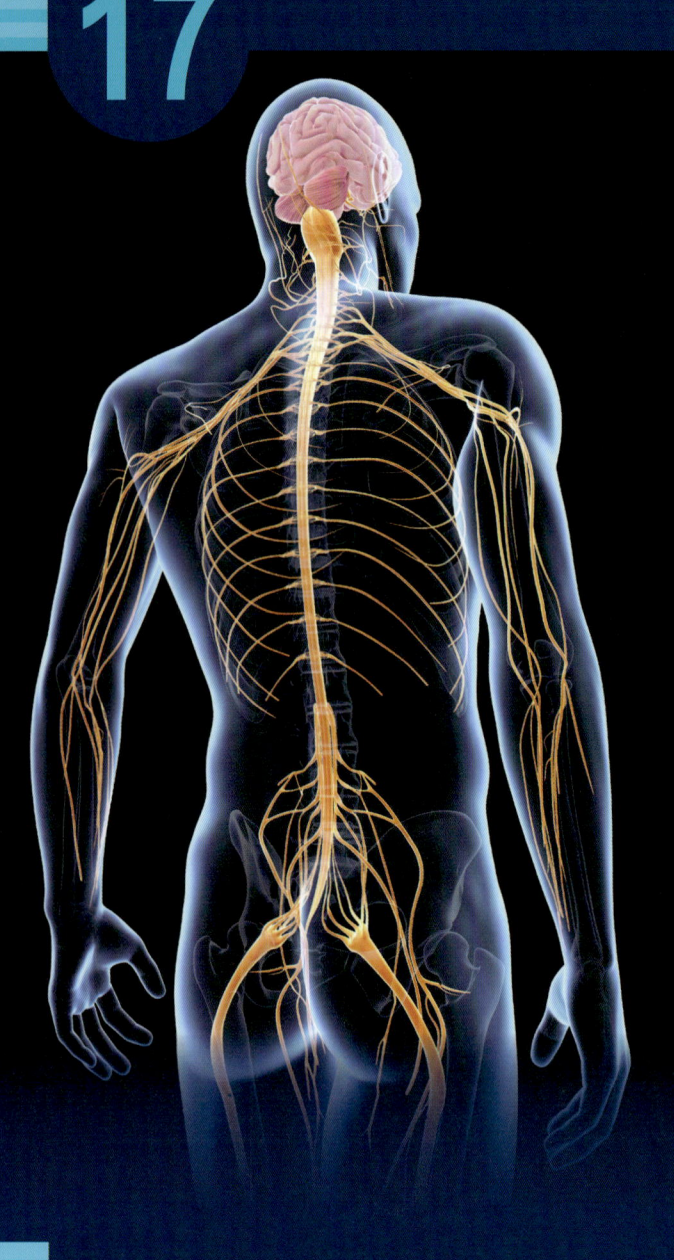

预测试

多项选择。选择正确答案，在每个题号的左侧写上你选择的字母。

____ 1. The basic cell of the nervous system is a(n)
   a. myofiber
   b. neuron
   c. osteoblast
   d. chondrocyte

____ 2. The largest part of the brain is the
   a. cerebrum
   b. adrenal
   c. cortex
   d. pituitary

____ 3. The midbrain, pons, and medulla oblongata make up the
   a. ventricle
   b. spinal cord
   c. cerebellum
   d. brainstem

____ 4. Involuntary responses are controlled by the
   a. somatic nervous system
   b. voluntary nervous system
   c. autonomic nervous system
   d. diaphragm

____ 5. A simple response that requires few cells is a
   a. reflex
   b. mutation
   c. sensation
   d. stimulus

____ 6. A disorder, often of unknown cause, characterized by seizures is called
   a. cystic fibrosis
   b. spina bifida
   c. epilepsy
   d. thyrotoxicosis

____ 7. An instrument used to study the electric activity of the brain is the
   a. electrocardiograph
   b. electroencephalograph
   c. CT scanner
   d. sonograph

____ 8. An extreme, persistent fear is a(n)
   a. palliative
   b. prognosis
   c. analgesic
   d. phobia

学习目标

学完本章后，应该能够：

1 ▶ 描述神经系统的组成部分。
2 ▶ 描述神经元的结构。
3 ▶ 简单描述脑部的各个区域及其功能。
4 ▶ 描述中枢神经系统是如何被保护的。
5 ▶ 描述脊髓的结构。
6 ▶ 列举简单反射的组成部分。
7 ▶ 比较交感神经系统和副交感神经系统。
8 ▶ 识别并使用与神经系统相关的单词组成部分。
9 ▶ 描述影响神经系统的 8 种主要疾病。
10 ▶ 描述 5 种主要的行为障碍。
11 ▶ 定义神经病学使用的缩略语。
12 ▶ 分析案例研究中涉及神经系统的医学术语。

Case Study: B.C.s's Pediatric Brain Tumor
案例研究：B. C. 的儿童脑肿瘤

Chief Complaint

B. C., a previously healthy and active 6-year-old, woke up one morning complaining that his head hurt. He had a few episodes of vomiting early in the morning, and he was not able to walk straight when he got out of bed. His parents took him to the pediatrician, who, after noting the headache, morning emesis, and progressive loss of muscle coordination (ataxia), conducted a brief examination and then made an immediate referral to a neurologist.

Examination

Before talking with the patient, the neurologist spoke with B. C.'s parents to obtain a prior medical history. They stated that he had a healthy childhood thus far with normal illnesses such as earaches, a few colds, and sore throats. The parents indicated that B. C. is a first grader and attends a public elementary school. They said he loves school and baseball. The latter is his favorite extracurricular activity.

The neurologist spoke with B. C. and explained what he was going to do. Next he performed a thorough neurologic examination. Then he offered to B.C. a simple explanation of the tests he was going to order. Finally he answered all of the patient's and parents' questions.

Clinical Course

B. C.'s parents took him to the radiology department of the hospital for a scheduled MRI. The radiologist reported the scan revealed some dense tissue indicating a suspicious mass. A lumbar puncture (LP) was performed, which revealed some suspicious cells in the cerebrospinal fluid (CSF).

B. C. had a craniotomy with tumor resection five days later. The cerebellar tumor was found to be noninfiltrating and was enclosed within a cyst, which was totally removed. B. C. spent two days in the neurologic intensive care unit (NICU) because he was on seizure precautions and monitoring for increased intracranial pressure (ICP). A regimen of focal radiation followed after recovery from surgery. His spine was also treated because of the potential spread of tumor cells in the CSF. B. C. did not have chemotherapy because of the danger that hydrocephalus might develop, which generally requires a ventriculoperitoneal (VP) shunt.

主诉

B. C. 是一名健康活跃的 6 岁男孩，一个早晨醒来后他主诉头痛。他早上有几次呕吐，下床时他不能直走。他的父母带他去看儿科医生，医生在记录了头痛、早晨呕吐和肌肉协调进行性丧失（共济失调）之后，做了一个简单的检查，然后立即转诊给神经科医生。

检查

在与患者交谈之前，神经科医生与 B. C. 的父母谈话以获得以前的病史。他们说 B. C. 有一个健康的童年，迄今为止只有一些常见的疾病，如耳痛、几次感冒和喉咙痛。父母表示 B. C. 是一个公立小学的一年级学生，热爱学校和棒球，棒球是他最喜欢的课外活动。

神经科医生与 B. C. 交谈，并解释了他将要做什么。接下来他进行了彻底的神经系统检查，然后简单地向 B. C. 说明了他要做的测试。最后，他回答了患者及其父母的所有问题。

临床病程

B. C. 的父母带他到医院的放射科进行预约的 MRI。放射科医生报告扫描显示了一些致密的组织，表明有可疑的肿块。进行腰椎穿刺（LP），结果显示脑脊液（CSF）中有一些可疑细胞。

5 天后，B. C. 做了肿瘤切除开颅手术。发现小脑肿瘤是非浸润性的，被封闭在囊肿内，被完全去除。因为要预防癫痫和监测颅内压力（ICP）的升高，B. C. 在神经重症监护病房（NICU）中呆了 2 天。手术恢复后，又做了局灶性辐射治疗。因为肿瘤细胞在 CSF 中的潜在扩散，脊髓也做了治疗。B. C. 没有做化疗，因为可能出现脑积水的危险，这通常需要腹膜腔内（VP）分流。

简介

神经系统（nervous system）与内分泌系统共同协调并控制身体，调节身体对环境的反应并维持体内平衡（homeostasis）。内分泌系统通过激素循环发挥功能，神经系统则通过电脉冲（electric impulse）以及在局部释放被称为神经递质（neurotransmitter）的化学物质发挥功能。

神经系统的构成

为研究方便，神经系统可以根据结构分为两个部分：

- 中枢神经系统（central nervous system，CNS），由大脑和脊髓组成（图 17-1）。
- 周围神经系统（peripheral nervous system，PNS），由大脑和脊髓以外的所有神经组织构成。

根据功能，神经系统可以被分为：

- 躯体神经系统（somatic nervous system），控制骨骼肌肉。
- 内脏或自主神经系统（visceral or autonomic nervous system，ANS），控制平滑肌、心肌和腺体。自主神经系统调节对压力的反应，并协助维持体内平衡。

神经系统中有两类细胞。神经元（neurons），或神经细胞，构成神经系统的传导组织。神经胶质（neuroglia）是支撑并保护神经组织的细胞。

神经元

神经元是神经系统的基本功能单元（图 17-2）。每个神经元都有从细胞体延伸出来的两种纤维：

- 树突（dendrite）向细胞体传送脉冲。
- 轴突（axon）将脉冲带离细胞体。

一些轴突被微白的脂肪性物质髓磷脂（myelin）

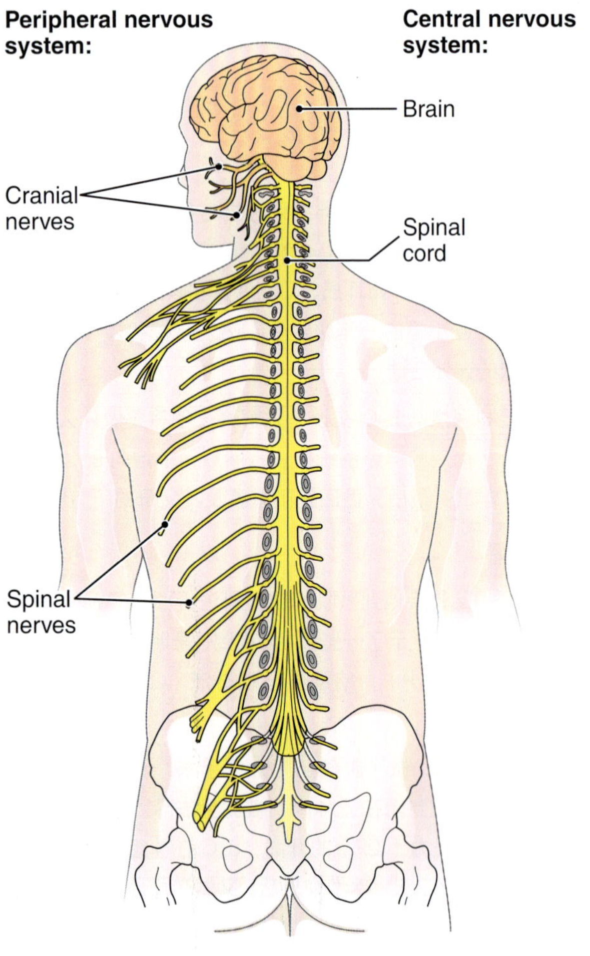

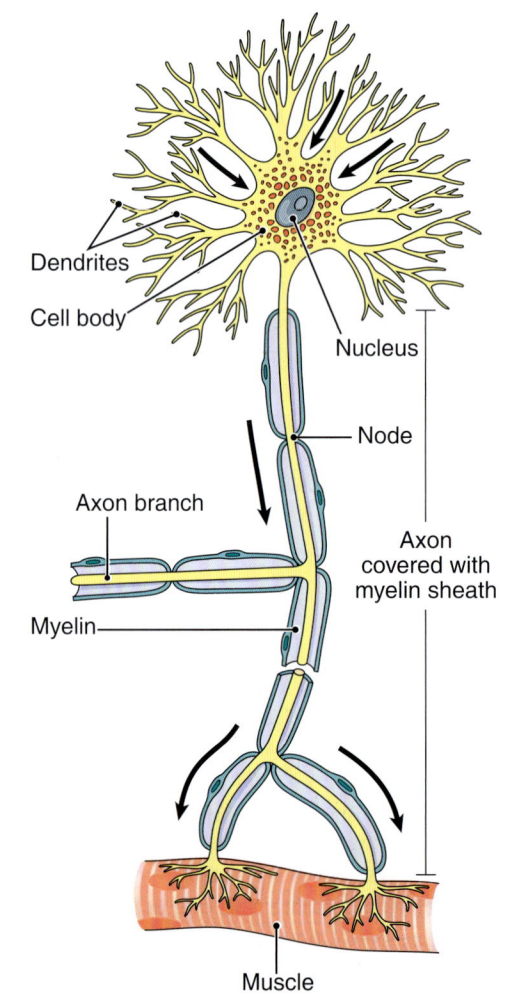

图 17-1 神经系统的解剖划分

图 17-2 运动神经元。轴突中的断裂表示长度，箭头表示神经脉冲的方向

覆盖，这种物质隔离并保护轴突，还会尽快电传导。被覆盖的轴突被描述为有髓鞘的（myelinated），它们构成了神经系统的白质（white matter）。无髓鞘的的组织构成神经系统的灰质（gray matter）。

每个神经元都是神经系统传送信息通道的一个组成部分。发送脉冲到中枢神经系统的神经元是感觉神经元（sensory neuron），或传入（afferent）神经元；将脉冲传送离开中枢神经系统的神经元是运动神经元（motor neuron），或传出（efferent）神经元。中枢神经系统内的连接细胞被称为中间神经元（interneuron）。

突触（synapse）是两个神经元之间的接触点。能量通过突触从一个细胞传送到另一个细胞，通常是通过神经递质，有时直接传送电流。

神经

单个的神经纤维集中在神经束（bundle）中，就像电线在电缆中一样。如果这个束是周围神经系统的一部分，就被称为一根神经。神经通道周围细胞体的集合被称为神经节（ganglion）。一些神经（感觉神经）只包含感觉神经元，还有一些神经（运动神经）只包含运动神经元，但大多数神经包含两种神经纤维，被称为混合神经。

脑

脑是头颅中的神经组织，由大脑（cerebrum）、间脑（diencephalon）、脑干（brainstem）和小脑（cerebellum）组成。大脑是脑补部最大的部分（图 17-3）；主要由白质构成，外面有一层很薄的灰质大脑皮层（cerebral cortex）。脑的较高级功能，如记忆、推理和抽象，都发生在大脑皮层。大脑的独特表面由脑沟（sulcus，复数 sulci）和脑回（gyrus，复数 gyri）组成，这种结构提供了额外的表面面积（图 17-4）。大脑由一个深沟分为两个半球，这个深沟被称为纵裂（longitudinal fissure）。每个半球进一步分为特定功能的叶（图 17-4），这些叶根据覆盖它们的颅骨命名。

脑的其他部分：

- 间脑包含丘脑（thalamus）、下丘脑（hypothalamus）和垂体腺（图 17-3）。丘脑接受感觉信息，并将其引导到大脑皮层的适当部分。下丘脑控制垂体，并在内分泌和神经系统之间形成链接。

- 脑干（图 17-3）由以下部分组成：

  - 中脑（midbrain），包含改善视觉和听力的反射中心。

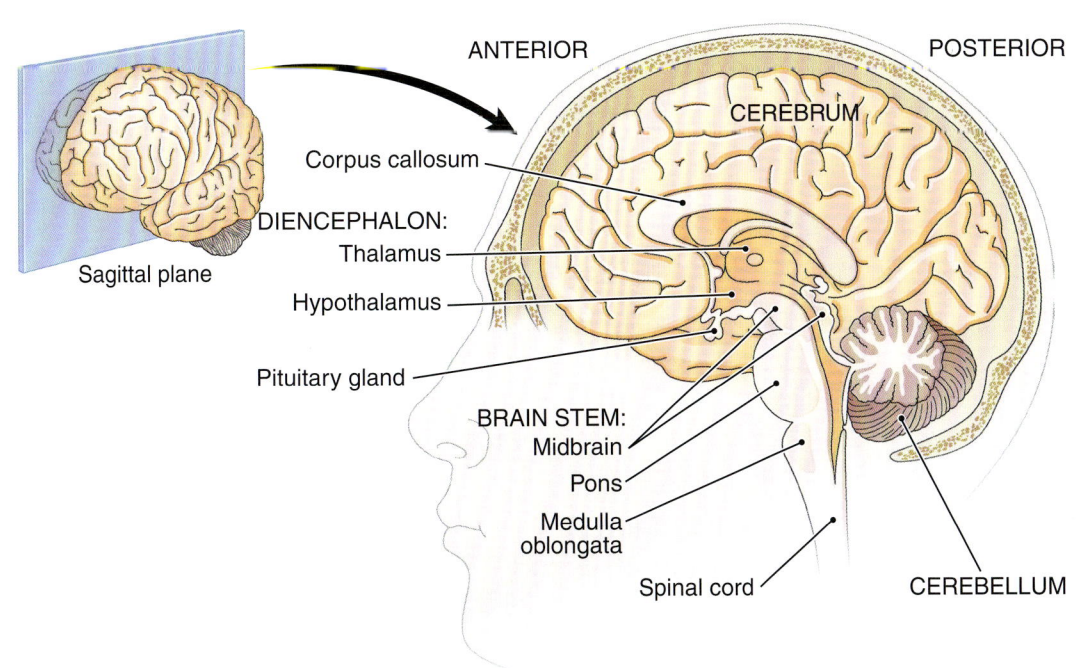

图 17-3　脑部，矢状截面

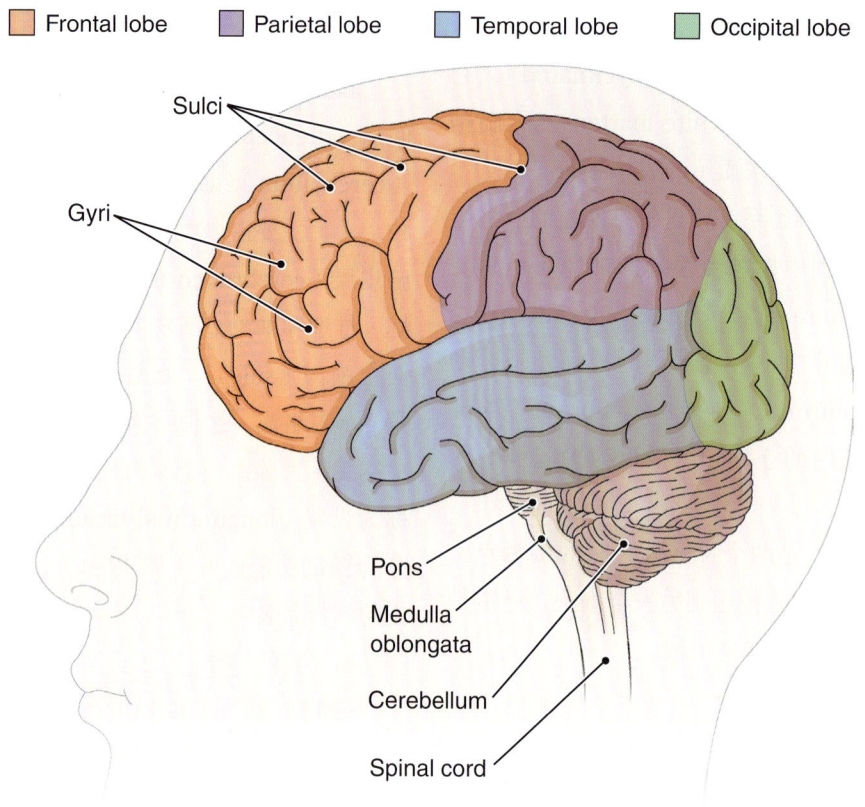

图 17-4 脑部的外表面，侧视图。图中显示了大脑的叶和表面特征，以及脑和脊髓的其他部分

- 脑桥（pons），在脑干的前表面形成一个凸出部分，包含连接脑部不同区域的纤维。
- 延髓（medulla oblongata），连接脑部和脊髓，由脑部发出或接收的脉冲都要经过这一区域。延髓还有控制心率、呼吸和血压的生命中枢。

小脑在大脑之下，脑桥和延髓背后（图 17-3）。与大脑一样，小脑也分为两个半球。小脑协助控制随意肌的运动，保持体位、协调和平衡。

保护大脑

头颅内有四个室（腔体），其中充满脑脊液（cerebrospinal fluid，CSF）。脑脊液在脑部和脊髓中循环，作为这些组织的保护性缓冲。覆盖脑部和脊髓的是三个保护层，共同被称为脑脊膜（meninges）（图 17-5）。它们都由意为"母亲"的希腊单词 mater 命名，以指示它们的保护功能。它们是：

- 硬脑膜（dura mater），最外和最硬的一层。dura 意为"硬"。
- 蛛网膜（arachnoid mater），很薄的蛛网样的中间层。名称源自于拉丁语蜘蛛的单词，意为它看起来像蜘蛛网。
- 软脑膜（pia mater），很薄的脉管内层，直接附着在脑部和脊髓组织上。pia 意为"柔软"。

有 12 对颅神经连接脑部（图 17-6）。这些神经有罗马数字编号和各自的名称，框 17-1 给出了相关信息。

脊髓

脊髓起始于延髓，在第一和第二腰椎之间变细截止（图 17-7）。脊髓在颈部和腰部区域有扩张，手臂和腿部的神经在扩张部位分别加入脊髓。在截面图中（图 17-8），脊髓中央是灰质，外围是白质，灰质向前后突出形成背角和腹角。白质包含上升和下降束（纤

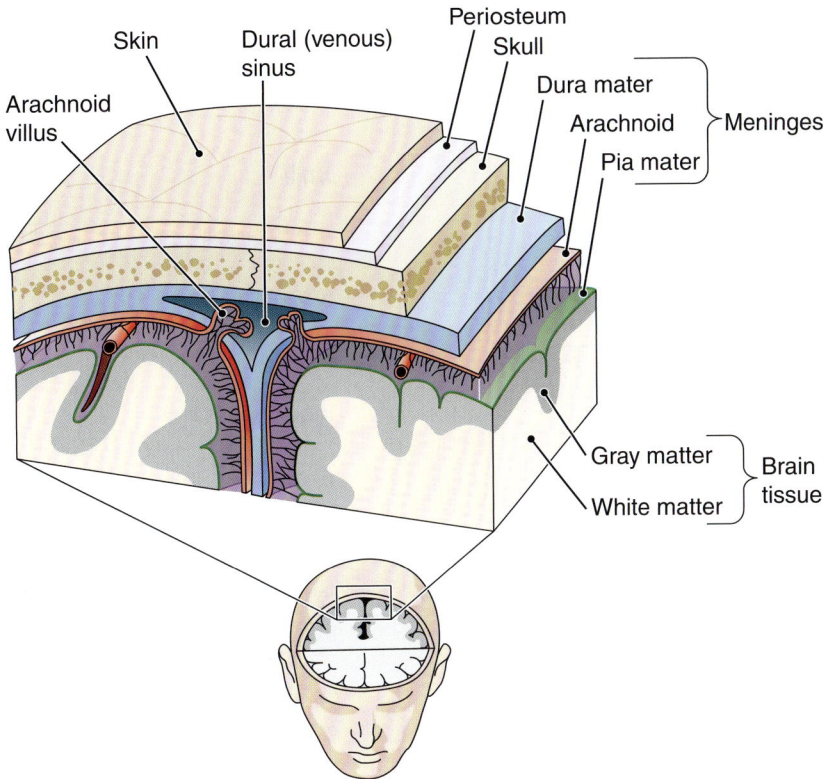

图 17-5　脑脊膜。图中示出了头前部的 3 个保护层和相邻的组织

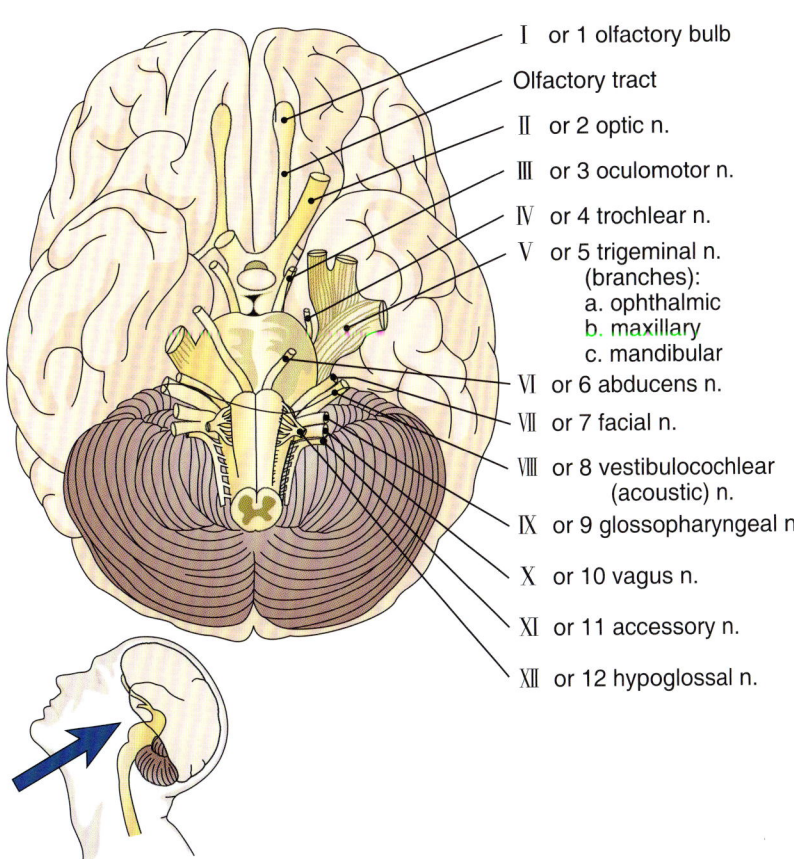

图 17-6　颅神经。在下视图的一侧示出了 12 跟颅神经

供你参考
颅神经

框 17-1

罗马数字	名称	功能
I	olfactory ［ɒlˈfæktəri］嗅觉神经	传送嗅觉脉冲
II	optic ［ˈɒptik］视觉神经	传送视觉脉冲
III	oculomotor ［ˌɒkjʊləˈməʊtə］眼动神经	控制眼睛肌肉的运动
IV	trochlear ［ˈtrɒkliə］滑车神经	控制一块眼球肌肉
V	trigeminal ［traiˈdʒeminl］三叉神经	传送来自于面部的感觉脉冲，控制咀嚼肌
VI	abducens ［æbˈdju:sənz］外展神经	控制一块眼球肌肉
VII	facial ［ˈfeiʃl］面部神经	控制面部表情肌肉、唾液腺和泪腺，传导一些味觉脉冲
VIII	vestibulocochlear ［ˈvestibjʊləʊkəʊkliəər］前庭神经	传导听觉和平衡脉冲，也被称为听觉神经（auditory or acoustic nerve）
IX	glossopharyngeal ［ˌglɒsəʊfəˈrindʒiəl］舌咽神经	传导来自于舌与咽的感觉脉冲，刺激腮腺唾液腺，并部分控制吞咽功能
X	vagus ［ˈveigəs］迷走神经	支配胸部和腹部的大多数器官，控制消化分泌
XI	spinal accessory ［əkˈsesəri］副神经	控制颈部肌肉
XII	hypoglossal ［ˌhaipəˈglɒsəl］舌下神经	控制舌头肌肉

维束），传送脑部发出和接收的脉冲。髓管（central canal）中包含脑脊液。

脊髓神经

有 31 对脊髓神经连接脊髓（图 17-7），这些神经在脊髓的不同部分分组为：

- 颈椎神经：8 对
- 胸椎神经：12 对
- 腰椎神经：5 对
- 骶椎神经：5 对
- 尾椎神经：1 对

每根神经通过两个根加入脊髓（图 17-8）。背根将感觉脉冲传入脊髓，腹根将运动脉冲带离脊髓到肌肉或腺体。背根的扩张是背根神经节，感觉神经元的细胞体将脉冲传导到中枢神经系统（图 17-8）。

反射

只需要几个神经元的简单反应是反射（图 17-9）。在脊髓反射中，脉冲只通过脊髓，并不到达脑部。这种反应的一个例子是用于体格检查的膝跃反射（knee-jerk reflex）。不过，大多数神经反应涉及中枢神经系统中很多神经元之间复杂的相互作用。

自主神经系统

自主神经系统（autonomic nervous system，ANS）是控制肌肉和腺体无意识活动的神经系统部分（图 17-10），其自身也分为两个部分：

- 交感神经系统（sympathetic nervous system）激发我们的应激反应，即所谓的战或逃反应（fight-or-flight response）。它会提升心跳和呼吸的速率，刺激肾上腺，将更多的血压输送

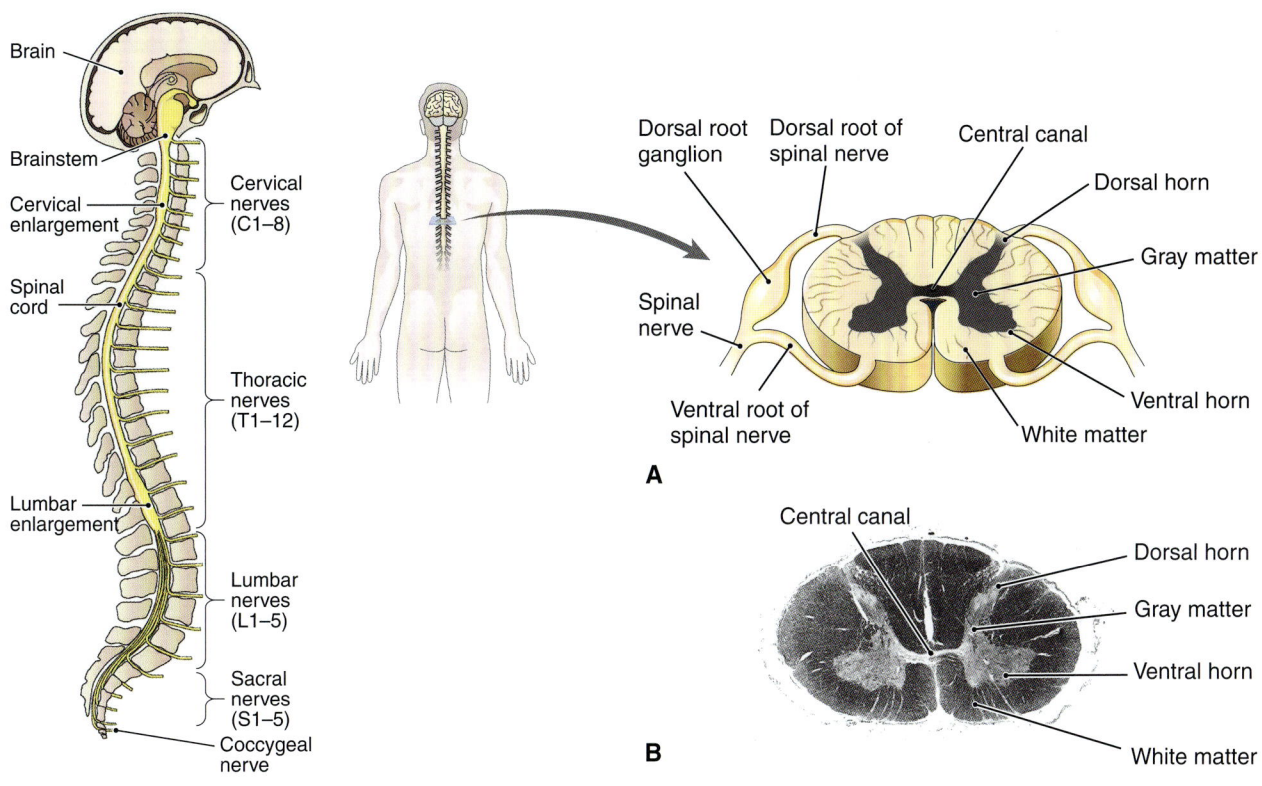

图 17-7 脊髓，侧视图。图中显示了脊神经的划分

图 17-8 脊髓，横断面。A. 图显示灰质和白质的组织和脊神经的根；B. 脊髓横切面的显微图（放大 5 倍）

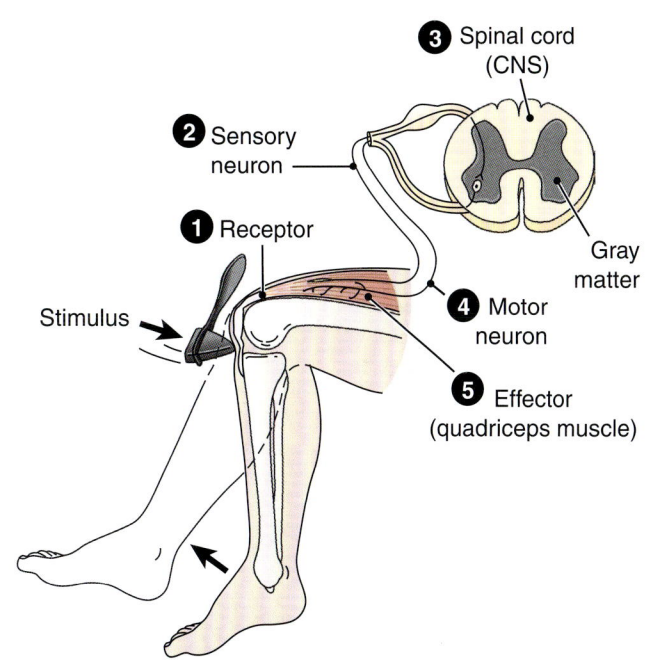

图 17-9 反射通道（弧）。图示的为膝反射，数字表示脉冲的顺序

到骨骼肌。

- 副交感神经系统（parasympathetic nervous system）将身体恢复到稳定状态，并刺激维护活动，例如食物消化。大多数器官同时受这两个系统的控制，一般而言，两个系统对一个给定器官的作用相反。

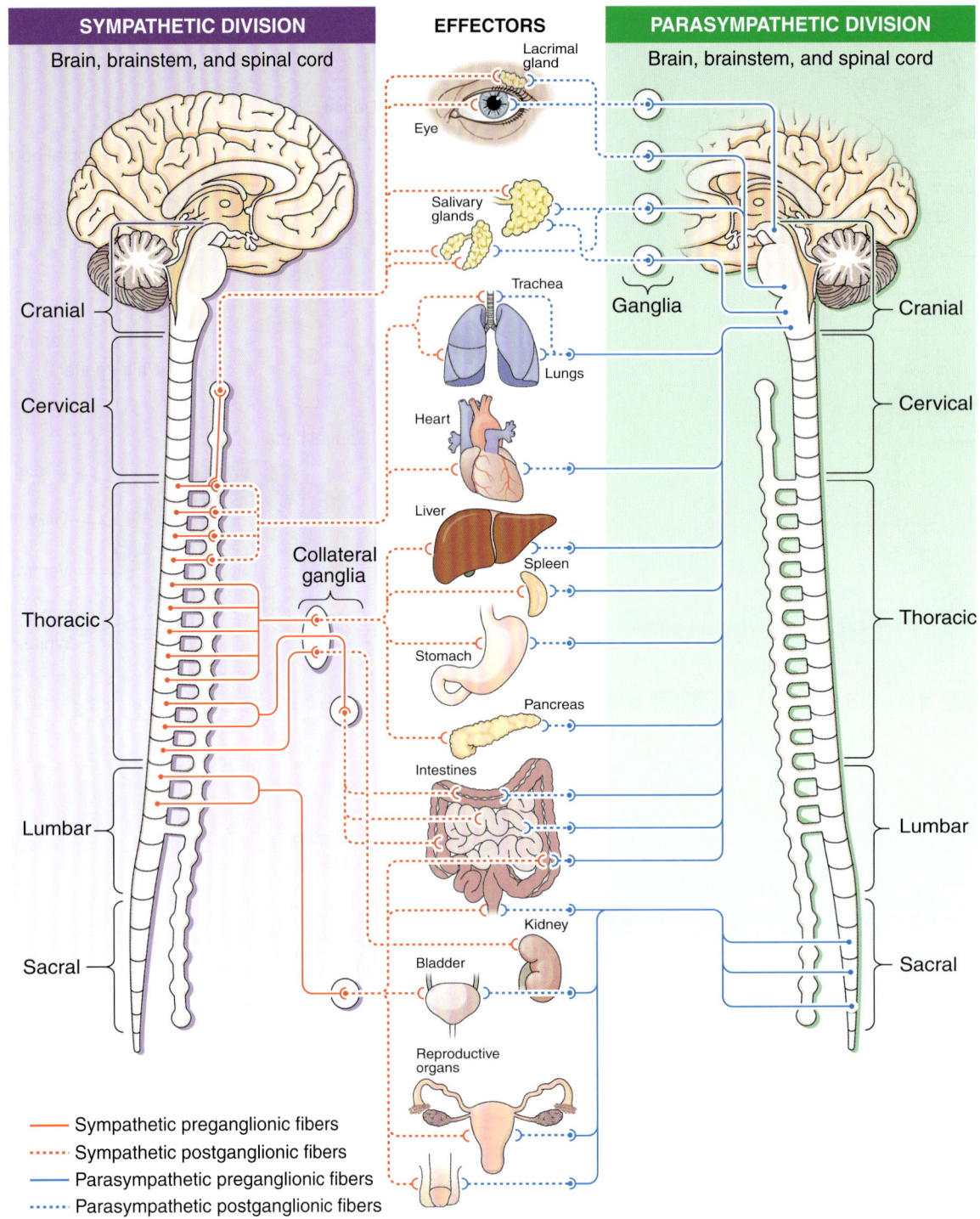

图 17-10 自主神经系统（ANS）。每个 ANS 通道具有两个神经元，如实线和虚线所示。图中仅显示了身体一侧的每个分区（交感神经和副交感神经）

Terminology 关键术语

正常结构与功能

afferent	[ˈæfərənt]	传入的，传送到一个给定的点，例如感觉神经元和神经将脉冲传送到中枢神经系统（词根：fer 意为"传送"）

Terminology 关键术语

arachnoid mater [əˈræknɔid]	蛛网膜，脑膜的中间层（源自于希腊语蜘蛛的单词，意为蛛网膜组织看起来像一个蜘蛛网）
autonomic nervous system ANS	自主神经系统，协调无意识活动的部分神经系统，控制平滑肌、心肌和腺体；也被称为内脏神经系统（visceral nervous system）
axon [ˈæksɒn]	轴突，将脉冲传导出细胞体的神经纤维
brain	脑部，颅骨内的神经组织，由大脑、间脑、脑干和小脑构成（词根：encephal/o）
brainstem	脑干，脑部的一部分，由中脑、脑桥和延髓构成
central nervous system (CNS)	中枢神经系统，脑部和脊髓
cerebellum [ˌserəˈbeləm]	小脑，脑部的后面部分，在脑桥和延髓的背后；帮助协调运动，并维持平衡和体外（词根：cerebell/o）
cerebral cortex [ˈserəbrəl ˈkɔːteks]	大脑皮层，大脑的灰质薄表面层（词根：cortic/o）
cerebrum [səˈriːbrəm]	大脑，脑部很大的上部；被纵裂分为两个半球（词根：cerebr/o）
cerebrospinal fluid (CSF) [ˌseribrəuˈspainl]	脑脊液，在脑部和脊髓中循环的起保护作用的水样液体
cranial nerves [ˈkreiniəl]	颅神经，与脑部相连的 12 对神经
dendrite [ˈdendrait]	树突，将脉冲传导到细胞体的神经纤维
diencephalon [ˌdaienˈsefəlɒn]	间脑，脑部的一部分，包含丘脑、下丘脑和垂体腺；位于大脑和脑干之间
dura mater [ˈdjʊərə]	硬脑膜，脑膜的强壮、坚韧的最外层
efferent [ˈefərənt]	传出的，传送离开一个给定的点，例如运动神经元和神经将脉冲传出中枢神经系统（词根：fer 意为"传送"）
ganglion [ˈgæŋgliən]	神经节，中枢神经系统外神经元细胞体的集合（复数：ganglia；词根：gangli/o, ganglion/o）
gray matter	灰质，神经系统中无髓鞘的组织
gyrus [ˈdʒairəs]	脑回，大脑表面突起的褶积（图 17-4）（复数：gyri）
hypothalamus [ˌhaipəˈθæləməs]	下丘脑，脑部控制垂体腺和维持体内平衡的部分
interneuron [ˌintəˈnjʊərɒn]	中间神经元，神经通道中位于感觉神经元和运动神经元之间的神经元，例如在中枢神经系统中发送脉冲的神经元
medulla oblongata [miˈdʌlə ɒblɒŋˈgɑːtə]	延髓，脑部连接脊髓的部分，包含控制呼吸、心率和血压的生命中枢（词根：medull/o）。通常简称为 medulla
meninx [ˈmiːniŋks] 脑脊膜	覆盖脑部和脊髓的三层膜（图 17-5，复数：meninges，词根：mening/o, meninge/o）
midbrain	中脑，脑干中间脑和脑桥之间的部分，包含协调视觉和听觉反射的中心

Terminology 关键术语

motor	运动的，描述传出神经元和神经将脉冲传导出中枢神经系统
myelin [ˈmaiəlin]	髓磷脂，包围神经系统特定轴突的微白色脂肪物质
neuroglia [njʊəˈrɒgliə]	神经胶质，神经系统的支持细胞，也被称为胶质细胞（glial cells，源自于意为"胶水"的单词，glia 词根：gli/o）
neuron [ˈnjʊərɒn]	神经元，神经系统的基本单元，也被称为神经细胞
neurotransmitter [ˈnjʊərəʊtrænzmitə]	神经递质，跨越突触传递能量的一种化学物质，例如去甲肾上腺素（norepinephrine）、乙酰胆碱（acetylcholine）、血清素（serotonin）和多巴胺（dopamine）
nerve	神经，中枢神经系统外的一束神经纤维（词根：neur/o）
parasympathetic nervous system	副交感神经系统，自主神经系统的一部分，翻转应激反应，恢复体内平衡。它会降低心率和呼吸频率，刺激消化、排尿和生殖活动
peripheral nervous system (PNS)	周围神经系统，中枢神经系统以外的神经系统
pia mater [ˈpaiə ˈmeitə]	软脑膜，脑脊膜的最内层
pons [pɒnz]	脑桥，脑干腹面上的一个圆形区域，包含连接脑部区域的纤维；形容词为 pontine
reflex [ˈriːfleks]	反射，对刺激的简单、快速和自动的反应
root	根，连接脊髓的脊髓神经分支；背根连接脊髓的背灰质角，腹根连接脊髓的腹灰质角（词根：radicul/o）
sensory	感觉的，描述传出神经元和神经将脉冲传导到中枢神经系统
somatic nervous system	躯体神经系统，控制骨骼肌的部分神经系统
spinal cord	脊髓，脊柱中包含的神经组织，从延髓延续到第二腰椎（词根：myel/o）
spinal nerves	脊髓神经，与脊髓相连的 31 对神经
sulcus [ˈsʌlkəs]	脑沟，大脑表面的浅沟（图 17-4，复数：sulci）
sympathetic nervous system	交感神经系统，启动应激反应的部分自主神经系统，会加快心率和呼吸，为骨骼肌提供更多的血液
synapse [ˈsainæps]	突触，两个神经元之间的结合点；运动神经元与肌肉或腺体之间的结合点
thalamus [ˈθæləməs]	丘脑，脑部的一部分，接收除嗅觉之外的所有感觉脉冲，并将脉冲引导到大脑皮层适当部位（词根：thalam/o）
tract	束，中枢神经系统内的神经纤维束
ventricle [ˈventrikl]	室，小腔体，例如脑部充满脑脊液的脑室（词根：ventricul/o）
visceral nervous system	内脏神经系统，自主神经系统
white matter	白质，有髓鞘的神经组织

与神经系统相关的单词组成部分

参见表 17-1 至表 17-3

表 17-1　神经系统和脊髓的词根

词根	含义	示例	示例定义
neur/o, neur/i	神经系统、神经组织、神经	neurotrophin [njʊərəʊt'rɒfin]	神经营养因子（troph/o 意为"营养"）
gli/o	神经胶质	glial ['glaiəl]	神经胶质的
gangli/o, ganglion/o	神经节	ganglioma [gæŋgli'əʊmə]	神经节瘤
mening/o, meninge/o	脑脊膜	meningocele [mə'niŋgəsi:l]	脑脊膜膨出
myel/o	脊髓	hematomyelia [hi:mətəʊmai'i:liə]	脊髓出血
radicul/o	脊髓神经根	radiculopathy [ræ'dikjʊləʊpəθi]	脊髓神经根疾病

练习 17-1

定义下列形容词。

1. neural
   ['njʊərəl]　pertaining to a nerve or the nervous system＿＿＿＿＿＿＿＿
2. neuroglial
   [n'jʊərəʊgliəl]　＿＿＿＿＿＿＿＿
3. radicular
   [ræ'dikjʊlə(r)]　＿＿＿＿＿＿＿＿
4. meningeal
   [mə'nindʒiəl]　＿＿＿＿＿＿＿＿
5. ganglionic
   [ˌgæŋgli'ɒnik]　＿＿＿＿＿＿＿＿

填空。

6. A meningioma [minindʒi'əʊmə] is a tumor affecting the＿＿＿＿＿＿＿＿.
7. A neurotropic [ˌnjʊərə'trɒpik] dye has an affinity for the＿＿＿＿＿＿＿＿.
8. Meningococci [məˌniŋgə'kɒki] are bacteria (cocci) that infect the＿＿＿＿＿＿＿＿.
9. Myelodysplasia [maiələʊdi'spleiziə] is abnormal development of the＿＿＿＿＿＿＿＿.

定义下列术语。

10. ganglionectomy
    [gæŋgliɒn'ektəmi]　＿＿＿＿＿＿＿＿
11. polyradiculitis
    [pɒlirədikjʊ'laitis]　＿＿＿＿＿＿＿＿
12. neurolysis
    [njʊə'rɒlisis]　＿＿＿＿＿＿＿＿

练习 17-1

13. radiculalgia
[rædikjʊ'ældʒə] _____

14. myelography
[mai'lɒgrəfi] _____

写出下列定义的单词。

15. tumor of glial cells _____
16. x-ray image of the spinal cord _____
17. pain in a nerve _____
18. inflammation of the spinal cord _____
19. any disease of the nervous system _____

表 17-2   脑部的词根

词根	含义	示例	示例定义
encephal/o	脑部	anencephaly [ænən'sefəli]	无脑畸形
cerebr/o	大脑（脑部）	infracerebral [infrə'serəbrəl]	脑下的
cortic/o	大脑皮层	corticospinal [kɔ:ti'kɒspinl]	皮质脊髓的
cerebell/o	小脑	supracerebellar [sju:p'reisrbelə]	小脑上的
thalam/o	丘脑	thalamotomy [θælə'mɒtəmi]	丘脑切开术
ventricul/o	腔、室	intraventricular [ˌintrəven'trikjʊlə]	室内的
medull/o	延髓（脊髓）	medullary ['medəlari]	延髓的
psych/o	心理	psychogenic [ˌsaikəʊ'dʒenik]	源于心理的
narc/o	昏迷、失去意识	narcosis [nɑːˈkəʊsis]	麻醉
somn/o, somn/i	睡眠	somnolence ['sɒmnələns]	嗜睡

练习 17-2

填空。

1. Somnambulism [sɒm'næmbjəlizəm] means walking during _____.
2. The term decerebrate [di:'seribreit] refers to functional loss in the _____.
3. The hypothalamus [ˌhaipə'θæləməs] is below the _____.
4. A psychoactive [ˌsaikəʊ'æktiv] drug has an effect on the _____.
5. A narcotic [nɑːˈkɒtik] is a drug that causes _____.
6. An electroencephalogram [iˌlektrəʊin'sefələgræm] (EEG) is a record of the electric activity of the _____.

练习 17-2

7. The term cerebrovascular [ˌserəbrəʊ'væskjələ] refers to blood vessels in the _____.

写出下列定义的形容词，请注意词尾。

8. pertaining to (-ic) the mind _____
9. pertaining to (-al) the cerebral cortex _____
10. pertaining to (-ic) the thalamus _____
11. pertaining to (-al) the cerebrum _____
12. pertaining to (-ar) a ventricle _____

定义下列单词。

13. encephalopathy [enˌsefə'lɒpəθi] _____
14. insomnia [in'sɒmniə] _____
15. psychology [sai'kɒlədʒi] _____
16. cerebrospinal [ˌseribrəʊ'spainəl] _____
17. extramedullary [ekstrəmi'dʌləri] _____
18. ventriculotomy [ventrikjʊ'ləʊtəʊmi] _____

写出下列定义的单词。

19. radiograph of a ventricle _____
20. pertaining to the cerebral cortex and the thalamus _____
21. within the cerebellum _____
22. inflammation of the brain _____
23. above the cerebrum _____

表 17-3　神经系统的后缀

后缀	含义	示例	示例定义
-phasia	说话	heterophasia [hetərəʊ'feisiə]	异语症
-lalia	说话、学语	coprolalia [kɒprə'leiljə]	秽语症（copro- 意为"粪便"）
-lexia	阅读	bradylexia [b'reidileksiə]	阅读过慢
-plegia	麻痹、瘫痪	tetraplegia [tetrə'pli:dʒə]	四肢麻痹
-paresis*	部分麻痹、虚弱	hemiparesis [hemipə'ri:sis]	轻偏瘫

表 17-3　神经系统的后缀

后缀	含义	示例	示例定义
-lepsy	发作	narcolepsy ['nɑ:kəʊlepsi]	嗜睡发作
-phobia*	持续、不合理的害怕	agoraphobia [ˌægərə'fəʊbiə]	广场恐惧症
-mania*	兴奋状态、强迫	megalomania [ˌmegələ'meiniə]	自大狂

* 可以作为一个单词使用

练习 17-3

填空。

1. Epilepsy ['epilepsi] is a disease characterized by _____.
2. A person with alexia [ə'leksiə] lacks the ability to _____.
3. Echolalia [ˌekəʊ'leiliə] refers to repetitive _____.
4. Another term for quadriplegia [ˌkwɒdri'pli:dʒə] is _____.
5. In myoparesis [maiəʊp'æeəsis], a muscle shows _____.

定义下列单词。

6. cardioplegia
   [kɑ:daiɒp'li:dʒə] _____
7. aphasia
   [ə'feiziə] _____
8. alexia
   [ə'leksiə] _____
9. pyromania
   [ˌpairəʊ'meiniə] _____
10. gynephobia
    [ˌdʒaini'fəʊbiə] _____
11. quadriparesis
    [kwɒd'raipæeəsis] _____

写出下列定义的单词。

12. fear of (or abnormal sensitivity to) light _____
13. fear of night and darkness _____
14. paralysis of one side (hemi-) of the body _____
15. slowness in speech (-lalia) _____

神经系统的临床表现

血管疾病

脑血管意外（cerebrovascular accident，CVA）或脑卒中（stroke）是指任何致使脑部组织缺氧的事件。这些事件包括为脑部供血的血管堵塞、血管破裂或一些会导致脑内出血的伤害。脑卒中是发达国家第四大死因，并且是瘫痪（paralysis）和其他神经残疾的首要起因。脑卒中的风险因素包括高血压、动脉粥样硬化、心脏病、糖尿病和吸烟，遗传也是一个因素。

血栓

血栓（thrombosis）是指在血管中形成了血凝块（blood clot）。通常，在脑卒中的情况下，血栓发生在为脑部供血的颈部大血管颈动脉。被来自于身体其他部位的阻塞物突然堵塞被称为栓塞（embolism）。脑卒中时，栓塞通常源自于心脏。

利用 X 线无法穿透（radiopaque）的染色剂，CT 扫描和其他 X 线技术的脑血管造影能够发现这些阻塞物。在血栓形成的情况下，可以手术切除堵塞部分的血管，并插入一个移植物。如果涉及通向脑部的颈动脉，需要进行颈动脉内膜切除术（carotid endarterectomy）以打开血管。溶解这种血凝块的溶栓（thrombolytic）药物也可供使用。

动脉瘤

动脉瘤（aneurysm）是血管的局部扩张（图 17-11），可能破裂并引起出血。动脉瘤可能是先天的，也可能是其他原因引起的，特别是削弱血管壁的动脉粥样硬化。

根据造成伤害的程度，脑血管出血的影响可能是重大功能损失，也可能是轻微的感觉或运动功能受损。失语症（aphasia），语言交流能力损失或受损是常见的滞后效应。受伤害对侧的偏瘫（hemiplegia）也不少见。研究发现，出血与其他形式的脑部伤害一样，及早进行的习服疗法（retraining therapy）有助于恢复损失的功能。

创伤

脑挫伤（cerebral contusion）是脑部表面的撞伤，通常是对头部的打击所致。血液从局部血管中漏出，但伤害并不大。

更严重的伤害可能引起脑脊膜内或周围出血，导致血肿。颅骨骨折造成的动脉伤害通常在头部的一侧，可能是硬脑膜外血肿（epidural hematoma）引起的（图 17-12），会出现在硬脑膜和颅骨之间。快速

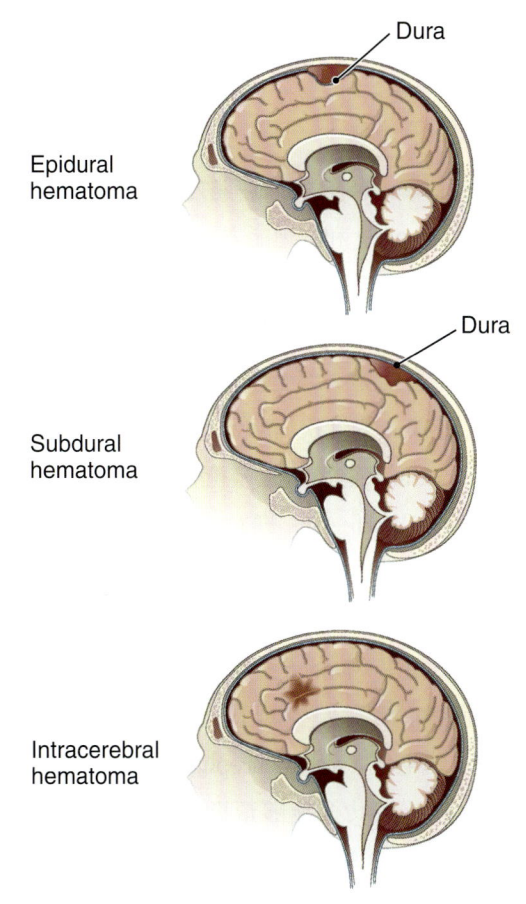

图 17-12 颅血肿。图中显示了硬膜外、硬膜下和脑内血肿的位置

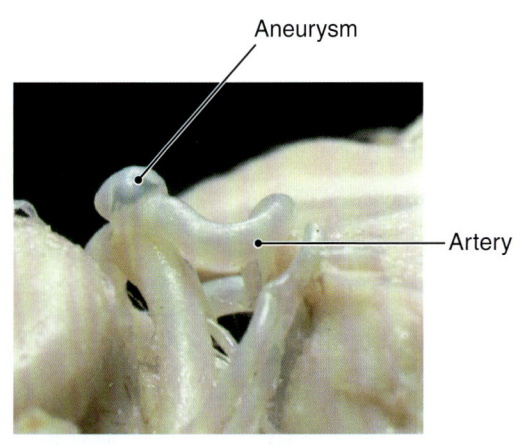

图 17-11 动脉瘤。薄壁动脉瘤从动脉突出

积累的出血会对局部血管造成压力，阻断脑部的血流。会导致头痛。意识损失或受伤对侧偏瘫。CT 扫描和核磁共振能够进行诊断。如果压力不能在 1~2d 内缓解，会导致死亡。

硬脑膜下血肿（图 17-12）通常是对头部前面或后面的打击所致，因为移动的头部会撞击静止的物体。打击的力量会使硬脑膜与其下的蛛网膜分离，来自于受损血管（通常是静脉）的血液会慢慢进入这一空间。血液逐渐积累会对脑部造成压力，引起头痛、虚弱和痴呆（dementia）。如果继续出血，会导致死亡。图 17-12 还显示了脑部组织自身的出血，形成了脑内血肿（intracerebral hematoma）。

脑震荡（cerebral concussion）是由头部被打击或跌落所致，通常伴随暂时的意识损失和短暂的失忆症（amnesia）。脑震荡的滞后效应可能包括头痛、头昏、呕吐、乏力甚至瘫痪，还有其他一些症状。发生在被打击对侧的脑部损伤被称为对冲性伤害（contrecoup injury）（源自于法语，意为"反击"）。

其他伤害可能直接损害脑部。对脑底部的伤害可能涉及延髓的生命中枢，妨碍呼吸和心脏功能。

意识混乱与昏迷

意识混乱（confusion）是理解能力（comprehension）、一致性（coherence）和推理能力（reasoning ability）下降导致对环境刺激产生不适当反应的状态，可能会恶化到语言能力损失、记忆损失、警觉降低和情绪变化。意识混乱可能是头部受伤、药物中毒、大手术、器官衰竭、感染或变性疾病所致。

昏迷（coma）是无法被唤醒的意识损失状态。昏迷的起因包括脑部受伤、癫痫、中毒、代谢失衡（例如糖尿病的酮酸中毒或葡萄糖失衡），以及呼吸衰竭、肝衰竭或肾衰竭。

医疗人员使用不同的方法评估昏迷，例如对触觉、压力和轻度疼痛的反射行为和反应，比如轻轻的针刺。实验室测试、脑电图（electroencephalography，EEG），有时用 CT 和核磁共振能够帮助确定昏迷的起因。

感染

脑膜炎（meningitis）通常是通过耳朵、鼻子或

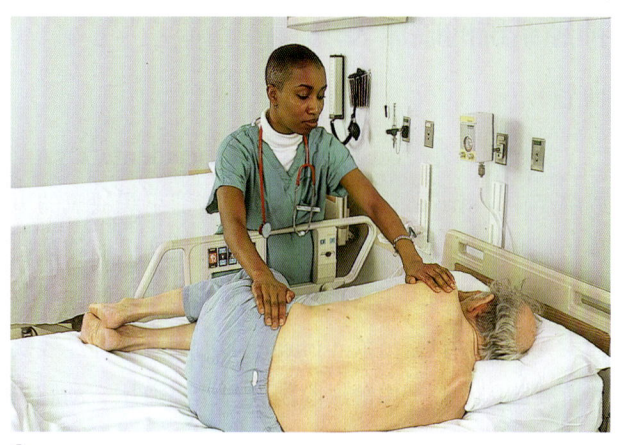

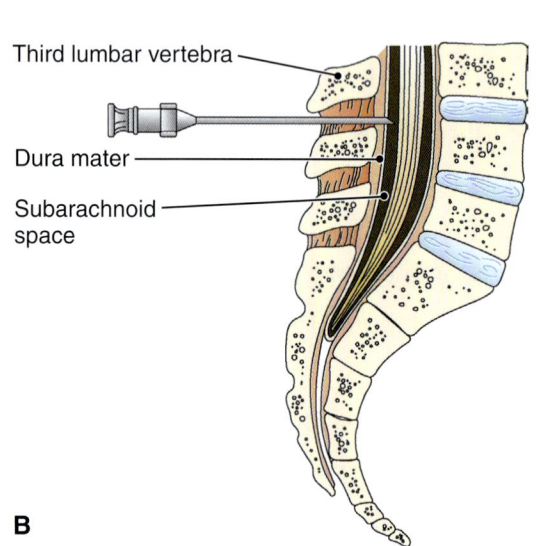

图 17-13　**腰椎穿刺**。A. 患者腰椎穿刺的位置；B. 从第三和第四或第四和第五腰椎之间的蛛网膜下空间中取出脑脊液

咽喉，或者是血液携带的细菌引起的。这些细菌之一是脑膜炎双球菌（meningococcus），也被称为脑膜炎奈瑟氏菌（Neisseria meningitidis），是密集人群脑膜炎流行的罪魁祸首。其他涉及脑膜炎病例的细菌包括流感嗜血杆菌（haemophilus influenzae）、肺炎双球菌（streptococcus pneumoniae）和大肠杆菌（escherichia coli）。脖子僵硬是常见症状，脊髓液中出现脓或淋巴细胞也是典型特征。

医生会通过腰穿抽取脊髓液进行分析诊断（图 17-13），即使用针头在腰部脊髓的脑脊膜中抽取脑脊液。实验室测试能够检验脑脊液中的白细胞和细菌进行脑膜炎诊断，检验红细胞进行脑部损伤或肿瘤诊断。还可以对抽出的脑脊液进行化学分析，正常的脑脊液是清澈透明的，包含葡萄糖和氯化物，但有非常少量的细胞，没有蛋白质。

其他能够引起脑膜炎和脑炎（encephalitis）的包括病毒感染、结核病和梅毒。可能感染中枢神经系统的病毒包括脊髓灰质炎病毒（poliovirus）、狂犬病病毒（rabies virus）、疱疹病毒（herpesvirus）、人类免疫缺陷病毒（HIV）和西尼罗河病毒这样的蜱和蚊媒病毒，以及普通的会引起麻疹和水痘等轻微疾病的病毒（比较罕见）。无菌性（aseptic）脑膜炎是一种由病毒引起的良性、非细菌的疾病。

引起水痘的水痘-带状疱疹（varicella-zoster）病毒也会导致带状疱疹（shingles），是一种神经感染。如果在儿童时期患过水痘，潜伏的病毒可能在以后被再次激活，并沿着周围神经系统扩散，引起瘙痒和水疱疹。带状疱疹的名称源自于拉丁语意为"带子"的单词，意为带状疱疹常常靠近或围绕腰部出现。超过60岁的人群有疫苗预防带状疱疹。

肿瘤

几乎所有起源于神经系统的肿瘤都是非传导支持细胞神经胶质的肿瘤。这种肿瘤被称为神经胶质瘤（glioma），可以根据涉及的特定细胞进行分类，例如星形细胞瘤（astrocytoma）或神经鞘瘤（neurilemmoma）。因为它们往往不会转移，这些肿瘤可以被描述为良性的。不过，它们会因为压迫脑组织而带来伤害（图17-14）。所引起的症状取决于它们的大小和位置，症状包括抽搐、头痛、呕吐、肌肉无力或特定感觉障碍，如视力或听力。如果出现水肿和脑积水，也是肿瘤引起的（图17-15）。

脑膜瘤（meningioma）是脑膜的肿瘤，因为不扩散并位于表面，手术可以完全切除它。

神经组织的肿瘤一般发生在童年时期，甚至可能起源于出生之前该组织快速增殖复制之时。还有，癌症可能从身体的其他部位转移到脑部。出于未知的原因，一些特定的癌症，如黑色素瘤、乳腺癌和肺癌往往会扩散到脑部。

退行性疾病

多发性硬化症（multiple sclerosis，MS）通常会在20~30岁发生，并且间断性地以不同的速度发展。该疾病涉及中枢神经系统中髓磷脂的片状损伤和组织硬化，症状包括视觉问题、四肢刺痛（tingling）或麻木（numbness）、尿失禁（urinary incontinence）、震颤（tremor）和步态僵硬（stiff gait）。多发性硬化症被认为是一种自身免疫性疾病，但确切原因不明。

当中脑的特定神经元出于不明原因不能分泌神经递质多巴胺时，就会发生震颤麻痹（帕金森症Parkinsonism），这会导致震颤、肌强直（muscle rigidity）、关节弯曲、运动不能（akinesia）和情绪问题。帕金森症需要每日服用左旋多巴（levodopa）进行治疗，

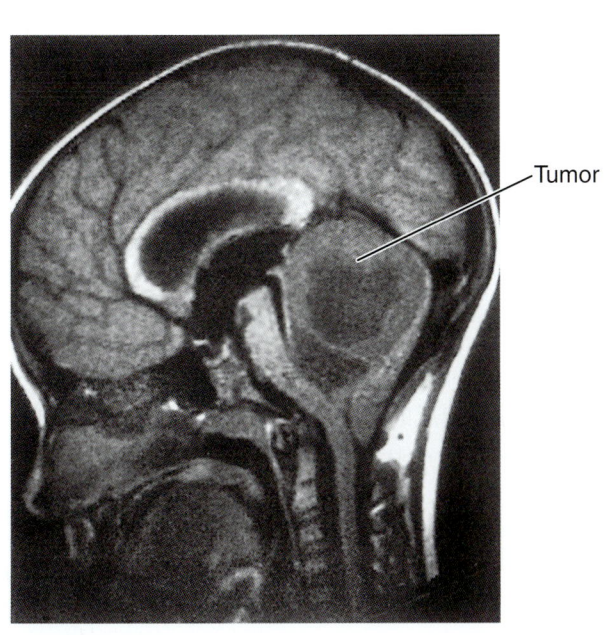

图 17-14 脑肿瘤。核磁共振显示大肿瘤从小脑中产生，并向前推动脑干

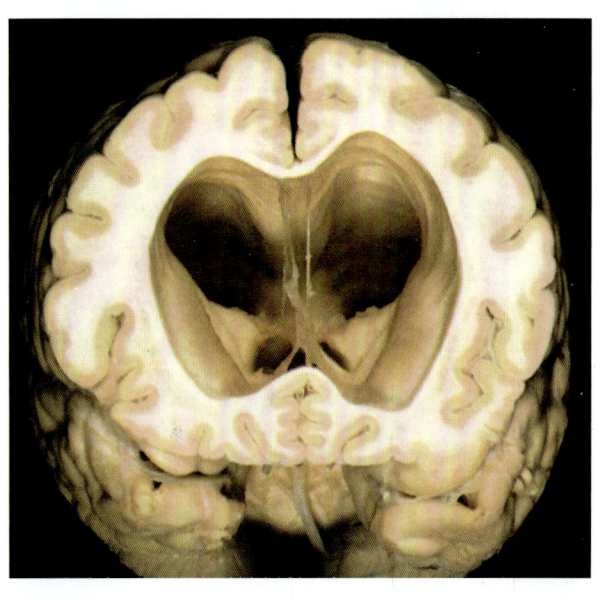

图 17-15 脑积水。脑的冠状切面图显示由阻碍脑脊液流动的肿瘤引起的明显的脑室增大

左旋多巴是一种通过循环能够进入脑部的多巴胺。

老年痴呆（阿尔茨海默病，Alzheimer disease，AD）由原因不明的神经元退化和大脑皮层萎缩（图17-16）所致。这些变化引起短期记忆力的进行性损失、意识混乱和性情改变。与老年痴呆相关的危险有受伤、感染、营养不良和食物或液体吸入肺部。最初被称为早老性痴呆（presenile dementia），只用于描述 50 岁之前的患者，现在这一术语也被用于老年患者。

老年痴呆可以通过 CT 或核磁共振诊断，并通过尸检确认。组织学研究显示，在组织上有被称为类淀粉蛋白（amyloid）的物质淤积，这种疾病可能是遗传性的。老年痴呆通常发生于唐氏综合征患者 40 岁之后，表明老年痴呆与染色体 21 异常有关，唐氏综合征也涉及该染色体。

多梗死性痴呆（multiinfarct dementia，MID）与老年痴呆相似，是一种进行性认知能力受损（cognitive impairment），伴随记忆力损失、判断力损失、运动障碍、运动和感觉功能改变、行为重复合社交技能损失。该疾病是由截断脑组织供血并使多个区域缺氧的多个小脑卒中引起的。

癫痫

癫痫（epilepsy）的一个主要特征是脑部异常电活动带来的反复发作（seizure）。这些发作形式各异，从短暂温和的失神发作（absence seizure，小发作，petit mal）到伴有意识损失、惊厥（convulsion）（间断性强烈的不自主肌肉收缩）和感觉障碍的严重强直阵挛性发作（tonic-clonic seizure，大发作，grand mal）。在其他情况下（痉挛发作，psychomotor seizures）会有 1~2 分钟的方向迷失。癫痫可能是肿瘤、受伤或神经疾病所致，但大多数病例的原因不明。

脑电图能够揭示脑部活动的异常，可被用于癫痫的诊断和治疗。这种疾病需要使用抗癫痫和抗惊厥药物控制发作，有时手术也有所帮助。如果发作不能得到控制，癫痫的患者应避免参与可能导致伤害的特定活动。

睡眠障碍

一般意义的睡眠障碍（dyssomnia）包括能够导致过度睡眠和难以开始或保持睡眠的多种可能的病症。这类病症的简单起因包括日程变更或跨时区旅行（时差，jet lag）。失眠（insomnia）是指尽管有充足的睡眠机会下的睡眠不足或睡眠不可恢复。失眠可能身体原因造成的，但更多地是与压力事件引起的情绪不安有关。嗜眠症（narcolepsy）的特征是在白天短暂的、无法控制的睡眠发作。这种病症需要兴奋剂、规律睡眠习惯和短暂的午休进行治疗。

睡眠呼吸暂停（sleep apnea）是指在睡眠期间出现暂短的不能呼吸。这通常是上呼吸道阻塞所致，常常与肥胖、饮酒或咽喉肌肉虚弱有关，还经常伴随带

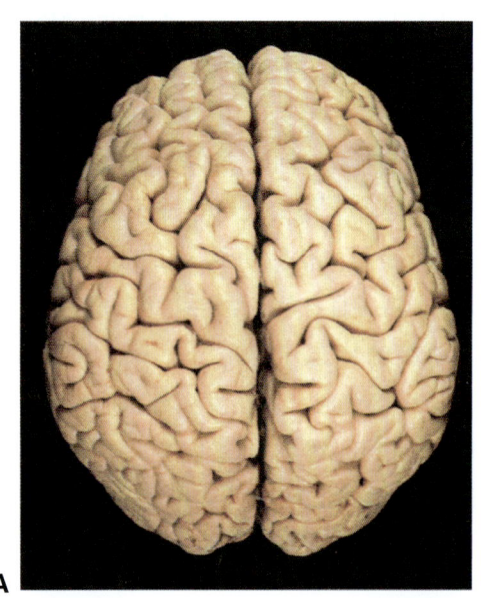

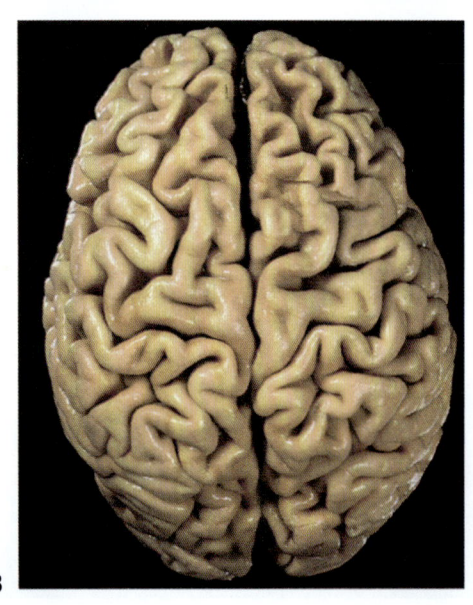

图 17-16　阿尔茨海默病的影响。A. 正常脑；B. 具有阿尔茨海默病的患者的脑，显示有皮质萎缩，脑回狭窄且脑沟扩大

健康职业 框 17-2

职业疗法的职业

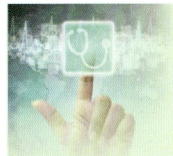

职业疗法（occupational therapy，OT）通过教导"生活技能"，帮助具有身体或精神残疾的人在家庭和工作中实现独立。许多人可以受益，包括：

- 从创伤例如骨折、截肢、烧伤、脊髓损伤、脑卒中和心脏病发作中恢复的人群。
- 有慢性病症如关节炎、多发性硬化、阿尔茨海默病和精神分裂症的人群。
- 有发育性障碍如唐氏综合征、脑性麻痹、脊柱裂、肌营养不良和自闭症的人群。

职业治疗师（occupational therapist，OT）作为多学科团队的一部分，包括但不限于医生、护士、物理治疗师、言语病理学家和社会工作者。职业治疗师还与家人密切合作，教育和指导他们如何协助患者取得进步。他们评估患者的能力并开发个性化治疗计划，帮助他们从伤害中恢复或补偿永久性残疾。治疗包括从工作任务到穿衣、烹饪和吃饭的教学活动，以及使用适应性设备，例如轮椅和计算机。

职业治疗师助理实施由职业治疗师开发的治疗计划，并针对目标的进展和可能的重新评估定期咨询职业治疗师。为了履行职责，职业治疗师和职业治疗师助手需要完整的科学教育和临床背景。在美国，当前的执业职业治疗师有学士或硕士学位。截至 2007 年，职业治疗师必须获得职业治疗硕士学位才能开业。毕业后，他们必须通过国家认证考试，并在必要的情况下，由国家许可才能执业。职业治疗师助理通常要参加两年的课程的培训，并参加认证考试。

职业治疗师及其助理在医院、诊所和护理机构工作，并访问家庭和学校。随着人口持续老龄化和对康复治疗的需求增加，就业前景仍然良好。美国职业治疗协会（American Occupational Therapy Association）在 www.aota.org 有更多关于职业治疗师职业的信息。

短暂沉静的大声打鼾。能够使舌头和颌部向前移动的齿科用具能够有助于防止睡眠呼吸暂停，其他方法包括手术矫正阻塞或通过面具提供正压通气。

睡眠障碍可以通过身体检查、睡眠史和睡眠习惯记录来诊断，睡眠习惯记录包括睡眠环境的细节和任何可能干扰睡眠的物质使用记录。也可能需要实验室研究构成的多导睡眠图（polysomnography）。

睡眠研究能够鉴定正常睡眠的两个组成部分，每个部分显示特定的脑电图模式。非快速眼动（nonrapid eye movement，NREM）睡眠有四个阶段，能够渐进地将一个人带入最深度的睡眠。如果发生梦游（sleepwalking，somnambulism），就会发生在该阶段。非快速眼动睡眠每隔大约一个半小时会有插入快速眼动（rapid eye movement，REM）睡眠，在快速眼动睡眠期间，眼球会快速转动，尽管眼睛是闭着的。做梦发生在快速眼动睡眠期，肌肉会失去张力，同时心率、血压和脑部活动都会上升。

其他

许多遗传性疾病都会影响神经系统，第 15 章中讨论了其中的一些。涉及神经系统的激素失衡在第 16 章进行了讨论。最后，药物、酒精、毒素和营养不足可能以不同的方式作用于神经系统。框 17-2 给出了关于职业治疗师的信息，他们经常参与治疗患有神经障碍的人。

行为障碍

本节介绍一些涉及神经系统的行为障碍。美国精神病学会（American Psychiatric Association）出版的《精神疾病诊断与统计手册（Diagnostic and Statistical Manual of Mental Disorders）》确定了行为障碍和精神疾病的临床诊断准则。

焦虑症

焦虑是一种畏惧、忧虑、不安或害怕的感觉，可能与身体问题或药物有关，常常被无助或损失自尊（selfesteem）的感觉引发。广泛性焦虑症（generalized anxiety disorder，GAD）的特征是对各种生活环境的长期过度和无法控制的忧虑，通常没有任何根据。可能会伴随肌肉绷紧（muscle tensing）、坐卧不安（restlessness）、呼吸困难、心悸（palpitation）、失眠、易怒（irritability）或疲乏。

恐慌症（panic disorder）也是一种形式的焦虑症，特征是强烈恐惧（intense fear）的发作。恐慌症的

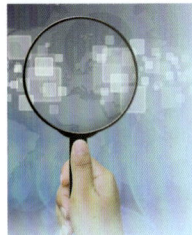

聚焦单词
恐惧症与狂躁症

框 17-3

恐惧症（phobias）与狂躁症（manias）的一些术语与其对应的行为一样奇怪和有趣。

广场恐惧症（agoraphobia）是畏惧处于公共场所，agora 在古希腊语中是的意思是市场。陌生恐惧症（xenophobia）是不合理地畏惧陌生人，源自于希腊语意为"陌生人或外国人"的词根 xen/o。恐高症（acrophobia）是畏惧高度，源自于词根 acro-，意为终点、最高处或最上面。在大多数医学术语中，这个词根都被用于表示末端，例如手足发绀（acrocyanosis）。恐水症（hydrophobia）是畏惧或嫌恶水（hydr/o），该术语也被用作狂犬病（rabies）的替代名称，因为感染这种麻痹性疾病的患者有吞咽口水和其他液体的困难。

拔毛狂（trichotillomania）是一种古怪的行为，强迫性地拔掉自己的头发以应对压力。这个单词源自于意为"头发"的词根 trich/o 加上意为"拔毛"的希腊语单词。盗窃狂（kleptomania）也被拼写为 cleptomania，源自于希腊语意为"贼"的单词，是指在没有需要的情况下不可抗拒的偷窃欲望。

患者可能会因为害怕恐慌发作或为应对发作而隔离自己或避免参加社交活动。

恐惧症（phobia）是对特定物体或情景的极端持续的恐惧（框 17-3）。恐惧的对象包括社交情景、特殊的物体（例如动物或血液）或活动（例如飞行或驾驶穿过隧道）。

强迫症（obsessive-compulsive disorder，OCD）的特征是持续侵入的干扰性思想或形象。为缓解对这些思想或形象的焦虑，强迫症患者会从事打乱正常生活活动的重复性行为，尽管患者知道这样的行为不合理。重复性行为模式包括重复清洗、执行某些仪式、重复一些单词或短语，以及排列、接触或计数一些物体。强迫症与完美主义（perfectionism）和行为刚性（rigidity in behavior）有关，一些专家认为与脑部神经递质 5-羟色胺（serotonin）水平低相关。强迫症需要行为疗法进行治疗，并使用抗抑郁药物提高脑部的 5-羟色胺水平（框 17-4）。

当压力巨大的灾难性事件导致持续的情绪问题时，这种情况被称为创伤后心理压力紧张综合征（posttraumatic stress disorder，PTSD）。被虐待、生活在威胁之中、目击犯罪、经历自然灾害的人，特别是战争退伍军人易患创伤后心理压力紧张综合征。反应包括愤怒、恐惧、睡眠障碍和一些身体症状，包括脑化学的变化和激素失衡。PTSD 常常与情绪问题

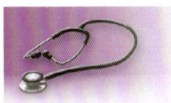

临床观点
精神活性药物：调节神经递质以改变情绪

框 4-2

目前使用的许多精神活性药物通过影响脑部神经递质的水平和活性来发挥作用，这些神经递质有 5-羟色胺、去甲肾上腺素和多巴胺。例如氟西汀（fluoxetine）及相关化合物被用于改变情绪。

氟西汀通过阻止 5-羟色胺再吸收提高其活性，即阻止将 5-羟色胺传送回突触的分泌细胞。与其他的选择性 5-羟色胺再吸收抑制剂（selective serotonin reuptake inhibitors，SSRI）一样，氟西汀延长在突触的神经递质的活性，产生一种提升情绪的效果。氟西汀被用于治疗抑郁、焦虑和强迫症。

其他的精神活性药物不像氟西汀这样有选择性。文拉法辛（venlafaxine）阻止 5-羟色胺和去甲肾上腺素的再吸收，被用于治疗抑郁和广泛性焦虑症。安非他酮（bupropion）阻止去甲肾上腺素和多巴胺的再吸收，被用于治疗抑郁和戒烟。另一类抗抑郁药物单胺氧化酶抑制剂（monoamine oxidase inhibitors，MAOI），能够阻止酶在突触分解 5-羟色胺，例如苯乙肼（phenelzine）和反苯环丙胺（tranylcypromine）。与选择性 5-羟色胺再吸收抑制剂一样，单胺氧化酶抑制剂能够提高突触对 5-羟色胺的获得量。

一些草药也被用于治疗抑郁。贯叶连翘（St. John's wort）包含活性成分金丝桃素（hypericin），能够非选择性地抑制 5-羟色胺的再吸收和阻止去甲肾上腺素和多巴胺的再吸收。在与其他任何药物一起使用贯叶连翘时，必须特别小心，特别是与其他抗抑郁药物组合时。使用的任何药物都要告知医护人员，包括正在服用的草药。

相关，例如抑郁（depression）、不合群（withdrawal）、药物滥用以及受损的社会和家庭关系。患者需要尽早治疗，包括情感支持、保护、心理疗法和药物治疗压抑与焦虑。

情绪障碍

抑郁症（depression）是一种以长时间感到悲伤（sadness）、空虚（emptiness）、无望（hopelessness）、不能集中注意力和缺少活动兴趣或快乐为特征的精神状态。抑郁症常常伴随失眠、食欲不振和自杀倾向，还常与其他身体或情绪问题共存。

心境恶劣障碍（dysthymia）是一种持续数月至数年的慢性情绪障碍，通常是由一个严重事件触发的。抑郁是常见症状，还有饮食失调、睡眠障碍、疲乏、注意力差、优柔寡断和感觉无望。

在双相情感障碍（bipolar disorder）（以前称为躁郁症 manic-depressive illness）中，正常情绪与抑郁症和狂躁症发作交替，狂躁时出于一种兴高采烈的状态，激动、过度兴奋或多动。双相情感障碍的治疗与抑郁症的治疗不同，包括情绪稳定药物和专门的精神健康疗法。

大多数用于治疗情绪障碍的药物都会影响脑部神经递质的水平，例如选择性5-羟色胺再吸收抑制剂会延长5-羟色胺的作用时间。

精神错乱

精神错乱（psychosis）是一种对现实有明显感知错误的精神状态。这种与现实的脱节可以通过患者的幻想（错误信念）得到证实，幻想（delusion）包括妄想、迫害或威胁幻想，或者幻觉（hallucination，想象中的感觉经历）。尽管患者的状态使其无法应对日常生活的需求，但却意识不到这种行为的不正常。

精神分裂症（schizophrenia）是一种形式的慢性精神错乱，可能包括古怪的行为、偏执（paranoia）、焦虑、幻想、不合群和自杀倾向。精神分裂症的诊断包含具有许多亚型的广泛类型的病症。精神分裂症的起因不明，但有证据显示与遗传因素和脑化学失衡有关。

注意力缺陷多动障碍

注意力缺陷多动障碍（attention deficit hyperactivity disorder，ADHD）很难诊断，因为它的许多症状与其他行为障碍的症状重叠或共存。不过在这些病例中注意力不集中和多动通常一起出现，其中之一可能是主要的。ADHD通常起始于儿童期，特点是注意力问题、容易厌烦（easy boredom）、缺乏耐心（impatience）和冲动性行为（impulsive behavior）。通过其坐立不安（fidgeting）、身体扭动（squirming）、快速动作或多话的表现可以明显地显现出相关的多动症。在成年，ADHD可能会与其他病症混淆，例如情绪障碍、药物滥用和内分泌问题。

ADHD与脑部结构和新陈代谢相互关联，治疗需要精神疗法（psychotherapy）或行为疗法，以及特定的药物疗法。传统上会给患ADHD的儿童处方使用兴奋剂哌甲酯（methylphenidate），但近来抗抑郁剂阿托莫西汀（atomoxetine）的使用效果不错。

广泛性发育障碍

广泛性发育障碍（pervasive developmental disorder，PDD）这一术语是指出现在生命早期并影响社交技能的损伤。有些形式的PDD通常与一定程度的精神发育迟缓（mental retardation）有关，不过，一个有PDD的人可能有正常或者高于平均水平的智力，甚至非常卓越。每个有PDD的儿童都是独特的，有其自己特定的需求。这些病症与自闭症（autism）和阿斯伯格综合征（Asperger syndrome）都属于同一系列。

自闭症是一种起因不明的复杂病症，通常好发于2~6岁没有达到适当发育标准的儿童。自闭症的特征是自我专注（self-absorption），缺乏对社会接触和情感的反应。自闭症儿童可能智力低下且语言表达能力差，他们通常显得孤立和不合群。他们可能对外界刺激反应过度，并表现出自毁行为。还可能有重复性行为、出神（preoccupation）、情绪波动和拒绝改变。自闭症可能伴随神经问题、睡眠问题和饮食问题。自闭症患者可能需要精神健康专家、社会工作者和职业物理和语言治疗师的帮助。

阿斯伯格综合征的患者通常有很高的智力和语言能力，但在社会交流和理解他人行为方面有问题。因此，儿童患者通常会被孤立和欺负。这些儿童可能会发展出重复性行为，还可能对特定的事物有很强的兴趣。他们需要帮助学习解读社交提示，但通常能将他们的才能用于令其满足的职业。

治疗中使用的药物

精神治疗或精神活性药物是对精神状态起作用的药物，包括镇静剂（anxiolytics）、情绪稳定剂（mood stabilizer）、抗抑郁剂（antidepressant）和抗精神病药物（antipsychotic），也被称为神经松弛剂（neuroleptics）。许多这类药物都是通过提高脑部神经递质的水平而起作用。请注意，精神活性药物并不以同样的方式对每个人有效，通常必须试用不同的疗法，直至找到正确的药物。另外，药物产生作用可能需要数周的时间。更多信息请参见补充术语中特定类型精神活性药物的说明。

Terminology 关键术语

神经系统疾病

Alzheimer disease (AD)	阿尔茨海默病，老年痴呆症，因大脑皮层萎缩引起的一种痴呆症，也被称为早老性痴呆（presenile dementia，图 17-16）
amyloid [ˈæmiˈlɔid]	类淀粉蛋白，老年痴呆症和其他相关疾病患者脑部积累的一种成分部门的淀粉样物质
aneurysm [ˈænjərizəm]	动脉瘤，血管壁衰弱所致的局部血管异常膨胀（图 17-11），可能最终会破裂
aphasia [əˈfeiziə]	失语症，语言交流能力的损失或缺陷（源自于希腊语单词 phasis，意为"言语"）。在实践中，这个术语被广泛地用于一系列语言障碍，包括口头和书写两个方面。失语症可能影响对语言的理解（感觉性失语症，receptive aphasia）或者产生语言的能力（表达性失语症，expressive aphasia），完全性失语症（global aphasia）是这两种形式的组合
astrocytoma [ˌæstrəʊsaiˈtəʊmə]	星形细胞瘤，由星形胶质细胞构成的神经胶质瘤
cerebral contusion [ˈserəbrəl kənˈtjuːʒən]	脑挫伤，头部被击打后脑部表面的挫伤
cerebrovascular accident (CVA) [ˌserəbrəʊˈvæskjələ]	脑血管意外，大脑供血减少所致的脑部突然伤害，起因可能是动脉粥样硬化、血栓或动脉瘤破裂；通常被称为脑卒中（stroke）
coma [ˈkəʊmə]	昏迷，无法唤醒的深度意识损失状态
concussion [kənˈkʌʃn]	震荡，猛烈打击或冲击所致的伤害；脑震荡通常会导致意识损失
confusion [kənˈfjuːʒn]	意识混乱，理解力、一致性和推理能力下降的状态，会导致对环境刺激的不适反应
contrecoup injury [ˈkɒntrəkuː]	对冲性伤害，在头部被打击的对侧，由于脑部撞击颅骨造成的脑部伤害（源自于法语，意为"反击"）
convulsion [kənˈvʌlʃn]	惊厥，一系列强烈的、非自主的肌肉收缩。强直性惊厥是长时间的肌肉收缩；阵挛性惊厥是肌肉收缩和放松交替，在癫痫大发作（grand mal epilepsy）中，这两种惊厥都会出现
dementia [diˈmenʃə]	痴呆，逐渐且通常不可逆地损失智力功能

Terminology 关键术语（续表）

embolism [ˈembəlizəm]	栓塞，血管被血凝块或循环中携带的其他物质堵塞
encephalitis [enˌsefəˈlaitəs]	脑炎，脑部的炎症
epidural hematoma [ˌepiˈdjuərəl ˌhiːməˈtəumə]	硬脑膜外血肿，在硬脑膜空间（硬脑膜与颅骨之间）的血液积累
epilepsy [ˈepilepsi]	癫痫，涉及脑部电活动突然爆发的一种慢性疾病，会导致惊厥发作
glioma [glaiˈəumə]	神经胶质瘤，神经胶质细胞的肿瘤
hemiparesis [hemipəˈriːsis]	轻偏瘫，身体一侧部分瘫痪或虚弱
hemiplegia [ˌhemiˈpliːdʒiə]	偏瘫，身体一侧瘫痪
hydrocephalus [ˈhaidrəʊsefələs]	脑积水，因流动阻塞所致的脑部周围脑脊液积累增加，可能是肿瘤、炎症、出血或先天畸形所致
insomnia [inˈsɒmniə]	失眠症，有充足的睡眠机会条件下的睡眠不足或无法恢复睡眠
meningioma [minindʒiˈəumə]	脑脊膜瘤，脑脊膜的肿瘤
meningitis [ˌmeninˈdʒaitis]	脑膜炎，脑膜的炎症
multiinfarct dementia (MID)	多梗死性痴呆，由多次小脑卒中所致的长期大脑局部缺血引起的痴呆。会导致进行性认知功能、记忆和判断能力的损失，以及运动和感觉功能的变化
multiple sclerosis (MS) [skləˈrəʊsis]	多发性硬化症，涉及中枢神经系统髓磷脂流失的一种慢性进行性疾病
narcolepsy [ˈnɑːkəʊlepsi]	嗜眠症，日间短暂的、无法控制的睡眠发作
neurilemmoma [nɜːraiˈleməumə]	神经鞘瘤，周围神经鞘的肿瘤；又称为许旺氏细胞瘤（schwannoma）
paralysis [pəˈræləsis]	瘫痪，暂时或永久性的功能损失。迟缓性瘫痪（flaccid paralysis）涉及肌肉张力和反射的损失和肌变性。痉挛性瘫痪（spastic paralysis）涉及肌肉张力和反射过度，但没有肌变性
Parkinsonism	帕金森症，起源于脑部基底神经节的一种病症，特点是行动缓慢、震颤、僵硬和假面状面容。也被称为 Parkinson disease
seizure [ˈsiːʒə(r)]	突然发作，癫痫突然发作。最常见的发作形式是强直阵挛性发作（tonic-clonic seizure）或大发作（grand mal，源自于法语，意为"大病"）、失神发作（absence seizure）或小发作（petit mal，源自于法语，意为"小病"）和精神运动性发作（psychomotor seizure）
shingles [ˈʃiŋglz]	带状疱疹，沿着神经通道发生是急性病毒感染，会引起皮肤上的小病变。起因是引起水痘的病毒复活。也被称为 herpes zoster [ˌhɜːpiːz ˈzɒstə(r)]
sleep apnea [æpˈniːə]	睡眠呼吸暂停，睡眠期间短暂的呼吸停止
stroke [strəʊk]	脑卒中，一根或多根脑血管血流突然中断，导致脑组织损失氧气和坏死；起因是血管中的血凝块（缺血性脑卒中 ischemic stroke）或血管破裂（出血性脑卒中 hemorrhagic stroke），也被称为脑血管意外（cerebrovascular accident，CVA）
subdural hematoma [sʌbˈdjuərəl]	硬脑膜下血肿，硬脑膜之下的血压积累（图17-12）

Terminology 关键术语（续表）

thrombosis [θrɒmˈbəʊsɪs]	血栓形成，血管内血凝块的发展
tremor [ˈtremə(r)]	震颤，震动或不自主的运动

诊断与治疗

carotid endarterectomy [enˌdɑːtəˈrektəmɪ]	颈动脉内膜切除术，手术切除颈动脉内膜，颈动脉是颈部为脑部供血最大的血管
cerebral angiography [ændʒɪˈɒɡrəfɪ]	脑血管造影术，在注射造影剂后通过X线研究脑血管
electroencephalography (EEG) [ɪˈlektrəʊensefəˈlɒɡrəfɪ]	脑电图学，脑电图，放大、记录并解读脑部的电活动
L-dopa	左旋多巴，用于治疗帕金森症的药物，也拼写为 levodopa
lumbar puncture	腰椎穿刺，穿透腰部脊髓的蛛网膜下腔抽出脊髓液进行分析诊断或注射麻醉剂（图17-13）；也被称为脊椎穿刺（spinal tap）
polysomnography [ˌpɒlɪːsɒmnəʊˈɡrəfɪ]	多导睡眠图，为诊断睡眠障碍，在睡眠期间同时监测不同的生理功能

行为障碍

anxiety [æŋˈzaɪətɪ]	焦虑，恐惧、担心、不安或害怕的感觉
Asperger syndrome	阿斯伯格综合征，一种自闭症的连续性行为状况，对社交互动和理解有困难，对特定事物有强烈的兴趣和重复性行为
attention deficit hyperactivity disorder (ADHD)	注意力缺陷多动症，一种起始于童年的病症，特点是注意力问题、易烦躁、冲动性行为和多动
autism [ˈɔːtɪzəm]	自闭症，一种起因不明的病症，自我专注、缺乏对社交和情感的反应、出神、重复性行为和拒绝改变（源自于 auto-，意为"自我"和 -ism，意为"状态"）
bipolar disorder [baɪˈpəʊlə]	双相情感障碍，一种带有狂躁（兴奋状态）发作的抑郁症；又称为躁狂抑郁症（manic depressive illness）
delusion [dɪˈluːʒn]	妄想，与认识和经验不一致的错误信念
depression [dɪˈpreʃn]	抑郁症，一种长时间感觉悲伤、空虚、无望和缺少活动的兴趣和乐趣的精神状态
dysthymia [dɪsˈθaɪmɪə]	心境恶劣障碍，一种温和的抑郁症，通常是从对一个严重的生活事件的反应发展而来的（源自于前缀 dys- 和希腊语 thymos，意为"精神，情感"）
hallucination [həˌluːsɪˈneɪʃn]	幻觉，与现实或外部刺激不相关的虚假的感觉
mania [ˈmeɪnɪə]	躁狂症，一种兴奋状态，可能包括激动、过度兴奋或多动（形容词：manic）
obsessive-compulsive disorder (OCD)	强迫症，一种与反复侵入的意念、形象和为缓解焦虑所进行的重复性行为相关的病症
panic disorder	恐慌症，一种形式的焦虑症，特点是强烈恐惧的发作
paranoia [ˌpærəˈnɔɪə]	妄想狂，一种以嫉妒、迫害或感觉威胁或伤害妄想为特征的精神状态

Terminology	关键术语（续表）
phobia ['fəʊbiə]	恐惧症，对特定物体或情景的极度持续恐惧
posttraumatic stress disorder (PTSD)	创伤后应激障碍，暴露于威胁生命的灾难性事件（例如创伤、虐待、自然灾害和战争）后的持续的情感障碍
psychosis [saɪˈkəʊsɪs]	精神错乱，精神障碍极度严重，以致于引起对现实的带有妄想和幻觉的总体错觉
schizophrenia [ˌskɪtsəˈfriːniə]	精神分裂症，一组了解甚少的严重精神疾病，特征是精神错乱、妄想、幻觉和孤僻或古怪的行为（schizo 意为"分裂"，phren 意为"精神"）

Terminology	补充术语
正常结构与功能	
acetylcholine (ACh) [ˌæsɪtɪlˈkɒliːn]	乙酰胆碱，一种神经递质；涉及乙酰胆碱的活动胆碱能的（cholinergic）
basal ganglia	基底神经节，在大脑和上脑干中四个涉及运动和协调的灰质团
blood–brain barrier	血脑屏障，循环血液与脑部之间的一种特殊的膜，能够防止有害物质进入脑组织
Broca area	布罗卡区，大脑左前叶控制言语生成的区域
circle of Willis	韦利斯氏环，几根为脑部供血的动脉环，位于大脑底部；又称为大脑动脉环（cerebral arterial circle）
contralateral [ˌkɒntrəˈlætərəl]	对侧的，影响身体相对的一侧
corpus callosum [ˈkɔːpəs kɑːˈləʊsəm]	胼胝体，两个大脑半球之间的连接纤维带
dermatome [ˈdɜːmətəʊm]	皮区，植皮刀，脊髓神经支配的皮肤区域；植皮时用于切割皮肤的器械（参见第 21 章）
ipsilateral [ˌɪpsɪˈlætərəl]	同侧的，身体的同一侧
leptomeninges [ˈleptəʊmenɪŋz]	柔脑膜，软脑膜和蛛网膜一起
norepinephrine [ˌnɔːrepɪˈnefrɪn]	去甲肾上腺素，一种在化学成分和功能上与肾上腺素非常相似的神经递质，也拼写为 noradrenaline
nucleus [ˈnjuːkliəs]	神经核，中枢神经系统中神经细胞的集合
plexus [ˈpleksəs]	丛，神经或血管的网络
pyramidal tracts [ˈpɪrəmɪdl]	锥体束，一组协调很好运动神经束。这些锥体束中的大多数神经纤维穿过延髓到达脊髓的对侧，并影响对侧的身体。不在锥体束中的纤维被称为锥体束外的（extrapyramidal）
reticular activating system (RAS)	网状激活系统，脑部中广泛分布的负责维持清醒的系统
Schwann cells	施万细胞，在周围轴突产生髓磷脂鞘的细胞

Terminology 补充术语（续表）

Wernicke area	韦尼克区，颞叶中与语言理解相关的区域
症状与病症	
amyotrophic lateral sclerosis (ALS) [eimaiə'trɒfik]	肌萎缩性脊髓侧索硬化症，一种疾病，特点是因运动神经元变形引起的肌肉虚弱、痉挛和夸张反射；也被称为卢伽雷病（Lou Gehrig disease）
amnesia [æmˈniːziə]	失忆症，记忆损失（起源于希腊语单词 mneme 意为"记忆"和否定性前缀 a-）
apraxia [eiˈpræksiə]	失用症，不能有目的地运动或正确使用物体
ataxia [əˈtæksiə]	共济失调，缺乏肌肉协调；也被称为协同失调（dyssynergia）
athetosis [əˈðetəʊsis]	手足徐动症，手臂非自主、缓慢、扭曲的运动，特别是手和手指
Bell palsy [ˈpɔːlzi]	贝尔麻痹，面部神经麻痹
berry aneurysm [ˈænjərizəm]	颅内小动脉瘤，脑动脉的小囊样动脉瘤
catatonia [ˌkætəˈtəʊniə]	紧张症，精神分裂症的一个阶段，在该阶段中，患者很迟钝，倾向于保持固定的位置，不动或不说话
cerebral palsy	脑性瘫痪，一种非进行性神经肌肉疾病，通常是接近出生时中枢神经系统损伤引起的。症状可能包括痉挛、非自主运动或共济失调
chorea [kəˈriə]	舞蹈症，一种以四肢或面部肌肉非自主扭动为特征的神经病症
claustrophobia [ˌklɔːstrəˈfəʊbiə]	幽闭恐惧症，害怕被关在密封的空间（源自于拉丁语单词 claudere，意为"关闭"）
compulsion [kəmˈpʌlʃn]	强迫症，为缓解压力而进行的一种重复性的、固定不变的行为
Creutzfeldt-Jakob disease (CJD)	克罗伊茨费尔特-雅各布病，一种由感染性蛋白质朊病毒引起的缓慢发展的脑变性疾病。与牛绵状脑病（bovine spongiform encephalopathy，BSE）有关
delirium [diˈliriəm]	谵妄，一种突然、暂时的精神混乱状态，特征是兴奋、坐卧不安和语无伦次
dysarthria [disˈɑːθriə]	构音障碍，缺乏必要的肌肉控制引起的语言发音缺陷
dysmetria [disˈmetriə]	辨距障碍，在主动运动中步伐和四肢位置混乱。在运动范围不足症（hypometria），四肢伸展不足；在运动范围过度症（hypermetria），四肢伸展超过目标
euphoria [juːˈfɔːriə]	欣快症，一种夸张的幸福感觉，兴高采烈
glioblastoma [ˌgliəʊblæˈstəʊmə]	恶性胶质瘤，恶性星形细胞瘤
Guillain-Barré syndrome	格林-巴利综合征，一种急性多神经炎，伴有病毒感染后发生的进行性肌无力。大多数病例能够完全康复，但需要数月至数年的时间
hematomyelia [hiːmətəʊmaiˈiːliə]	脊髓出血，脊髓中出血，例如来自于受伤
hemiballism [ˈhemibəlaizəm]	偏侧抽搐，一侧身体的痉挛和扭动
Huntington disease	亨廷顿病，一种中枢神经系统的遗传疾病，通常出现在30~50岁。患者显示进行性痴呆和舞蹈症，10~15年内会发生死亡

Terminology 补充术语（续表）

hypochondriasis [ˌhaipəkɒnˈdraiəsis]	疑病症，对自己的健康异常焦虑
ictus [ˈiktəs]	猝发，冲击或突然发作，例如癫痫发作
lethargy [ˈleθədʒi]	昏睡，一种迟钝或昏迷状态
migraine [ˈmiːgrein]	偏头痛，慢性强烈的跳动性头痛，可能是脑动脉血管变化所致。可能的起因包括遗传因素、压力、外伤和激素波动。头痛可能由视觉障碍、恶心、畏光和刺痛感觉引起的
neurofibromatosis [njʊəˈrəʊfaibrəʊmətəʊsis]	多发性神经纤维瘤，周围神经多个肿瘤的病症
neurosis [njʊəˈrəʊsis]	神经衰弱，一种由未解决的冲突引起的情绪障碍，以焦虑为主要特征
paraplegia [ˌpærəˈpliːdʒə]	截瘫，腿和下半身麻痹
parasomnia [ˌpærəsɒmniə]	深眠状态，在睡眠期间发生不希望发生的事，例如做恶梦，或者不希望发生的事在睡眠期间变得更糟
quadriplegia [ˌkwɒdriˈpliːdʒə]	四肢麻痹，四肢瘫痪（tetraplegia）
Reye syndrome	瑞氏综合征，一种罕见的急性脑病，发生在儿童病毒感染后。可能涉及肝、肾和心脏。与病毒性疾病期间服用阿司匹林相关
sciatica [saiˈætikə]	坐骨神经痛，以坐骨神经及其分支的严重疼痛为特征的神经炎
somatoform disorders [səˈmɑːtɔːfɔːm]	躯体形式障碍，与身体疾病症状相关的病症，例如疼痛、高血压或慢性疲劳，但无器质性疾病
somnambulism [sɒmˈnæmbjəlizəm]	梦游症，在睡眠时离床走动或执行其他运动功能；也常用 sleepwalking
stupor [ˈstjuːpə(r)]	昏迷，无意识状态或失去反应能力的嗜睡
syringomyelia [siriŋɡəʊmaiˈiːliə]	脊髓空洞症，一种以在脊髓中形成充满液体的腔为特征的进行性疾病
tic [tik]	抽搐，非自主、痉挛性、复发性和无目的运动或发声
tic douloureux [ˌduːləˈruː]	三叉神经痛，在三叉神经区域的极度疼痛发作；也常用 trigeminal neuralgia
tabes dorsalis [ˈteibiːz dɔːˈseilis]	脊髓痨，脊髓的背（后）部分破坏，伴随感觉和身体位置意识的丧失，如在梅毒的高级病例中所见
Tourette syndrome	妥瑞综合征，具有间歇性运动和声音表现的抽搐疾病，从儿童期开始。也可能有强迫和强迫行为、多动和注意力不集中
transient ischemic attack (TIA)	短暂性脑缺血发作，突然、短暂和暂时的脑功能障碍，通常会引起流向大脑的血液中断
Wallerian degeneration	沃勒变性，远端神经因受伤而产生的退化
whiplash [ˈwiplæʃ]	颈部过度屈伸受伤，由快加速和快减速引起的颈椎受伤，导致肌肉、韧带、椎间盘和神经的损伤

Terminology 补充术语（续表）

第 18 章和第 20 章中还有一些与神经症状相关的词汇

诊断与治疗

Babinski reflex	巴宾斯基反射，当脚底被抚摸时，外脚趾的扩展和大脚趾在超过其他脚趾的延伸。这种反应在婴儿中是正常的，但对成人表明一种特定运动神经的病变（图 17-17）
evoked potentials [iˈvəʊkt pəˈtenʃəls]	诱发电位，感觉刺激后记录的脑部电活动。包括视觉诱发电位（visual evoked potentials，VEP）、脑干听觉诱发电位（brainstem auditory evoked potentials，BAEP）和通过刺激手或腿获得的体感诱发电位（somatosensory evoked potentials，SSEP）。这些检查被用于评估中枢神经系统的功能
Glasgow Coma Scale	格拉斯哥昏迷量表，通过为眼睛开度、运动反应和言语反应分别分配一个分数来评估意识水平的系统
positron emission tomography (PET)	正电子发射断层扫描成像，使用放射性葡萄糖或另一种代谢活性物质产生组织生化活性图像。用于研究活的健康或患病的大脑，也用于心脏内科。图 17-18 比较了脑部 CT、核磁共振和 PET 扫描的图像
Romberg sign	龙贝格征，当闭上眼睛且双脚靠拢时不能保持平衡
sympathectomy [ˌsimpəˈθektəmi]	交感神经切除术，用手术或化学方法阻断交感神经传输
trephination [ˌtrefiˈneiʃən]	环钻术，从头颅上切下一块骨骼；也指用于环钻术的装置

精神活性药物

antianxiety agent [æntiːənˈzaiəti]	抗焦虑剂，通过对中枢神经系统的平静、镇静作用来缓解焦虑；例如氯氮卓（chlordiazepoxide）、地西泮（diazepam）和阿普挫仑（alprazolam）；也常用 anxiolytic
antidepressant [ˌæntidiˈpresnt]	抗抑郁药，（不同于下面单独分类的药物）阻断神经递质如 5-羟色胺、去甲肾上腺素和多巴胺单独或组合的再摄取，例如安非他酮（bupropion）、米塔扎平（mirtazapine）、奈法唑酮（nefazodone）、文拉法辛（venlafaxine）、阿托西汀（atomoxetine）
monoamine oxidase inhibitor (MAOI) [ˌmɔnəuˈæmiːn ˈɔksideis]	单胺氧化酶抑制剂，阻断分解去甲肾上腺素和 5-羟色胺从而延长其作用的酶，例如苯乙肼（phenelzine）、反苯环丙胺（tranylcypromine）、异卡波肼（isocarboxazid）
neuroleptics [njʊərəʊˈleptiks]	精神松弛剂，用于治疗精神病的药物，包括精神分裂症，例如氯氮平（clozapine）、氟哌啶醇（haloperidol）、利培酮（risperidone）、奥氮平（olanzapine）；也被称为抗精神病药（antipsychotic）。作用机制未知，但可能干扰神经递质
selective serotonin reuptake inhibitors (SSRI)	选择性 5-羟色胺再摄取抑制剂，阻断脑部对 5-羟色胺的再摄取，从而提供 5-羟色胺水平，例如氟西汀（fluoxetine）、西酞普兰（citalopram）、帕罗西汀（paroxetine）、舍曲林（sertraline）
stimulant [ˈstimjʊlənt]	兴奋剂，促进活动性和幸福感，例如哌甲酯（methylphenidate）、右旋安非他明（methylphenidate、）安非他命+右旋安非他明
tricyclic antidepressants [traiˈsaiklik]	三环抗抑郁药，阻断去甲肾上腺素、5-羟色胺或两者的再摄取，例如阿米替林（amitriptyline）、氯米帕明（clomipramine）、丙咪嗪（imipramine）、多塞平（doxepin）、曲米帕明（trimipramine）

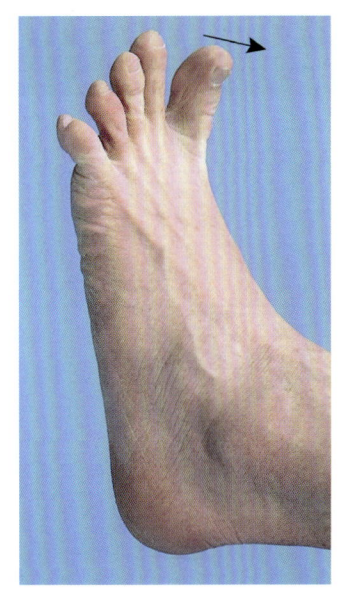

图 17-17 巴宾斯基反射。在脚底被抚摸时,大脚趾向后弯曲,其他脚趾展开。这种反应在婴儿中是正常的,但在成人则表示有运动损伤

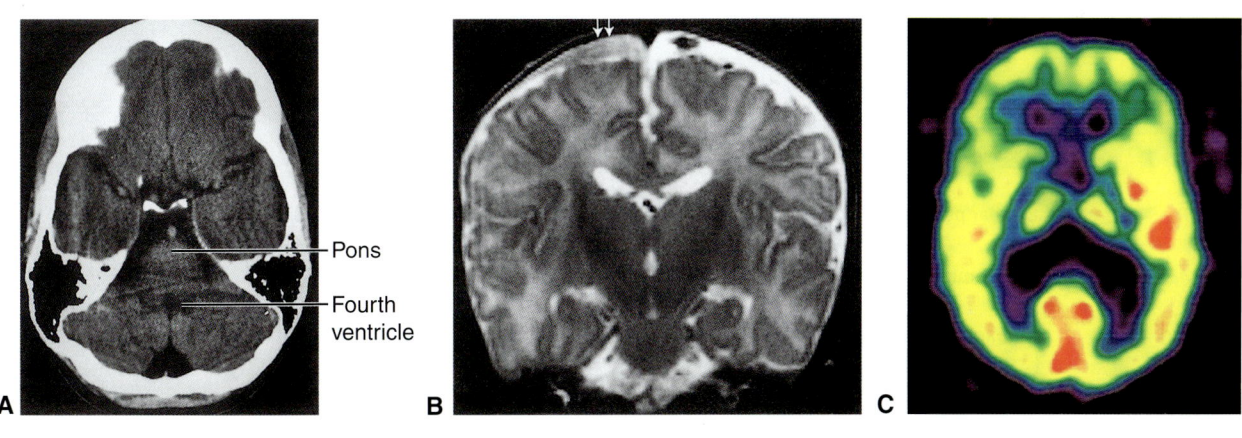

图 17-18 脑图像。A. 正常成人脑的 CT 扫描;B. 脑部核磁共振显示硬膜下血肿(箭头);C. PET 扫描显示不同代谢活性的区域

Terminology	缩略语	
ACh	Acetylcholine	乙酰胆碱
AD	Alzheimer disease	阿尔茨海默病
ADHD	Attention deficit hyperactivity disorder	注意力缺陷障碍
ALS	Amyotrophic lateral sclerosis	肌萎缩性脊髓侧索硬化症
ANS	Autonomic nervous system	自主神经系统
BAEP	Brainstem auditory evoked potentials	脑干听觉诱发电位
CBF	Cerebral blood flow	脑血流

Terminology 缩略语（续表）

CJD	Creutzfeldt-Jakob disease	克罗伊茨费尔特-雅各布病
CNS	Central nervous system	中枢神经系统
CP	Cerebral palsy	脑瘫
CSF	Cerebrospinal fluid	脑脊液
CVA	Cerebrovascular accident	脑血管意外
CVD	Cerebrovascular disease; also cardiovascular disease	脑血管疾病；心血管疾病
DSM	Diagnostic and Statistical Manual of Mental Disorders	精神障碍诊断与统计手册
DTR	Deep tendon reflexes	深腱反射
EEG	Electroencephalogram; electroencephalograph(y)	脑电图；脑电描记术
GAD	Generalized anxiety disorder	广泛性焦虑症
ICP	Intracranial pressure	颅内压
LMN	Lower motor neuron	下运动神经元
LOC	Level of consciousness	意识水平
LP	Lumbar puncture	腰椎穿刺
MAOI	Monoamine oxidase inhibitor	单胺氧化酶抑制剂
MID	Multiinfarct dementia	多梗死性痴呆
MS	Multiple sclerosis	多发性硬化症
NICU	Neurologic intensive care unit; also neonatal intensive care unit	神经重症监护病房；新生儿重症监护病房
NPH	Normal pressure hydrocephalus	压力脑积水
NREM	Nonrapid eye movement (sleep)	非快速眼动（睡眠）
OCD	Obsessive–compulsive disorder	强迫症
PDD	Pervasive developmental disorder	广泛性发育障碍
PET	Positron emission tomography	正电子发射断层成像
PNS	Peripheral nervous system	外围神经系统
PTSD	Posttraumatic stress disorder	创伤后应激障碍
RAS	Reticular activating system	网状激活系统
REM	Rapid eye movement (sleep)	快速眼动（睡眠）
SSEP	Somatosensory evoked potentials	体感诱发电位

Terminology 缩略语（续表）

SSRI	Selective serotonin reuptake inhibitor	选择性 5- 羟色胺再吸收抑制剂
TBI	Traumatic brain injury, thrombotic brain infarction	创伤性脑损伤，脑梗死溶栓
TCA	Tricyclic antidepressant	三环抗抑郁药
TIA	Transient ischemic attack	短暂性脑缺血发作
UMN	Upper motor neuron	上运动神经元
VEP	Visual evoked potentials	视觉诱发电位

Case Study Revisited 案例研究再访

B. C.'s Follow-Up

B. C. was discharged six days after his surgery with mild hemiparesis, which was expected to resolve within the next few weeks. He was scheduled for six weeks of outpatient rehabilitation, and his prognosis was good. The pediatric physical and occupational therapists were able to motivate B. C. by playing therapeutic games with him, including using a baseball and having him "walk and run the bases." B. C. was looking forward to rejoining his baseball team next season.

B. C. 的随访

B. C. 在手术后第 6 天出院，轻度偏瘫，预计在未来几周内解决。他预定了 6 个星期的门诊康复，预后良好。通过与他一起玩治疗游戏，儿科物理和职业治疗师能够激励 B. C.，包括使用棒球和让他"走动和跑垒"。B. C. 期待下个赛季重新加入他的棒球队。

CHAPTER 17 复习

标记练习

神经系统的解剖划分

在对应的下划线上写出每个编号部分的名称。

4 _____   1 _____

Brain   Peripheral nervous system
Central nervous system Spinal cord
Cranial nerves   Spinal nerves

1. _____
2. _____
3. _____
4. _____
5. _____
6. _____

运动神经元

在对应的下划线上写出每个编号部分的名称。

Axon branch   Muscle
Axon covered with myelin sheath   Myelin
Cell body   Node
Dendrites   Nucleus

1. _____
2. _____
3. _____
4. _____
5. _____
6. _____
7. _____
8. _____

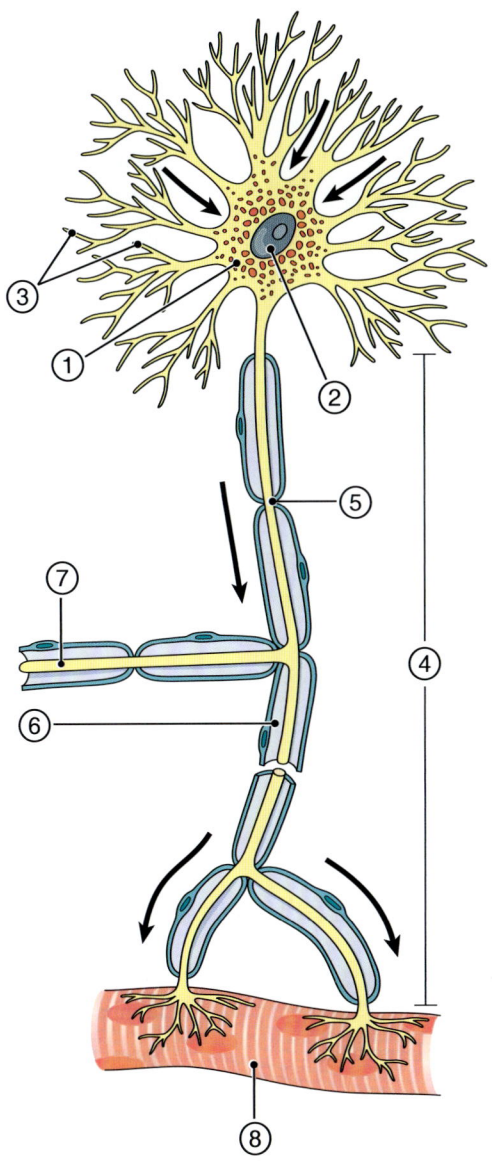

脑部外表面

在对应的下划线上写出每个编号部分的名称。

Cerebellum　　　　　　Parietal lobe
Frontal lobe　　　　　　Pons
Gyri　　　　　　　　　Spinal cord
Medulla oblongata　　　Sulci
Occipital lobe　　　　　Temporal lobe

1. _____
2. _____
3. _____
4. _____
5. _____
6. _____
7. _____
8. _____
9. _____
10. _____

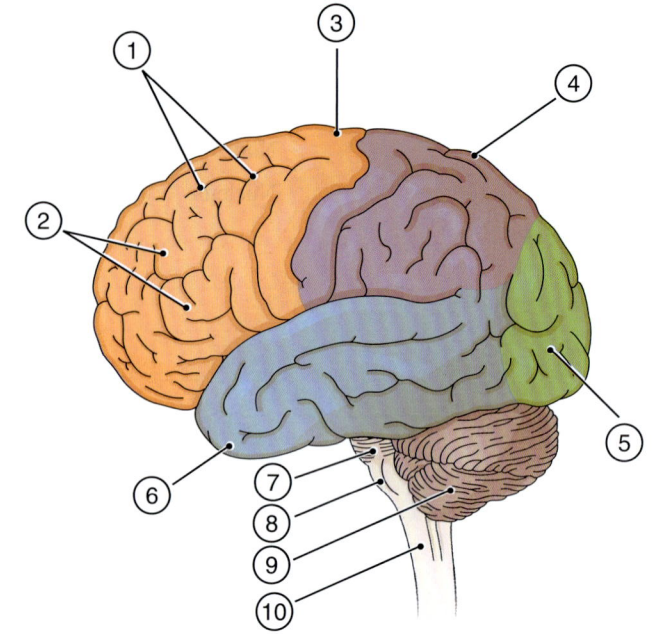

脊髓，侧视图

在对应的下划线上写出每个编号部分的名称。

Brain　　　　　　　　　Lumbar enlargement
Brainstem　　　　　　　Lumbar nerves
Cervical enlargement　　Sacral nerves
Cervical nerves　　　　　Spinal cord
Coccygeal nerve　　　　Thoracic nerves

1. _____
2. _____
3. _____
4. _____
5. _____
6. _____
7. _____
8. _____
9. _____
10. _____

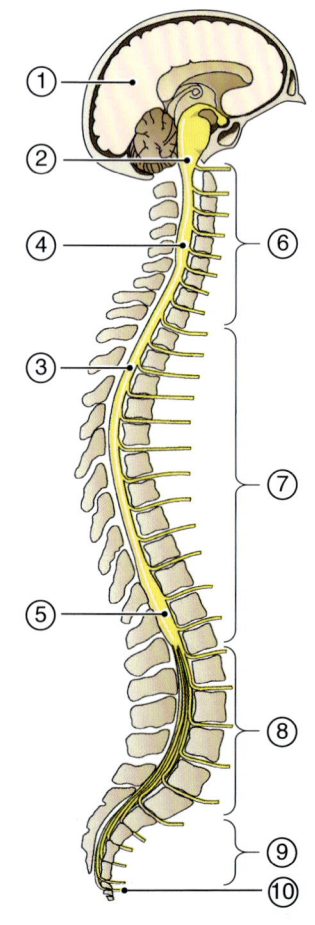

脊髓，横截面

在对应的下划线上写出每个编号部分的名称。

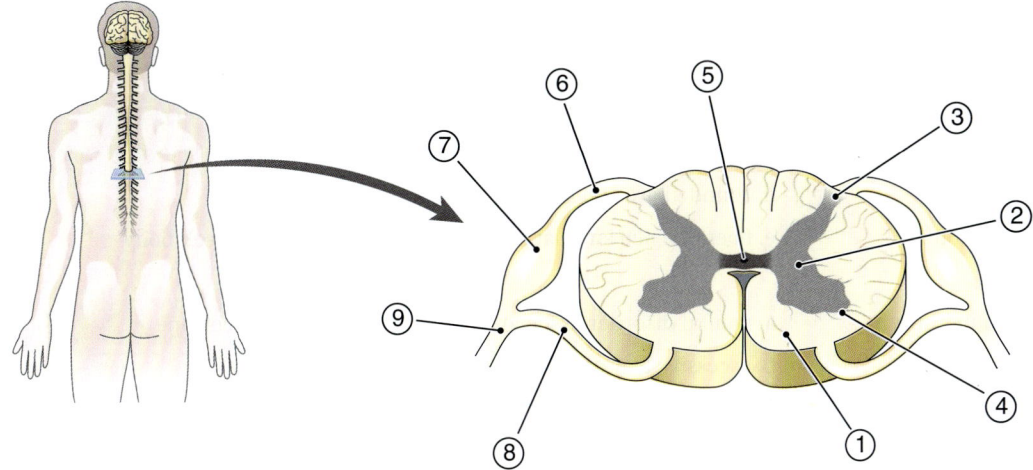

Central canal
Dorsal horn
Dorsal root ganglion
Dorsal root of spinal nerve
Gray matter

Spinal nerve
Ventral horn
Ventral root of spinal nerve
White matter

1. _____
2. _____
3. _____
4. _____
5. _____
6. _____
7. _____
8. _____
9. _____

反射通道

在对应的下划线上写出每个编号部分的名称。

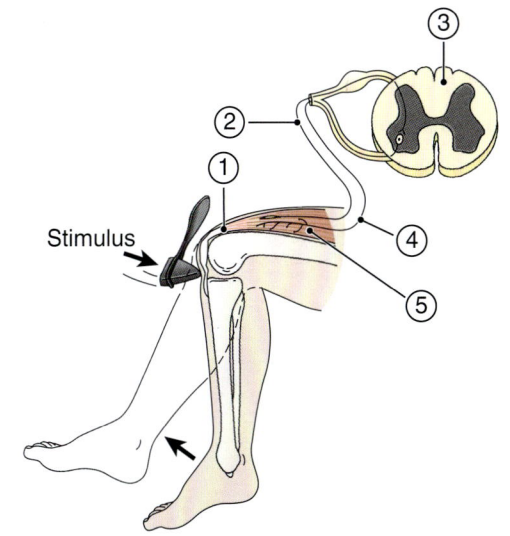

Effector
Motor neuron
Receptor

Sensory neuron
Spinal cord (CNS)

1. _____
2. _____
3. _____
4. _____
5. _____

术语

匹配

匹配下列术语，在每个题号左侧写上适当的字母。

____ 1. dendrite   a. region that connects the brain and spinal cord
____ 2. medulla oblongata   b. part of the brain that contains the thalamus and pituitary
____ 3. pons   c. whitish material that covers some axons
____ 4. myelin   d. rounded area on the ventral surface of the brainstem
____ 5. diencephalon   e. fiber of a neuron that conducts impulses toward the cell body

____ 6. contrecoup injury   a. mental disorder associated with delusions of persecution
____ 7. aphasia   b. excessive fear of pain
____ 8. hydrocephalus   c. loss of speech communication
____ 9. paranoia   d. accumulation of CSF in the brain
____ 10. odynophobia   e. damage to the brain on the side opposite the point of a blow

____ 11. cystoplegia   a. partial paralysis or weakness
____ 12. paresis   b. paralysis of the bladder
____ 13. meningomyelocele   c. series of violent, involuntary muscle contractions
____ 14. convulsion   d. localized dilation of a blood vessel
____ 15. aneurysm   e. hernia of the meninges and spinal cord

补充术语

____ 16. plexus   a. a sudden blow or attack
____ 17. ipsilateral   b. a neurotransmitter
____ 18. dermatome   c. area of skin supplied by a spinal nerve
____ 19. acetylcholine   d. on the same side; unilateral
____ 20. ictus   e. network

____ 21. amnesia   a. fear of being enclosed
____ 22. euphoria   b. state of sluggishness
____ 23. claustrophobia   c. loss of memory
____ 24. ataxia   d. lack of muscle coordination
____ 25. lethargy   e. sense of elation

____ 26. REM   a. type of psychoactive drug
____ 27. SSRI   b. eye movement during sleep
____ 28. DSM   c. mental disturbances that follow trauma
____ 29. PTSD   d. procedure to remove fluid from the spinal column
____ 30. LP   e. reference for diagnosis of mental disorders

填空

31. The largest part of the brain is the _____.

32. The fluid that circulates around the central nervous system is _____.
33. The support cells of the nervous system are the _____.
34. The junction between two nerve cells is a(n) _____.
35. The scientific name for a nerve cell is _____.
36. The membranes that cover the brain and spinal cord are the _____.
37. A simple, rapid, automatic response to a stimulus is a(n) _____.
38. The sympathetic and parasympathetic systems make up the _____.
39. A chemical that acts at a synapse is a(n) _____.
40. The posterior portion of the brain that coordinates muscle movement is the _____.
41. The strong, fibrous, outermost cover of the brain and spinal cord is the _____.

定义

定义下列单词。

42. corticothalamic [kɔːtikəθæˈlæmik] _____
43. polyneuritis [ˌpɒlinjʊˈraitis] _____
44. anencephaly [ænənˈsefəli] _____
45. hemiparesis [hemipəˈriːsis] _____
46. radicular [ræˈdikjʊlə(r)] _____
47. psychotherapy [ˌsaikəʊˈθerəpi] _____
48. panplegia [pænˈpliːdʒiə] _____
49. encephalomalacia [enˌsefələʊməˈleiʃiə] _____
50. dyssomnia [diˈsɒmniə] _____

写出下列定义的单词。

51. study of the nervous system _____
52. inflammation of the spinal cord and meninges _____
53. excision of a ganglion _____
54. any disease of the nervous system _____
55. creation of an opening into a brain ventricle _____
56. paralysis of one side of the body _____
57. within the cerebellum _____
58. difficulty in reading _____
59. fear of water _____
60. paralysis of one limb _____

拼写检查

在术语右侧的下划线上写出正确的拼写。

61. cerebim _____
62. neuroglia _____
63. ventricle _____
64. narcksis _____
65. thalmas _____

真假判断

判断下列语句。如果语句为真，在第一个空格上写上 T；如果语句为假，在第一个空格上写上 F，并通过在第二个空格上替换带下划线的单词更正语句。

	True or False	Correct Answer
66. <u>Sensory</u> fibers conduct impulses toward the CNS.	_____	_____
67. The spinal nerves are part of the <u>central</u> nervous system.	_____	_____
68. The cervical nerves are in the region of the <u>neck</u>.	_____	_____
69. Myelinated neurons make up the <u>gray</u> matter of the CNS.	_____	_____
70. CSF forms in the <u>ventricles</u> of the brain.	_____	_____
71. The fiber that carries impulses toward the neuron cell body is the <u>axon</u>.	_____	_____
72. There are <u>12</u> pairs of cranial nerves.	_____	_____
73. The innermost layer of the meninges is the <u>pia</u> mater.	_____	_____
74. Hyperlexia refers to increased skill in <u>reading</u>.	_____	_____

反义词

写出下列单词的反义词。

75. extramedullary _____
76. ipsilateral _____
77. postganglionic _____
78. tachylalia _____
79. motor _____
80. dorsal _____
81. afferent _____

形容词

写出下列单词的形容词形式。

82. ganglion _____
83. thalamus _____
84. dura _____
85. meninges _____
86. psychosis _____

复数

写出下列单词的复数形式。

87. ganglion _____
88. ventricle _____
89. meninx _____
90. embolus _____

排除

在下列每组中，为与其余不相配的单词加下划线，并说明你选择的理由。

91. CVA — lumbar puncture — embolism — thrombus — TIA

92. glioma — astrocytoma — meningioma — hematoma — neurilemmoma

93. gyri — sulci — mania — ventricles — lobes

94. MID — CNS — ADHD — OCD — GAD

单词构建

使用给出的单词组成部分写出下列定义的单词。

| -plegia | myel/o | -a- | -itis | dys- | brady- | my/o | tetra- | -paresis | -phasia | gangli/o | hemi- |

95. paralysis of the spinal cord
96. lack of speech
97. partial paralysis of one side of the body
98. muscle weakness
99. abnormal or difficult speech production
100. paralysis of a ganglion
101. paralysis of all four limbs
102. inflammation of the spinal cord
103. slowness of speech
104. paralysis of one side of the body
105. inflammation of a ganglion

单词分析

定义下列单词，并给出每个单词组成部分的含义。如果需要，可以使用词典。

106. hematomyelia ［hi:mətəʊmaiˈi:liə］
　　a. hemat/o
　　b. myel/o
　　c. -ia

107. myelodysplasia ［maiələʊdiˈspleiziə］
　　a. myel/o
　　b. dys
　　c. plas
　　d. -ia

108. polyneuroradiculitis ［pɒlinjʊərəʊræˈdikjʊlaitis］
　　a. poly
　　b. neur/o
　　c. radicul/o

d. -itis
109. dyssynergia ［di'sinɜ:dʒiə］
   a. dys
   b. syn
   c. erg
   d. -ia

Additional Case Studies
补充案例研究

Case Study 17-1: Cerebrovascular Accident (CVA)
案例研究 17-1：脑血管意外（CVA）

A. R., a 62 y/o man, was admitted to the ER with right hemiplegia and aphasia. He had a history of hypertension and recent transient ischemic attacks (TIAs), yet was in good health when he experienced a sudden onset of right-sided weakness. He arrived in the ER via ambulance within 15 minutes of onset and was received by a member of the hospital's stroke team. He had a rapid general assessment and neuro examination including a Glasgow Coma Scale (GCS) rating to determine his candidacy for fibrinolytic (clot-dissolving) therapy.

He was sent for a noncontrast CT scan to look for evidence of either hemorrhagic or ischemic stroke, postcardiac arrest ischemia, hypertensive encephalopathy, craniocerebral or cervical trauma, meningitis, encephalitis, brain abscess, tumor, and subdural or epidural hematoma. The CT scan, read by the radiologist, did not show intracerebral or subarachnoid hemorrhage. A.R. was diagnosed with probable acute ischemic stroke within one hour of the onset of symptoms and was cleared as a candidate for immediate fibrinolytic treatment.

He was admitted to the NICU for 48-hour observation to monitor his neuro status and vital signs. He was discharged after three days with a prognosis of full recovery.

A. R. 是一名 62 岁的男性，因右偏瘫和失语症被送入急诊室。他有高血压和近期短暂性脑缺血发作（TIA）的病史，在经历突然发作的右侧虚弱时，他的身体是健康的。在发病后 15 分钟内他被救护车送达急诊室，并被医院脑卒中医疗团队的一名成员接收。为他做了一个快速的总体评估和神经检查，包括格拉斯哥昏迷量表（GCS）评分，以确定他是否应当做血纤维蛋白溶解（凝块溶解）治疗。

他被送去进行无造影剂 CT 扫描，以寻找出血性或缺血性脑卒中、心肌梗死缺血、高血压性脑病、颅脑或颈部创伤、脑膜炎、脑炎、脑脓肿、肿瘤和硬膜下或硬膜外血肿的证据。放射科医生解读的 CT 扫描未显示脑内或蛛网膜下出血。A.R. 在症状发作后 1 小时内被诊断为可能的急性缺血性脑卒中，并被确认为立即溶纤治疗的候选者。

他被收入神经重症监护室观察 48 小时，以监测他的神经状态和生命体征。他 3 天后出院，预后完全康复。

Case Study 17-2: Neuroleptic Malignant Syndrome
案例研究 17-2：神经阻滞剂恶性综合征

J. N., a 21-year-old woman with chronic paranoid schizophrenia, was admitted to the hospital with a diagnosis of pneumonia. She was brought to the ER by her mother, who said J.N. had been very lethargic, had a temperature of 104°F, and had had muscular rigidity for three days. Her daily medications included Haldol (haloperidol) and Cogentin (benztropine mesylate). Her mother stated that J.N.'s psychiatrist had changed her neuroleptic medication the week before. Her secondary diagnosis was stated as neuroleptic malignant syndrome, a rare and life-threatening disorder associated with the use of antipsychotic medications. This drug-induced condition is usually characterized by alterations in mental status, temperature regulation, and autonomic and extrapyramidal functions.

J. N. was monitored for potential hypotension, tachycardia, diaphoresis, dyspnea, dysphagia, and changes in her level of consciousness (LOC). Her medications were discontinued, she was hydrated with IV fluids, and her body temperature was monitored for fluctuations. She was treated with bromocriptine, a dopamine antagonist, and dantrolene, a

J. N. 是一名 21 岁的慢性偏执型精神分裂症患者，因肺炎住进医院。J.N. 被她的母亲带到了急诊室，她说 J.N. 已经昏睡，体温为 104°F，肌肉僵硬已持续 3 天。她的日常药物包括 Haldol（氟哌啶醇）和 Cogentin（甲磺酸苯托品）。她的母亲说，J.N. 的精神科医生 1 周前改变了精神病药物。她的次要诊断为神经阻滞剂恶性综合征，是一种与使用抗精神病药物有关的罕见的危及生命的疾病。这种药物诱导的病症一般特征是精神状态、体温调节，以及自主神经和锥体外系功能的改变。

监测 J. N. 潜在的低血压、心动过速、发汗、呼吸困难、吞咽困难和意识水平（LOC）的变化。她的药物被停用，通过静脉输液补水，并且监测她的体温波动。治疗使用溴隐亭和丹曲林，溴隐亭是一种多巴胺拮抗剂，丹曲林

muscle relaxant and antispasmodic.

After five days, J. N. was transferred to a mental health facility and restarted on low-dose neuroleptics. She was monitored to prevent a recurrence of the syndrome. Both J. N. and her family were educated about neuroleptic malignant syndrome in preparation for her discharge back home in two weeks.

是一种肌肉松弛剂和解痉药。

5 天后，J. N. 被转移到精神健康病房，重新开始使用低剂量神经安定剂，并进行监测以防止该综合征的复发。J. N. 和她的家人接受了关于神经阻滞剂恶性综合征的教育，准备在 2 个星期内出院回家。

案例研究问题

多项选择。选择正确答案，在每个题号的左侧写上你选择的字母。

____ 1. Ischemic stroke is generally caused by
    a. hemorrhage
    b. hematoma
    c. thrombosis
    d. hemangioma

____ 2. Fibrinolytic therapy is directed toward
    a. stabilizing blood cells
    b. destroying RBCs
    c. triggering blood clotting
    d. dissolving a blood clot

____ 3. A general term for any disorder or alteration of brain tissue is
    a. encephalopathy
    b. neurocytoma
    c. dysencephaloma
    d. psychosomatic

____ 4. J. N. had disease manifestations related to involuntary functions and to movement controlled by motor fibers outside the pyramidal tracts. These functions are
    a. autonomic and neuroleptic
    b. autonomic and voluntary
    c. extrapyramidal and pyramidal
    d. autonomic and extrapyramidal

写出案例研究中下列含义的术语。

5. physician who treats psychiatric disorders_____

6. antipsychotic medications_____

7. pertaining to a lack of blood supply_____

8. inflammation of the meninges_____

9. collection of blood below the dura mater_____

10. pertaining to a perceived feeling of threat or harm_____

11. drug that relieves muscle spasms_____

12. inability to speak or understand speech_____

13. partial paralysis on one side_____

定义下列缩略语。

14. GCS_____

15. CT _____
16. NICU _____
17. CVA _____
18. TIA _____
19. LOC _____

CHAPTER

18 感觉系统

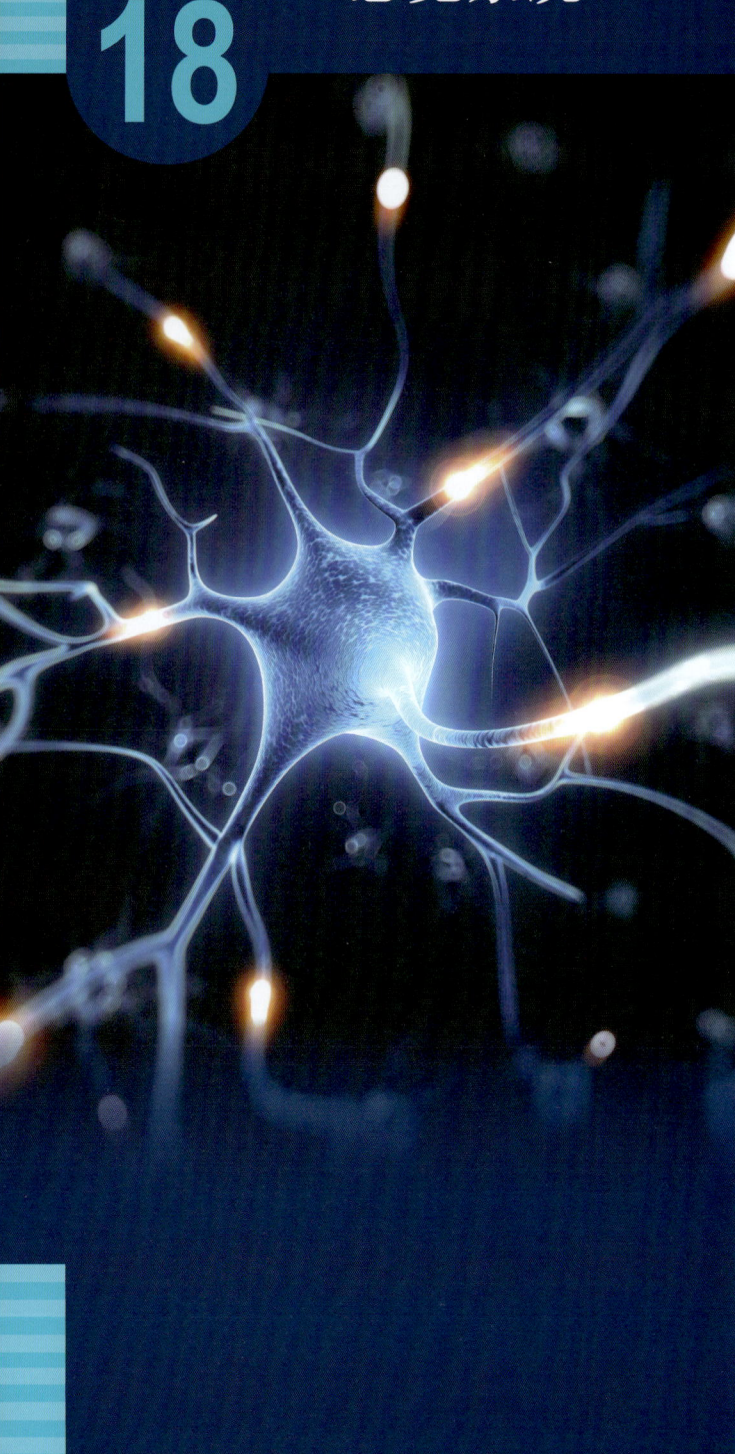

预测试

多项选择。选择正确答案，在每个题号的左侧写上你选择的字母。

____1. The scientific name for the sense of smell is
    a. osmosis
    b. olfaction
    c. gustation
    d. dialysis

____2. The term tactile refers to the sense of
    a. touch
    b. taste
    c. pain
    d. temperature

____3. The two senses located in the ear are
    a. hearing and pressure
    b. vision and hearing
    c. balance and taste
    d. hearing and equilibrium

____4. The receptor layer of the eye is the
    a. lens
    b. cornea
    c. retina
    d. pinna

____5. The scientific name for the white of the eye is
    a. pupil
    b. vitreous body
    c. sclera
    d. conjunctiva

____6. Clouding of the lens is termed
    a. vertigo
    b. cataract
    c. tinnitus
    d. glaucoma

学习目标

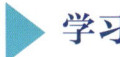

学完本章后，应该能够：

1. ▶ 说明感觉系统的作用。
2. ▶ 列出耳朵和眼睛的组成部分，并简要说明每个结构的功能。
3. ▶ 描述神经脉冲从耳朵到脑部的传输通道。
4. ▶ 描述视网膜和视神经在视觉中的作用。
5. ▶ 识别并使用与感觉相关的单词组成部分。
6. ▶ 描述与耳朵和眼睛相关的主要疾病。
7. ▶ 解释与耳朵和眼睛的研究中使用的缩略语。
8. ▶ 分析案例研究中与听觉和视觉相关的医学术语。

Case Study: K. L.'s Amblyopia
案例研究：K. L. 的弱视

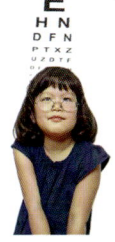

Chief Complaint

K. L., a recently adopted 7-year-old female, was seeing a pediatrician, Dr. McLaren, for the first time. Her new family was concerned that K. L. might have visual problems resulting in selfimage and schoolwork issues as one of her eyes appeared to deviate inward. Her physical examination was unremarkable except for the eye examination. Dr. McLaren explained to the parents that K.L. had a condition known as strabismic amblyopia, or a "lazy eye," and made a referral to an ophthalmologist.

Examination

Upon examining K. L., the ophthalmologist noted that the left eye deviated toward the medial canthus (angle). A complete visual examination was conducted, and the diagnosis was confirmed. K. L. did have amblyopia, in which one eye has lower visual acuity and is used less than the other eye. She also had slight hyperopia, commonly known as farsightedness. A treatment plan was devised and directed toward the development of normal visual acuity. It was discussed with the parents, who decided to move forward with the therapy.

Clinical Course

The ophthalmologist explained to K. L. that they wanted to make her weak eye stronger so she would see much better. This would be accomplished by putting a patch over the strong eye, which should correct the deviation. She would need to wear the patch for a prescribed number of hours each day, and she would also need to wear glasses. She would need to return to see the ophthalmologist so progress could be measured. While K.L. was not sure of the patch, she was excited about wearing glasses since her new mom and sister also wore glasses. She was fitted for glasses and provided with the "band aid" type of patch to apply over her right eye.

主诉

K. L. 是一名最近被收养的 7 岁女孩，第一次由儿科医生 Mdaren 博士看病。她的新家庭担心 K. L. 可能有视觉问题导致的自我认知和课外作业问题，因为她的一只眼睛似乎向内偏离。除了眼科检查外，她的体格检查无明显差异。McLaren 博士向她的父母说明 K. L. 有被称为斜视性弱视的病症，或称为"懒惰的眼睛"，并转诊给眼科医生。

检查

在检查 K.L. 时，眼科医生指出左眼偏向内角。进行了完整的视力检查，确认了诊断。K. L. 确实存在弱视，其中一只眼睛具有较低的视敏度，并且比另一只眼睛使用更少。她也有轻微的远视。医生制定了治疗计划，目标是正常视敏度的发展。与她的父母进行了讨论，他们决定向前推进治疗。

临床病程

眼科医生向 K. L. 说明他们想让她的弱视的眼睛变得更强，以便她有更好的视力。这将通过在视力较强的眼睛上戴一个眼罩，以矫正偏差。她每天需要在规定的时间内戴上眼罩，还需要戴眼镜。以后，她还要回到眼科医生那里，以便测试进展情况。虽然 K.L. 对眼罩不太确定，她很高兴戴眼镜，因为她的新妈妈和妹妹也戴眼镜。她配了眼镜，并附带"创可贴"式眼罩用于右眼。

简介

感觉系统（sensory system）是我们从内部和外部环境检测刺激的网络，它需要保持体内平衡，为我们提供压力，保护我们免受伤害。例如疼痛，是组织伤害的主要警告信号。产生于不同感觉接受器的信号必须传送到中枢神经系统进行解读。

感觉

感觉根据其是广泛分布还是局限于特定的感觉器官进行分类。一般的感觉接受器（receptor）遍布全身，许多都在皮肤上（图 18-1）。这些感觉包括：

- 疼痛，痛觉感受器在皮肤、肌肉、关节和内部器官上。
- 接触，触觉感受器在皮肤上。触觉的灵敏度取决于不同区域感受器的集中度，例如，在手指、嘴唇和舌头上高，在颈部背后和手背上低。
- 压力或深度接触，感受器在皮下和更深层的组织中。
- 温度，冷热感受器在皮肤上，在调节身体温的下丘脑中也有。
- 本体感受（proprioception）是对体位的知觉，感受器在协助判断体位和协调肌肉活动的肌肉、肌腱和关节中。

特殊感觉局限于头部复杂的感觉器官，这些感觉包括：

- 味觉（gustation）感受器位于舌头上的味蕾（taste bud）。这些感受器基本上只检测甜、酸、苦、咸和鲜味，鲜味是一种由在蛋白质和味精中含有的氨基酸触发的咸味。研究人员已经鉴定出碱和金属味道的感受器。嗅觉和味觉是化学感觉，也就是说，它们对溶液中的化学物质产生反应。

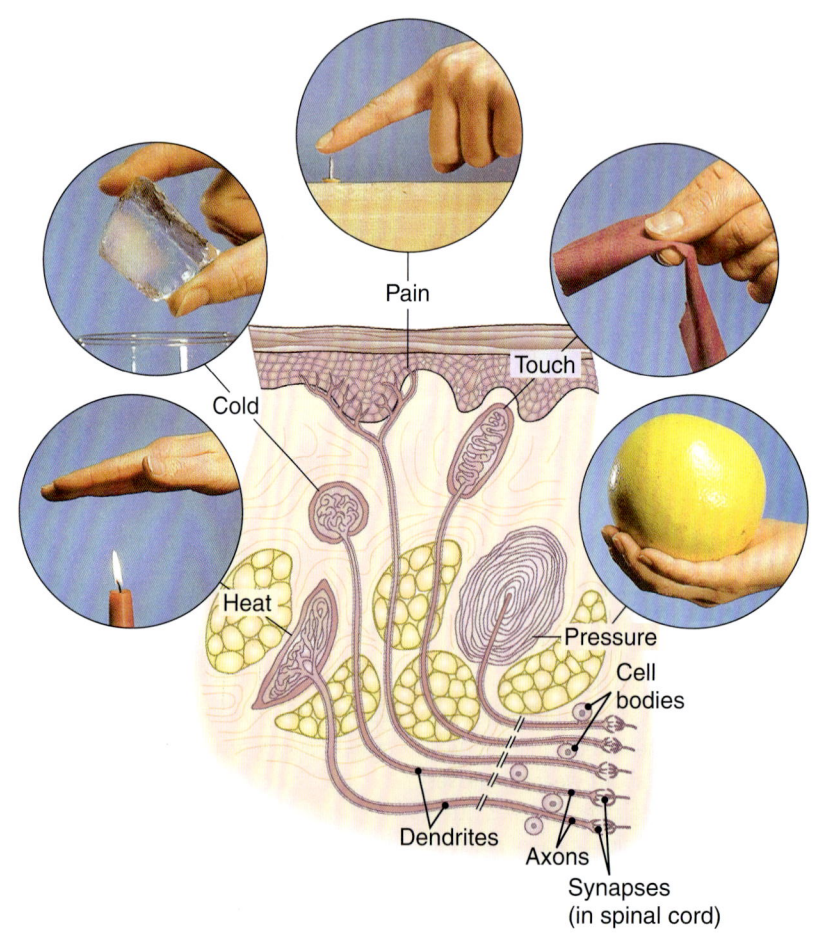

图 18-1 皮肤中一般感觉感受器。这些通路的突触在脊髓中

- 嗅觉（olfaction）感受器位于鼻中。嗅觉比味觉能够区别更多的化学物质，这两种感觉对刺激食欲和警告有害物质都很重要。
- 听觉（hearing）感受器位于耳中，这些感受器对声波在耳中传播所造成的运动产生反应。
- 平衡（equilibrium）感受器也位于耳内，这些感受器会被我们运动时耳内细胞位置的变化触发。
- 视觉（vision）感受器是光敏的，位于眼睛深部，由骨骼和其他支持结构保护。眼睛外部与内部肌肉的协调运动协助产生清晰的图像。

与感觉相关的后缀列于表 18-1 中。本章的其余部分将集中于临床最关注的听觉和视觉。

Terminology 关键术语

感觉系统

正常结构与功能

equilibrium [ˌi:kwiˈlibriəm]	平衡感，平衡的感觉
gustation [gʌsˈteiʃən]	味觉，味道的感觉；源自于拉丁语单词 geusis，意为"味道"
hearing [ˈhiəriŋ]	听觉，声音的感觉或感受
olfaction [ɒlˈfækʃn]	嗅觉，气味的感觉；词根 osm/o 意为"气味"
proprioception [ˌprəʊpriəˈsepʃən]	本体感觉，对体位、运动和平衡变化的知觉；感受器位于肌肉、肌腱和关节之中
sensory receptor	感觉感受器，感觉神经末端或与对刺激产生反应的感觉神经相关的特殊结构
tactile [ˈtæktail]	触觉的，与触觉相关的
vision [ˈviʒn]	视觉，通过物体发出的光感觉到它们的形状、大小和颜色的感觉

表 18-1　与感觉相关的后缀

后缀	含义	示例	示例定义
-esthesia	感觉	cryesthesia [kraiesθiːziə]	冷觉过敏
-algesia	疼痛	hypalgesia* [ˌhipælˈdʒiːziə]	痛觉迟钝
-osmia	嗅觉	pseudosmia [sˈjuːdəʊzmiə]	嗅幻觉
-geusia	味觉	parageusia [ˌpærəˈgjuːʒiə]	味觉异常（para-）

* 前缀 hyp/o.

练习 18-1

定义下列单词。

1. analgesia
   [ˌænəl'dʒi:ziə]

2. parosmia
   [pə'rɒsmiə]

3. ageusia
   ['idʒiəzə]

写出下列定义的单词。

4. muscular (my/o-) sensation
5. false sense of taste
6. sensitivity to temperature
7. excess sensitivity to pain
8. abnormal (dys-) sense of taste
9. lack (an-) of sensation

耳朵

耳内有听觉感受器和平衡感受器。为了研究方便，耳朵被分为三个部分：外耳、中耳和内耳（图 18-2）。

外耳由突出的耳廓（pinna，auricle）和外耳道（meatus）构成。耳道终止于鼓膜（tympanic membrane，eardrum），鼓膜将声音传送到中耳。外耳道的腺体产生蜡样的的物质耵聍（cerumen），能够保护耳道并协助预防感染。

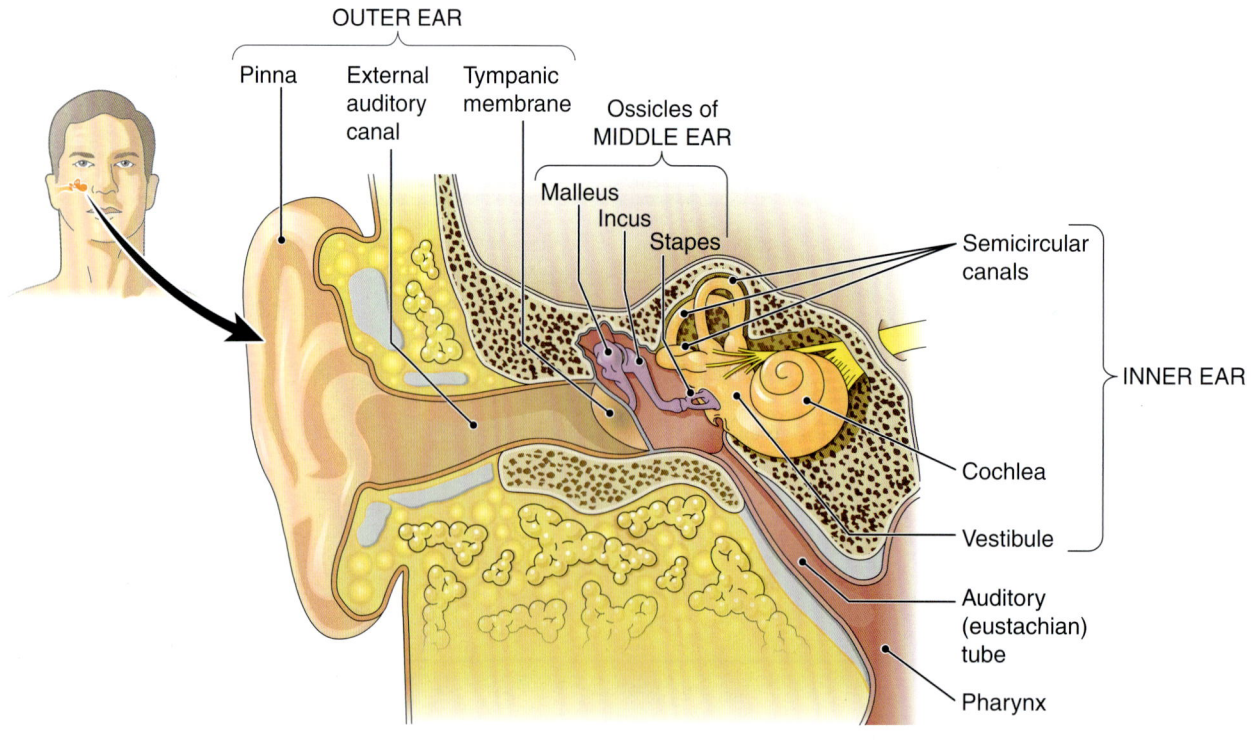

图 18-2　耳朵。图中示出了外耳、中耳和内耳

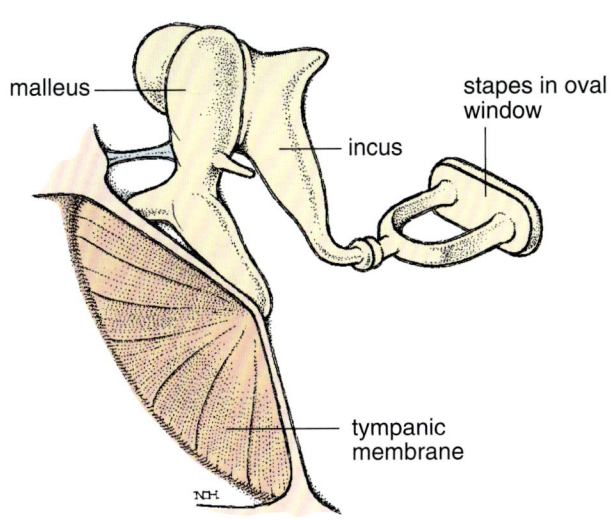

图 18-3　中耳的听小骨。锤骨与鼓膜接触。镫骨的基础与内耳的卵圆窗接触

因为内耳复杂的形状，被称为内耳迷路（labyrinth，图 18-4）。内耳由一个包含类似形状的膜通道的外骨架组成，整个迷路中充满液体。

耳蜗（cochlea）的形状像一个蜗牛壳，其中有与听觉相关的特殊的螺旋形器官（柯蒂氏器官 organ of Corti）。该感受器官中的细胞对通过耳蜗充满液体通道的声波产生反应。声波通过镫骨底部的一个开口卵圆窗（oval window）进入耳蜗，从另一个开口圆窗（round window）离开（图 18-4）。

平衡感局限于前庭器官（vestibular apparatus）。该结构包括室状前庭（chamber-like vestibule）和三个突出的半规管（semicircular canal）。前庭器官中的特殊细胞对运动产生反应（视觉和本体感觉对保持平衡也很重要。）。

神经脉冲通过前庭蜗神经（vestibulocochlear nerve）从耳朵传入脑部，前庭蜗神经是第八颅神经，也被称为听觉神经（acoustic nerve 或 auditory nerve）。该神经的耳蜗分支传送来自于前庭器官的与平衡相关的脉冲（图 18-4）。与耳朵和听觉相关的词根在表 18-2 中。

跨越中耳腔有三块小骨（ossicle），每块小骨根据其形状命名，分别是锤骨（malleus）、砧骨（incus）和镫骨（stapes）（图 18-3）。声波穿过三块小骨从镫骨的底部传入内耳。耳咽管（auditory tube）连接中耳与鼻咽，在外耳与中耳之间起压力平衡作用。

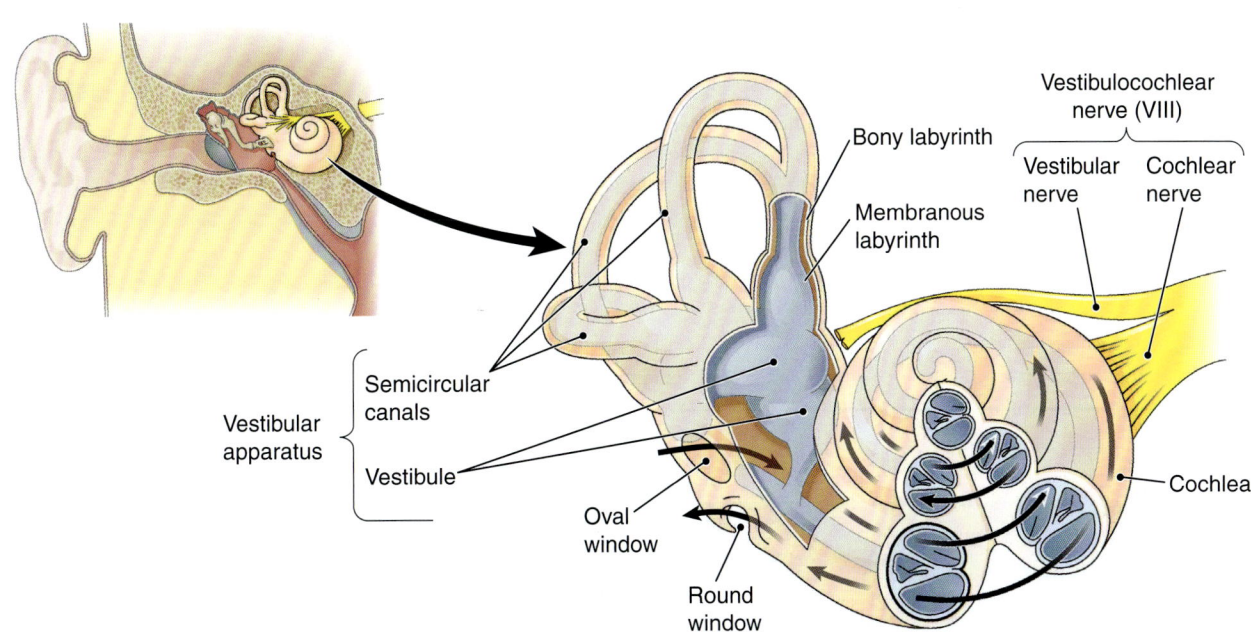

图 18-4　内耳。外骨迷路包含膜迷路。平衡感受器在前庭和半规管，听觉感受器——螺旋器在耳蜗。声波通过卵圆窗进入耳蜗，穿过耳蜗，然后通过圆窗出口。内耳中的前庭蜗神经（第八颅神经）将脉冲传入脑部

| Terminology | 关键术语 |

耳朵

正常结构与功能

auditory tube [ˈɔːditəri]	耳咽管，连接中耳与鼻咽的管道，在外耳与中耳之间起平衡压力的作用（词根：salping/o）；也被称为咽鼓管（pharyngotympanic tube），最初被称为欧氏管（eustachian tube）
cerumen [siˈruːmən]	耵聍，在外耳道中形成的褐色蜡样分泌物，能够保护耳道并预防感染；形容词形式为 ceruminous
cochlea [ˈkɒkliə]	耳蜗，内耳的螺旋部分，包含听觉感受器（词根：cochle/o）
external auditory canal	外耳道，从耳廓延伸至鼓膜的管道，也被称为 external auditory meatus
incus [ˈiŋkəs]	砧骨，耳内中间的小骨
labyrinth [ˈlæbərinθ]	内耳迷路，内耳，因其迷宫样复杂的结构而得名
malleus [ˈmæliəs]	锤骨，中耳内与鼓膜和砧骨接触的小骨
ossicle [ˈɒsikl]	小骨，中耳中的小骨，锤骨、砧骨和镫骨
pinna [ˈpinə]	耳廓，外耳的突出部分，也拼写为 auricle [ˈɔːrikl]
semicircular canal [ˌsemiˈsɜːkjələ(r)]	半规管，内耳中支撑平衡感受器的三根弯曲的管道
spiral organ	螺旋器，听觉感受器，位于内耳的耳蜗；又被称为柯蒂氏器官（organ of Corti）
stapes [ˈsteipiːz]	镫骨，与内耳相连的小骨（词根：staped/o, stapedi/o）
tympanic membrane [timˈpænik]	鼓膜，外耳道与中耳（鼓室）之间的膜，负责将声波传送到中耳的小骨（词根：myring/o, tympan/o）
vestibular apparatus [veˈstibjulə ˌæpəˈreitəs]	前庭器官，内耳中与平衡感受器连接的部分。由室状前庭和三个突出的半规管构成（词根：vestibule/o）
vestibule [ˈvestibjuːl]	前庭，内耳中支撑一些平衡感受器的室
vestibulocochlear nerve [ˈvestibjʊləʊkəʊkliəər]	前庭蜗神经，将听觉和平衡脉冲从耳朵传送到脑部的神经；是第八颅神经，也被称为听觉神经（auditory nerve 或 acoustic nerve）

表 18-1　与耳朵和听觉相关的词根

词根	含义	示例	示例定义
audi/o	听觉	audiology [ˌɔːdiˈɒlədʒi]	听力学
acous, acus, cus	声音，听觉	acoustic [əˈkuːstik]	声学的、听觉的

续表 18-1　与耳朵和听觉相关的词根

词根	含义	示例	示例定义
ot/o	耳朵	ototoxic [əʊtə'tɒksik]	耳毒性
myring/o	鼓膜	myringotome [miriŋ'gəʊtəʊm]	鼓膜刀
tympan/o	鼓室，鼓膜	tympanometry [timpə'nəʊmitri]	鼓室测压法
salping/o	咽鼓管	salpingoscopy ['sælpingəʊskəpi]	咽鼓管检查镜
staped/o, stapedi/o	镫骨	stapedioplasty [steipi:daiɒp'læsti]	镫骨成形术
labyrinth/o	内耳迷路	labyrinthitis [ˌlæbərin'θaitis]	迷路炎
vestibul/o	前庭，前庭器官	vestibulotomy [vestibjʊ'ləʊtəʊmi]	前庭切开术
cochle/o	耳蜗	retrocochlear ['retrəkəʊkliəər]	蜗后的

练习 18-2

填空。

1. Audition [ɔː'dɪʃ(ə)n] is the act of_____.
2. Hyperacusis [haipərə'kjuːsis] is abnormally high sensitivity to_____.
3. Otopathy [əʊtə'pæθi] means any disease of the_____.

定义以下形容词。

4. stapedial [stə'piːdiəl] _____
5. cochlear ['kɒkliə] _____
6. vestibular [ves'tibjʊlə] _____
7. auditory ['ɔːdətri] _____
8. labyrinthine [ˌlæbə'rinθain] _____
9. otic ['əʊtik] _____

写出下列定义的单词。

10. pain in the ear _____
11. incision of the labyrinth _____
12. endoscope for examining the auditory tube _____
13. instrument used to examine the ear _____
14. within the cochlea _____
15. pertaining to the vestibular apparatus and cochlea _____

练习 18-2

16. measurement of hearing (audi/o-) _____
17. plastic repair of the middle ear _____
18. excision of the stapes _____

定义下列单词。

19. tympanitis
    [ˌtɪmpəˈnaɪtɪs] _____

20. audiometer
    [ˌɔːdiˈɒmɪtə] _____

21. vestibulopathy
    [ˈvestɪbjʊləʊpəθi] _____

22. salpingopharyngeal
    [sælpɪŋəfæˈrɪndʒiːəl] _____

23. myringostapediopexy
    [mɪrɪŋəsteɪpiːdaɪɒˈpeksi] _____

听觉的临床表现

听力损失

听觉受损（hearing impairment）可能是疾病、受伤或影响耳朵自身或任何与听觉相关的神经通道的发育问题所致。

感音神经性（sensorineural）听力损失是内耳、第八颅神经或中枢听觉通道伤害所致。遗传、毒素、暴露于巨大的噪声和衰老都可能引起这种听力损失，损失的范围可以从听不到特定频率的声音到听力完全丧失（耳聋 deafness）。源于内耳的严重听力损失的人可以通过耳蜗移植（cochlear implant）获益。这种假体直接刺激耳蜗神经，绕过内耳的感受器细胞，使接受者能够听到中度到响亮的声音。

传导性（conductive）听力损失是内耳声波传输阻塞所致，起因包括堵塞、严重感染或中耳小骨固定。通常，医生能够成功治疗这些引起传导性听力损失的病症。

框 18-1 有关于听力学和听力障碍的研究和治疗职业的信息。

耳炎

耳炎（otitis）是耳朵的任何炎症。中耳炎（otitis

框 18-1

健康职业
听力专家

听力学家（audiologists）专门预防、诊断和治疗可能由损伤、感染、出生缺陷、噪音或衰老引起的听力障碍。他们记录完整的病史来诊断听力障碍，并使用专门的设备来测量听力敏锐度。听力学家设计和实施个性化治疗计划，其中可能包括为患者配备辅助听力装置，如助听器，或教授替代性沟通技巧，如唇读。听力学家还测量工作场所和社区的噪声水平，并教会公众如何预防听力损失。在过去，听力学家必须有硕士学位；现在，博士学位越来越成为在美国许可证颁发所需的学位。所有 50 个州都要求执业听力学家通过国家许可考试，并获得注册或许可。在一些州，分发助听器的听力学家必须具有助听器分配器许可证，该许可证与他们执业听力学的许可证是分离的。

听力学家在各种场合工作，例如医院、护理机构、学校、诊所和工业企业。因为听力学家的专业技能的需求将随着人口的增长而增加，因而工作前景是好的。美国听力科学院（American Academy of Audiology）在 www.audiology.org 有更多关于这个职业生涯的信息。

media）是指导致中耳腔积液的感染，起因之一是咽鼓管功能异常或阻塞，可能是过敏、腺样体肥大、受伤或先天畸形所致。另一个起因是扩散到中耳的感染，最常见是来自于上呼吸道。连续的感染可能导致脓液的积累和耳鼓穿孔。中耳炎通常会影响 5 岁以下的儿童，并可能导致听力损失。如果不用抗生素治疗，感染可能扩散到耳朵的其他区域和头部。鼓膜切开术（myringotomy）和在鼓膜放置一个管道能够帮助通气和排干中耳腔的积液。

外耳炎（otitis externa）是重复的真菌或细菌感染引起的外耳道炎症。外耳炎最常见于生活在热带气候的人群和游泳者，因而产生了一个替代性名称"游泳耳"。

耳硬化

在耳硬化（otosclerosis）中，内耳的骨结构恶化，然后重新形成可能最终硬化的海绵状骨组织。最常见的是镫骨固定在内耳之上不能震动，导致传导性听力损失。耳硬化症的起因不明，但一些病例是遗传所致。

一般可以通过手术切除受损的骨结构。在镫骨切除术（stapedectomy）中，镫骨被切除，人工骨被插入。

梅尼埃病

梅尼埃病（Ménière disease）是一种影响内耳的疾病，似乎涉及充满内耳的液体的产生与循环，但起因不明。症状包括眩晕（vertigo）、听力损失、耳鸣（tinnitus）和感觉耳中有压力。疾病的进程不均衡，症状可能随时间而减轻。梅尼埃病需要控制恶心和眩晕的药物进行治疗，例如用于治疗运动病的药物。如果病情严重，可以手术破坏内耳或部分第八颅神经。

听神经瘤

听神经瘤（acoustic neuroma）是发生于第八颅神经鞘的肿瘤。随着肿瘤的扩大，会挤压周围的神经，并干扰血液供应。这会导致耳鸣、头晕（dizziness）和进行性听力损失。随着肿瘤挤压脑干和其他颅神经，还会产生其他症状。通常，听神经瘤必须手术切除。

Terminology 关键术语	
耳朵	
疾病	
acoustic neuroma [əˈkuːstik njuˈrəumə]	听神经瘤，第八颅神经鞘的肿瘤，可能挤压周围的组织并产生症状
conductive hearing loss	传导性听力损失，因内耳声音传导阻塞所致的听力受损
Ménière disease	梅尼埃病，与内耳液体压力升高相关的疾病，特征是听力损失、眩晕和耳鸣
otitis externa [əʊˈtaitis]	外耳炎，外耳道的炎症，也被称为游泳耳（swimmer's ear）
otitis media	中耳炎，有浆液或黏液积累的中耳炎症
otosclerosis [ˌəʊtəskliˈrəʊsis]	耳硬化，耳中形成异常的，有时是硬化的骨组织。通常发生在卵圆窗周围或镫骨的底部，引起镫骨固定和进行性听力损失
sensorineural hearing loss [ˌsensəriˈnjʊərəl]	感音神经性听力损失，内耳、第八颅神经或内部听觉通道伤害所致的听力受损
tinnitus [ˈtinitəs]	耳鸣，一种耳中铃声或叮当声的感受
vertigo [ˈvɜːtigəʊ]	眩晕，因为身体在空间中运动或环境在身体周围移动而产生的一种运动幻觉，通常是前庭器官失调引起的。广泛地用于表示头晕目眩

Terminology 关键术语（续表）

耳朵

治疗

myringotomy [miriŋˈgɒtəmi]	鼓膜切开术，手术切开鼓膜，用于排干中耳腔的积液或将排液管插入鼓膜
stapedectomy [ˌseipiˈdektəmi]	镫骨切除术，手术切除镫骨，可能同时插入人工骨以矫正耳硬化症

Terminology 补充术语

正常结构与功能

aural [ˈɔːrəl]	耳的，听觉的，与耳相关或被耳感知的
decibel (dB) [ˈdesibel]	分贝，测量声音相对强度的单位
hertz (Hz) [hɜːts]	赫兹，测量声音频率的单位
mastoid process [ˈmæstɔid]	乳突，外耳道后面颞骨的小突起，由松散排列的骨质和小的充气腔构成
stapedius [steiˈpiːdjəs]	镫骨肌，附着在镫骨上的小肌肉。出现响亮的声音出现时，镫骨肌会收缩，产生听觉反射

症状与病症

cholesteatoma [kɒlistiːəˈtəʊmə]	胆脂瘤，包含胆固醇的囊样组织，常见于中耳和乳突区域；可能是慢性中耳感染的并发症
labyrinthitis [ˌlæbərinˈθaitis]	迷路炎，内耳迷路的炎症，也被称为 otitis interna
mastoiditis [ˌmæstɔiˈdaitis]	乳突炎，乳突气室的炎症
presbycusis [ˌprezbiˈkjuːsis]	老年性耳聋，因衰老引起的听力损失，也拼写为 presbyacusis

诊断与治疗

audiometry [ˌɔːdiˈɒmətri]	听力测定，测量听力
electronystagmography (ENG) [iˈlektrəʊnistægˈmɒgrəfi]	眼震电流描记法，一种通过电反应记录眼睛运动的方法；这种运动可能反应出前庭功能障碍
otorhinolaryngology (ORL) [ˌəʊtəʊrainəʊlæriŋˈgɒlədʒi]	耳鼻喉科学，研究耳、鼻、喉疾病的医学分支，也被称为 otolaryngology（OL）
otoscope [ˈəʊtəskəʊp]	耳镜，检查耳朵的设备（图 7-6）
Rinne test	林纳试验，通过比较骨传导和空气传导测量听力（图 18-5），骨传导通过耳后的乳突进行测试
spondee [ˈspɒndiː]	扬扬格，两个音节的单词，每个音节重音相同；用于听力测试，例如 toothbrush, baseball, cowboy, pancake
Weber test	韦伯试验，使用放置在头部中心的振动音叉来测试听力损失（图 18-6）

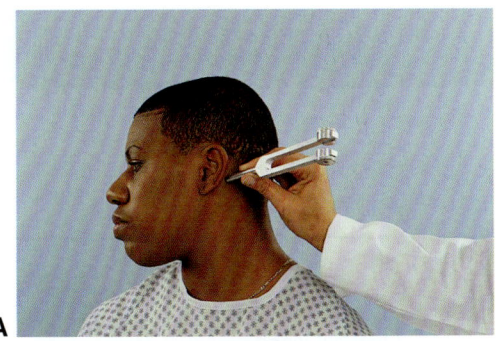
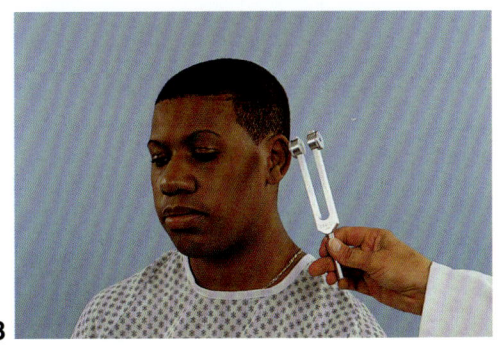

图 18-5 林纳试验。该测试评估声音在骨骼和空气中的传导。
A. 通过耳后乳突的骨传导测试；B. 空气传导试验

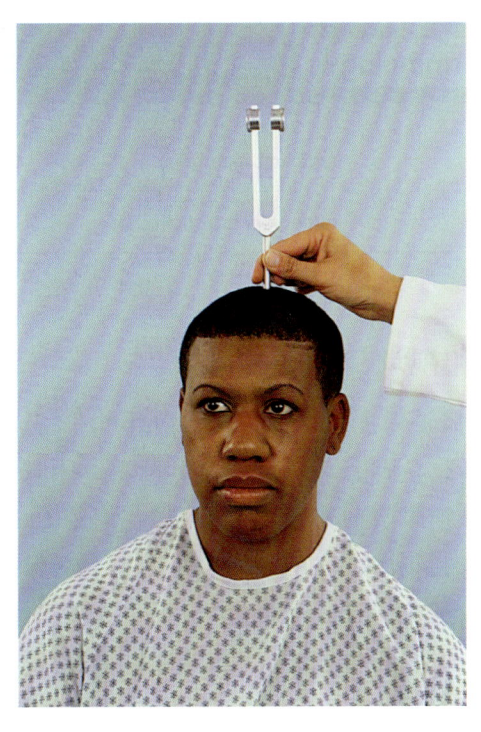

图 18-6 韦伯试验。该测试评估声音的骨传导

Terminology 缩略语

耳朵

ABR	Auditory brainstem response	听脑干反应
AC	Air conduction	空气传导
BAEP	Brainstem auditory evoked potentials	脑干听觉诱发电位
BC	Bone conduction	骨传导
dB	Decibel	分贝
ENG	Electronystagmography	眼震电流描记法
ENT	Ear(s), nose, and throat	耳鼻喉
HL	Hearing level	听力水平
Hz	Hertz	赫兹
OL	Otolaryngology	耳鼻喉科学
OM	Otitis media	中耳炎
ORL	Otorhinolaryngology	耳鼻喉科学
ST	Speech threshold	言语听阈

Terminology	缩略语（续表）	
TM	Tympanic membrane	鼓膜
TTS	Temporary threshold shift	暂时性阈移

眼睛和视觉

眼睛被保护在骨质的眼眶（orbit）之中，眼睑（eyelid）、眉毛（eyebrow）和睫毛（eyelash）也都有保护眼睛的作用（图18-7）。泪腺（lacrimal gland）用于润滑液持续冲刷和清洗眼睛。保护性的结膜（conjunctiva）是眼睑内壁的一层薄膜，能够覆盖眼睛的前部。结膜折起后在眼球和眼睑之间形成一个狭窄的空间，眼药水和眼药膏可以渗入这个结膜囊。眼睛分为三层（图18-8），从最外层到最内层分别命名为：

1. 巩膜（sclera），通常被称为白眼球，是韧性的表面保护层。巩膜延伸至眼睛的前部，成为透明的角膜（cornea）。

2. 色素层（uvea）是中间层，由三部分构成：

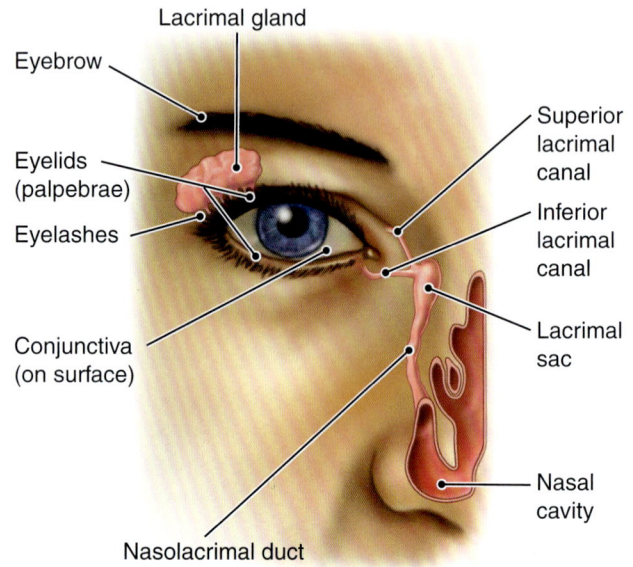

图18-7 眼睛的保护结构。泪腺产生流经眼睛并流入泪道的泪液

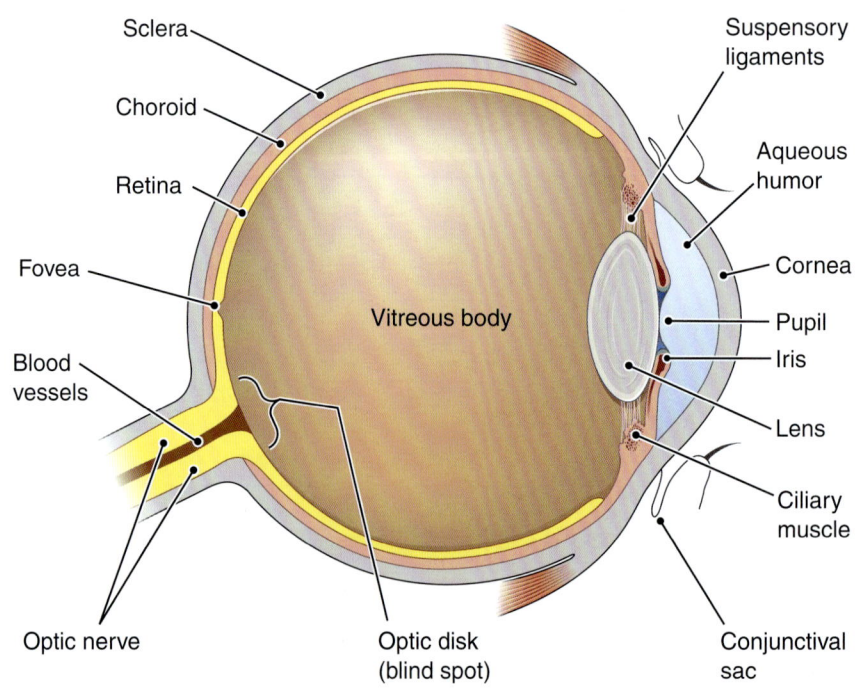

图18-8 眼睛。图中示出了眼球的三个层和视觉中涉及的其他结构

- 脉络膜（choroid），位于眼球前部的血管和色素层。脉络膜为视网膜（retina）提供营养。
- 睫状体（ciliary body），包含控制晶状体（lens）形状的肌肉。通过控制晶状体的形状，眼睛能够获得近处和远处的视觉，这一过程被称为视觉调节（accommodation）（图18-9）。为了观察近物，晶状体必须变得更圆。
- 虹膜（iris），控制瞳孔（pupil）大小的肌肉环，能够控制进入眼睛的光线（图18-10）。由基因控制的虹膜色素决定眼睛的颜色。

3. 视网膜是最内层，是实际的视觉感受器。视网膜由两种对光线产生反应的特殊细胞构成：
- 视杆细胞（rods）在微弱的光线下工作，提供较低的视敏度，对颜色没有反应。
- 视锥细胞（cones）在明亮的光线下工作，有较高的视敏度，对颜色有反应。

适当的视觉需要光线在穿过眼睛时产生折射（refraction），以聚焦在视网膜特定的位置。视杆细胞和视锥细胞产生的脉冲通过视神经（第二颅神经）传送到脑部。在视神经与视网膜的连接点上没有视杆细胞和视锥细胞，这一点没有视觉感受，被称为视盘（optic disk）或盲点（blind spot，图18-8）。中央凹（fovea）是视网膜靠近视神经处的一个小凹陷，集中了大量的视锥细胞，是最大时间敏锐度的一点。中央凹周围的黄色斑点被称为黄斑（macula）（图18-11）。

眼球（eyeball）是一个充满胶状物质的玻璃体（图18-9），能够协助维持眼睛的形状，并折射光线。眼

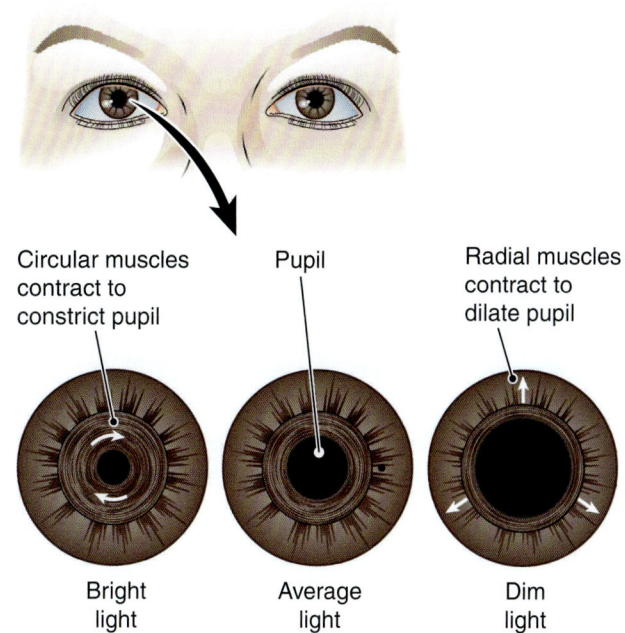

图18-10 虹膜的功能。在明亮的光线下，虹膜中的肌肉收缩瞳孔，限制进入眼睛的光。在昏暗的光线中，虹膜扩张瞳孔以允许更多的光进入眼睛

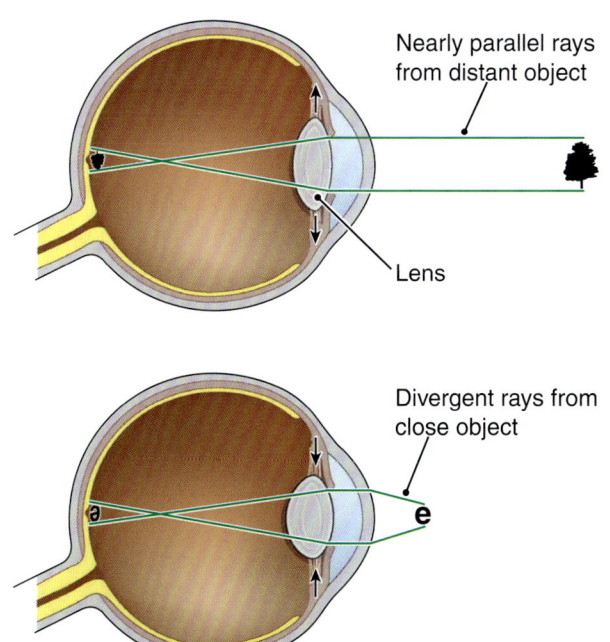

图18-9 近视的视力调节。观察近物体时，透镜必须变得更圆，以将光线聚焦在视网膜上

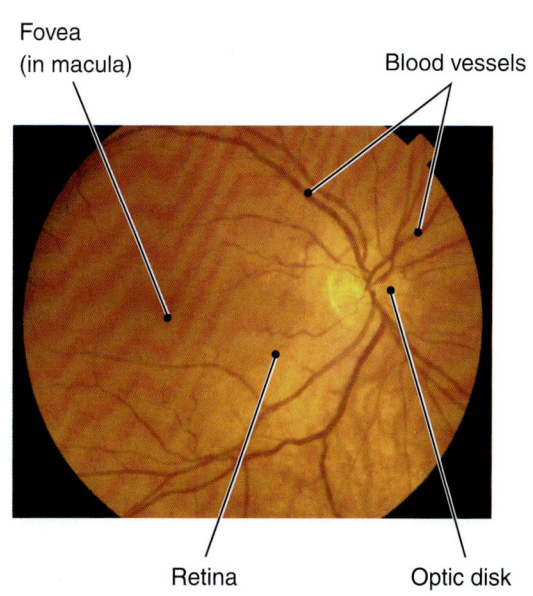

图18-11 通过检眼镜看到的眼底。图中示出视网膜中的视盘（盲点）和中央凹——视力最敏锐的点

框 18-2

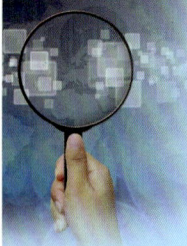

聚焦单词
希腊语的影响力

一些最美丽（最难拼写和最难发音）的单词源自于希腊语。esthesi/o 意为"感觉"，出现在单词 anesthesia（麻醉）之中，麻醉是缺乏感觉的状态，特别是疼痛感。它还出现在单词 esthetics（美学）之中（也拼写为 aesthetics），是关于美丽、艺术和外观的。在单词 presbycusis（老年性耳聋）和 presbyopia（老花眼）中，前缀 presby- 意为"老的"，这些病症都出现在老年人身上。词根 cycl/o 是与眼睛环状的睫状体有关的，源自于希腊语意为"圆环或车轮"的单词，这一词根也出现在单词 bicycle（自行车）和 tricycle（三轮车）之中。另一个与眼睛相关的术语 iris（虹膜）在希腊语中意为"彩虹"，虹膜是眼睛中有颜色的部分。

词根 sthen/o 意为"力量"，出现在单词 asthenia 中，意为缺乏力量或虚弱。Neurasthenia 是一个表示"神经衰弱"的旧术语，现在被用于指涉及一般性乏力、焦虑和疼痛的病症。该词根还与意为"美丽"的词根 cali 一起出现在单词 calisthenics（健美操）中，所以，在健美操中所做的节奏加强和调节锻炼通过力量显示出了美丽。

希腊语词根 steth/o 意为"胸"，但 stethoscope（听诊器）不仅用于听胸部的声音，也用于听身体其他部位的声音。

Asphyxia（窒息）源自于希腊语意为"脉搏"的词根 sphygm/o，其字母的意思是"脉搏停止"，这在一个人窒息时发生。该词根还出现在 sphygmomanometer（血压计）中，是测量血压的装置。看着这个单词并试图将其念出来的人马上就明白了为什么大多数人都把该装置称为 blood pressure cuff（血压袖带）！

房水（aqueous humor）充满眼前部至晶状体的液体，能够维持角膜的形状并折射光线。这种液体会持续产生，并从眼中排出。

每只眼睛外部附着六块肌肉，协调眼睛的运动以实现集合（convergence），即协调眼睛的运动，使两只眼睛凝视同一个点。

框 18-2 介绍了一些医学单词的希腊语起源，包括一些与眼睛相关的单词

Terminology 关键术语

眼睛

正常结构与功能

术语	释义
accommodation [əˌkɒməˈdeɪʃn]	视觉调节，调整晶状体的曲率以便获得不同距离的视觉
aqueous humor [ˈeɪkwiəs ˈhjuːmə]	眼房水，充满眼前部至晶状体的液体
choroid [ˈkɔːrɔɪd]	脉络膜，眼睛的深色血管形成的中层（词根：chori/o, choroid/o），是色素层的一部分
ciliary body [ˈsɪliəri ˈbɒdi]	睫状体，色素层围绕晶状体的肌肉部分，负责调节晶状体的形状以获得远和近的视觉（词根：cycl/o）
cone [kəʊn]	视锥细胞，视网膜中对光产生反应的特殊细胞；视锥细胞具有高视敏度，在强光下工作，对颜色有反应
conjunctiva [ˌkɒndʒʌŋkˈtaɪvə]	结膜，眼睑内壁的黏膜，覆盖眼球的前表面
convergence [kənˈvɜːdʒəns]	汇聚，协调眼睛的运动，凝视同一个点
cornea [ˈkɔːniə]	角膜，巩膜前面透明的部分（词根：corne/o, kerat/o）
fovea [ˈfəʊviːə]	中央凹，视网膜的微小凹陷，是视觉最锐利的点；也被称为 fovea centralis, central fovea

Terminology	关键术语
iris ['airis]	虹膜，晶状体与角膜之间有颜色的肌肉环；通过改变在其中心的瞳孔的大小调节进入眼睛的光线（词根：ir, irid/o, irit/o）；复数形式为 irides ['iəri‚di:z]
lacrimal gland ['lækriml]	泪腺，分泌泪水的腺体（词根：lacrim/o, dacry/o）
lens [lenz]	晶状体，眼睛前部透明的双凸结构，能够折射光线并进行视觉调节（词根：lent/i, phak/o）
macula ['mækjʊlə]	黄斑，视网膜上包含中央凹的黄色斑点
optic disk	视盘，视神经与视网膜的结合点，在该点没有视杆细胞和视锥细胞；也被称为盲点（blind spot）或视乳头（optic papilla）
orbit ['ɔ:bit]	眼眶，包含眼球的骨腔
palpebra ['pælpəbrə]	眼睑，闭合在眼睛前表面上的保护性折皱（上部或下部）（词根：palpebr/o, blephar/o）；形容词形式为 palpebral，复数形式为 palpebrae；也常用 eyelid
pupil ['pju:pl]	瞳孔，虹膜中心的开口（词根：pupil/o）
refraction [ri'frækʃn]	折射，光线通过眼睛时弯曲聚焦于视网膜上特定的点；也指眼屈光不正的诊断和矫正
retina ['retinə]	视网膜，眼睛最内部的感光层，包含特殊的视觉感受器视杆细胞和视锥细胞（词根：retin/o）
rod [rɒd]	视杆细胞，视网膜上对光产生反应的特殊细胞；视杆细胞的视敏度较低，在微光下工作，对颜色没有反应
sclera ['skliərə]	巩膜，眼睛的白色韧性的纤维最外层；也被称为白眼球（词根：scler/o）
uvea ['ju:viə]	色素层，眼睛的中间血管层（词根：uve/o），由脉络膜、睫状体和虹膜构成
visual acuity ['viʒuəl ə'kjuiti]	视敏度，视觉的敏锐度
vitreous body ['vitri:əs 'bɒdi]	玻璃体，充满眼球主腔体的透明胶状物质，也被称为 vitreous humor

与眼睛和视觉相关的单词组成部分

参见表 18-3 至表 18-5

表 18-3　眼睛外部结构的词根

词根	含义	示例	示例定义
blephar/o	眼睑	symblepharon [sim'blefərɒn]	眼睑粘连
palpebr/o	眼睑	palpebral ['pælpibrəl]	眼睑的
dacry/o	泪液、泪器	dacryorrhea [deikri:ə'riə]	流泪

续表 18-3　眼睛外部结构的词根

词根	含义	示例	示例定义
dacryocyst/o	泪囊	dacryocystocele ［deikri:ə'sistəʊseli:］	泪囊突出
lacrim/o	泪液、泪器	lacrimation ［ˌlækrə'meiʃən］	泪液分泌

练习 18-3

定义下列单词。

1. nasolacrimal ［nə'sɒleikriml］
2. interpalpebral ［intɜ:'pælpibrəl］
3. blepharoplasty ［b'lefærəʊplæsti］
4. dacryocystectomy ［deikri:əsis'tektəmi］

使用给出的词根写出下列含义的单词。

5. paralysis of the eyelid (blephar/o)
6. stone in the lacrimal apparatus (dacry/o)
7. inflammation of a lacrimal sac

表 18-4　眼睛和视觉的词根

词根	含义	示例	示例定义
opt/o	眼睛、视觉	optometer ［ɒp'tɒmitə］	视力计
ocul/o	眼睛	sinistrocular ［sinis'trɒkjʊlə］	左眼的
ophthalm/o	眼睛	exophthalmos ［ˌeksɒf'θælməs］	眼球突出
scler/o	巩膜	episcleritis ［episkliə'raitis］	巩膜外层炎
corne/o	角膜	circumcorneal ［sɜ:kəm'kɔ:niəl］	角膜周的
kerat/o	角膜	keratoplasty ［'kerətəʊˌplæsti］	角膜移植术、角膜成形术
lent/i	晶状体	lentiform ［'lentifɔ:m］	晶状体形状的
phak/o, phac/o	晶状体	aphakia ［æ'feikjə］	无晶状体
uve/o	色素层	uveal ［'ju:viəl］	色素层的
chori/o, choroid/o	脉络膜	subchoroidal ［sʌbkɒ'rɔidl］	脉络膜下的

续表 18-4　眼睛和视觉的词根

词根	含义	示例	示例定义
cycl/o	睫状体	cycloplegic ［saiklə'pli:dʒik］	睫状肌麻痹剂
ir, irit/o, irid/o	虹膜	iridoschisis ［iri'dɒskaisis］	虹膜劈裂症
pupill/o	瞳孔	iridopupillary ［iridəʊp'ju:piləri］	虹膜瞳孔的
retin/o	视网膜	retinoscopy ［reti'nɒskəpi］	视网膜检影法

练习 18-4

填空。

1. In the opening case study, the medical specialist K.L. saw for her vision problems was a(n)_____.
2. Lenticonus is conical protrusion of the_____.
3. The oculomotor ［ˌɑkjʊlə'motɚ］ nerve controls movements of the_____.
4. The science of orthoptics ［ɔː'θɒptiks］ deals with correcting defects in_____.
5. The term phacolysis ［fə'kɔlisis］ means destruction of the_____.
6. A keratometer ［ˌkɛrə'tɒmitə(r)］ is an instrument for measuring the curves of the_____.

识别并定义下列单词与眼睛相关的词根。

	Root	Meaning of Root
7. optometrist ［ɒp'tɒmətrist］	_____	_____
8. microphthalmos ［maikrəf'θælməʊz］	_____	_____
9. interpupillary ［intə'pju:piləri］	_____	_____
10. retrolental ［ˌretrəʊ'lentəl］	_____	_____
11. iridodilator ［'iəridədaileitər］	_____	_____
12. uveitis ［ˌjuːviˈaitis］	_____	_____
13. phacotoxic ［fəkə'tɒksik］	_____	_____

写出下列定义的单词。

14. inflammation of the uvea and sclera _____
15. hardening of the lens (use phac/o) _____
16. pertaining to the cornea _____
17. surgical fixation of the retina _____
18. inflammation of the ciliary body _____

练习 18-4

使用词根 ophthalm/o 写出下列定义的单词。

19. an instrument used to examine the eye
20. the medical specialty that deals with the eye and diseases of the eye

使用词根 orid/o 写出下列定义的单词。

21. surgical removal of (part of) the iris
22. paralysis of the iris

定义下列单词。

23. dextrocular
   [ˈdekstrəkjʊlə]
24. lenticular
   [lenˈtikjʊlə]
25. iridocyclitis
   [iridəʊsiˈklaitis]
26. chorioretinal
   [ˈkɔːriəritinəl]
27. keratitis
   [ˌkerəˈtaitis]
28. cyclotomy
   [saiˈklɒtəmi]
29. optical
   [ˈɒptikl]
30. sclerotome
   [ˈskliərətəʊm]
31. retinoschisis
   [retiˈnɒskisis]

表 18-5　眼睛和视觉*的后缀

后缀	含义	示例	示例定义
-opsia	视觉	heteropsia [hetəˈrɒpsiə]	双眼不等视
-opia	眼睛、视觉	hemianopia [ˌhemiənˈəʊpiə]	偏盲

* 组合后缀 -ops（眼睛）+ -ia.

练习 18-5

使用后缀 –opsia 写出下列定义的单词。

1. a visual defect in which objects seem larger (macr/o) than they are_____
2. lack of (a-) color (chromat/o) vision (complete color blindness)_____

使用后缀 –opia 写出下列定义的单词。

3. double vision_____
4. changes in vision due to old age (use the prefix presby- meaning "old")_____
5. In the opening case study, K.L. was diagnosed with "lazy eye," technically known as_____.

后缀 -opia 加在词根 metr/o（意为"测量"）之后构成的单词与眼睛的屈光能力有关。请在 -metropia 上加上前缀构成下列单词。

6. a lack of refractive power in the eye_____
7. unequal refractive powers in the two eyes_____

视觉的临床表现

屈光不正

如果眼球太长，影像就会形成在视网膜之前。为使聚焦清晰，必须把物体移到距眼睛更近的位置。这种情况在技术上被称为近视（myopia, nearsightedness）（图 18-12）。与之相反的情况是远视（hyperopia, farsightedness），也就是眼球太短，影像形成在视网膜之后，为清晰聚焦必须把物体移到距眼睛更远的位置。伴随年龄增长发生的老花眼（presbyopia）也会产生这样的效果。晶状体失去弹性，不再能够调节近视力，人就变得越来越远视。散光（astigmatism）是角膜或晶状体的弯曲不规律，扭曲了进入眼睛的光线，并模糊了视觉。

眼镜能够补偿大多数屈光缺陷，如图 18-12 所示的近视和远视。框 18-3 给出了矫正屈光（refractive error）不正的手术技术。

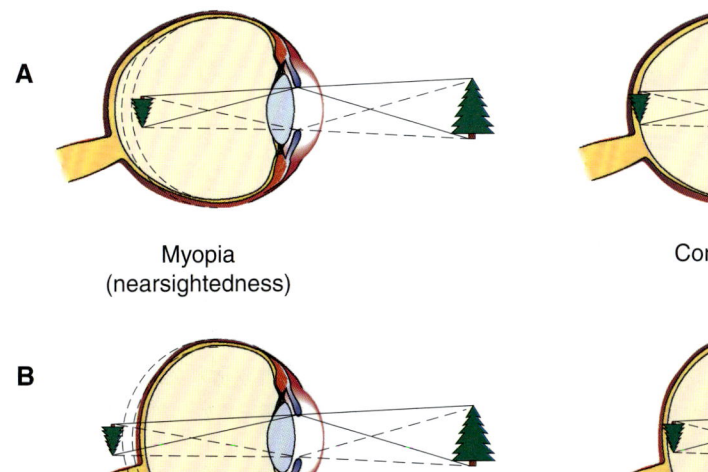
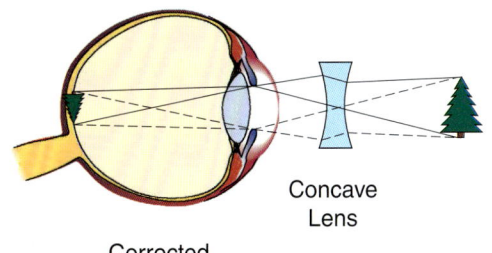
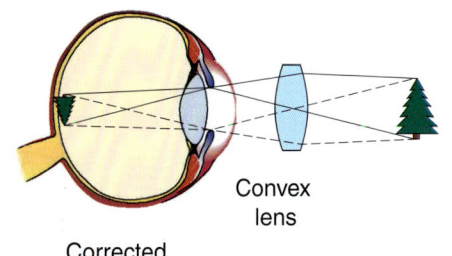

图 18-12 **屈光不正。** A. 近视；B. 远视。凹面（向内弯曲）透镜校正近视；凸（向外弯曲）透镜校正远视

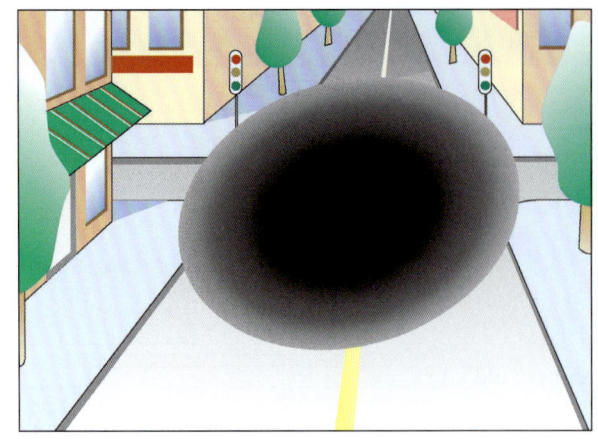

图 18-13　视网膜脱落

视网膜障碍

视网膜脱落（retinal detachment）是视网膜与眼睛的下层（脉络膜）分离，可能是肿瘤、出血或眼睛受伤所致（图 18-13）。这种情况会妨害视觉，通常可用激光进行修复。

黄斑变性（degeneration of the macula）是老年人视觉问题的常见起因。涉及衰老时，这种变性被称为老年性黄斑变性（age-related macular degeneration，AMD）。在一种形式的黄斑变性（干性）中，物质会在视网膜上积累，维生素 C 与维生素 E、β-胡萝卜素（beta carotene）和锌补充剂能够延缓这一过程。在另一种形式的新生血管性（湿性）黄斑变性中，视网膜下生长出异常的血管，造成视网膜脱落。激光手术能够阻止这些血管的生长，并延缓视力损失。最近，眼科医生使用常规眼内注射抑制血管生成的药物，成功地延缓了湿性黄斑变性进程。黄斑变性通常会影响中心视觉，但不影响周边视觉（图 18-14B）。黄斑变性的其他起因是药物毒素和遗传因素。

与糖尿病相关的循环问题会最终引起视网膜的变化，被称为糖尿病视网膜病变（diabetic retinopathy）。除血管伤害外，还有一种黄色蜡状高脂蛋白渗出物。随着时间发展，会生成新的血管并渗入玻璃体，引起出血、视网膜脱落和失明。糖尿病性视网膜病变的视觉效果如图 18-14C 所示。

感染

一些微生物能够引起静脉炎（conjunctivitis），这是一种高度传染性疾病，通常被称为"红眼病（pink eye）"。

沙眼衣原体（Chlamydia trachomatis）会引起颗粒性结膜炎，是角膜和结膜的炎症，会导致瘢痕。这种疾病在美国和其他发达国家很少见，但在不发达国家是一种常见的致盲原因，尽管用磺胺药物和抗生素很容易治愈。

淋病通常会引起新生儿急性结膜炎，被称为新生儿眼炎（ophthalmia neonatorum）。常规给新生儿使用抗生素药膏来预防这种眼镜感染。

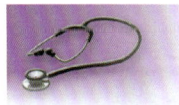

临床观点
眼睛手术：高技术一瞥

框 18-3

白内障（cataracts）、青光眼（glaucoma）和屈光不正是常见的眼睛疾病。在过去，白内障和青光眼的治疗集中在控制疾病。屈光不正使用眼镜和新近的隐形眼镜矫正。现在，使用激光和微手术技术，眼科医生能够切除白内障，减轻青光眼，并使屈光不正的人们摆脱眼镜和隐形眼镜。这些高技术方法包括：

· 准分子激光原位角膜磨镶术（laser in situ keratomileusis，LASIK）矫正屈光不正。在这种方法中，医生使用激光改造角膜，以便使光线直接折射到视网膜，而不是折射到视网膜之前或之后。用微型角膜刀（microkeratome）在角膜的外层切下一个皮片，在用计算机控制的激光雕刻角膜的中层，然后再将切下的皮片放回原处。这个过程只需几分钟，患者能够快速恢复视力，通常只有很小的术后疼痛。

· 超声乳化白内障吸出术（Phacoemulsification）消除白内障。在这种方法中，医生通过巩膜在接近角膜外边缘处做一个小切口（约 3mm），将超声波探头从这个切口插入晶状体中心。探头使用声波乳化晶状体的中心核，然后将其吸出。再将一个人工晶状体永久植入到晶状体囊中（图 18-15）。这种方法通常是无痛的，患者在术后一两天中可能会感觉不适。

· 激光小梁成形术（laser trabeculoplasty）治疗青光眼。这种方法使用激光帮助将液体排出眼睛，降低眼压。激光瞄准位于角膜和虹膜之间的排泄通道，通过烧灼打开通道，改善液体排出。这种方法通常也是无痛的，只需要几分钟即可。

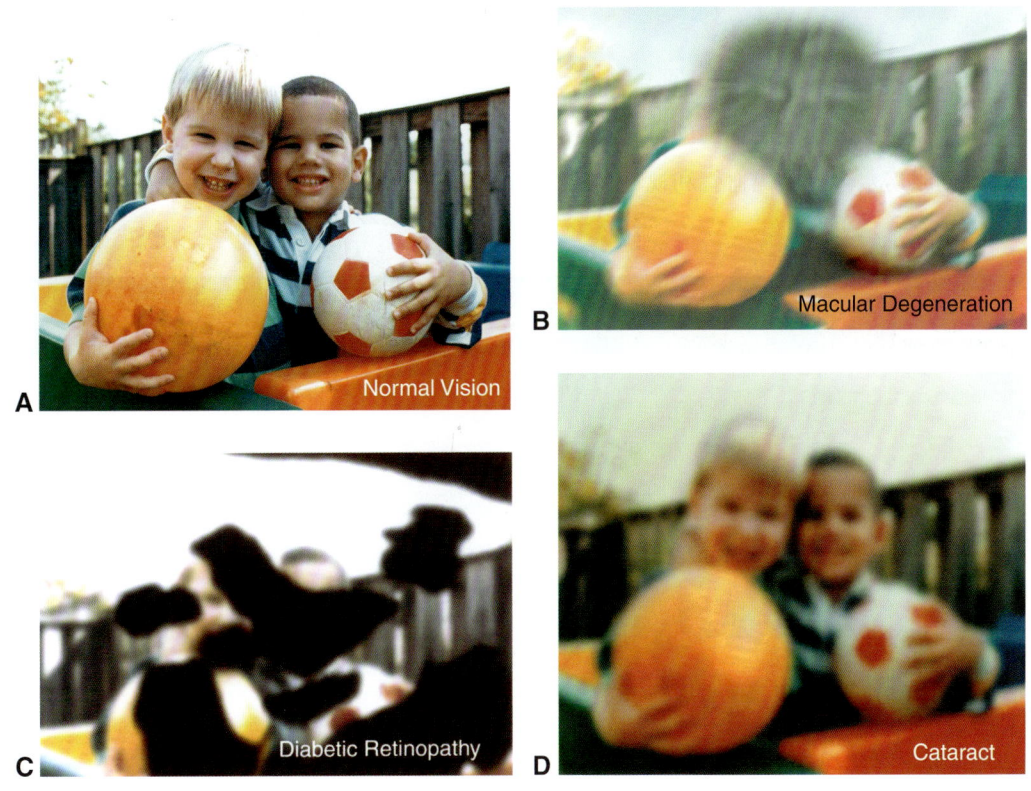

图 18-14 视觉障碍

白内障

白内障（cataract）是晶状体的不透明（混浊）部分（图 18-14D）。白内障的起因包括疾病、受伤、化学物质和暴露于物理因素，特别是阳关的紫外辐射。白内障常常出现在老年人身上，能够使暴露于环境因素和衰老引起的退化变性所致。

未来防止失明，眼科医生必须手术切除混浊的晶状体。通常，晶状体前囊会与白内障一起切除，保留后囊（图 18-15）。在超声乳化白内障吸出术（phacoemulsification）中，高频超声波将晶状体破碎，并通过一个小切口（框 18-3）吸出。白内障切除后，通常会植入人工晶状体（artificial intraocular lens，IOL）来补偿失去的晶状体。最初的移植只能提供固定距离内的视觉，最新的移植被设计容许进行远近视觉调节。替代性的选择是佩戴隐形眼镜或特殊眼镜。

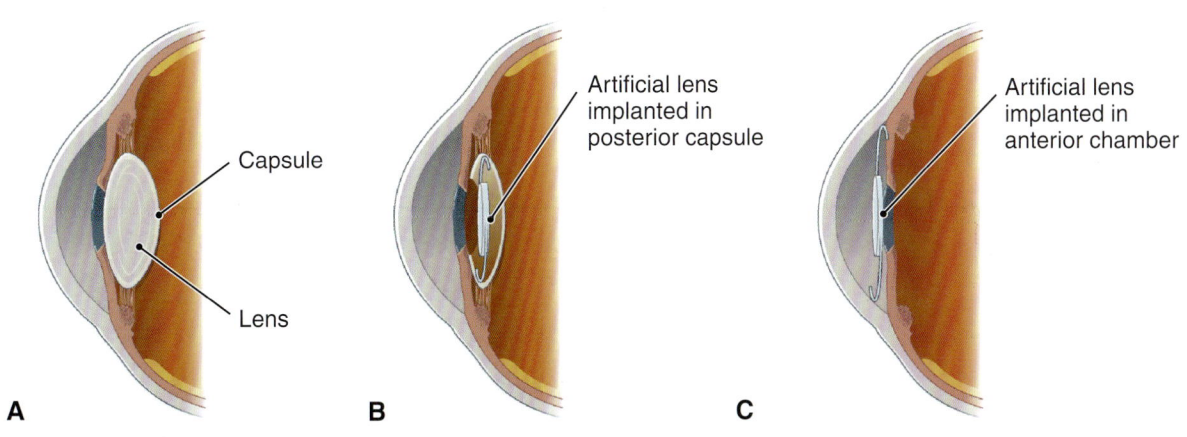

图 18-15 白内障摘除手术。A. 正常眼解剖的横截面；B. 囊外晶状体摘除涉及去除晶状体，但留下完整的后囊以接收合成的人工晶状体；C. 囊内晶状体摘除涉及移除晶状体和晶状体囊并且在前房中植入人工晶状体

青光眼

青光眼（glaucoma）是眼内压力的一种异常升高，如果眼房水的产生多于能够被眼睛排出的量，就会发生青光眼。多余的眼房水会对眼内血管和视觉神经产生压力，会导致失明。青光眼起因很多，排查该疾病是日常眼睛检查的一部分。妊娠早期胎儿风疹感染可能会引起青光眼、白内障以及听力损失。青光眼的治疗通常使用降低眼压的药物，偶尔需要手术（框 18-3）。

Terminology 关键术语

眼睛

疾病

age-related macular degeneration(AMD)	老年性黄斑变性，与衰老相关的黄斑变性；黄斑变性会损害中央视觉
astigmatism [əˈstɪgmətɪzəm]	散光，一种由角膜或晶状体曲率不规则引起的屈光不正
cataract [ˈkætərækt]	白内障，眼睛晶状体混浊
conjunctivitis [kənˌdʒʌŋktɪˈvaɪtɪs]	结膜炎，结膜的炎症；红眼病
diabetic retinopathy [ˌdaɪəˈbetɪk retɪˈnɔpəθi]	糖尿病视网膜病变，与糖尿病相关的视网膜退行性病变
glaucoma [glɔːˈkəʊmə]	青光眼，眼压升高引起的一种眼睛疾病，会损害视盘并引起视觉损失。通常是眼前部液体排出问题所致
hyperopia [ˌhaɪpəˈrəʊpɪə]	远视，光线被聚焦于视网膜后，只有远离眼睛的物体才能被看清的一种屈光不正；也常用 farsightedness 或 hypermetropia
myopia [maɪˈəʊpɪə]	近视，光线被聚焦于视网膜前，只有靠近眼睛的物体才能被看清的一种屈光不正；也常用 nearsightedness
ophthalmia neonatorum [ɒfˈθælmɪə niːɒnæˈtɔːrʌm]	新生儿眼炎，出生时淋球菌感染引起的严重的结膜炎
phacoemulsification [fəkəʊemʌlsɪfɪˈkeɪʃn]	超声乳化白内障吸除术，通过超声波破坏并吸出晶状体来去除白内障
presbyopia [ˌprezbɪˈəʊpɪə]	老花眼，眼睛在老年时发生的变化；晶状体失去了弹性，无法调节近视
retinal detachment	视网膜脱落，视网膜从其下面的脉络膜分离
trachoma [trəˈkəʊmə]	颗粒性结膜炎，沙眼衣原体引起的感染，会导致炎症贺文角膜和结膜的瘢痕。在不发达国家是常见的致盲因素

Terminology　补充术语

眼睛

正常结构与功能

canthus	[ˈkænθəs]	眼角，在眼睑之间的狭缝的两端的角
diopter	[daiˈɒptə]	屈光度，晶状体折射能力的测量
emmetropia	[ˌeməˈtrəʊpiə]	正视眼，眼睛屈光正常的状态，平行的光线会准确聚焦在视网膜上
fundus	[ˈfʌndəs]	底部，底部或基底，距一个结构的开口最远的部位。眼底是用眼膜曲率镜（ophthalmoscope）能够看到眼内后部
meibomian gland		睑板腺，眼睑分泌脂肪的腺体
tarsus	[ˈtɑːsəs]	睑板，给眼睛赋予形状的致密的结缔组织结构；也常用 tarsal plate
zonule	[ˈzəʊnjuːl]	晶状体悬韧带，支撑晶状体的纤维系统，也被称为 suspensory ligaments

症状和病症

amblyopia	[ˌæmbliˈəʊpiə]	弱视，儿童两眼视敏度不相同飞状况（前缀 ambly- 意为"模糊"）。如果不矫正，不使用较弱的眼睛会导致失明。也被称为"懒惰眼 lazy eye"
anisocoria	[ænisəʊˈkɔːriə]	瞳孔不等，两个瞳孔（词根：cor/o）大小不等的状况
blepharoptosis	[blefæˈrɒptəʊsis]	眼睑下垂，上眼睑下垂无力
chalazion	[kəˈleiziən]	睑板腺囊肿，炎症和睑板腺堵塞所致的眼睑上的小团块
drusen	[dˈruːzn]	脉络膜疣，出现在眼睛视网膜下的微小黄色斑点样的小瘤，通常岁年龄增长而发生，但也因特定的异常状况而发生
floater	[ˈfləʊtə(r)]	飞蚊症，在视野中有一个源自于玻璃体的小运动物体。浮游物出现为斑点或螺纹，是玻璃体的良性变性或胚胎沉积物在视网膜上投射的阴影
hordeolum	[hɔːˈdiːələm]	眼睑炎，眼睑睑板腺的炎症；也被称为麦粒肿（sty）
keratoconus	[kerətəʊˈkəʊnəs]	圆锥角膜，角膜中心的锥形突出
miosis	[maiˈəʊsis]	瞳孔缩小，瞳孔的异常收缩（源自于希腊语，意为"缩小"）
mydriasis	[miˈdraiəsis]	瞳孔散大，瞳孔明显或异常的扩大
nyctalopia	[ˌniktəˈləʊpiə]	夜盲症，无法在微弱对光线或夜间有良好的视觉（词根：nyct/o），通常是因为缺乏维生素 A，维生素 A 被用于产生微弱光线视觉所需的色素
nystagmus	[nisˈtægməs]	眼球震颤，眼球快速、非自主、有节奏地运动；可能发生于神经系统疾病或内耳前庭器官的疾病
papilledema	[pæpiliˈdiːmə]	视神经乳头水肿，视盘肿胀；也常用 choked disk
phlyctenule	[flikˈtenjʊl]	小水泡，角膜或结膜上的小水泡或小结节
pseudophakia	[sjuːdəʊˈfɑːkjə]	假晶状体，白内障的晶状体被去除并植入人工晶状体的状态

Terminology 补充术语（续表）

retinitis [ˌreti'naitis]	视网膜炎，视网膜的炎症，起因包括全身疾病、感染、出血和暴露于强光
retinitis pigmentosa	色素性视网膜炎，一种开始于童年早期的遗传性视网膜慢性变性疾病，视神经发生萎缩，视网膜上有色素聚集
retinoblastoma [retinəʊblæs'təʊmə]	视网膜母细胞瘤，一种恶性视网膜神经胶质瘤，通常出现在儿童早期，有时是遗传性的；如果不治疗会致命，但目前的治愈率很高
scotoma [skə'təʊmə]	暗点，视野中视觉减退的区域
strabismus [strə'bizməs]	斜视，每只眼睛的视线不同时指向相同对象的眼睛偏离。也被称为 heterotropia 或 squint。不同的偏离形式用 -tropias 加上一个代表方向的前缀来表示，例如内斜视（esotropia）、外斜视（exotropia）、上斜视（hypertropia）和下斜视（hypotropia）。也使用后缀 -phoria，如 esophoria（内隐斜视）
synechia [si'nekiə]	虹膜粘连，虹膜与晶状体或角膜的粘连（复数形式为 synechiae）
xanthoma [zæn'θəʊmə]	黄色瘤，通常出现在眼睑上的柔软、轻微凸起的黄色斑块或结节；多发于老年人，也被称为睑黄瘤（xanthelasma）

诊断与治疗

canthotomy ['kænθəʊtəmi]	眦切开术，手术切开眼角
cystotome [sis'təʊtəʊm]	晶状体囊刀，切开晶状体囊的工具
electroretinography (ERG) [iˌlektrəʊˌretə'nɒgrəfi]	视网膜电描记法，研究视网膜对光刺激的电反应
enucleation [enˈjuːkliːʃən]	眼球摘除术，手术摘除眼球
gonioscopy [gəʊniːəʊsˈkɒpi]	前房角镜检查，检查角膜与虹膜之间的夹角（前房角，词根：goni/o 意为"角度"），液体通过该角从眼睛中排出
keratometer [kerə'tɒmitə(r)]	角膜曲率计，测量角膜曲率的仪器
mydriatic [ˌmidri'ætik]	扩瞳药，引起瞳孔扩张的药物
phorometer ['fʌrɒmitər]	隐斜测量计，确定斜视的程度和种类的仪器
retinoscope ['retinəskəʊp]	视网膜镜，用于确定眼睛屈光不正的仪器，也被称为影检镜（skiascope）
slit-lamp biomicroscope	裂隙灯显微镜，放大检查眼睛的仪器
Snellen chart ['snelən]	斯内伦视力表，打印的由尺寸逐渐减小的字母用于测试视力的图表，测试时要被测试者在设定距离观察并辨识图表上的字母；测试结果为在 20 英尺的距离处受试者的视力与正常视力相比的分数
tarsorrhaphy [tɑːˈsɒrəfi]	睑缘缝合术，部分或整个上下眼睑缝合
tonometer [təʊˈnɒmitə]	眼压计，测量眼睛液体压力的仪器

Terminology 缩略语

眼睛

A, Acc	Accommodation		视觉调节
AMD	Age-related macular degeneration		老年性黄斑变性
ARC	Abnormal retinal correspondence		异常视网膜对应
As, AST	Astigmatism		散光
cc	With correction		有矫正
Em	Emmetropia		正视眼
EOM	Extraocular movement, muscles		眼球外运动,眼外肌
ERG	Electroretinography		视网膜电描记法
ET	Esotropia		内斜视
FC	Finger counting		眼前数指
IOL	Intraocular lens		人工晶体
IOP	Intraocular pressure		眼压
NRC	Normal retinal correspondence		正常视网膜对应
NV	Near vision		近视力
sc	Without correction		没有矫正
VA	Visual acuity		视敏度
VF	Visual field		视野
XT	Exotropia		外斜视

Case Study Revisited 案例研究再访

K. L.'s Follow-Up

K. L. started wearing the patch on her right eye during waking hours. She progressed to wearing it four to five hours a day as ordered by the ophthalmologist. The glasses she obtained from the optician were helping her to focus, and she was able to read her schoolwork. She had adjusted well to the treatment plan and showed improved vision. The family was satisfied with results from the therapeutic plan.

K. L. 的随访

K. L. 开始在醒着的时间为右眼佩戴眼罩。她按照眼科医生的指示,每天戴 4~5 小时。她从眼镜商那里得到帮助她聚焦的眼镜,使她能够看清家庭作业。她很好地适应了治疗计划,并显示出视力改善。家人对治疗计划的结果感到满意。

CHAPTER 18 复习

标记练习

耳朵

在对应的下划线上写出每个编号部分的名称。

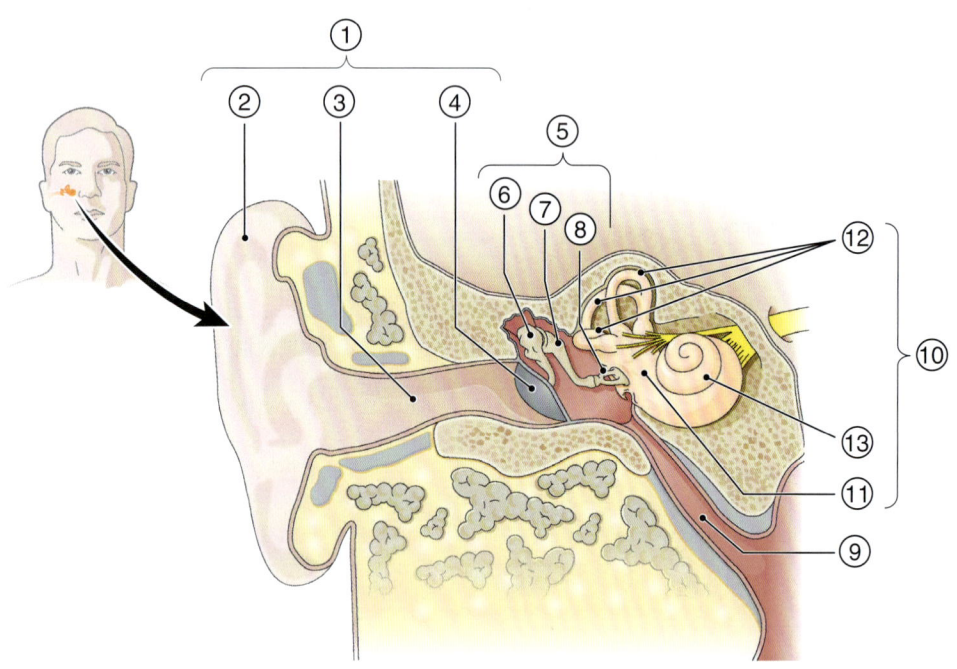

Cochlea
Auditory (Eustachian) tube
External auditory canal
Incus
Inner ear
Malleus
Ossicles (of middle ear)

Outer ear
Pinna
Semicircular canals
Stapes
Tympanic membrane
Vestibule

1. _____
2. _____
3. _____
4. _____
5. _____
6. _____
7. _____
8. _____
9. _____
10. _____
11. _____
12. _____
13. _____

眼睛

在对应的下划线上写出每个编号部分的名称。

Aqueous humor
Choroid
Ciliary muscle
Conjunctival sac
Cornea
Fovea
Iris

Lens
Optic disk (blind spot)
Optic nerve
Pupil
Retina
Sclera
Vitreous body

1. _____
2. _____
3. _____
4. _____
5. _____
6. _____
7. _____
8. _____
9. _____
10. _____
11. _____
12. _____
13. _____
14. _____

术语

匹配

匹配下列术语，在每个题号左侧写上适当的字母。

____ 1. palpebra
____ 2. ossicle
____ 3. rods and cones
____ 4. vestibular apparatus
____ 5. lens

a. small bone
b. structure that changes shape for near and far vision
c. an eyelid
d. location of equilibrium receptors
e. vision receptors

____ 6. tactile
____ 7. tinnitus
____ 8. hyperesthesia
____ 9. fovea
____ 10. hemianopia

a. increased sensation
b. blindness in half the visual field
c. point of sharpest vision
d. pertaining to touch
e. sensation of noises in the ear

____ 11. anacusis
____ 12. ophthalmoplegia
____ 13. phacomalacia
____ 14. parosmia
____ 15. keratoplasty

a. corneal transplant
b. abnormal smell perception
c. paralysis of an eye muscle
d. softening of the lens
e. total loss of hearing

补充术语

____ 16. diopter
____ 17. mastoid process
____ 18. stapedius
____ 19. canthus
____ 20. decibel

a. angle between the eyelids
b. small muscle attached to an ear ossicle
c. projection of the temporal bone
d. unit of sound intensity
e. unit for measuring the refractive power of the lens

____ 21. emmetropia
____ 22. nystagmus
____ 23. mydriasis
____ 24. drusen
____ 25. amblyopia

a. abnormal dilation of the pupil
b. small growths beneath the retina
c. rapid, involuntary eye movements
d. normal refraction of the eye
e. commonly called "lazy eye"

____ 26. AMD
____ 27. Hz
____ 28. AST
____ 29. ENT
____ 30. IOL

a. irregularity in the curve of the eye
b. an implanted lens
c. otorhinolaryngology
d. eye disorder associated with aging
e. a unit for measuring pitch of sound

填空

31. The scientific name for the eardrum is_____.
32. The type of hearing loss resulting from damage to the eighth cranial nerve is described as_____.
33. The ossicle that is in contact with the inner ear is the_____.
34. The outermost layer of the eye wall is the_____.
35. The bending of light rays as they pass through the eye is_____.
36. The innermost layer of the eye that contains the receptors for vision is the_____.
37. The transparent extension of the sclera that covers the front of the eye is the_____.
38. The sense of awareness of body position is_____.

定义

定义下列单词。

39. audiologist [ˌɔːdiˈɒlədʒist]
40. ophthalmometer [ˌɒfθælˈmɒmitə]
41. aphakia [æˈfeikjə]
42. subscleral [ˈsʌbsklrəl]
43. iridotomy [iriˈdɒtəmi]
44. myringoscope [miˈriŋəskəup]
45. perilental [pəriˈlentl]
46. dacryorrhea [deikriːəˈriə]
47. presbycusis [prezbiˈkjuːsis]
48. keratoiritis [kerətɔiəˈraitis]

写出下列定义的单词。

49. softening of the lens _____

50. measurement of the pupil _____

51. surgical removal of the stapes _____

52. drooping of the eyelid _____

53. plastic repair of the ear _____

54. pertaining to the vestibular apparatus and cochlea _____

55. any disease of the retina _____

56. absence of pain _____

57. pertaining to tears _____

58. excision of (part of) the ciliary body _____

59. endoscopic examination of the auditory tube _____

60. technical name for farsightedness _____

形容词

写出下列单词的形容词形式。

61. cochlea _____

62. palpebra _____

63. choroid _____

64. uvea _____

65. cornea _____

66. sclera _____

67. pupil _____

反义词

写出下列单词的反义词。

68. hyperesthesia _____

69. hypalgesia _____

70. cc _____

71. hyperopia _____

72. mydriasis _____

73. esotropia _____

单词构建

使用给出的单词组成部分写出下列定义的单词。

-pexy -ia osm/o kerat/o -al -schisis -scopy pseud/o- retin/o an- -plasty salping/o sub -myring/o

74. false sense of smell _____

75. plastic repair of the tympanic membrane _____

76. examination of the retina _____

77. examination of the auditory tube _____

78. absence of the sense of smell_____
79. splitting of the retina_____
80. examination of the tympanic membrane_____
81. beneath the retina_____
82. surgical fixation of the retina_____
83. examination of the cornea_____

真假判断

检查以下语句。如果语句为真，则在第一个空格写入 T；如果语句为假，则在第一个空格中写入 F，并通过在第二个空格中替换带下划线的单词来更正语句。

	True or False	Correct Answer
84. The spiral organ is located in the <u>vestibule</u> of the inner ear.		
85. An osmoceptor is a receptor for the sense of <u>smell</u>.		
86. The malleus is located in the <u>middle ear</u>.		
87. Gustation is the sense of <u>taste</u>.		
88. Hypergeusia is an abnormal increase in the sense of <u>touch</u>.		
89. In bright light the pupils <u>dilate</u>.		
90. A myringotomy is incision of the <u>stapes</u>.		
91. The lacrimal gland produces <u>aqueous humor</u>.		

排除

在下列每组中，为与其他不相配的单词加下划线，并说明你选择的理由。

92. pressure — temperature — smell — touch — pain
_____

93. cochlea — pinna — vestibule — oval window — semicircular canals
_____

94. incus — lacrimal gland — eyelash — conjunctiva — palpebral
_____

95. glaucoma — myopia — cataract — macular degeneration — presbycusis
_____

单词分析

定义下列单词，并给出每个单词组成部分的含义。如果需要，可以使用词典。

96. asthenopia ［æsθi'nəupiə］_____
    a. a_____
    b. sthen/o_____
    c. -op(s)_____
    d. -ia_____

97. pseudophakia ［sju:dəʊ'fɑ:kjə］_____
    a. pseudo_____
    b. phak/o_____

    c. -ia
98. cholesteatoma [kəʊlistiːəˈtəʊmə]
    a. chol/e
    b. steat/o
    c. -oma
99. exotropia [ˌeksəˈtrəʊpiə]
    a. ex/o
    b. trop/o
    c. -ia
100. anisometropia [ænisəʊˈmetrəʊpiə]
    a. an
    b. iso
    c. metr/o
    d. op(s)
    e. –ia

Additional Case Studies
补充案例研究

Case Study 18-1: Audiology Report
案例研究 18-1：听力报告

S. R., a 55 year-old man, reported decreased hearing sensitivity in his left ear for the past three years. In addition to hearing loss, he was experiencing tinnitus and aural fullness. Pure-tone test results revealed normal hearing sensitivity for the right ear and a moderate sensorineural hearing loss in the left ear. Speech thresholds were appropriate for the degree of hearing loss noted. Word recognition was excellent for the right ear and poor for the left ear when the signal was present at a suprathreshold level. Tympanograms were characterized by normal shape, amplitude, and peak pressure points bilaterally. The contralateral acoustic reflex was normal for the right ear but absent for the left ear at the frequencies tested (500 to 4,000 Hz). The ipsilateral acoustic reflex was present with the probe in the right ear and absent with the probe in the left ear. Brainstem auditory evoked potentials (BAEPs) were within normal range for the right ear. No repeatable response was observed from the left ear. A subsequent MRI showed a 1-cm acoustic neuroma.

S. R. 是一名 55 岁的男人，报告在过去 3 年中左耳的听力敏感性下降。除了听力损失之外，他还经历了耳鸣和耳闷。纯音测试结果显示右耳听力敏感性正常，左耳感觉神经性听力中度损失。语言阈值与所述的听力损失程度相符。当信号以超阈值水平存在时，右耳单词识别很好，而左耳较差。鼓室图的特征是双侧形状、振幅和峰值压力点正常。在测试频率（500~4000Hz）下，对侧声反射在右耳正常，在左耳不存在。探针在右耳中同侧声反射存在，而探针在左耳中不存在。右耳的脑干听觉诱发电位（BAEP）在正常范围内。左耳没有观察到可重复的反应。随后的核磁共振显示有1cm的听神经瘤。

Case Study 18-2: Phacoemulsification with Intraocular Lens Implant
案例研究 18-2：晶状体乳化加人工晶体植入

W. S., a 68 y/o, was scheduled for surgery for a cataract and relief from "floaters," which she had noticed in her visual field since her surgery for a retinal detachment the previous year. She reported to the ambulatory surgery center an hour before her scheduled procedure. Before transfer to the operating room, she spoke with her ophthalmologist, who reviewed the surgical plan. Her right eye was identified as the operative eye, and it was marked with a "yes" and the surgeon's initials on the lid. She was given anesthetic drops in the right eye and an intravenous bolus of 2 mg of midazolam (Versed).

In the OR, W. S. and her operative eye were again identified by the surgeon, anesthetist, and nurses. After anesthesia and akinesia were achieved, the eye area was prepped and draped in sterile sheets. An operating microscope with video system was positioned over her eye. A 5-0 silk suture was placed through the superior rectus muscle to retract the eye. A lid speculum was placed to open the eye. A minimal conjunctival peritomy was performed, and hemostasis was achieved with wet-field cautery. The anterior chamber was entered at the 10:30 o'clock position. A capsulotomy was performed after Healon was placed in the anterior chamber. Phacoemulsification was carried out without difficulty. The remaining cortex was removed by irrigation and aspiration.

An intraocular lens (IOL) was placed into the posterior chamber. Miochol was injected to achieve papillary miosis, and the wound was closed with one 10-0 suture. Subconjunctival Celestone and Garamycin were injected.

W. S. 是一名 68 岁的女性，预约了白内障手术和"飞蚊症"缓解，去年治疗视网膜脱离的手术后她的视野中出现了飞蚊症。她在预约手术前1小时向流动手术中心报到。在转移到手术室之前，她与她的眼科医生交谈，她的眼科医生评估了手术计划。她的右眼被确认为手术眼，并在眼睑上标有"是"和外科医生的缩写。她的右眼被给予麻醉滴剂，静脉内推注2mg咪达唑仑（Versed）。

在手术室，外科医生、麻醉师和护士再次确认了 W. S. 和她的手术眼。在实现麻醉和失去运动能力后，眼睛区域被准备好，并由无菌单子覆盖。将具有视频系统的手术显微镜放置在她的眼睛上。将 5-0 丝缝线穿过上直肌放置以缩回眼睛，用眼睑扩张器打开眼睛。进行了最小结膜周围切除术，并且用湿场烧灼术实现止血。前房在 10:30 的位置进入，在前房放置透明质酸钠后进行囊切开术。晶状体乳化顺利进行，通过灌洗和抽吸除去剩余的皮质。

将人工晶体（IOL）置入后房。注射氯化乙酰胆碱以实现乳头状瞳孔缩小，并用一个10-0缝合线闭合伤口。结膜下注射倍他米松和加瑞霉素，去除眼睑控制器并回

The lid speculum and retraction suture were removed. After application of Eserine and Bacitracin ointments, the eye was patched, and a shield was applied. W.S. left the OR in good condition and was discharged to home for four hours later.

缩缝线。在使用毒扁豆碱和杆菌肽软膏后，眼睛被罩上，并施加屏蔽。W.S. 离开手术室时处于良好状态，4 小时后被送到家里。

案例研究问题

多项选择。选择正确答案，在每个题号左侧写上你选择的字母。

____ 1. The study of hearing is termed
    a. acousticology
    b. radio frequency
    c. audiology
    d. otology

____ 2. Sensorineural hearing loss may result from
    a. damage to the second cranial nerve
    b. damage to the eighth cranial nerve
    c. otosclerosis
    d. otitis media

____ 3. The term that means "on the same side" is
    a. contralateral
    b. bilateral
    c. distal
    d. ipsilateral

____ 4. Another name for an acoustic neuroma is
    a. macular degeneration
    b. acoustic neurilemmoma
    c. auditory otosclerosis
    d. acoustic glaucoma

____ 5. Ultrasound destruction and aspiration of the lens is called
    a. catarectomy
    b. phacoemulsification
    c. stapedectomy
    d. radial keratotomy

____ 6. The term akinesia means
    a. movement
    b. lack of sensation
    c. washing
    d. lack of movement

写出案例研究中下列含义的单词。

7. above a minimum level _____

8. pertaining to or perceived by the ear _____

9. record obtained by tympanometry _____

10. pertaining to sound or hearing _____

11. physician who specializes in conditions of the eye _____

12. perception of sounds, such as ringing or tinkling in the ear _____

13. a circular incision through the conjunctiva _____

14. within the eye _____

15. abnormal contraction of the pupil _____

16. below the conjunctiva _____

定义下列缩略语。

17. Hz _____

18. BAEP _____

19. IOL _____

CHAPTER 19

骨骼系统

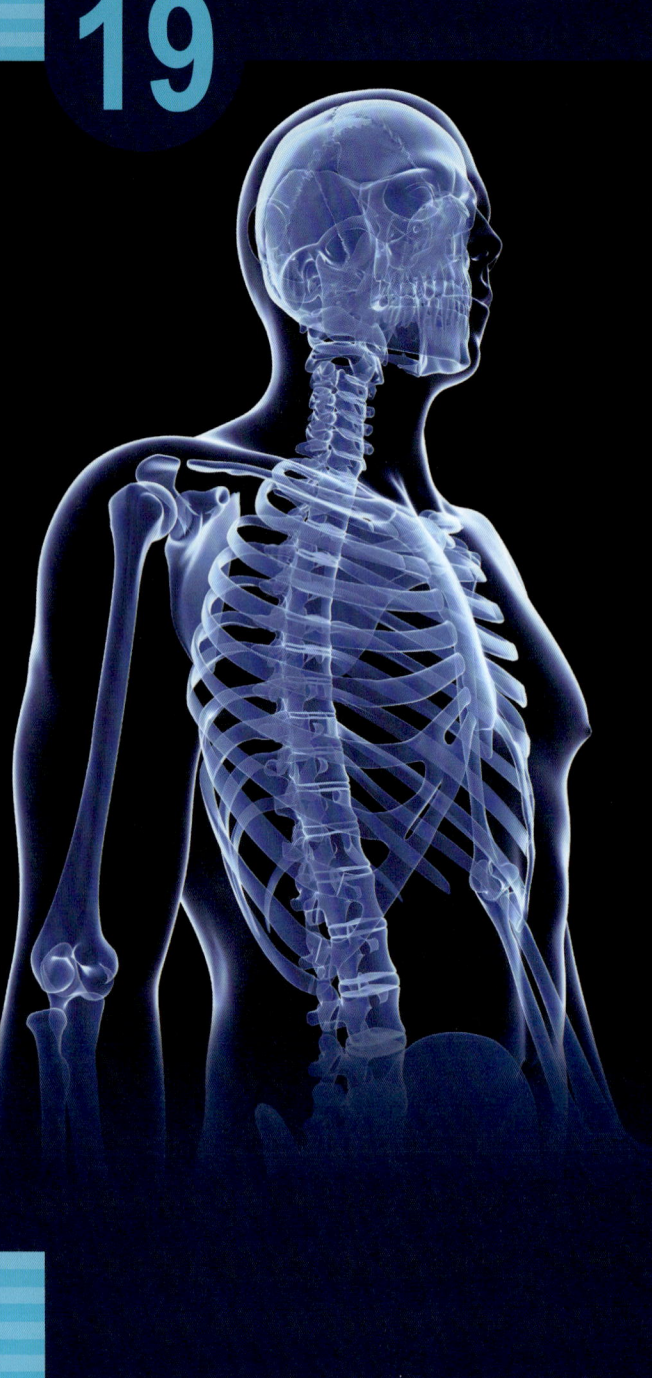

预测试

多项选择。选择正确答案，在每个题号左侧写上你选择的字母。

_____ 1. The root oste/o means
a. cartilage
b. fat
c. heart
d. bone

_____ 2. The root myel/o refers to the spinal cord. Used in reference to bones it means
a. bone marrow
b. joint
c. bone shaft
d. membrane

_____ 3. A bone of the spinal column is a
a. ventricle
b. cortex
c. labyrinth
d. vertebra

_____ 4. The large, flared superior bone of the pelvis is the
a. phalange
b. ilium
c. thorax
d. duodenum

_____ 5. The bones of the wrist are the
a. digits
b. cervices
c. carpals
d. ribs

_____ 6. The bone of the thigh is the
a. patella
b. cranium
c. umbilicus
d. femur

_____ 7. A general term for inflammation of a joint is
a. arthritis
b. conjunctivitis
c. epididymitis
d. myocarditis

_____ 8. Chondrosarcoma is a tumor that originates in
a. adipose tissue
b. bone
c. cartilage
d. muscle

▶ 学习目标

学完本章后，应该能够：

1. ▶ 比较中轴骨骼和附肢骨骼。
2. ▶ 简述骨组织的生成。
3. ▶ 描述长骨的结构。
4. ▶ 比较骨缝、骨联合与滑膜关节。
5. ▶ 描述滑膜关节的结构。
6. ▶ 识别并使用与骨骼相关的词根。
7. ▶ 描述影响骨骼和关节的六种主要疾病。
8. ▶ 分析案例研究中与骨骼相关的医学术语。

Case Study: L. R.'s Idiopathic Adolescent Scoliosis
案例研究：L. R. 的特发性青少年脊柱侧弯

Chief Complaint

Four years ago, L. R., a 15-year-old female, had a posterior spinal fusion (PSF) for correction of idiopathic adolescent scoliosis in a pediatric orthopedic hospital in another state. L.R. is a gifted musician, and her favorite pastime is playing the piano, guitar, and other musical instruments. Lately she has experienced considerable back pain that she attributed to long hours at the piano or playing the guitar. It was time for her routine follow-up orthopedic visit, and now she presents with a significant prominence of the right scapula and back pain in the mid- and lower back.

Examination

A history was taken and medical records were reviewed followed by a physical examination. The medical records indicated that the patient's spinal curvature had been surgically corrected with the insertion of bilateral laminar and pedicle hooks and two 3/16-inch rods. A bone autograft was taken from L.R.'s right posterior superior ilium and applied along the lateral processes of T4 to L2 to complete the fusion. The physical examination was normal except for surgical scarring along the spine, a projecting right scapula, and asymmetry of the rib cage. During the history, L. R. denied numbness or tingling of the lower extremities, bowel or bladder problems, chest pain, or shortness of breath. The physician ordered a CT scan to determine if there had been continued growth on the anterior portion of the spine following the posterior fusion.

Clinical Course

The results of the CT scan of the upper thoracic spine showed a prominent rotatory scoliosis deformity of the right posterior thorax with acute angulation of the ribs. L. R.'s deformity is a common consequence of overcorrection of prior spinal fusion surgery, called crankshaft phenomenon.

L. R. was referred to the chief spinal surgeon of a local pediatric orthopedic hospital for removal of the spinal instrumentation, posterior spinal osteotomies from T4 to L2, insertion of replacement hooks and rods, bilateral rib resections, autograft bone from the resected ribs, partial scapulectomy and possible bone allograft, and bilateral chest tube placement. The surgical plan was explained to her and her mother, and consent was obtained and signed. The surgical procedure and the potential benefits versus risks were discussed. L. R. and her parents stated that they fully understood and provided consent to proceed with the plan for surgery.

主诉

4 年前，15 岁的女性 L. R. 在另一个州的儿科骨科医院做了后侧脊柱融合术（PSF），用于矫正特发性青少年脊柱侧凸弯。L.R. 是一个天才的音乐家，她最喜欢的娱乐是弹钢琴、吉他和玩儿其他乐器。最近她经历了严重的背痛，她将背痛归因于长时间弹钢琴或吉他。现在是她常规随访矫形外科时候，她的右肩胛骨显着突出，中后腰背部疼痛。

检查

记录了病史，审查了医疗记录，随后体格检查。医疗记录表明，患者的脊柱弯曲已经通过插入双侧椎板和椎弓根钩和 2 个 3/16 英寸的拉杆做了手术矫正。骨髓自体移植取自于后右上髂骨，应用于 T4 至 L2 的外侧突起以完成融合。体格检查查正常，除了沿脊柱的手术瘢痕，突出的右肩胛骨和肋骨不对称。在病史上，L. R. 说没有下肢麻木或麻痹、肠或膀胱问题以及胸痛或呼吸急促。医生指示做 CT 扫描以确定在后部融合之后脊柱的前部是否在持续生长。

临床病程

上胸椎的 CT 扫描结果显示，右后胸部有明显的旋转性脊柱侧弯畸形，肋骨有剧烈弯曲。L. R. 的畸形是以前的脊柱融合手术过度矫正的常见结果，称为曲轴现象。

L. R. 被转诊给当地儿科矫形医院的首席脊柱外科医生，去除脊柱内固定，做 T4 到 L2 的后脊柱截骨术，插入替换的钩和杆，双侧肋骨切除，从切除的肋骨做自体骨移植，部分肩胛骨切除和可能同种异体骨移植和双侧胸管放置。向她和她母亲解释了手术计划，并获得了已签字的同意书。讨论了外科手术和潜在的受益与风险。L. R. 和她的父母说他们完全理解并同意执行手术计划。

简介

骨骼构成了身体的架构，保护重要器官，并于肌肉系统一起在关节产生运动。成人的骨骼（skeleton）有 206 块骨头，为研究方便分为两个部分。

骨骼的划分

中轴骨骼（axial skeleton）构成了人体骨架的中轴（图 19-1），包括：

- 头骨（skull），由 8 块颅骨和 14 块面骨构成（图 19-2）。除下颌骨与颞骨之间的关节（颞颌关节，temporomandibular joint，TMJ）外，头骨由不动关节（骨缝，suture）连接。
- 脊柱（spinal column）（图 19-3）由 26 块椎骨（vertebrae）构成。椎骨之间是增强脊柱力量和韧性的软骨（cartilage）盘。椎骨分为 5 组，从上到下分别为：

1. 颈椎（cervical vertebrae）（7 块），编号为 C1~C7。第一和第二颈椎还有特定的名称，分别是寰椎（atlas）和枢椎（axis）（图 19-3）。
2. 胸椎（thoracic vertebrae）（12 块），编号是 T1~T12。
3. 腰椎（lumbar vertebrae）（5 块），编号是 L1~L5。
4. 骶骨（sacrum S），由 5 块融合的骨头构成。
5. 尾骨（coccyx，Co），由 4~5 块融合的骨头构成。

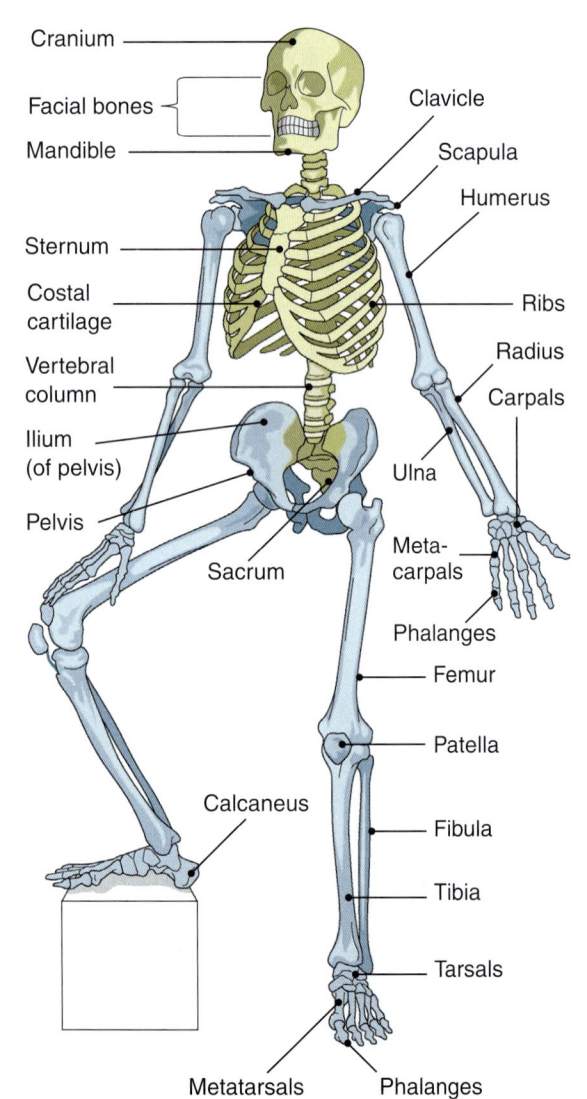

图 19-1 骨骼。中轴骨骼显示为黄色，附肢骨骼为蓝色

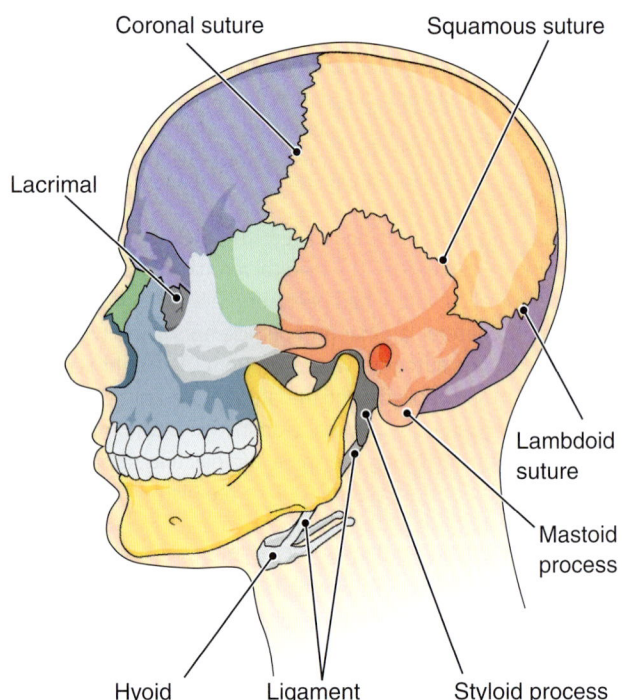

图 19-2 头骨，左视图。头骨内部可以看到一块额外的颅骨——筛骨。舌骨被认为是中轴骨骼的一部分，但不附着到任何其他骨骼。舌头和其他肌肉附着在舌骨上

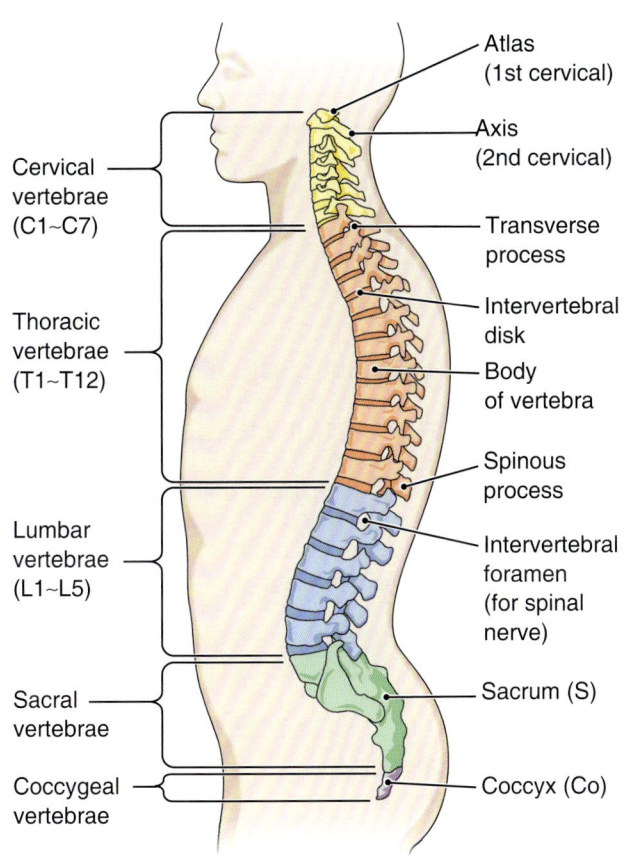

图 19-3　脊柱，左侧视图。图中显示了每组椎骨的编号和缩写，骶骨和尾骨由骨融合形成

- 胸廓（thorax）由 12 对通过软骨连接到胸骨（sternum）的肋骨（rib）构成。胸腔（rib cage）包围并保护胸部器官。

附肢骨骼（appendicular skeleton）附着于中轴骨骼（图 19-1），上部包括：

- 肩胛带（shoulder girdle）的骨骼，锁骨（clavicle）和肩胛骨（scapula）
- 上肢的骨骼，肱骨（humerus）、桡骨（radius）、尺骨（ulna）、腕骨（carpal）、掌骨（metacarpal）和指骨（phalanx）。

下部包括：

- 髋骨（pelvic bone）是与骶骨和尾骨连接形成骨盆的两块大骨头。每块髋骨由三块融合的骨头构成，分别是大喇叭形的髂骨（ilium）、坐骨（ischium）和耻骨（pubis）（图 19-4）。髋骨支撑股骨（femur）头的深窝是髋臼（acetabulum）。女性的骨盆比男性的宽，并有其他一些变形以适应分娩。
- 下肢的骨骼，股骨（femur）、髌骨（patella）、胫骨（tibia）、腓骨（fibula）、跗骨（tarsal）、

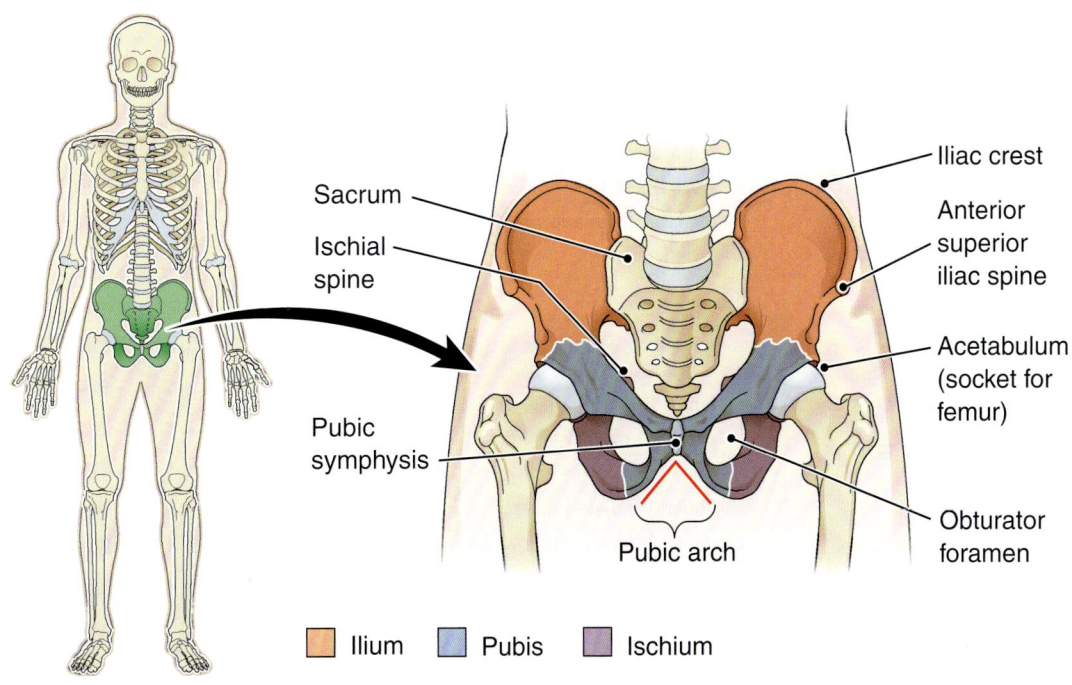

图 19-4　骨盆。髋骨是由髂骨、坐骨和耻骨融合形成，与骶骨和尾骨一起形成骨盆，髋臼是股骨的窝

> **供你参考** 框 19-1
> 骨骼

部位	骨骼	说明
axial skeleton [ˈæksiəl] 中轴骨		
SKULL [skʌl] 头骨		
cranium [ˈkreiniəm] 头颅	cranial bones 颅骨，8 块	包围脑部的室，覆盖耳朵，并形成眼窝
facial portion 面部	facial bones 面骨，14 块	形成脸面和包围感觉器官的室
hyoid [ˈhaiɔid] 舌骨		下颚骨（mandible）之下的 U 形骨骼，用于肌肉附着
ossicles [ˈɒsiklz] 听小骨	ear bones 耳骨，3 块	传送声波通过中耳
TRUNK [trʌŋk] 躯干		
vertebral column [ˈvəːtibrəl] 脊椎	vertebrae [ˈvɜːtibriː] 椎骨，26 块	包围脊髓
thorax [ˈθɔːræks] 胸廓	sternum [ˈstɜːnəm] 胸骨 ribs [rib] 肋骨，12 对	胸廓的前骨 包围胸部器官
appendicular skeleton [ˌæpənˈdikjʊlə] 附肢骨骼		
UPPER DIVISION 上部		
shoulder girdle [ˈgɜːdl] 肩胛带	clavicle [ˈklævikl] 锁骨 scapula [ˈskæpjʊlə] 肩胛骨	前面的，在胸骨和肩胛骨之间 后面的，锚挂运动手臂的肌肉
upper extremity 上肢	humerus [ˈhjuːmərəs] 肱骨 ulna [ˈʌlnə] 尺骨 radius [ˈreidiəs] 桡骨 carpal [ˈkɑːpl] 腕骨，8 块 metacarpal [ˌmetəˈkɑːpl] 掌骨，5 块 phalanx [ˈfælæŋks] 指骨，14 块	近端臂骨 前臂的内侧骨 前臂的侧骨 手腕骨 手掌骨 手指骨
LOWER DIVISION 下部		
pelvic bones 髋骨	os coxae [ˈkɒksiː] 髋骨，2 块	与脊椎的骶骨和尾骨连接形成骨盆
lower extremity 下肢	femur [ˈfiːmə(r)] 股骨 patella [pəˈtelə] 髌骨 tibia [ˈtibiə] 胫骨 fibula [ˈfibjələ] 腓骨 tarsal [ˈtɑːsl] 跗骨，7 块 metatarsal [ˌmetəˈtɑːsl] 跖骨，5 块 phalanx [ˈfælæŋks] 趾骨，14 块	大腿骨 膝盖骨 腿的内侧骨 侧腿骨 踝骨，大的足跟骨是跟骨 脚背骨 脚趾骨

跖骨（metatarsal）和趾骨（phalanx）。形成脚跟（heel）的大跗骨是跟骨（calcaneus）（图19-1）。

所有这些骨骼群，以及下颌的舌骨（hyoid）和耳小骨都按发音顺序列在框19-1中。

骨生成

骨骼是通过向一种致密的结缔组织软骨逐渐添加钙盐和磷盐而生成的。这一成骨（ossification）过程起始于出生前，并持续到成年。虽然骨骼看起来是惰性的（inert），但实际上是活的组织，在其整个生命中不断地被替换和重塑。在这些变化中涉及3类细胞：

- 成骨细胞（osteoblast），产生骨骼的细胞。
- 骨细胞（osteocyte），成熟的骨骼细胞，帮助维护骨组织。
- 破骨细胞（osteoclast），涉及骨组织的分解，释放所需的矿物质或允许改造和修复。

骨骼破坏以便其成分能够进入循环的过程被称为再吸收（resorption）。这一过程持续发生，并通常与骨生成（bone formation）保持平衡。在疾病状态，再吸收可能比骨生成发生得更快或更慢。

长骨的结构

典型的长骨（图19-5）有一个由紧密的骨组织构成的骨干（shaft或diaphysis）。在骨干中是包含黄色骨髓的髓腔（medullary cavity），骨髓含有很高的脂肪。两端不规则的骨骺（epiphyses）是由较不密集的海绵状（松质骨cancellous）骨组织构成（图19-6）。

海绵骨中的空隙包含造血的红骨髓。一层软骨覆盖着骨骺（epiphysis），以保护关节处的骨骼表面。一层薄纤维组织骨膜（periosteum）覆盖骨骼的外表面，营养并保护骨骼，并为生长和修复生产新的骨骼细胞。

在每端骨干与骨骺之间的区域被称为干骺端（metaphysis），是生长区或骺板（epiphyseal plate）。在整个童年期间，长骨的这一区域一直生长。当骨骼停止延伸时，这个区域就变得完全钙化，但仍保留可见的骨骺线（epiphyseal line，图19-5）。

在胳膊、腿、手和脚中都有长骨。其他的骨骼有：

- 扁骨（flat bone），例如颅骨、肋骨和肩胛骨等。

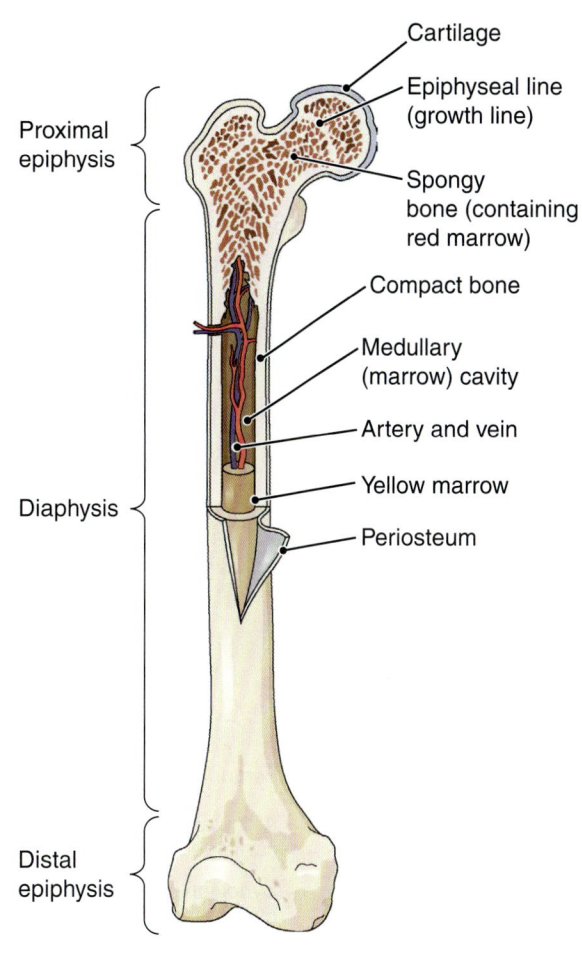

图 19-5　长骨的结构

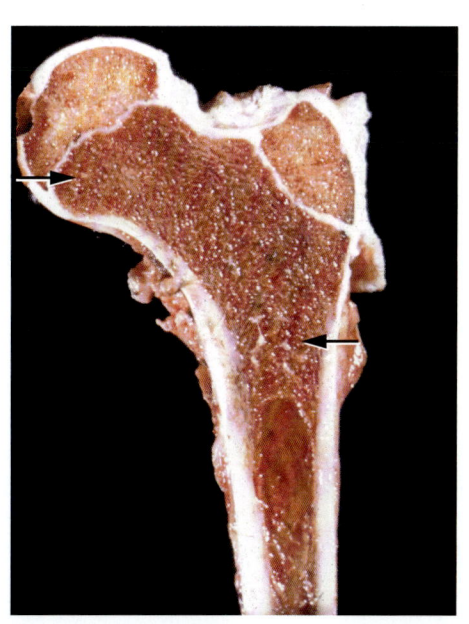

图 19-6　骨组织，纵切面。该长骨的骨骺（末端）具有紧凑骨的外层。组织的其余部分是海绵状（松质骨）骨，如箭头所示。横向的生长线也是可见的

- 短骨（short bone），例如腕骨和踝骨。
- 不规则骨（irregular bone），例如面骨、脊椎骨等。

关节

关节（joint 或 articulation）根据它们所容许的运动程度分类：

- 骨缝（suture）是由纤维结缔组织固定在一起的关节，如头骨之间的骨缝（图 19-2）。
- 骨联合（symphysis）使用纤维软骨连接的能够轻微移动的关节，例如脊椎骨之间（图 19-3）和耻骨之间的关节（图 19-4）。
- 滑膜关节（synovial joint）或可动关节（diarthrosis）是能够自由运动的关节。这种关节容许大范围的运动，将在第 20 章讨论。肌腱将肌肉附着于骨骼之上，能够在关节处产生运动。

可动关节会受到磨损（wear）和撕裂（tear），它们因此会有一些保护性特征（图 19-7）。可动关节腔包含滑膜液（synovial fluid），能够缓冲并润滑关节。滑膜液是关节腔内壁的滑膜产生的。关节连接骨骼的末端由软骨缓冲和保护，一个与骨膜连接的纤维囊包围着整个关节。滑膜关节由连接关节骨骼的韧带（ligament）稳定和加强。滑囊是一个充满滑膜液的小囊，处于肌腱（tendon）、韧带（ligament）和骨骼之间的应力点处，能够缓冲关节周围的区域。

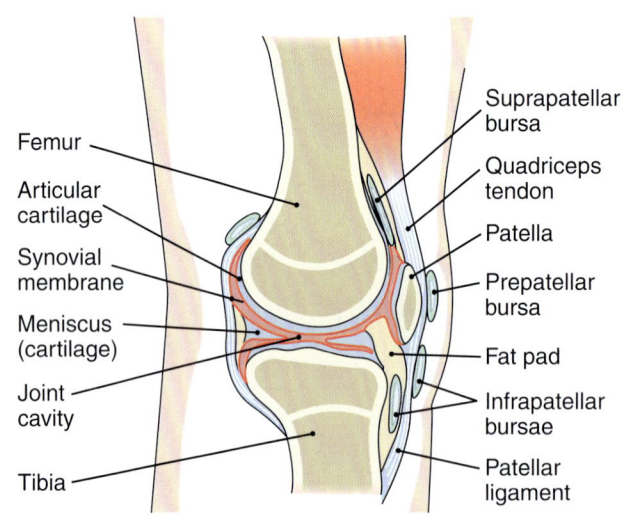

图 19-7　膝关节，矢状截面。膝关节是一个可自由移动的滑膜关节，也称为动关节。滑液充满关节腔。图中还示出了其他保护结构，例如软骨、关节囊、韧带和滑囊

Terminology　关键术语

正常结构与功能

acetabulum [ˌæsəˈtæbjʊləm]	髋臼，髋骨承载股骨头的骨窝（源自于拉丁语意为"醋"的单词，意为髋臼的形状像醋瓶）
articulation [ɑːˌtɪkjuˈleɪʃn]	关节，参见 joint；形容词形式为 articular
atlas [ˈætləs]	寰椎，第一颈椎（图 19-3）（词根：atlant/o）
axis [ˈæksɪs]	枢椎，第二颈椎（图 19-3）
bone [bəʊn]	骨骼，骨头，一种钙化的紧密的结缔组织；骨组织；也是由这种组织构成的骨架的个体单元（词根：oste/o）

Terminology 关键术语（续表）

bone marrow [bəun ˈmærəʊ]	骨髓，充满骨腔的软物质。黄骨髓充满长骨的中腔；血液细胞是在红骨髓中生成的，红骨髓位于海绵骨组织（词根：myel/o）
bursa [ˈbɜːsə]	滑囊，充满液体的囊，能够降低关节附件的摩擦阻力（词根：burs/o）
cartilage [ˈkɑːtilidʒ]	软骨，骨架、喉咙、气管和支气管中的一种紧密的结缔组织，是大多数骨组织的前体（词根：chondr/o）
diarthrosis [ˌdaiɑːˈθrəʊsis]	动关节，可以自由活动的关节；也被称为滑膜关节（synovial joint）（形容词 diarthrotic）
diaphysis [daiˈæfəsis]	骨干，长骨的骨体
epiphyseal plate [epiˈfisˈiəl]	骨骺板，长骨的生长区；位于干骺端，骨干与骨骺之间。当骨骼停止生长时，这一区域表现为骨骺线。也拼写为 epiphysial
epiphysis [iˈpifisis]	骨骺，长骨不规则形状的末端
ilium [ˈiliəm]	髂骨，髋骨的大喇叭形的上部（词根：ili/o）（形容词：iliac）
joint [dʒɔint]	关节，两块骨骼之间的接合部；也被称为 articulation（词根：arthr/o）
ligament [ˈligəmənt]	韧带，连接两块骨骼的强壮的结缔组织带
metaphysis [miˈtæfisis]	干骺端，长骨骨干与骨骺之间的区域；在发育期，是长骨的生长区
ossification [ɔsifiˈkeiʃən]	骨化，形成骨组织（源自于拉丁语 os，意为"骨骼"）
osteoblast [ˈɒstiəblæst]	成骨细胞，生产骨组织的细胞
osteoclast [ˈɒstiəklæst]	破骨细胞，破坏骨组织的细胞
osteocyte [ˈɒstiəsait]	骨细胞，成熟的骨骼细胞，营养并维护骨组织
pelvis [ˈpelvis]	骨盆躯，体下部的大骨环。由两块髋骨（ossa coxae）与骶骨和尾骨联合构成（复数：pelves）每块髋骨由三块骨骼构成，髂骨、坐骨（ischium）和耻骨（pubis）
periosteum [ˌperiˈɒstiəm]	骨膜，覆盖骨骼表面的纤维膜
resorption [riˈsɔːpʃən]	再吸收，将骨组织分解并吸收进入循环
skeleton [ˈskelitn]	骨骼，人体的骨骼由 206 块骨头构成（词根：skelet/o）。中轴骨部分（80块）有头骨、脊柱、肋骨和胸骨构成；附肢骨架（126块）由四肢、肩胛和骨盆构成
suture [ˈsuːtʃə(r)]	骨缝，固定关节，例如头盖骨之间的关节
symphysis [ˈsimfəsis]	骨联合，可轻微移动的关节
synovial fluid [saiˈnəʊviəl]	滑膜液，自由移动关节中包含的液体；也常用 synovia（词根：synov/i）
tendon [ˈtendən]	肌腱，连接肌肉与骨骼的结缔组织纤维带
thorax [ˈθɔːræks]	胸廓，躯干颈部与腹部之间的部分，由 12 对肋骨和胸骨构成

与骨架、骨骼和关节相关的词根

参见表 19-1 和 19-2

表 19-1　骨骼和关节的词根

词根	含义	示例	示例定义
oste/o	骨骼	osteopenia [ˌɒstiːəʊˈpiːniə]	骨质减少
myel/o	骨髓、脊髓	myeloid [ˈmaɪəlɔɪd]	骨髓的或像骨髓的
chondr/o	软骨	chondroblast [ˈkɒndrəʊblɑːst]	成软骨细胞
arthr/o	关节	arthrosis [ɑːˈθrəʊsɪs]	关节、影响关节的病症
synov/i	滑膜液、关节	asynovia [æsɪˈnəʊvaɪə]	滑液缺乏
burs/o	滑囊	peribursal [ˌperiːbɜːˈsæl]	滑囊周的

练习 19-1

填空。

1. Arthrodesis [ɑːθrəʊˈdiːsɪs] is fusion of a(n) _____.
2. Myelogenous [maɪəˈlɒdʒənəs] means originating in _____.
3. Osteolysis [ˌɒstiˈɒlɪsɪs] is destruction of _____.
4. A chondrocyte [ˈkʌdrɒsɪt] is a cell found in _____.
5. A bursolith [ˈbɜːsɒlɪθ] is a stone in a(n) _____.

定义下列单词。

6. arthrocentesis
   [ˌɑːθrəʊsənˈtiːzɪs] _____
7. myelopoiesis
   [ˌmaɪələʊpɔɪˈiːsɪs] _____
8. chondrodynia
   [ˌkɒndrəʊˈdɪniə] _____
9. osteoid
   [ˈɒstiɔɪd] _____
10. bursitis
    [ˌbɜːˈsaɪtɪs] _____
11. synovial
    [saɪˈnəʊvɪəl] _____

写出下列定义的单词。

12. inflammation of bone and bone marrow　_____
13. a bone-forming cell　_____
14. pertaining to or resembling cartilage　_____

练习 19-1 （续表）

15. any disease of a joint _____
16. inflammation of a synovial membrane _____
17. radiography of the spinal cord _____
18. incision of a bursa _____
19. tumor of bone marrow _____
20. instrument for examining the interior of a joint _____

单词 ostosis 意为"骨生长"。将该单词用作后缀，写出下列单词。

21. excess growth of bone _____
22. abnormal growth of bone _____

表 19-2 骨骼的词根

词根	含义	示例	示例定义
crani/o	颅骨，头颅	craniometry [ˌkreini'ɒmitri]	颅骨测量法
spondyl/o	脊椎	spondylolysis [spɒndi'lɒlisis]	椎骨脱离
vertebr/o	脊椎，脊柱	paravertebral [pɑː'reivɜːtibrəl]	椎旁的
rachi/o	脊柱	rachischisis [rə'kiskəsis]	脊柱裂
cost/o	肋骨	costochondral [kɒstəʊ'kɒndrəl]	肋骨及其软骨的
sacr/o	骶骨	presacral [p'resəkrəl]	骶骨前的
coccy, coccyg/o	尾骨	coccygeal* [kɒk'sidʒiəl]	尾骨的
pelvi/o	骨盆	pelviscope ['pelviskəʊp]	盆腔镜
ili/o	髂骨	iliopelvic [iliəʊ'pelvik]	髂盆的

* 注意拼写

练习 19-2

写出下列定义的形容词。

1. pertaining to (-al) the skull _____
2. pertaining to (-al) a rib _____
3. pertaining to (-ic) the pelvis _____
4. pertaining to (-ac) the ilium _____
5. pertaining to (-al) the spinal column _____

练习 19-2 （续表）

6. pertaining to (-al) the sacrum _____

定义下列单词。

7. craniotomy
   [ˌkreini'ɒtəmi] _____
8. prevertebral
   [pri'vɜ:tibrəl] _____
9. spondylodynia
   [ˌspɒndiləʊ'dinjə] _____
10. pelvimetry
    [pel'vimitri] _____

写出下列定义的单词。

11. fissure of the skull _____
12. above the pelvis _____
13. pertaining to the cranium and sacrum _____
14. pertaining to the sacrum and ilium _____
15. surgical puncture of the spine; spinal tap _____
16. surgical excision of a rib _____
17. plastic repair of a vertebra (use vertebr/o) _____
18. inflammation of the vertebrae (use spondyl/o) _____
19. around the sacrum _____
20. below the ribs _____
21. pertaining to the ilium and coccyx _____
22. excision of the coccyx _____

骨骼的临床表现

骨骼疾病通常会涉及周围的组织——韧带、肌腱和肌肉，并被作为肌肉骨骼系统（musculoskeletal system）疾病进行研究（肌肉系统将在第 20 章进行讨论）。聚焦于骨骼和肌肉系统疾病的医学专科是骨科（orthopedics）。物理治疗师和职业治疗师也必须了解这些系统（框 19-2）。框 19-3 给出了一些描述肌肉骨骼系统异常的丰富多彩的术语。

骨骼和关节的大多数异常会显示在简单的 X 线片上（图 19-8 为正常关节的 X 线片），放射性骨扫描、CT

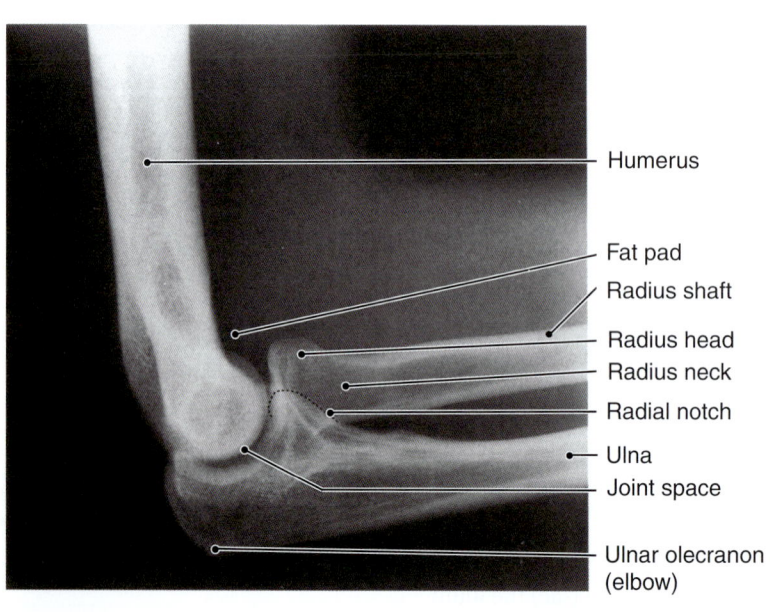

图 19-8 正常左肘关节的 X 线片，侧视图。肘突是近端尺骨扩大形成的肘部骨突出

框 19-2

健康职业
物理疗法的职业

物理疗法（physical therapy）能够恢复移动性并减轻关节炎或肌肉骨骼损伤的疼痛，从神经肌肉、心血管、肺和皮肤伤害事件中恢复的个体也是物理疗法的候选者。示例包括创伤性脑损伤（traumatic brain injury, TBI）、心肌梗死（myocardial infarction, MI）、慢性阻塞性肺疾病（chronic obstructive pulmonary disease, COPD）和烧伤。

物理治疗师（physical therapist, PT）与医生、护士、职业治疗师和其他专职医疗保健专业人员密切合作。一些人治疗广泛的疾病，而其他人关注特定的年龄组、医疗领域或运动医学。无论什么专科，物理治疗师都负责检查患者并开发个性化治疗计划。检查包括病史和力量、移动性、平衡、协调和耐力测试。治疗计划可以包括伸展和锻炼以改善移动性；热敷、冷敷和按摩以减轻疼痛；以及使用拐杖、假肢和轮椅。

物理治疗师助理（physical therapy assistant, PTA）在物理治疗师直接的监督下工作。物理治疗师助理负责实施预先建立的治疗计划，教导患者如何进行锻炼和使用设备，并将结果报告给物理治疗师。

虽然在美国许多执业物理治疗师有学士或硕士学位，现在大多数认可的物理治疗学校提供博士课程需要 3 年的研究生后教育。美国的物理治疗师通常从社区学院毕业并获得副学士学位，并且必须通过考试。物理治疗师和物理治疗师助理在医院和诊所执业，也可以访问家庭和学校。随着美国人口持续老龄化，对康复治疗的需求增加，物理治疗师就业前景良好。有关物理治疗职业的更多信息请联系美国物理治疗协会（American Physical Therapy Association），网址为 www.apta.org。

和核磁共振也经常使用。病症的指示是血液中钙和碱性磷酸酶（alkaline phosphatase）水平的变化，碱性磷酸酶是骨骼钙化所需要的一种酶。

感染

骨髓炎（osteomyelitis）是由进入伤口或血液中携带的脓液形成的细菌引起的骨髓炎症。通常血液丰富的长骨末端会被侵犯，然后感染会扩散到其他区域，例如骨髓，甚至关节。使用抗生素能够得到降低骨髓炎的威胁。结核病可能会扩散到骨骼，特别是四肢的长骨、手腕和脚踝的骨骼。

脊柱结核病被称为波特病（Pott disease）。被感染的椎骨被削弱并可能塌陷，引起疼痛、畸形和脊髓压力。只要菌株还没有产生耐药性而且患者没有被其他疾病所削弱，抗生素能够控制结核病。

骨折

骨折（fracture）是骨骼断裂，通常是外伤所致。骨折的影响取决于断裂的位置和严重性、相关的损伤、可能的并发症（例如感染）和成功的愈合（可能需要

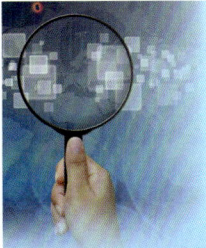

框 19-3

聚焦单词
名副其实

一些病症由非常描述性的术语命名。在骨科中，不同类型滑囊炎的名称是基于导致发炎的重复性压力。例如，"裁缝屁股（tailor's bottom）"涉及骨盆的坐骨，因为像裁缝那样坐着缝纫可能会引起坐骨发炎。"女佣膝盖（housemaid's knee）"来自于长时间用手和膝盖擦洗地板，"网球肘（tennis elbow）"是因为网球运动是其最常见起因而被命名。"学生肘（student's elbow）"起源于学习时倾斜着看书，尽管现在的学生以为在计算机上学习而更容易发生颈部和腕部问题。

术语 knock-knee（敲膝）描述膝外翻（genu valgum），膝盖异常靠近，两踝之间距离过宽。膝内翻（genu varum）正相反，两膝远离，脚跟靠近，由此产生了术语弓形腿 bowleg（弓形腿）。dowager's hump（贵妇的驼背）是由于骨质疏松症而出现在两肩之间的背部，在老年妇女中最常见。

支持手臂的神经根部的损伤可能导致手臂轻微外展并向内旋转，手腕弯曲且手指指向后方，这一状况被形象地命名为"侍者小费体位（waiter's tip position）"。"大力水手的肩膀（Popeye's shoulder）"是二头肌肌腱头部分类撕裂的迹象，受影响的手臂在肘关节弯曲的条件下外展时，上臂会显露出凸起——就像大力水手的肩膀。

供你参考
骨折的类型
框 19-3

骨折类型	说明
closed 闭合性	没有开发伤口的简单骨折
Colles 柯雷氏骨折	带有手向后位移的桡骨远端骨折
comminuted 粉碎性骨折	骨骼破裂或压碎的骨折
compression 压缩骨折	由骨骼两端受力引起的骨折，例如脊椎骨
greenstick 青枝骨折	骨骼一侧断裂，另一侧弯曲
impacted 嵌入骨折	骨骼的一个断片被打入另一个断片之中
oblique 斜形骨折	断裂发生在横跨骨骼的一个角度，通常是一个断片滑过另一个
open 开放性骨折	带有开放性伤口的骨折，或者断裂的骨骼穿过皮肤出来
Pott 波特骨折	有胫骨关节受损的腓骨远端骨折
spiral 螺旋形骨折	螺旋形或 S 形骨折，通常是扭伤引起的
Transverse 横向骨折	与骨骼长轴成直角的断裂

数月的时间）。在闭合性（closed）或简单骨折中，皮肤没有破裂。如果骨折带有皮肤伤口，则被称为开放性骨折（open fracture）。各种不同形式的骨折列在框 19-4，并显示在图 19-9 之中。

骨折的复位（reduction）是指将折断的骨骼重新对齐。如果不需要手术，复位被称为闭合性的；开放性复位需要手术将骨骼置于适当的位置。为确保适当愈合，可能需要钢钉（rod）、钢板（plate）或螺丝钉（screw）。为了在愈合期间固定骨骼，通常需要夹板（splint）或管型石膏夹（cast）。牵引（traction）是指在愈合期间使用滑轮和重物来维持骨折的骨骼对准。牵引装置可以附接到皮肤上，或通过销或丝线附接于骨骼本身。

代谢性骨骼疾病

骨质疏松（osteoporosis）是导致骨骼弱化的骨质损失（图 19-10）。绝经后雌性激素的下降使得大多数超过 50 岁的女性易受此疾病的影响。预防骨质疏松的方法包括健康的饮食、服用钙和维生素 D，以及参加定期的负重锻炼，例如步行、跑步、有氧运动（aerobics）和重量训练。这些锻炼能够刺激骨骼生长，也对预防跌倒所必需的平衡和肌肉力量有所贡献。准更年期激素替代疗法（hormone replacement therapy，HRT）能够预防骨质疏松，但是出于安全性的考虑，这种疗法正在被重新评估。一些药物能够降低骨骼再吸收和提高骨密度，包括二磷酸盐（bisphonate）和第 15 章讨论过的选择性雌激素受体调节剂（selective estrogen receptor modulator，SERM）。

骨质疏松要使用双能 X 线吸收测量（dual-energy x-ray absorptiometry，DEXA）扫描进行诊断和监测，双能 X 线吸收测量扫描是一种测量骨骼无机物密度（bone mineral density，BMD）的成像技术。诊断术语骨质减少（osteopenia）是指骨密度低于平均值，这并不被认为是异常的。骨质减少可能会发展成为骨质疏松，但不一定需要治疗。

其他可能导致骨质疏松的情况包括营养不良、不被使用（disuse，如偏瘫和在石膏管中固定）和肾上

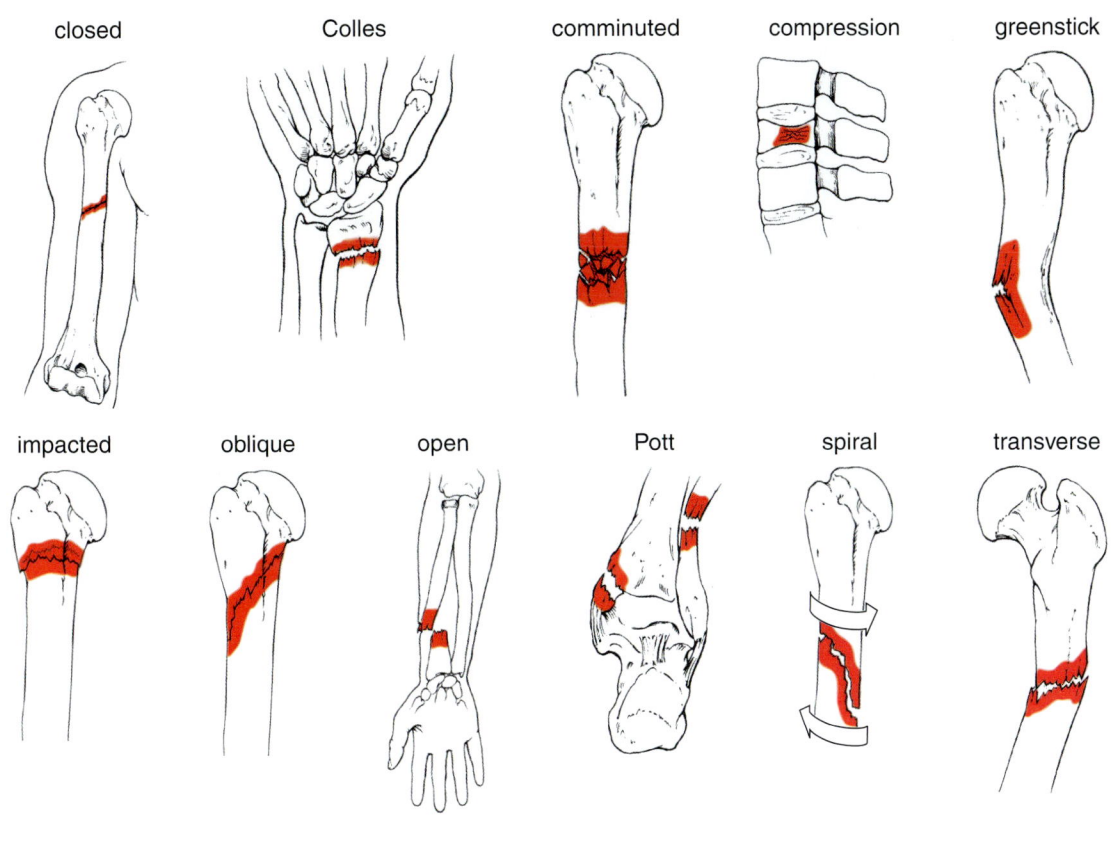

图 19-9 骨折的类型

腺皮质激素过多。甲状旁腺过于活跃也会导致骨质疏松，因为甲状旁腺激素会使钙从骨骼中释放提高血液的钙水平。特定的药物、吸烟、缺乏锻炼和大量摄入酒精、咖啡因和蛋白质也会促进骨质疏松的发展。

在骨软化症（osteomalacia）中，因为钙盐形成的减少发生工作组软化。可能的起因包括缺乏维生素 D、肾病、肝病和特定的肠道疾病。当骨软化症发生在儿童时，该疾病被称为软骨病（rickets，图 19-11）。软骨病通常是由缺乏维生素 D 引起的。

畸形性骨炎（osteitis deformans）被称为佩吉特病（Paget disease），是一种骨骼畸形过度生长变厚的老年性疾病（图 19-12）。这种疾病会导致长骨成弓形和扁骨扭曲，例如头盖骨。畸形性骨炎通常涉及中轴骨的骨骼，引起疼痛、骨折和听力损失。随着时间发展，可能会有神经系统的症状、心力衰竭和骨癌的倾向。

肿瘤

骨原性肉瘤（osteogenic sarcoma）或骨肉瘤（osteosarcoma）最常见于骨骼的生长区，特别是膝盖周围，这是一种高度恶性的肿瘤，通常需要截肢（amputation），这种肿瘤通常会转移到肺部。

软骨肉瘤（chondrosarcoma）通常发生在中年。如其名称所示，这种肿瘤发生于软骨。软骨肉瘤可能需要截肢，而且通常会转移到肺部。

在恶性骨骼肿瘤病例中，早期手术切除对预防扩散非常重要。骨骼肿瘤的症状是疼痛、容易骨折和血清钙和碱性磷酸酶（alkaline phosphatase）水平的

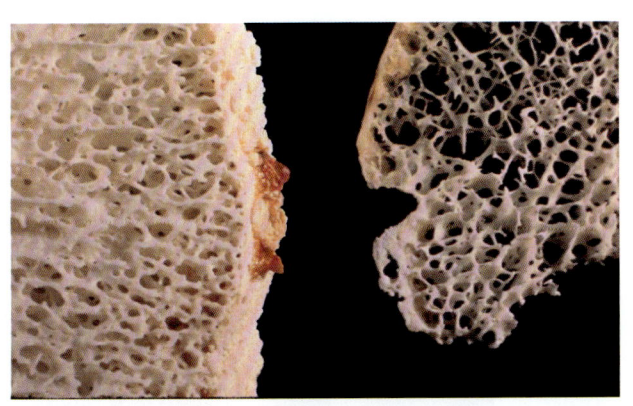

图 19-10 骨质疏松症。图中显示的股骨头骨质疏松症（右）与正常对照（左）的对比

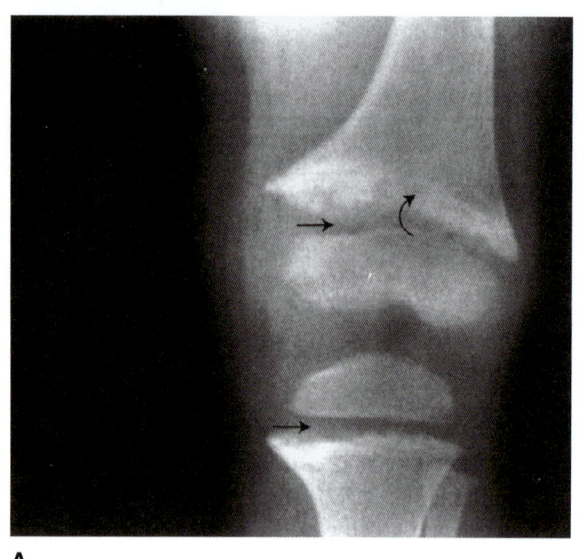
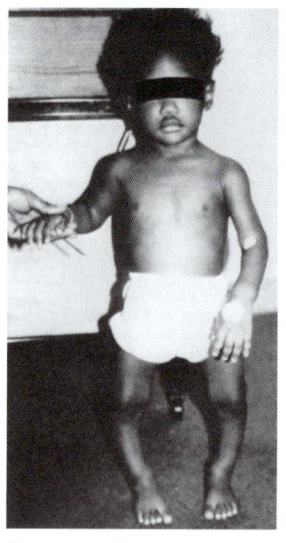

图 19-11 软骨病。A. 左膝关节的X线成像显示骨的生长区扩大（箭头）；B. 显示软骨病的幼儿

上升。除了原发性肿瘤，身体其他部位的肿瘤常常会转移到骨骼，最常见的是转移到脊柱。

关节疾病

关节疾病的一些起因包括先天畸形、关节或邻近骨骼的感染、导致变性的伤害和因丧失供血所致的坏死。关节炎（arthritis）这一术语被广泛地用于指任何关节的炎症，基于这一原因，关节炎可以分为几类。

关节炎

最常见的关节炎是骨关节炎（osteoarthritis，OA）或退行性关节病（degenerative joint disease，DJD）（图 19-13）。这种疾病涉及因磨损和撕裂造成的关节软骨的逐渐退化变性。骨关节炎的发病诱因是年龄、遗传、受伤、先天骨骼畸形和内分泌失调，通常发生在中年和中年以后，涉及承重关节，如膝、髋和手指关节。X线片显示关节腔狭窄和骨骼增厚。软骨可能破裂并脱离，引起关节炎并使下面的骨骼暴露。

骨关节炎治疗需要用镇痛剂缓解疼痛，使用皮质激素抗炎药和非甾体抗炎药，以及物理疗法。可以将类固醇直接注射到发炎的关节中，但因为可能会最终引起软骨损伤，1年内只能每隔几个月注射一次。治疗还可能包括通过关节穿刺术（arthrocentesis）从关节中抽出过多的液体。使用冰敷、抬升和针刺也有助于缓解疼痛。

风湿性关节炎（rheumatoid arthritis，RA）是全身性关节炎性疾病，通常发生于年轻的女性。确切的起因不明，可能涉及免疫反应。一组被称为类风湿因子（rheumatoid factor）的抗体常常出现在血液中，但它们并不总是风湿性关节炎特异性的，也会发生在其他全身性疾病之中。关节腔内部的滑囊膜会有增生，这种增生会覆盖并破坏关节软骨，滑膜液会积累，引起关节肿胀（图 19-14）。下面的骨骼会变性，最终

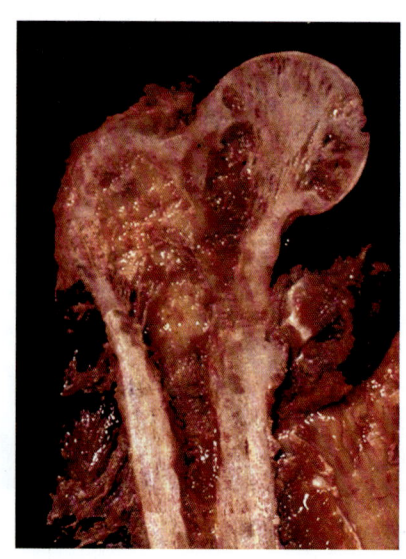

图 19-12 佩吉特病。图中股骨的一部分骨骺过度生长

引起关节强直（ankylosis）治疗包括休息、物理疗法、镇痛和抗炎药物。

痛风（gout）是血液中尿酸水平升高引起的，尿酸的盐会沉积在关节中。这种疾病通常发生于中年男性，并且疼痛几乎总是涉及大脚趾根部。痛风可能是原发性代谢紊乱所致，或者是其他疾病的继发影响，例如肾病。治疗需要使用抑制尿酸形成或提升其排泄的药物。

关节修复

骨科医生（orthopedist）使用一种被称为关节镜（arthroscope）的内窥镜检查关节内部，并在需要时进行手术修复（图 19-15）。使用关节镜可以切除或改造关节软骨，修复或置换肌腱。

如果保守治疗不能缓解，骨科医生可能建议做关节成形术（arthroplasty）。这一术语广义为任何关节改造，但通常用于全部或部分关节置换。髋、膝、肩和其他关节都可以用假体置换，以消除疼痛和恢复

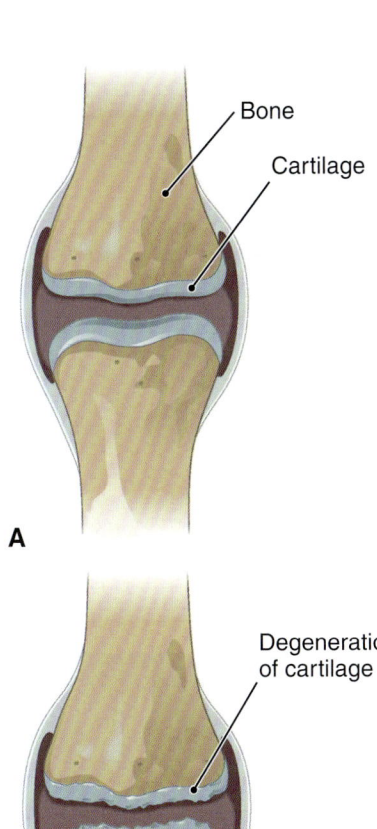

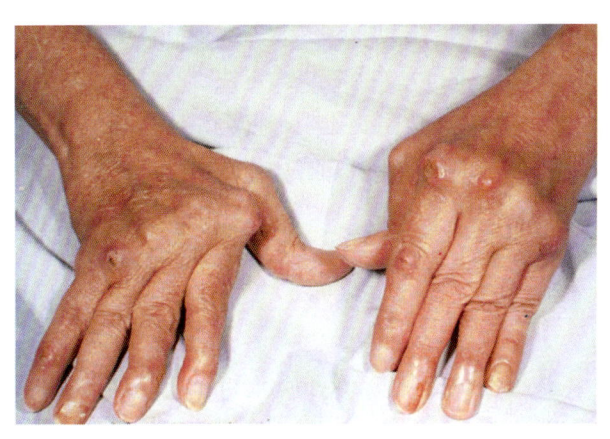

图 19-14 晚期类风湿性关节炎。手显示出关节肿胀和手指偏移

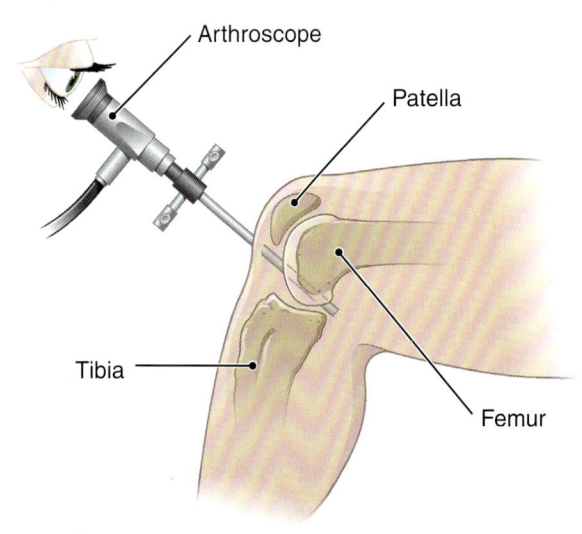

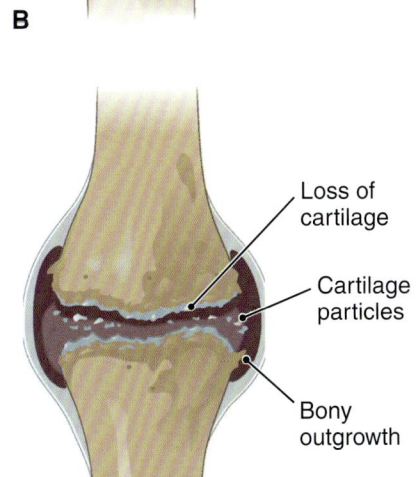

图 19-13 骨关节炎。A. 正常关节；B. 骨关节炎的早期阶段。C. 疾病的晚期

图 19-15 膝关节镜检查。将关节镜（一种类型的内窥镜）插入在股骨末端的突出部之间以观察膝盖的后部

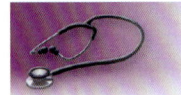

临床观点

框 19-5

关节成形术：为更好生活的仿生部件

自从 1960 年代早期第一例完全髋关节置换术患者以来，已经成功进行了数百万关节置换术，或称为关节成形术（arthroplasty）。大多数关节成形术是为了在尝试了减轻体重、物理疗法和药物疗法之后，使患有骨关节炎或其他慢性退行性骨骼疾病的老年人减轻关节疼痛。最常见的是修复髋关节和膝关节，在美国每年要做 30 万例髋关节成形术和 50 万例膝关节置换。骨科医生也能够置换肩、肘、腕、手、踝和足关节。

人造的或假体（prosthetic）关节被设计得坚固、无毒、耐腐蚀（corrosion-resistant）并且能够牢固地与患者结合。现在，计算机控制的机器能够用比过去更短的时间和更低的价格生产出个性化的人造关节。类似于那些用于完全髋关节置换的球窝关节假体，由一个杯、一个球和一根拉杆组成。杯置换髋臼（acetabulum），用螺丝钉或胶固定在骨盆上。杯通常是塑料的，但也可以制成更为持久耐用的陶瓷或金属的。球由金属或陶瓷制成，置换股骨头，并连接在置换了股骨干的拉杆上。拉杆是由不同的金属合金制成的，通常用胶固定。被设计得能够促进骨骼生长进入其中的拉杆常被用于更年轻、更活跃的患者，因为这种拉杆被认为能够更持久地保持牢固的连接。

直到最近，关节成形术很少用于年轻人，因为假体的生命周期大约只有 10 年。现在的材料和手术技术能够将这一时间延长到 20 年或更长，经受关节成形术的年轻人在术后需要的置换就更少了。这一改进非常重要，因为年轻成年人运动相关的关节受伤事件越来越多了。

活动性，如框 19-5 所示。

缓解疼痛和为关节提供稳定性的最终替代办法是关节固定术（arthrodesis），这会导致完全丧失关节活动性。医生使用钢钉和骨移植物固定关节，并使骨骼表面粘连。

脊柱疾病

强直性脊柱炎（ankylosing spondylitis）是一种主要发生在男性的脊柱疾病。关节软骨被破坏，椎骨之间的椎间盘钙化并且骨骼发生融合（ankylosis）（图 19-16）。病变起始于低位的脊柱并向上发展，会限制活动性。

脊椎前移（spondylolisthesis）是指一块椎骨在其下面的椎骨上向前滑动（-listhesis，意为"滑动"）（图 19-17）。继续发展就会形成椎骨脱离（spondylolysis），正常稳定椎骨的关节结构发生变性。脊椎前移最常发生于腰部承重的脊柱，引起后背疼痛，有时因刺激脊髓神经根导致腿部疼痛。

椎间盘突出

在椎间盘突出（herniated disk）病例中（图 19-18），椎间盘的中心块（髓核，nucleus pulposus）通过椎间盘的弱化外环（纤维环，annulus fibrosus）突出到椎管中。这通常发生在脊柱的腰骶或颈部区域，是受伤或提重物所致。突出或滑动的椎间盘对脊髓或脊髓神经造成压力，常常会引起坐骨神经痛（sciatica）。

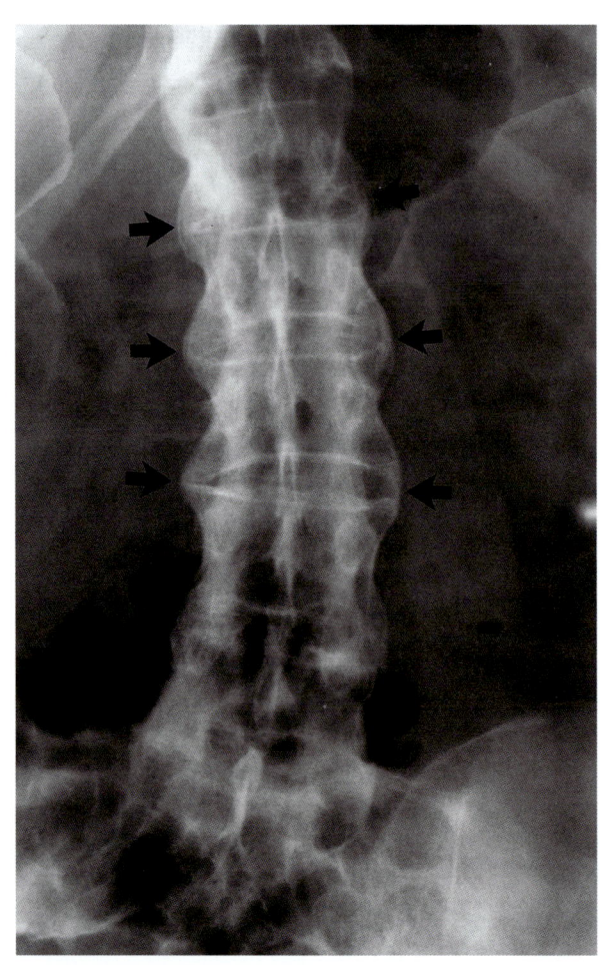

图 19-16 强直性脊柱炎。正面腰部 X 线片显示骨生成正在桥接椎间盘空间（箭头）并融合椎骨

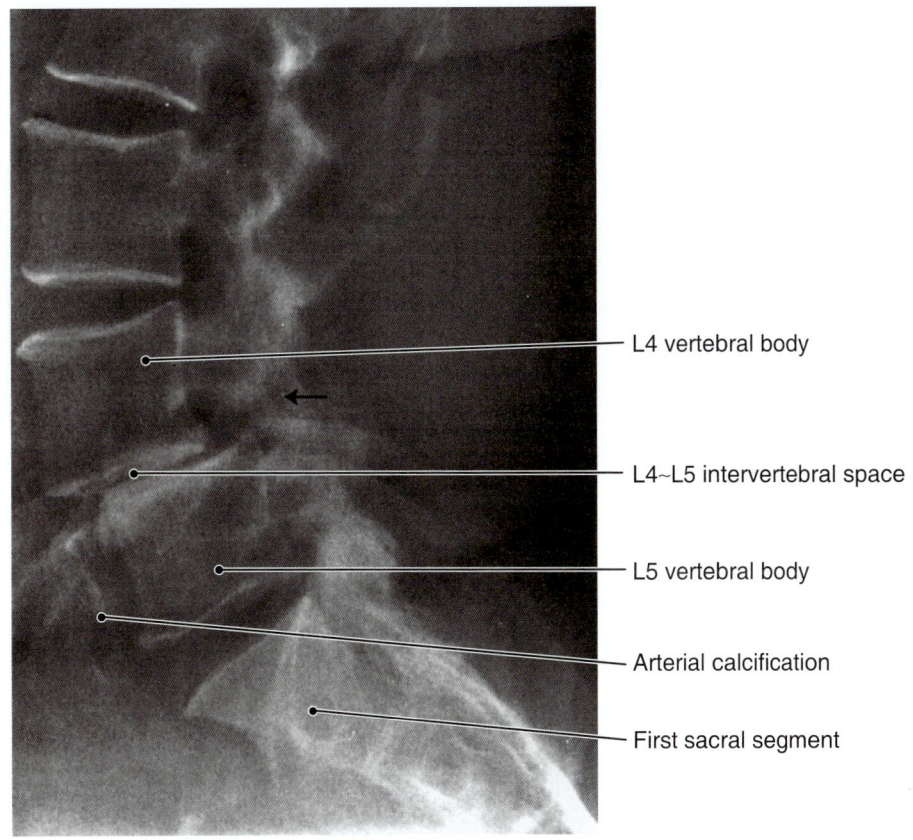

图 19-17　**脊椎前移**。L4 椎体在 L5 上向前滑动，L4~L5 椎间盘空间明显变窄

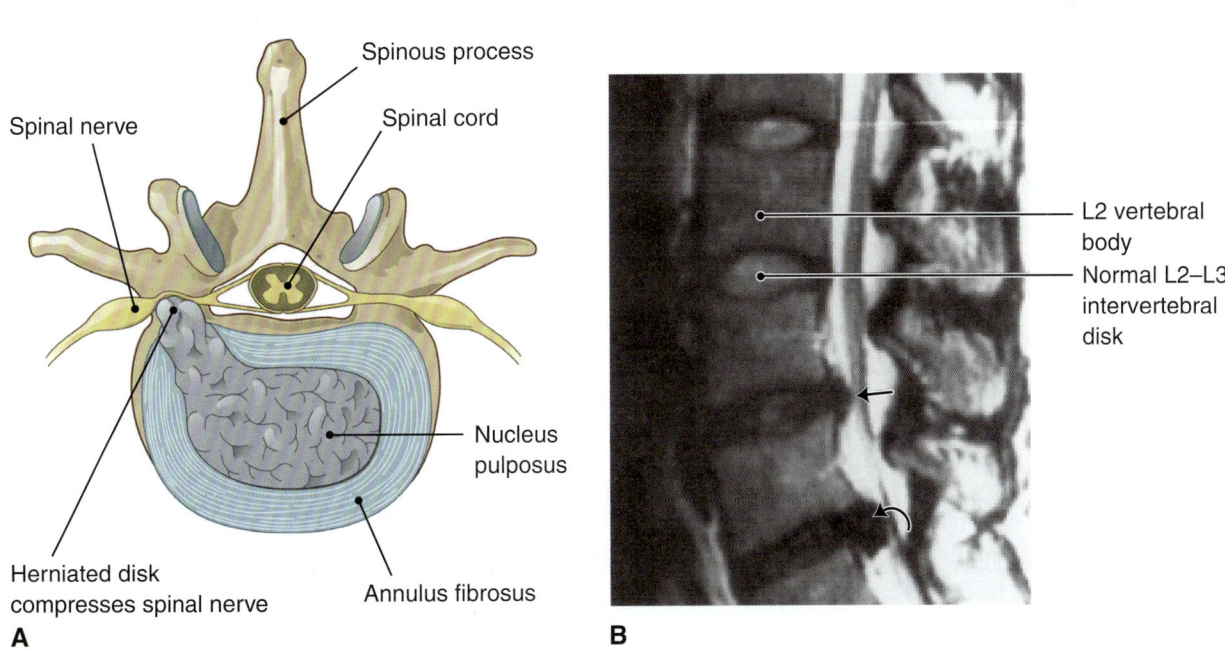

图 19-18　**椎间盘突出**。A. 椎间盘的中心块突出进入椎管，对脊神经产生压力；B. 腰椎的磁共振图像矢状切面显示在多层次的椎间盘突出。在 L3~L4 椎间盘（直箭头）隆起，L4~L5 腰椎间盘挤出（弯曲的箭头）

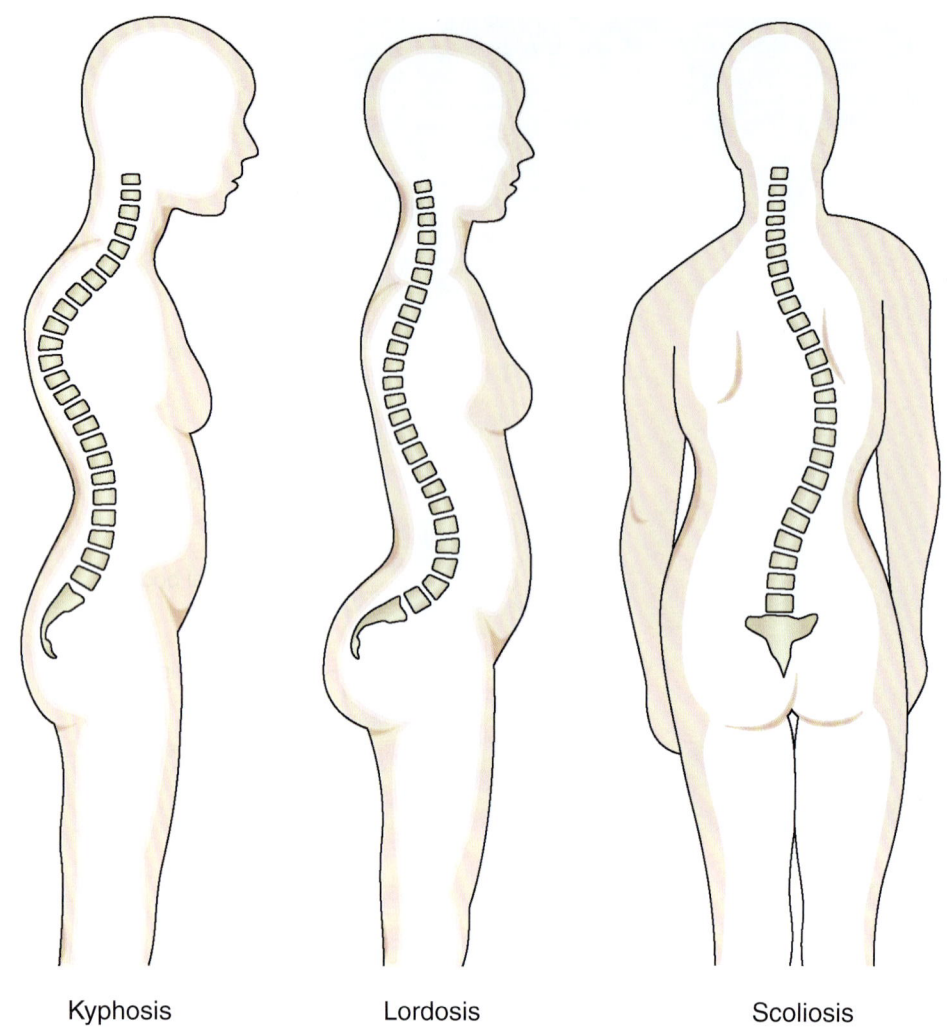

Kyphosis　　　　　Lordosis　　　　　Scoliosis

图 19-19　脊柱弯曲。脊柱后凸是胸部弯曲过大；脊柱前凸是腰部弯曲过大；脊柱侧弯是任何区域的侧向弯曲

背部肌肉会产生痉挛，可能导致残疾。

椎间盘突出可以通过脊髓造影术（myelography）、CT 扫描、核磁共振和神经肌肉测试（neuromuscular test）进行诊断。治疗包括卧床休息和降低疼痛、肌肉痉挛和炎症的药物，随后是一个加强核心和相关肌肉的锻炼计划。对严重的病例，可能需要执行切除椎间盘的椎间盘切除术（diskectomy），有时还要用骨移植物做椎骨融合以稳定脊椎。使用微创手术技术（在放大镜下通过微小的切口进行手术），现在可以精确地切除突出的椎间盘组织，而不是整个椎间盘。

脊柱弯曲

脊柱有四个正常的弯曲——两个在颈部和腰部向前，两个在胸部和骶部向后（图 19-3）。这些弯曲的任何夸大或偏离被称为脊柱弯曲（curvature of the spine）。图 19-19 给出了三类常见的脊柱弯曲：

- 脊柱后凸（kyphosis）是夸大的胸部弯曲，被通俗地称为"驼背（hunchback）"。
- 脊柱前弯（lordosis）是夸大的腰部弯曲，被通俗地称为"塌背（swayback）"。
- 脊柱侧弯（scoliosis）是任何部位的侧向弯曲。

脊柱弯曲可能是先天的，也可能是因肌肉虚弱、偏瘫、姿态不良、关节问题、椎间盘变性、极度肥胖或者脊髓结核、软骨病或骨质疏松等疾病所致。极度严重的病例可能引起疼痛、呼吸问题或退行性变化。

童年期拉伸脊柱可能有助于矫正脊柱弯曲。如果需要手术，椎骨融合以及骨移植和植入物被用于稳定脊柱。目前，医生有时可以借助内窥镜进行这些矫正。

Terminology 关键术语

疾病

ankylosing spondylitis [ˌæŋkiˈləʊzɪŋ ˌspɒndɪˈlaɪtɪs]	强直性脊柱炎，涉及脊柱关节和周围软组织的慢性、进行性炎性疾病，最常见于年轻男性；也被称为类风湿性脊柱炎（rheumatoid spondylitis）
ankylosis [ˌæŋkɪˈləʊsɪs]	关节强直，关节固定不能活动
arthritis [ɑːˈθraɪtɪs]	关节炎，关节的炎症
chondrosarcoma [ˌkɒndrəʊsɑːˈkəʊmə]	软骨肉瘤，软骨的恶性肿瘤
curvature of the spine [ˈkɜːvətʃə(r)]	脊柱弯曲，夸大的脊柱弯曲，例如脊柱侧弯（scoliosis）、脊柱前弯（lordosis）和脊柱后凸（kyphosis）（图19-19）
degenerative joint disease (DJD)	退行性关节疾病，骨关节炎，参见下面的osteoarthritis
fracture [ˈfræktʃə(r)]	骨折，骨骼断裂。在闭合性或简单骨折中，断裂的骨骼没有穿透皮肤；在开放性骨折中，会伴有皮肤伤口（图19-9）
gout [ɡaʊt]	痛风，一种急性关节炎，通常起始于膝盖或足部，是尿酸盐在关节中积累引起的
herniated disk [ˈhɜːnieɪtɪd]	椎间盘突出，椎间盘的中心块（髓核，nucleus pulposus）通过椎间盘的弱化外环（纤维环annulus fibrosus）突出到椎管中；又称为破裂的或"滑动"椎间盘（ruptured or "slipped" disk）
kyphosis [kaɪˈfəʊsɪs]	脊柱后凸，胸部脊柱的夸大弯曲；俗称为驼背（hunchback, humpback，图19-19）
lordosis [lɔːˈdəʊsɪs]	脊柱前弯，腰部脊柱的夸大弯曲；俗称为塌背（swayback，图19-19）
osteoarthritis (OA) [ˌɒstiəʊɑːˈθraɪtɪs]	骨关节炎，关节软骨的进行性退化变质，在关节内及周围会长出新的骨骼和软组织；是最常见的关节炎类型，因磨损、受伤或疾病所致；也被称为退行性关节疾病（degenerative joint disease，DJD）
osteogenic sarcoma [ˌɒstiəʊˈdʒenɪk sɑːˈkəʊmə]	骨原性肉瘤，恶性骨骼肿瘤；又称为骨肉瘤（osteosarcoma）
osteomalacia [ˌɒstiəʊməˈleɪʃə]	骨软化症，因缺乏维生素D或其他疾病引起的骨骼软化和弱化
osteomyelitis [ˌɒstiəʊˌmaɪəˈlaɪtɪs]	骨髓炎，因感染，通常是细菌感染引起的骨骼和骨髓炎症
osteopenia [ˌɒstiːəʊˈpiːniə]	骨质减少，骨密度低于平均水平，可能预示骨质疏松
osteoporosis [ˌɒstiəʊpəˈrəʊsɪs]	骨质疏松症，以骨密度降低为特征的病症，最常见于绝经后的白人女性；发病诱因包括饮食不良、缺少活动和雌激素水平低
Paget disease	佩吉特病，老年人的骨骼疾病，特点是骨骼增厚并变形，长骨成弓形；也被称为畸形性骨炎（osteitis deformans）
Pott disease	波特病，椎骨的炎症，通常是结核病引起的
rheumatoid arthritis (RA) [ˈruːmətɔɪd]	风湿性关节炎，起因不明的慢性自身免疫性疾病，导致外围关节及相关结构的炎症；女性患者多于男性患者
rheumatoid factor	类风湿因子，风湿性关节炎和其他全身性疾病患者血液中发现的一组抗体

Terminology	关键术语（续表）
rickets ['rikits]	软骨病，儿童骨形成不良，通常是缺乏维生素 D 引起的
sciatica [sai'ætikə]	坐骨神经痛，腿部延坐骨神经走向的严重疼痛，通常与脊髓神经根刺激相关
scoliosis [ˌskəʊli'əʊsis]	脊柱侧弯，任意部位的脊柱侧向弯曲（图 19-19）
spondylolisthesis [spɒndiləʊlis'θi:sis]	脊柱前移，一块椎骨在另一块椎骨上的前向位移（-listhesis 意为"滑动"）
spondylolysis [spɒndi'lɒlisis]	椎骨脱离，椎骨关节部分的变性，造成脊柱扭曲，特别是腰部

治疗

alkaline phosphatase ['ælkəlin 'fɒsfəteis]	碱性磷酸酶，骨形成所需要的一种酶；这种酶的血清活性可用于诊断
arthrocentesis [ɑ:θrəʊ'səntizis]	关节穿刺术，通过针头穿刺从关节中吸出液体
arthrodesis [ɑ:θ'rəʊdi:sis]	关节融合术，手术固定关节；人工关节强直
arthroplasty ['ɑ:zrəˌplæsti]	关节成形术，使用假体或完全置换关节
arthroscopy [ɑ:'θrɒskəpi]	关节镜检查，用内窥镜检查关节内部或在关节做手术（图 19-14）；使用的设备是关节镜（arthroscope）
diskectomy [dis'kektəmi]	椎间盘切除术，手术切除突出的椎间盘；也拼写为 discectomy
orthopedics [ˌɔ:θə'pi:diks]	骨科，研究和治疗骨骼、肌肉及其相关结构的疾病的医学专科；字面的含义是"直立的"（ortho）"儿童"（ped）；也拼写为 orthopaedics
reduction of a fracture	骨折复位，将断裂的骨骼恢复原位；可能是闭合性的（不需要手术）或开放性的（需要手术）
traction ['trækʃn]	牵引，拉伸的过程，例如在治疗颈椎受伤时牵引头部

药物

antiinflammatory agent	抗炎药，减轻炎症的药物，包括甾体和非甾抗炎药（NSAID）
bisphosphonate [bis'fɒsfəʊneit]	双磷酸盐，用于预防和治疗骨质疏松的药物；通过减少骨转换提高骨密度。例如阿仑膦酸钠（alendronate）、利塞膦酸钠（risedronate）和伊班膦酸钠（ibandronate）
nonsteroidal antiinflammatory drug (NSAID)	非甾抗炎药，不是甾体化合物减轻炎症的药物，包括阿司匹林、布洛芬和其他前列腺素阻滞剂，前列腺素是自然产生的促进炎症的物质
selective estrogen receptor modulator (SERM)	选择性雌激素受体调节剂，作用于雌激素受体的药物。雷洛昔芬（raloxifene）被用于预防绝经后骨质疏松。其他选择性雌激素受体调节剂被用于预防和治疗对雌激素敏感的乳腺癌

Terminology 补充术语

正常结构与功能

annulus fibrosus [ˈænjʊləs faiˈbrəʊsəs]	纤维环，椎间盘外部环样的部分（图 19-17）
calvaria [kælˈveəriə]	颅盖，头颅的圆顶状上部
coxa [ˈkɒksə]	髋，髋部
cruciate ligaments [ˈkruːʃieit]	十字韧带，在膝关节交叉处连接胫骨和腓骨的韧带。有前十字韧带（anterior cruciate ligament，ACL）和后十字韧带（posterior cruciate ligament，PCL）。Cruciate 意为"形状像十字"
genu [ˈdʒenʊː]	膝，膝部
glenoid cavity [ˈgliːnɔid]	肩胛盂，肩胛骨的骨窝，与肱骨头形成关节
hallux [ˈhæləks]	蹰趾，大脚趾
malleolus [məˈliːələs]	踝，胫骨和腓骨在脚踝两侧的突出部分
meniscus [məˈniskəs]	半月板，特定关节中的半月形软骨盘，例如在膝关节。在膝部，内侧半月板和外侧半月板分离胫骨和股骨；复数形式为 menisci；meniscus 意为"新月"
nucleus pulposus [ˌnjuːkliəs pʌlˈpəʊsəs]	髓核，椎间盘的中心块（图 19-17）
olecranon [əʊˈlekrənɒn]	肘突，尺骨形成的肘部突起
os [ɒs]	骨（拉丁语）；复数形式为 ossa
osseous [ˈɒsiəs]	骨的，与骨骼相关的
symphysis pubis [ˈsimfəsis ˈpjuːbis]	耻骨联合，前骨盆关节，由两块耻骨联合构成（图 19-4）；也常用 pubic symphysis

* 参见框 19-5 骨标记列表

症状与病症

achondroplasia [eiˌkɒndrəˈpleiʒə]	软骨发育不全，长骨生长区的软骨生长减少，导致侏儒症；是一种遗传性疾病
Baker cyst	贝克氏囊肿，因慢性刺激所致的滑囊膨胀和滑膜液过多造成的膝关节囊肿
bunion [ˈbʌnjən]	滑囊肿，大脚趾跖骨关节的炎症和肿大，通常带有大脚趾朝向其他脚趾的位移
bursitis [ˌbɜːˈsaitis]	滑囊炎，滑囊的炎症，起因包括受伤、刺激和关节疾病；肩、髋、肘和膝关节是常见的发病部位
carpal tunnel syndrome [ˌkɑːpl ˈtʌnl]	腕管综合征，正中神经在通过腕骨形成的隧道时出生的压力引起手的麻木和虚弱
chondroma [kɒnˈdrəʊmə]	软骨瘤，一种软骨的良性肿瘤
Ewing tumor	尤文瘤，一种通常发生于 5~15 岁儿童的骨骼肿瘤。这种肿瘤起始于一块骨骼的骨干，并迅速扩散到其他骨骼。放疗可能有效，但会复发。也被称为尤文肉瘤（Ewing sarcoma）

Terminology 补充术语（续表）

exostosis [ˌeksɒs'təʊsis]	外生骨疣，从骨骼表面生出的骨质赘生物
giant cell tumor	骨巨细胞瘤，通常发生于儿童和青年人的骨骼肿瘤。骨骼的两端被大量不会转移的物质破坏，通常在膝部
hammertoe ['hæmətəʊ]	槌状趾，趾关节位置改变，以致于脚趾呈现爪状外观，第一关节向上突出，在步行时产生刺激和疼痛
hallux valgus ['hæləks 'vælgəs]	跚趾外翻，涉及大脚趾在跖关节横向位移的痛苦病症。还会有跖骨头扩大和囊肿形成
Heberden nodes	希伯登骨节，骨关节炎患者手指远端骨节软骨中形成的小硬结
hemarthrosis [heˈmɑːθrəʊsis]	关节出血，关节腔出血
Legg-Calvé-Perthes disease leg	股骨头缺血性坏死病腿，股骨近端的生长中心的变性（骨软骨病，osteochondrosis）。骨骼最终能够恢复，但可能会有畸形和虚弱。最常见于青年男性
myeloma [ˌmaiəˈləʊmə]	骨髓瘤，一种骨髓中造血细胞的癌症（参见第 10 章）
neurogenic arthropathy [njʊərəʊˈdʒenik ɑːˈθrɔpəθi]	神经性关节病，神经刺激受损引起的退行性关节疾病；最常见的起因是糖尿病；也被称为夏科氏关节病（Charcot arthropathy）
Osgood-Schlatter disease	胫骨粗隆骨软骨病，胫骨近端的生长中心的变性（骨软骨病），在膝盖处会引起疼痛和肌腱炎
Osteochondroma [ˌɒstiəʊkɒnˈdrəʊmə]	骨软骨瘤，由骨骼和软骨构成的良性肿瘤
osteochondrosis [ˌɒstiəʊkɒnˈdrəʊsis]	骨软骨病，儿童骨骼生长中心的疾病，组织变性后会发生再钙化
osteodystrophy [ˌɒstiˈɔːdistrəʊfi]	骨营养不良，骨骼发育异常
osteogenesis imperfect (OI) [ˌɒstiəˈdʒenəsis ˌimpəˈfektə]	成骨不良症，一种会导致形成容易断裂的脆骨的遗传性疾病。胶原合成有缺陷，胶原是结缔组织中的主要结构性蛋白质
osteoma [ˌɒstiˈəʊmə]	骨瘤，一种通常较小且局限的良性骨骼肿瘤
Reiter syndrome	赖特综合征，慢性多发性关节炎，通常影响年轻男性；发生于细菌感染之后，常见于 HIV 感染者；可能会涉及眼睛和泌尿生殖系统
spondylosis [spɒndiˈləʊsis]	椎关节强直，脊椎变形并强直，会导致对脊髓和脊髓神经根的压力；通常被用于指任何脊柱退行性损伤
subluxation [sʌblʌkˈseiʃən]	半脱位，部分脱位
talipes [ˈtælipiːz]	畸形足，足部畸形，特别是先天性的；也被称为马蹄内翻足（clubfoot）
valgus [ˈvælgəs]	外翻，向外弯曲
varus [ˈveərəs]	内翻，向内弯曲
von Recklinghausen disease	范 - 瑞克林豪森氏病，由甲状旁腺激素增加引起的骨组织丢失；骨骼变得脱钙、变形并容易断裂

Terminology 补充术语（续表）

诊断与治疗

allograft [ˌæləˈgrɑːft]	同种异体移植，相同物种但不同遗传组成的个体之间的组织移植；也常用同种移植（homograft）、同种异基因移植（allogeneic graft）（参见 autograft）
arthroclasia [ɑːθrəʊˈkleizjə]	关节活动术，手术打破强直的关节，以提供活动性
aspiration [ˌæspəˈreiʃn]	吸出，通过吸力移除，例如将液体从体腔中吸出
autograft [ˈɔːtəʊgrɑːft]	自体移植，从接受移植物的人身体上或身体内的部位取出的组织移植；也常用同体移植（autologous graft，参见 allograft）
chondroitin [kənˈdrɔitin]	软骨素，在结缔组织中发现的一种复杂的多糖；通常与氨基葡萄糖（glucosamine）一起被用作膳食补充剂，治疗关节疼痛
glucosamine [gluːkəʊˈsæmiːn]	氨基葡萄糖，一种被用于治疗关节疼痛的膳食补充剂
goniometer [ˌgəʊniˈɒmitə]	测角仪，一种测量关节角度和运动的设备（词根：goni/o 意为"角度"）
iontophoresis [aiɒntəfəˈriːsis]	离子电渗疗法，通过电流将给定药物的离子引入组织；用于治疗肌肉骨骼疾病
laminectomy [ˌlæmiˈnektəmi]	椎板切除术，切除椎骨的后弓（椎板，lamina）
meniscectomy [miʊiˈsektəmi]	半月板切除术，手术切除膝关节的新月形软骨（半月板）
myelogram [ˈmaiələʊgræm]	骨髓 X 线造影，注射不透射线染料后的脊柱 X 线片；被用于评估椎间盘突出
osteoplasty [ˈɒstiəplæsti]	骨整形术，从关节中刮除受损的骨骼
prosthesis [prɒsˈθiːsis]	假体，人工器官或部件，例如人工假肢

供你参考

骨标记 框 19-6

标记	说明
condyle [ˈkɒndil] 骨节	在一个关节冠凸起窄脊上的平滑、圆形的突起（图 19-4 中的髂嵴，iliac crest）
epicondyle [ˌepiˈkɒndail] 上髁	骨节之上的突起
facet [ˈfæsit] 小面	骨骼的小（平）面
foramen [fəʊˈreimən] 孔	骨骼中的孔（图 19-3 中的脊髓神经孔）
fossa [ˈfɒsə] 窝	空腔
meatus [miˈeitəs] 道	通道或管道，例如骨骼内的长通道；也是管道的外开口，例如尿道突起（图 19-2 中的乳状和柱状突起）
sinus [ˈsainəs] 窦	一个空间或通道，例如某些颅骨中充满空气的空间（图 19-20）
spine [spain] 棘	尖突起（图 19-4 中的坐骨棘）

> **供你参考**
> 骨标记
>
> | 标记 | 说明 |
> |---|---|
> | trochanter ［trəʊˈkæntə］转子 | 股骨顶部大的钝突起 |
> | tubercle ［ˈtjuːbəkl］结节 | 小的圆形突起 |
> | tuberosity ［tjuːbəˈrɒsiti］隆起 | 大的圆形突起 |

续框 19-6

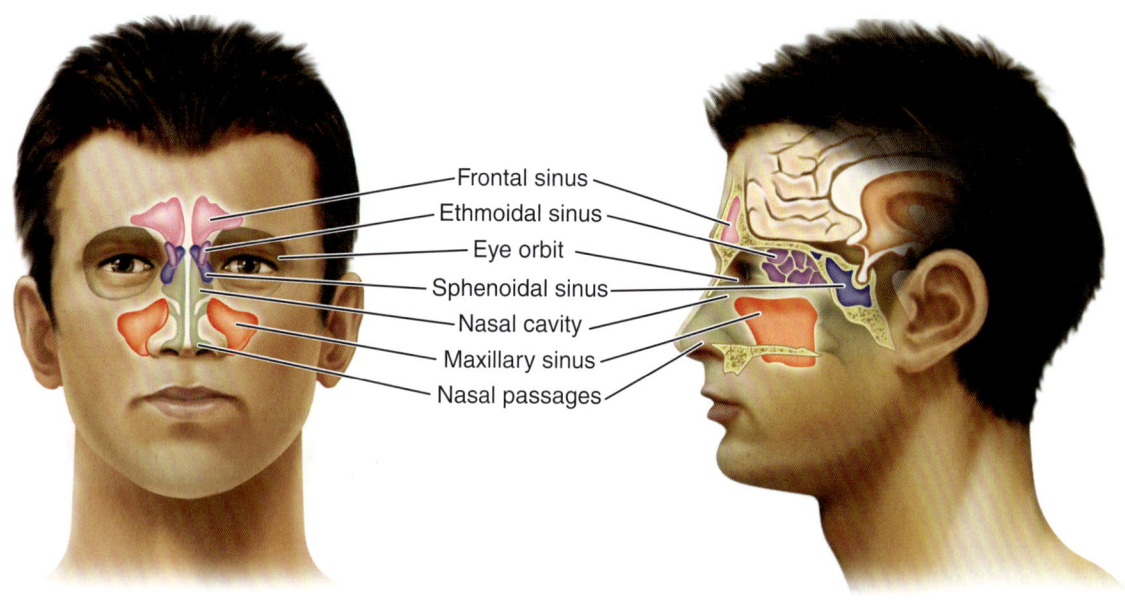

A Frontal View　　　**B** Lateral View

图 19-20　鼻窦。窦是腔或中空空间，例如在某些颅骨中充满空气的腔室，以减轻颅骨的重量。A. 头的前视图显示鼻窦；B. 侧视图

Terminology　缩略语

ACL	Anterior cruciate ligament	前十字韧带
AE	Above the elbow	肘上
AK	Above the knee	膝上
ASF	Anterior spinal fusion	前路脊柱融合
BE	Below the elbow, also barium enema	肘下，钡灌肠
BK	Below the knee	膝下
BMD	Bone mineral density	骨密度
C	Cervical vertebra; numbered C1 to C7	颈椎，编号 C1~C7

Terminology 缩略语（续表）

Co	Coccyx; coccygeal	尾骨，尾骨的
DEXA	Dual-energy x-ray absorptiometry (scan)	双能 X 线吸收计量法（扫描）
DIP	Distal interphalangeal (joint)	远端指间（关节）
DJD	Degenerative joint disease	退行性关节疾病
Fx	Fracture	骨折
HNP	Herniated nucleus pulposus	脱出的髓核
IM	Intramedullary, also intramuscular	髓内的，肌内的
L	Lumbar vertebra; numbered L1 to L5	腰椎，编号 L1~L5
MCP	Metacarpophalangeal (joint)	掌指（关节）
MTP	Metatarsophalangeal (joint)	跖趾（关节）
NSAID(s)	Nonsteroidal antiinflammatory drug(s)	非甾体抗炎药
OA	Osteoarthritis	骨关节炎
OI	Osteogenesis imperfecta	成骨不全症
ORIF	Open reduction internal fixation	切开复位内固定
ortho, ORTH	Orthopedics	骨科
PCL	Posterior cruciate ligament	后十字韧带
PIP	Proximal interphalangeal (joint)	近端指间（关节）
PSF	Posterior spinal fusion	后路脊柱融合
RA	Rheumatoid arthritis	风湿性关节炎
S	Sacrum; sacral	骶骨，骶骨的
SERM	Selective estrogen receptor modulator	选择性雌激素受体调节剂
T	Thoracic vertebra; numbered T1 to T12	胸椎，编号 T1~T12
THA	Total hip arthroplasty	全髋关节置换术
TKA	Total knee arthroplasty	全膝关节置换术
TMJ	Temporomandibular joint	颞下颌关节
Tx	Traction	牵引

Case Study Revisited
案例研究再访

L. R.'s Follow-Up

L. R. underwent a successful surgical procedure and was transferred to the pediatric ICU. Her postoperative course progressed well. She was discharged with orders for continued physical therapy and follow-up visits to the see the surgeon. L.R. had excellent compliance with all postoperative instructions and was able to resume her musical activities sooner than expected.

L. R. 的随访

L. R. 的外科手术进行成功并转移到儿科 ICU。她的术后进展良好，出院后继续接受物理治疗并随访外科医生。L. R. 完全遵守所有的术后指示，并能够比预期更快地恢复她的音乐活动。

CHAPTER 19 复习

标记练习

骨骼

在对应的下划线上写出每个编号部分的名称。

Calcaneus	Patella
Carpals	Pelvis
Clavicle	Phalanges
Cranium	Radius
Facial bones	Ribs
Femur	Sacrum
Fibula	Scapula
Humerus	Sternum
Ilium	Tarsals
Mandible	Tibia
Metacarpals	Ulna
Metatarsals	Vertebral column

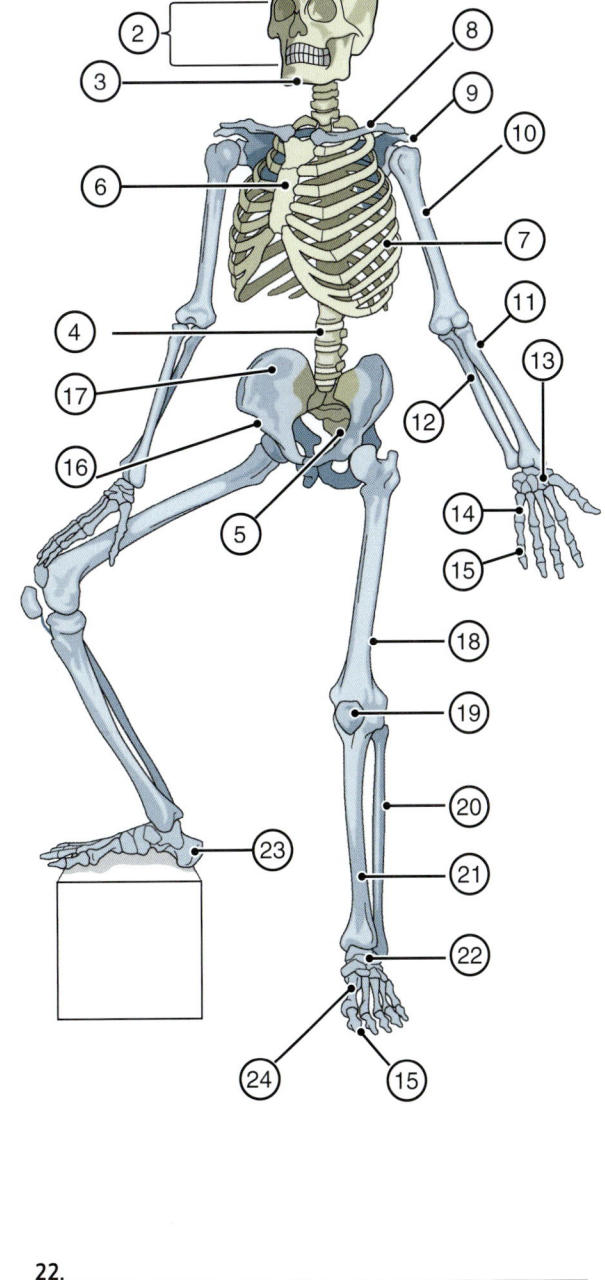

1. _____
2. _____
3. _____
4. _____
5. _____
6. _____
7. _____
8. _____
9. _____
10. _____
11. _____
12. _____
13. _____
14. _____
15. _____
16. _____
17. _____
18. _____
19. _____
20. _____
21. _____
22. _____
23. _____
24. _____

头骨，左视图

在对应的下划线上写出每个编号部分的名称。

Frontal
Hyoid
Lacrimal
Mandible
Maxilla
Nasal
Occipital
Parietal
Sphenoid
Temporal
Zygomatic

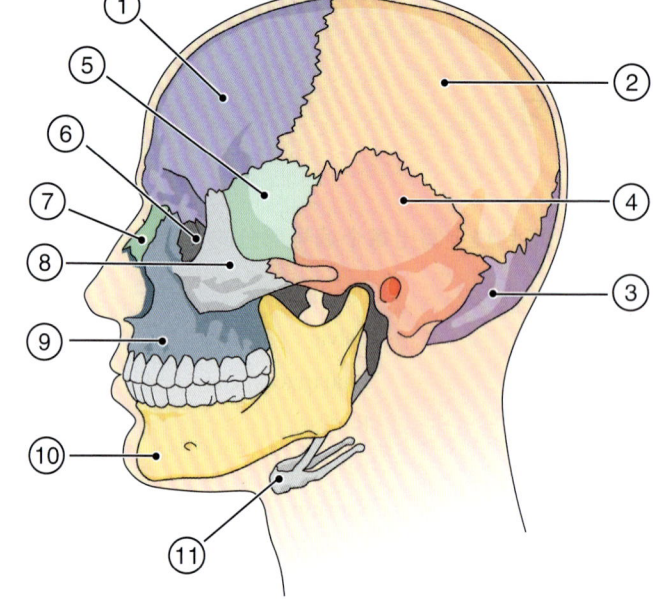

1. _____
2. _____
3. _____
4. _____
5. _____
6. _____
7. _____
8. _____
9. _____
10. _____
11. _____

脊柱

在对应的下划线上写出每个编号部分的名称。

Body of vertebra
Cervical vertebrae
Coccyx
Intervertebral disk
Lumbar vertebrae
Sacrum
Thoracic vertebrae

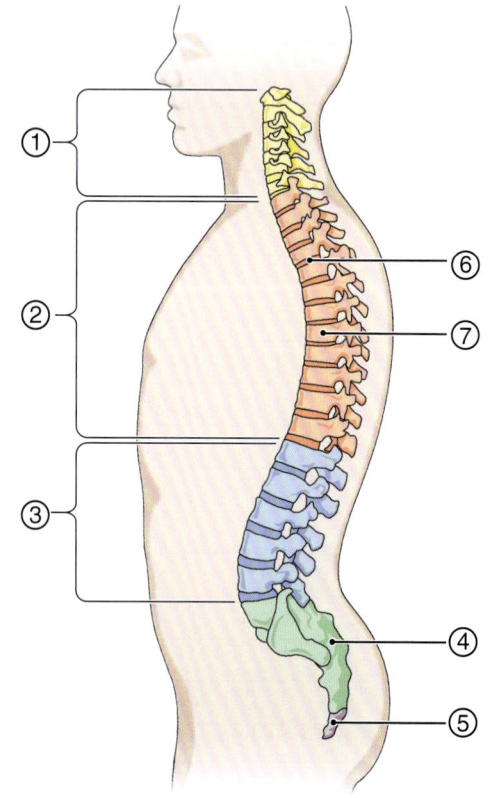

1. _____
2. _____
3. _____
4. _____
5. _____
6. _____
7. _____

骨盆

在对应的下划线上写出每个编号部分的名称。

Ilium　　　　　　　　Pubic symphysis
Ischium　　　　　　　Acetabulum
Pubis　　　　　　　　Sacrum

1. _____
2. _____
3. _____
4. _____
5. _____
6. _____

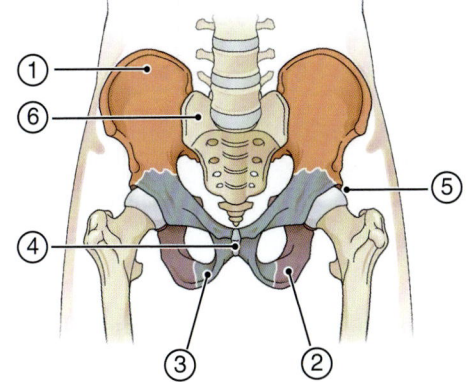

长骨的结构

在对应的下划线上写出每个编号部分的名称。

Artery and vein　　　　Medullary cavity
Cartilage　　　　　　　Periosteum
Compact bone　　　　　Proximal epiphysis
Diaphysis　　　　　　　Spongy bone (containing red marrow)
Distal epiphysis　　　　Yellow marrow
Epiphyseal line (growth line)

1. _____
2. _____
3. _____
4. _____
5. _____
6. _____
7. _____
8. _____
9. _____
10. _____
11. _____

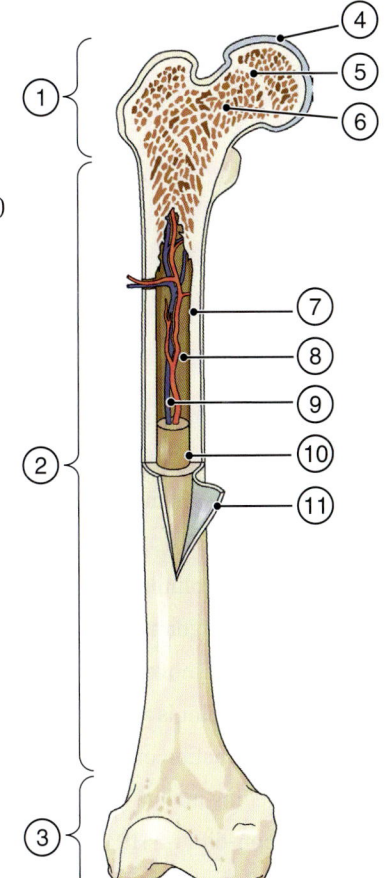

术语

匹配

匹配下列术语，在每个题号左侧写上适当的字母。

____ 1. periosteum   a. an immovable joint

____ 2. epiphysis   b. breakdown and removal of tissue

____ 3. suture   c. cell that breaks down bone

____ 4. osteoclast   d. membrane that covers a bone

____ 5. resorption   e. end of a long bone

____ 6. osteopenia   a. immobility of a joint

____ 7. ankylosis   b. spinal tap

____ 8. kyphosis   c. displacement of a vertebra

____ 9. spondylolisthesis   d. exaggerated curve of the thoracic spine

____ 10. rachiocentesis   e. deficiency of bone tissue

补充术语

____ 11. laminectomy   a. great toe

____ 12. chondroitin   b. dietary supplement for treatment of joint pain

____ 13. subluxation   c. excision of part of a vertebra

____ 14. hallux   d. part of the ulna that forms the elbow

____ 15. olecranon   e. partial dislocation

填空

21. A fibrous band of connective tissue that connects a muscle to a bone is a(n)_____.

22. The type of tissue that covers the ends of the bones at the joints is_____.

23. The study and treatment of disorders of the skeleton, muscles, and associated structures is_____.

24. The part of the vertebral column that articulates with the ilium is the_____.

25. Chondrosarcoma is a malignant tumor of_____.

26. The fluid that fills a freely movable joint is_____.

27. A fluid-filled sac near a joint is a(n)_____.

28. Myelogenesis is the formation of_____.

29. Hemarthrosis is bleeding into a(n)_____.

30. Spondylarthritis (spon-dil-ar-THRI-tis) is arthritis of the_____.

31. Rachischisis (ra-KIS-kih-sis) is fissure of the_____.

定义

定义下列单词。

32. myelitis ［ˌmaɪəˈlaɪtɪs］_____

33. ossification ［ɔsɪfɪˈkeɪʃən］_____

34. arthrodesis ［ɑːθrəʊdiːsɪs］_____

35. synovectomy ［sɪnəˈvektəmɪ］_____

36. chondrocyte ['kʌndrɒsit] _____
37. subcostal [sʌb'kɒstəl] _____
38. coccydynia [kɒk'saidiniə] _____
39. spondylitis [ˌspɒndi'laitis] _____
40. polyarticular [pɒliɑ:'tikjʊlə(r)] _____
41. intraosteal [intrə'ɒzti:l] _____
42. peribursal [peri'bɜ:səl] _____

写出下列定义的单词。

43. formation of cartilage _____
44. surgical immobilization of a joint _____
45. measurement of the pelvis _____
46. tumor of bone and cartilage _____
47. narrowing of a joint _____
48. death (-necrosis) of bone tissue _____
49. stone in a bursa _____
50. incision into the cranium _____
51. near the sacrum _____
52. pertaining to the sacrum and ilium _____
53. surgical excision of the coccyx _____
54. endoscopic examination of a joint _____

在本章开头的 L.R. 案例研究中找出下列单词。

55. describing a disease with no known cause _____
56. a bone of the shoulder girdle _____
57. a bone of the pelvis _____
58. the area where T4 is located _____
59. incisions into bones _____
60. sideways curvature of the spine _____

形容词

写出下列单词的形容词形式。

61. sacrum _____
62. vertebra _____
63. coccyx _____
64. pelvis _____
65. ilium _____

真假判断

检查以下语句。如果语句为真，则在第一个空格写入 T；如果语句为假，则在第一个空格中写入 F，并通过在第二个空格中替换带下划线的单词来更正语句。

	True or False	Correct Answer
66. The growth region of a long bone is in the <u>diaphysis</u>.	_____	_____
67. The tarsal bones are found in the <u>ankle</u>.	_____	_____
68. A slightly moveable joint is a <u>symphysis</u>.	_____	_____
69. The femur is part of the axial <u>skeleton</u>.	_____	_____
70. The <u>cervical</u> vertebrae are located in the neck.	_____	_____
71. The cells that produce cartilage are <u>chondroblasts</u>.	_____	_____
72. Blood cells are formed in yellow bone <u>marrow</u>.	_____	_____
73. An exaggerated lumbar curve of the spine is <u>scoliosis</u>.	_____	_____
74. The term varus means bent <u>inward</u>.	_____	_____

排除

在下列每组中，为与其余不相配的单词加下划线，并说明你选择的理由。

75. trochanter — process — hyoid — meatus — condyle
_____

76. lambdoid — occipital — parietal — frontal — sphenoid
_____

77. sacr/o — rachi/o — spondyl/o — vertebr/o — cost/o
_____

78. Pott — sciatic — impacted — comminuted — greenstick
_____

79. T — C — L — Co — OA
_____

单词构建

使用给出的单词组成部分写出下列单词。

spondyl/o   -plasty   arthr/o   -lysis   -odynia   oste/o   -tome

80. pain in a joint _____
81. destruction of a vertebra _____
82. pain in a vertebra _____
83. loosening or separation of a joint _____
84. instrument for cutting bone tissue _____
85. plastic repair of a joint _____
86. pain in a bone _____
87. instrument for incising a joint _____
88. destruction of bone tissue _____
89. plastic repair of a bone _____

单词分析

定义下列单词，并给出每个单词组成部分的含义。如果需要，可以使用词典。

90. osteochondrosis ［ɒstiəʊkɒn'drəʊsis］ _____

    a. oste/o _____

    b. chondr/o _____

    c. -sis _____

91. spondylosyndesis ［spɒndi'ləʊsindizis］ _____

    a. spondyl/o _____

    b. syn _____

    c. -desis _____

92. exostosis ［ˌeksɒs'təʊsis］ _____

    a. ex/o _____

    b. ost(e)/o _____

    c. -sis _____

93. achondroplasia ［eiˌkɒndrə'pleiʒə］ _____

    a. a _____

    b. chondr/o _____

    c. plas _____

    d. -ia _____

94. osteoporosis ［ˌɒstiəʊpə'rəʊsis］ _____

    a. osteo _____

    b. poro _____

    c. -sis _____

Additional Case Studies
补充案例研究

Case Study 19-1: Arthroplasty of the Right TMJ
案例研究 19-1：右颞下颌关节的关节成形术

S. A., a 38 YO teacher, was admitted for surgery for degenerative joint disease (DJD) of her right temporomandibular joint (TMJ). She has experienced chronic pain in her right jaw, neck, and ear since her automobile accident the previous year. S. A.'s diagnosis was confirmed by CT scan and was followed up with conservative therapy, which included a bite plate, NSAIDs, and steroid injections. She had also tried hypnosis in an attempt to manage her pain but was not able to gain relief. Her doctor referred her to an oral surgeon who specializes in TMJ disorders. S. A. was scheduled for an arthroplasty of the right TMJ to remove diseased bone on the articular surface of the right mandibular condyle.

On the following day, she was transported to the OR for surgery. She was given general endotracheal anesthesia, and a vertical incision was made from the superior aspect of the right ear down to the base of the attachment of the right earlobe. After appropriate dissection and retraction, the posterior-superior aspect of the right zygomatic arch was bluntly dissected anteroposteriorly. With a nerve stimulator, the zygomatic branch of the facial nerve was identified and retracted from the surgical field with a vessel loop. The periosteum was then incised along the superior aspect of the arch. An inferior dissection was then made along the capsular ligament and retracted posteriorly. With a Freer elevator, the meniscus was freed, and a horizontal incision was made to the condyle. With a Hall drill and saline coolant, a high condylectomy of approximately 3 mm of bone was removed while conserving function of the external pterygoid muscle. The stump of the condyle was filed smooth and irrigated copiously with NS. The lateral capsule, periosteum, subcutaneous tissue, and skin were then closed with sutures. The facial nerve was tested before closing and confirmed to be intact. A pressure pack and Barton bandage were applied. The sponge, needle, and instrument counts were correct. Estimated blood loss (EBL) was approximately 50 mL.

S.A. was discharged on the second postoperative day with instructions for a soft diet, daily mouth-opening exercises, an antibiotic (Keflex 500 mg po q6h), Tylenol no. 3 po q4h PRN for pain, and four weekly postoperative appointments.

S. A. 是一名 38 岁的教师，住院做她的右颞下颌关节（TMJ）的退行性关节病（DJD）手术。自从去年的汽车事故以来，她经历了右下巴、颈部和耳朵的慢性疼痛。S. A. 的诊断被 CT 扫描证实，采取保守治疗，包括咬合板、非甾体抗炎药和类固醇注射。她也试图通过催眠治疗疼痛，但不能得到缓解。她的医生将她转诊给专门治疗右颞下颌关节疾病的口腔外科医生。S. A. 被安排进行右颞下颌关节的关节成形术以消除右下颌髁突关节表面上患病的骨头。

第 2 天，她被送到手术室进行手术。给她做了常规的气管内麻醉，并且从右耳的上方向下到右耳垂的基部进行垂直切口。在适当的切割和收缩后，右颧弓的后上方被前后切开。使用神经刺激器，确认面部神经的颧分支，并用血管袢使其从手术区域缩回。然后沿着弓的上部切开骨膜，然后沿着囊韧带进行下层切割并向后缩回。使用弗里尔提肌释放半月板，并且对髁髁状突做水平切口。使用霍尔钻和盐水冷却剂，通过高位骨节切除术去除了大约 3mm 骨头，同时保留外翼肌的功能。髁状突的残部被锉平，并用生理盐水冲洗，然后用缝合线封闭侧囊、骨膜、皮下组织和皮肤。在缝合前测试面神经，并确认其是完整的。使用压力包和巴尔通绷带。海绵、针头和器械计数正确。估计失血量（estimated blood loss，EBL）约为 50ml。

S.A. 在术后第 2 天出院，被指示食用软饮食，每日做开口锻炼，口服抗生素（头孢氨苄 500mg 口服，每 6 小时一次），扑热息痛口服，每 4 小时一次，根据疼痛需要服用，以及每周 4 次的术后随访。

Case Study 19-2: Osteogenesis Imperfecta
案例研究 19-2：成骨不全

M. H., a 3-year-old boy with osteogenesis imperfecta (OI) type III, was admitted to the pediatric orthopedic hospital for treatment of yet another fracture. Since birth he has had 15 arm and leg fractures as a result of his congenital disease. This latest fracture occurred when he twisted at the hip while standing in his wheeled walker. He has been in a research study and receives a bisphosphonate infusion every two months. He is short in stature with short limbs for his age and has bowing of both legs.

M. H. was transferred to the OR and carefully lifted to the OR table by the staff. After he was anesthetized, he was positioned with gentle manipulation, and his left hip was elevated on a small gel pillow. After skin preparation and sterile draping, a stainless steel rod was inserted into the medullary canal of his left femur to reduce and stabilize the femoral fracture. The muscle, fascia, subcutaneous tissue, and skin were sutured closed. Three nurses gently held M. H. in position on a pediatric spica box while the surgeon applied a hip spica (body cast) to stabilize the fixation, protect the leg, and maintain abduction. M. H. was transferred to the postanesthesia care unit (PACU) for recovery. The surgeon dictated the procedure as an open reduction internal fixation (ORIF) of the left femur with intramedullary (IM) rodding and application of spica cast.

M. H. 是一名 3 岁的患有Ⅲ型成骨不全（osteogenesis imperfecta，OI）的男孩，住入小儿骨科医院治疗另一个骨折。自出生以来，由于先天性疾病，他有 15 次手臂和腿的骨折。站在轮椅中扭曲臀部时，导致了最新的骨折。他一直在被研究中，每 2 个月接受一次双膦酸盐注射。他的身材矮小，四肢短，双腿成弓形。

M. H. 被转诊到手术室，并由工作人员小心地抬上手术台。在被麻醉后，他被轻柔地固定体位，左髋由一个小凝胶枕头抬高。在皮肤准备和无菌遮盖之后，将不锈钢杆插入其左股骨的髓管中以减小和稳定股骨骨折。将肌肉、筋膜、皮下组织和皮肤缝合闭合。三名护士轻轻握住在儿科人字形绷带箱中的 M. H.，让外科医生使用髋人字石膏以稳定固定，保护腿，并保持外展。M. H. 被转移到麻醉后护理病房（postanesthesia care unit，PACU）进行康复。外科医生口述该手术为使用髓内（intramedullary，IM）插管和人字石膏的左股骨切开复位内固定（open reduction internal fixation，ORIF）。

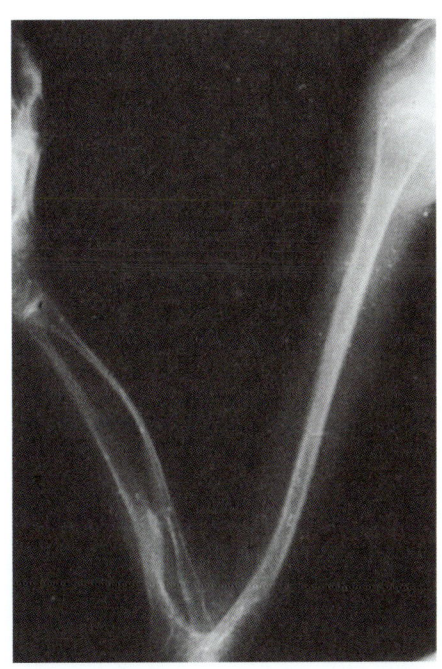

成骨不全。上肢的 X 线成像显示胶原蛋白生产缺损导致的薄骨和骨折

案例研究问题

多项选择。选择正确的答案，在每个题号左侧写上你选择的字母。

____ 1. A condylectomy is
    a. removal of a joint capsule
    b. removal of a rounded bone protuberance
    c. enlargement of a cavity
    d. removal of a tumor

____ 2. The articular surface of a bone is located
    a. under the epiphysis
    b. at a joint
    c. at a muscle attachment
    d. at a tendon attachment

____ 3. The dissection directed anteroposteriorlywas done
    a. posterior – superior
    b. circumferentially
    c. front to back
    d. top to bottom

____ 4. Another term for bow-legged is
    a. knock-kneed
    b. adduction
    c. varus
    d. valgus

____ 5. An IM rod is placed
    a. inferior to the femoral condyle
    b. into the acetabulum
    c. within the medullary canal
    d. lateral to the epiphysial growth plates

写出案例研究中下列含义的术语。

6. pertaining to the cheek bone _____

7. the membrane around a bone _____

8. a crescent-shaped cartilage in a joint _____

9. plastic repair of a joint _____

10. formation of bone tissue _____

11. a break in a bone _____

12. present at birth _____

13. the thigh bone _____

定义下列缩略语。

14. DJD _____

15. NS _____

16. TMJ _____

17. OI _____

18. ORIF _____

19. EBL _____

CHAPTER 20 肌肉系统

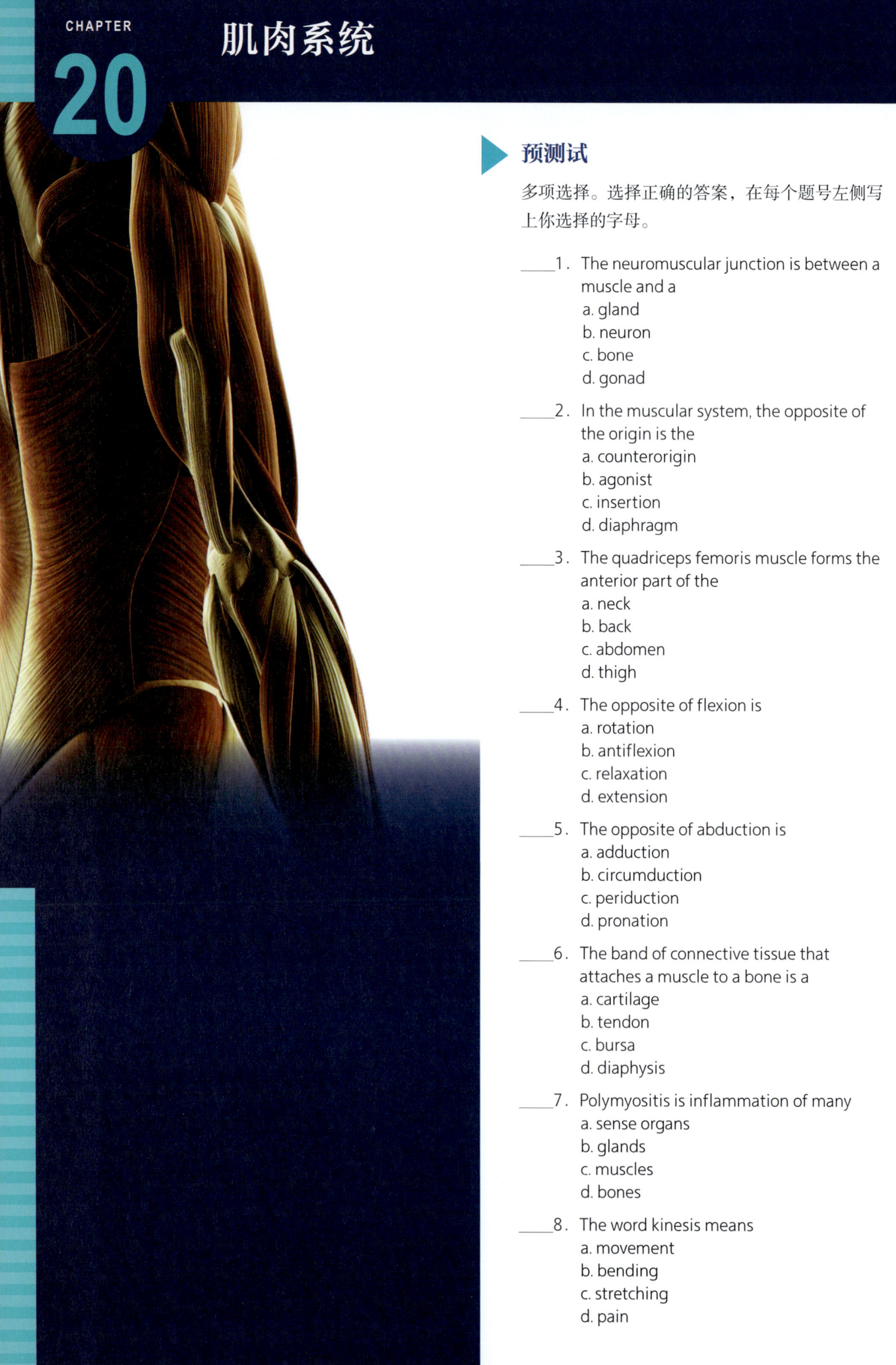

预测试

多项选择。选择正确的答案，在每个题号左侧写上你选择的字母。

____ 1. The neuromuscular junction is between a muscle and a
a. gland
b. neuron
c. bone
d. gonad

____ 2. In the muscular system, the opposite of the origin is the
a. counterorigin
b. agonist
c. insertion
d. diaphragm

____ 3. The quadriceps femoris muscle forms the anterior part of the
a. neck
b. back
c. abdomen
d. thigh

____ 4. The opposite of flexion is
a. rotation
b. antiflexion
c. relaxation
d. extension

____ 5. The opposite of abduction is
a. adduction
b. circumduction
c. periduction
d. pronation

____ 6. The band of connective tissue that attaches a muscle to a bone is a
a. cartilage
b. tendon
c. bursa
d. diaphysis

____ 7. Polymyositis is inflammation of many
a. sense organs
b. glands
c. muscles
d. bones

____ 8. The word kinesis means
a. movement
b. bending
c. stretching
d. pain

学习目标

学完本章后,应该能够:

1. ▶ 比较平滑肌、心肌和骨骼肌的位置和功能。
2. ▶ 描述骨骼肌的典型结构。
3. ▶ 简述肌肉收缩的机制。
4. ▶ 说明肌肉如何配合产生运动。
5. ▶ 描述肌肉产生的主要运动类型。
6. ▶ 列出一些肌肉命名的规则,并给出示例。
7. ▶ 识别并使用与肌肉系统相关的词根。
8. ▶ 描述至少 7 种影响肌肉的疾病。
9. ▶ 解释与肌肉相关的缩略语。
10. ▶ 分析几个涉及肌肉的案例研究。

Case Study: T. D.'s Brachial Plexus Injury
案例研究: T. D. 的臂丛神经损伤

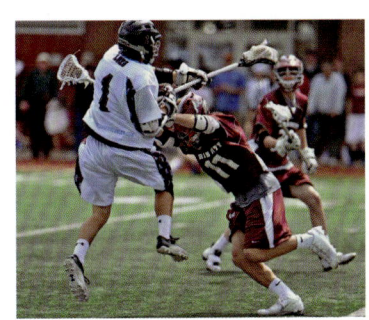

Chief Complaint

T. D., a 16-year-old high school student, had a severe lacrosse accident that resulted in a flail arm. He had sustained right brachial plexus injury and had no recovery. He has continued to take medication for neurologic pain. He was scheduled to see his orthopedic surgeon for a possible brachial plexus exploration.

Examination

The orthopedic surgeon examined T. D. and noted that there had not been any change in his condition since the previous visit. T. D. still had no feeling or motion in his right shoulder or arm. He had atrophy over the supraspinatus and infraspinatus muscles and also subluxation of his shoulder and deltoid atrophy. He had no active motion of the right upper extremity and no sensation. The rest of his orthopedic exam showed full ROM of his hips, knees, and ankles with intact sensation and palpable distal pulses as well as normal motor function. He was diagnosed with a possible middle trunk brachial plexus injury from C7.

Clinical Course

T. D. and his parents had previous discussions with the surgeon and were aware of the prognosis and treatment plan. With middle trunk brachial plexus injury, damage to the subscapular nerve will interrupt conduction to the subscapularis and teres major muscles. Damage to the long thoracic nerve prevents conduction to the serratus anterior muscles. Injury to the pectoral nerves affects the pectoralis major and minor muscles.

T. D. was scheduled for an EMG, nerve conduction studies, and somatosensory evoked potentials (SSEPs). His diaphragm was examined under fluoroscopy to R/O phrenic nerve injury. The results of the diagnostic studies indicated that T. D. had most likely sustained a middle trunk brachial plexus injury. T. D. was scheduled for a brachial plexus exploration with possible nerve graft, nerve transfer, bilateral sural (calf) nerve harvest, or gracilis muscle graft from his right thigh.

主诉

T. D. 是一名 16 岁的高中生,一个严重的长曲棍球事故导致连枷臂。他患有右臂丛神经损伤,没有恢复。他继续服用药物治疗神经性疼痛。他计划去看骨科医生进行臂丛神经探查。

检查

骨科医生检查了 T. D.,并注意到自从上次访视以来他的病情没有任何变化。T. D. 的右肩或手臂仍然没有感觉或不能运动。他的冈上肌和冈下肌萎缩,肩部半脱位,三角肌萎缩。他的右上肢不能主动运动,没有感觉。骨科检查的其余部分显示他的臀部、膝盖和脚踝的运动范围(ROM)充分,感觉未受损,有可触知的远端脉搏,运动功能正常。他被诊断为可能的从 C7 开始的中间躯干臂丛神经丛损伤。

临床病程

T. D. 和他的父母以前与医生讨论过,并知道预后和治疗计划。随着中间躯干臂丛神经损伤,对肩胛下神经的损伤会中断向肩胛下肌和大圆肌的传导。对胸长神经的损伤会阻止向前锯肌的传导,对胸神经的损伤会影响胸大肌和胸小肌。

T. D. 被安排做肌电图(EMG)、神经传导分析和测量体感诱发电位(somatosensory evoked potential, SSEP)。隔膜荧光透视检查排除了膈神经损伤。诊断分析结果表明 T. D. 很可能是持续的中间躯干臂丛神经损伤。T. D. 被安排做臂丛探查,同时进行可能的神经移植、神经移位、双侧腓肠(小腿)神经移植,或从他的右大腿做股薄肌移植。

简介

肌肉（muscle）组织的主要特征是其收缩能力。当受到刺激时，肌肉缩短产生骨骼、血管壁或内部器官的运动，还能维持部分收缩以保持体态。另外，肌肉收缩产生的热量是体热的主要来源。

肌肉的类型

人体中有三种类型的肌肉组织（图 20-1）：

- 平滑肌（内脏的 visceral）（smooth muscle）成中空器官的内壁，例如胃、肠道、子宫，和导管的内壁，例如血管和细支气管。平滑肌非自主地运动，负责蠕动并推动物质通过系统。
- 心肌（cardiac muscle）构成心壁的心肌层。心肌非自主地发挥作用，负责心脏的泵血动作。
- 骨骼肌（skeletal muscle）连接骨骼，负责自主运动。骨骼肌还能保持体态，并产生大部分体热。所有自主肌肉共同构成肌肉系统。

骨骼肌

下面的讨论描述了骨骼肌的特征，骨骼肌是三种肌肉类型中最广泛研究的。

肌肉结构

肌肉由单个细胞组成，通常被称为纤维，因为它们是长线状的。这些细胞通过结缔组织保持在束（bundle）中（图 20-2）。覆盖每块肌肉的是结缔组织的鞘（sheath）或筋膜（fascia）。这些支持性组织合并形成连接肌肉与骨骼的肌腱（tendon）。

肌肉动作

骨骼肌通过神经系统的运动神经元刺激收缩（图 20-3）。在肌肉神经接点（neuromuscular junction，NMJ），神经元的分支在突触（synapse）遇到肌肉细胞，神经递质乙酰胆碱（acetylcholine，ACh）从小囊（vesicle）释放到一个轴突分支。乙酰胆碱与肌肉细胞膜相互作用激起细胞收缩。肌肉细胞中的两种特殊蛋白丝——肌动蛋白（actin）和肌球蛋白（myosin）相互作用产生收缩。这一反应需要细胞的能量成分（ATP）和钙。框 20-1 讨论了使用类固醇提高肌肉的发育和力量。

除非刺激继续，大多数骨骼肌快速收缩然后快速放松。有时骨骼肌会保持稳定的部分收缩状态，以维持体态。这种稳定的状态被称为紧张（强直性痉挛），或肌张力（muscle tone）。

肌肉成对工作，在关节产生运动。当一块肌肉，主动肌（agonist），收缩时，与其相对的肌肉，拮

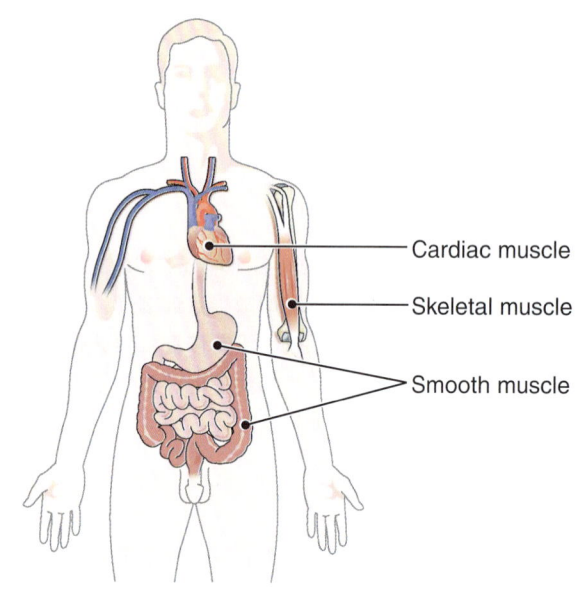

图 20-1 肌肉类型。平滑肌组成管道和中空器官的壁，例如胃和肠；心肌组成心壁；骨骼肌附着于骨骼

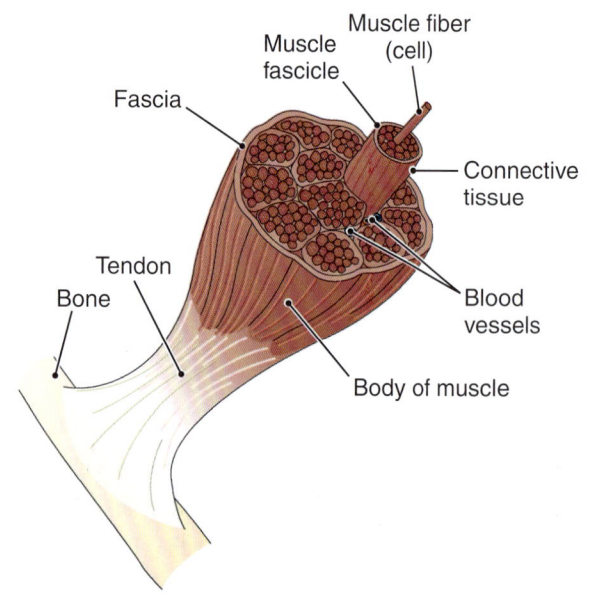

图 20-2 骨骼肌的结构。图中所示的结缔组织是将肌肉连接到骨骼的肌腱

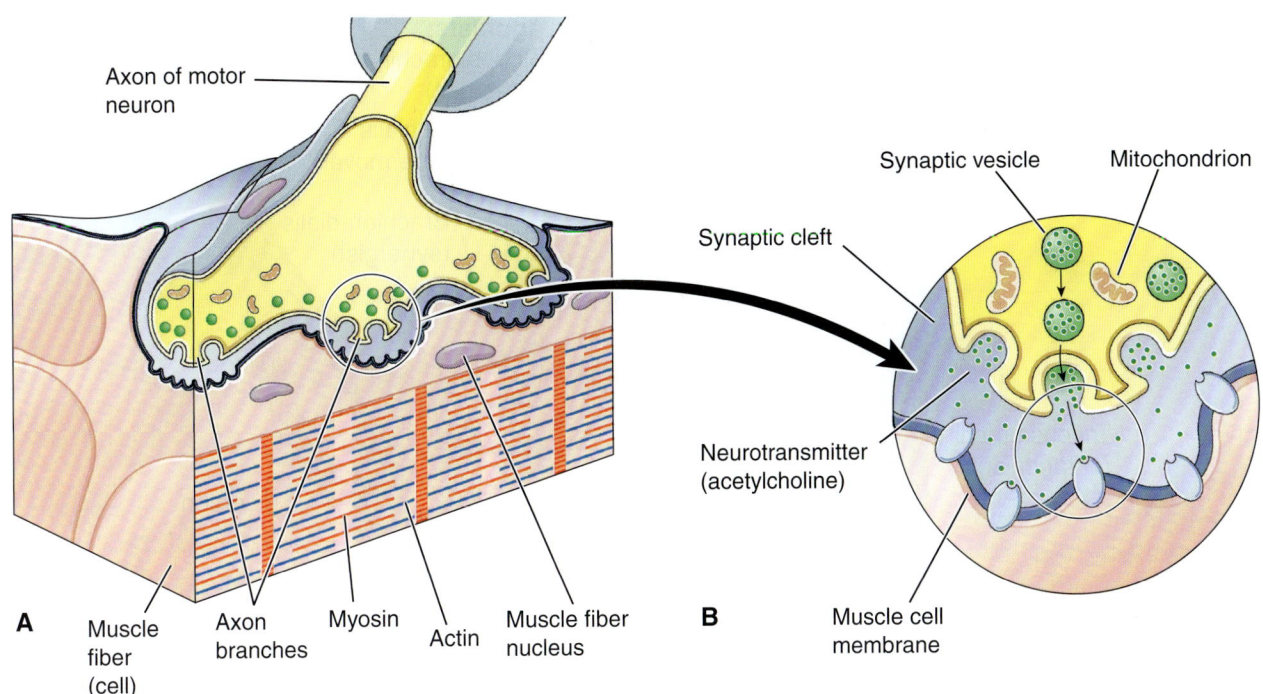

图 20-3 神经肌肉接点（NMJ）。A. 运动神经元的分支末端与肌纤维（细胞）膜接触。B. 神经肌肉接点的放大视图，显示从神经元释放的神经递质（乙酰胆碱）及其对肌细胞膜的附着。线粒体产生 ATP，是细胞的能量复合物

抗肌（antagonist），必须放松。例如，当上臂前表面上的肱肌（brachialis）收缩以弯曲臂时，后表面上的肱三头肌（triceps brachii）必须松弛（图 20-4）。当上臂伸展时，这些动作被反转；肱三头肌收缩，肱肌必须放松。任何有助于主动肌产生作用的肌肉称为协作肌（synergist）。例如，肱二头肌（biceps brachii）（当手臂屈曲时在前表面上看的最清楚）和肱桡肌（brachioradialis）帮助肱肌屈曲手臂。

肌肉的命名

肌肉可以根据其所在的位置（例如靠近的骨骼）、纤维的方向或其大小、形状或附着点的数量（如后缀 -ceps 表示的）命名（图 20-4）；也可以根据其动作，在动作的词根上加后缀 -or 命名。例如，产生关节弯曲的肌肉被称为屈肌（flexor）。请查阅图 20-6 和图 20-7 中肌肉的图形，看看你能在肌肉名称中发现几项准则。请注意，有时在命名时应用了不只一项准则。

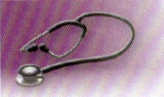

框 20-1
临床观点
合成类固醇：不惜代价获胜？

通过促进代谢和刺激生长，合成类固醇（anabolic steroids）能够模仿雄性激素的作用。这些药物被合法以处方使用，以促进肌肉再生和防止因手术后停用产生的萎缩。然而，运动员也会非法购买并使用它们，以增加肌肉的生长和力量并提高耐力。

当类固醇被非法用于提高运动员的成绩时，所需的剂量大到足以产生严重的不良反应。它们会提高血液胆固醇的水平，可能导致心脏病、肾衰竭和脑卒中。类固醇会损害肝脏，使其易患疾病和癌症。类固醇抑制免疫系统，增加感染和癌症的风险。对于男性，类固醇会引起阳痿、睾丸萎缩、精子计数低、不育和女性特征发育，例如乳腺发育（男性乳房发育症，gynecomastia）。对女性，类固醇会打乱排卵和月经，并产生男性特征，例如乳房萎缩、阴蒂肥大、体毛增多和声音低沉。对于男性和女性，类固醇都会提高秃顶的风险，特别是男性，它们会引起情绪波动、抑郁和暴力。在给定的运动中，肌肉附着在骨骼稳定部分的点是起端（origin）；肌肉附着在骨骼运动部分的点是附着点（insertion）（图 20-4）。

框 20-2 描述了关节不同类型的运动，这些运动示于图 20-5。框 20-3 给出了运动健身职业的信息。

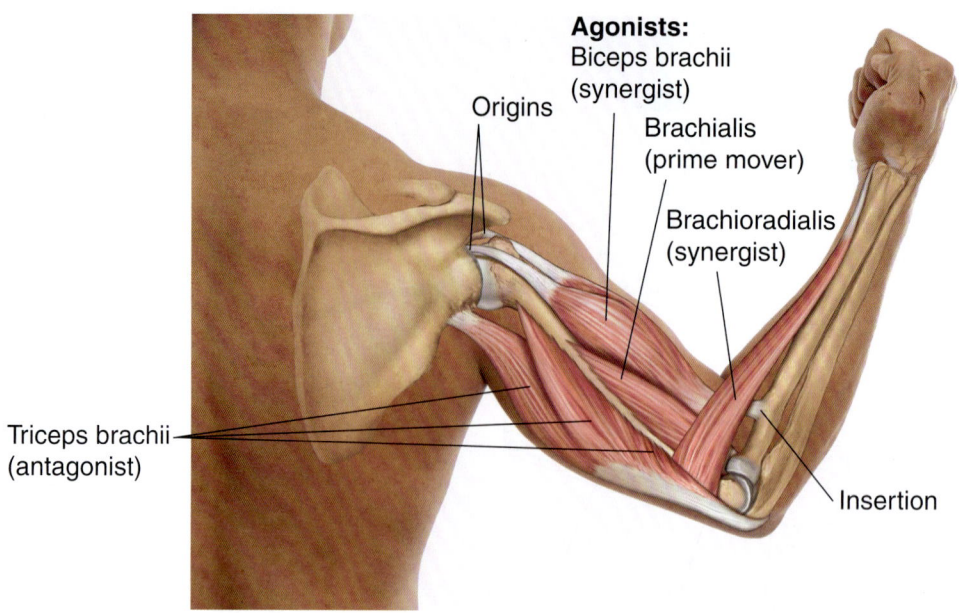

图 20-4 肌肉合作。当肱肌主动肌主导弯曲手臂时，肱三头肌是对抗肌，必须放松。协作肌，肱二头肌和肱桡肌，协助这一行动。当手臂伸展时，这些肌肉的动作反转。该图还示出了肱二头肌的三个附着体，两个起端和一个附着点

供你参考
运动的类型

框 20-2

运动	定义	示例
flexion［'flekʃn］弯曲	关闭关节的角度	膝或肘关节的弯曲
extension［ik'stenʃn］伸展	打开关节的角度	伸直膝或肘关节
abduction［æb'dʌkʃn］外展	远离身体中线的运动	手臂在肩关节向外运动
adduction［ə'dʌkʃən］内收	朝向身体中线的运动	将抬起的手臂收回来
rotation［rəʊ'teiʃn］旋转	一个身体部分在其自身轴上的转动	前臂从肘部转动
circumduction［sɜːkəm'dʌkʃən］环形	围绕中心点的圆周运动	用伸直手臂的画圈
pronation［prəʊ'neiʃən］下转	向下转	手掌向下转动
supination［ˌsjuːpi'neiʃən］上转	向上转	手掌向上转动
eversion［i'vɜːʃən］外翻	向外转	脚掌向外转动
inversion［in'vɜːʃn］内翻	向内转	脚掌向内转动
dorsiflexion［dɔːsi'flekʃən］背屈	向后弯曲	移动脚使脚趾朝上，远离脚掌
plantar flexion［'plæntə］跖屈	脚掌弯曲	使脚趾朝下

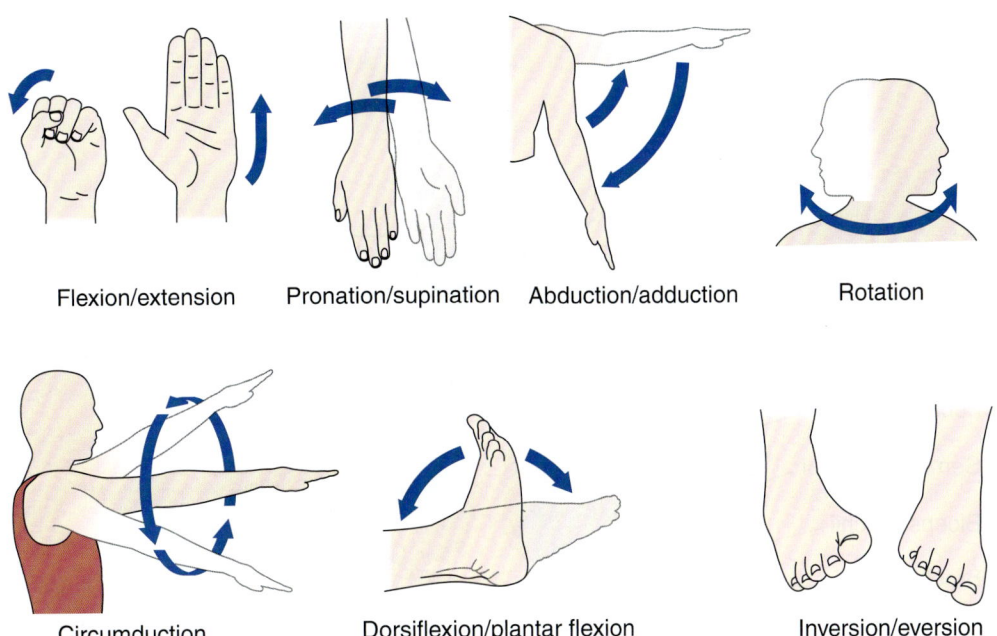

图 20-5　运动的类型。肌肉收缩在关节处产生运动。一些肌肉由它们产生的运动类型命名，例如屈肌、伸张肌和内收肌

框 20-3

健康职业

锻炼和健身的职业

有几个相关的职业涉及治疗、健康维护和休闲锻炼计划的管理。美国运动医学学院（American College of Sports Medicine，ACSM）的网站 www.acsm.org 有关于这些领域的信息和一些认证项目。

· 运动生理学家（exercise physiologist，EP）研究体育运动涉及的机制和身体对运动的生理反应。他们为残疾人或疾病患者，如心血管和呼吸道疾病患者，设计综合健康、运动和康复计划。他们可以在临床环境、私人企业、健康俱乐部或教育机构中与医生合作。大多数运动生理学家有硕士学位，但有些工作可能只需要学士学位，教学或研究需要博士学位。运动生理学家可以通过美国运动医学学院或运动生理学中心（Center for Exercise Physiology，CEP）认证。美国运动生理学家协会（American Society of Exercise Physiologists）在 www.asep.org 有关于这个职业的信息。

· 运动训练师（athletic trainer）专门从事肌肉骨骼损伤的预防和治疗。他们建议客户正确地使用锻炼设备和装置，例如支具，以帮助防止受伤。他们与私人机构、医疗机构、运动员和运动队的医生合作。运动训练师的工作可以有确定的时间表，但如果是运动队的工作，则可能需要较长的、不规律的时间。大多数运动训练师都有硕士以上学历位。医疗和教学方面的就业机会预计会很好，虽然有运动队的工作有限。国家运动训练师协会（National Athletic Trainers' Association）在 www.nata.org 有更多关于这个职业的信息。

· 健身工作者（fitness worker）包括各种职业活动，如私人教练以及团体健身、瑜伽和普拉提教练。在各种类型的锻炼活动中，这些专业人员引导、指导和激励个人或团体。传统上，他们在工作室、健身俱乐部或私人住宅工作，但他们越来越多地出现在工作场所，组织和指导员工的健身计划。他们的工作也可能涉及管理责任。私人教练必须获得认证，其他健身专业人员也被鼓励进行认证。考生必须具有高中毕业文凭和心肺复苏术（CPR）证书，并且必须通过书面考试，有时还要通过实践考试。越来越多地需要学士学位，希望进入管理工作的人可能需要更高的学位。专门从事特定运动方式的教练，如普拉提或瑜伽，必须通过自己的培训标准。这些领域的就业机会预计随着人口老龄化和对健康和身体健康的日益关注而增加。全国认证机构委员会（National Commission for Certifying Agencies）在 credentialingexcellence.org 可以帮助找到认可的健身认证项目。

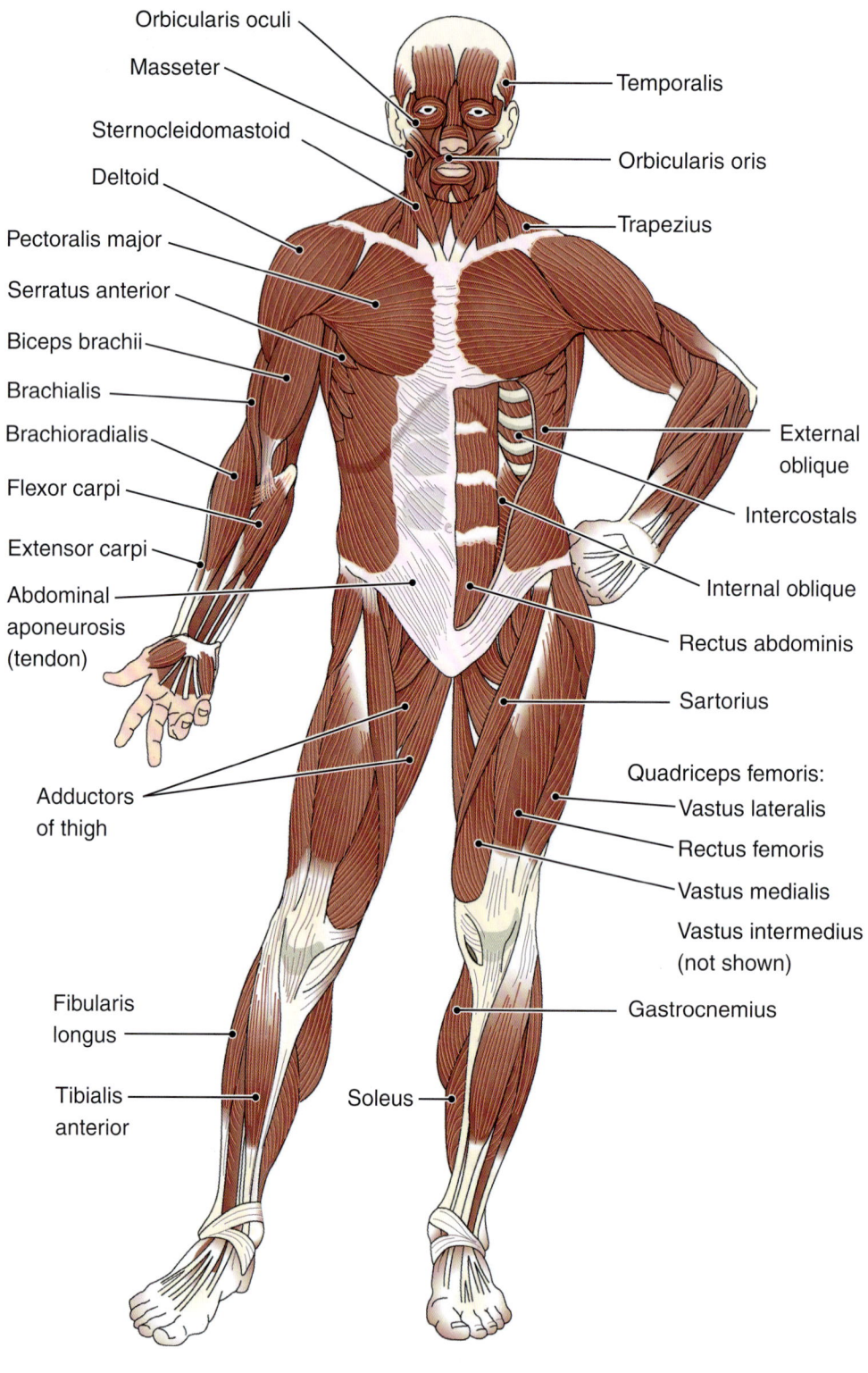

图 20-6 浅表肌肉，前视图

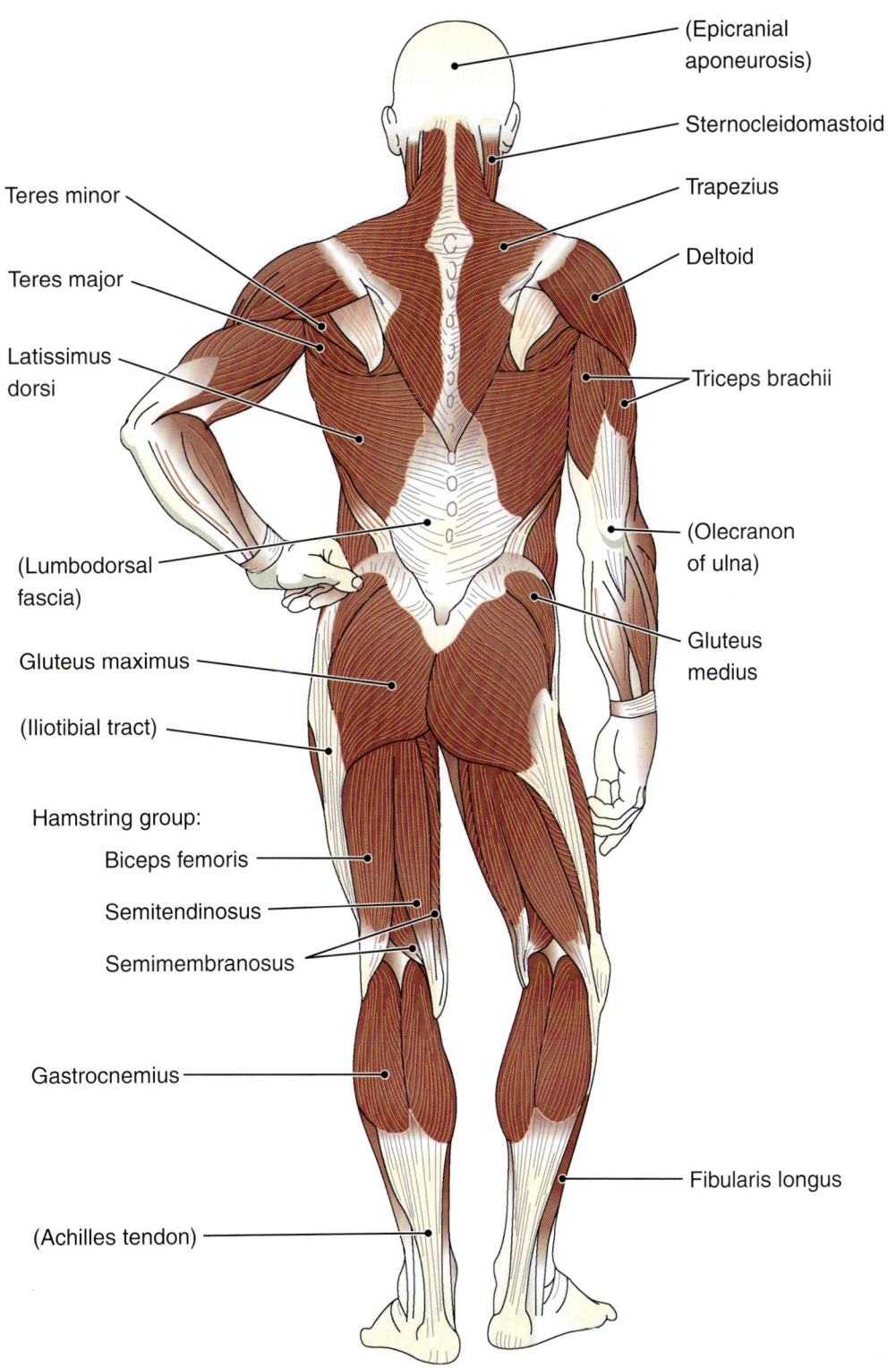

图 20-7 浅表肌肉，后视图。相关组织标记在括号中

Terminology 关键术语

正常结构与功能

acetylcholine (ACh)　[ˌæsitil'kɒli:n]	乙酰胆碱，一种刺激骨骼肌收缩的神经递质
actin　['æktin]	肌动蛋白，肌肉细胞中的两种收缩蛋白之一；另一种是肌球蛋白
agonist　['ægənist]	主动肌，执行给定运动的肌肉（源自于希腊语 agon 意为"竞赛"、"奋斗"）
antagonist　[æn'tægənist]	对抗肌，与主动肌相对的肌肉，在主动肌收缩时它必须放松
cardiac muscle	心肌，构成心脏壁的非自主肌肉
fascia　['feiʃə]	筋膜，覆盖肌肉的结缔组织纤维鞘（词根：fasci/o）；复数形式为 fasciae
fascicle　['fæsikl]	肌束，肌肉或神经纤维的小束
insertion　[in'sɜːʃn]	附着点，在给定的运动中，肌肉在骨骼的运动部分的附着点
muscle　['mʌsl]	肌肉，通过收缩产生运动的器官；也指构成这种器官的组织（词根：my/o, muscul/o）
myosin　['maiəsin]	肌球蛋白，肌肉细胞中的两种收缩蛋白之一；另一种是肌动蛋白
neuromuscular junction (NMJ)	神经肌肉接点，运动神经元分支与肌肉细胞直接的接触点，或突触
origin　['ɒridʒin]	起端，在给定运动中，肌肉在骨骼的稳定部分的附着点
skeletal muscle　['skelitl]	骨骼肌，运动骨骼并保持体态的自主肌肉
smooth muscle　[smuːð]	平滑肌，构成中空器官、血管和导管内壁的非自主肌肉
synergist　['sinədʒist]	协作肌，协助主动肌产生给定运动的肌肉
tendon　['tendən]	肌腱，连接肌肉与骨骼的结缔组织纤维带（词根：ten/o, tendin/o）
tonus　['təʊnəs]	紧张，肌肉部分收缩保持稳固的稳定状态；又称为肌肉紧张（muscle tone，词根：ton/o）

与肌肉相关的词根

参见表 20-1

表 4-1　与肌肉相关的词根

词根	含义	示例	示例定义
my/o	肌肉	myositis*　[maiəʊ'saitis]	肌炎
muscul/o	肌肉	musculature　['mʌskjələtʃə(r)]	肌肉组织
in/o	肌肉纤维	inotropic　[ˌiːnə'trɒpik]	作用于肌肉纤维的

续表 4-1　与肌肉相关的词根

词根	含义	示例	示例定义
fasci/o	筋膜	fasciodesis [fæˈʃiːəʊdiːsis]	筋膜固定术
ten/o, tendin/o	肌腱	tenostosis [tenɒsˈtəʊsis]	腱骨化
ton/o	肌肉紧张	cardiotonic [kɑːdiəʊˈtɒnik]	强心剂
erg/o	工作	ergonomics [ˌɜːgəˈnɒmiks]	工效学
kin/o-, kine, kinesi/o, kinet/o	运动	kinesis [kiˈniːsis]	运动（复数 kinetic）

* 请注意，该词根在后缀 -itis 前增加了一个 s

练习 20-1

定义下列形容词。

1. muscular
2. fascial
3. kinetic
4. tendinous
5. tonic

写出下列定义的单词。

6. incision into a muscle
7. inflammation of a muscle with its tendon
8. study of movement
9. excision of fascia
10. pain in a tendon

填空。

11. Myoglobin [ˈmaiəˌgləʊbin] is a type of protein (globin) found in_____.
12. Inosclerosis [inɒskləˈrəʊsis] is hardening of tissue from an increase in_____.
13. Fasciitis [ˌfæʃiˈaitis] is inflammation of_____.
14. Dystonia [disˈtəʊniə] is abnormal muscle_____.
15. An ergograph [ˈɜːgəʊgrɑːf] is an instrument for recording muscle_____.
16. Kinesia [kaiˈniːziə] is a term for sickness caused by_____.
17. Myofibrils [maiɔːˈfaibrilz] are small fibers found in_____.
18. The muscularis layer in the wall of a hollow organ or duct is composed of_____.

练习 20-1 （续表）

定义下列术语。

19. hypermyotonia [haipəmaiə'təuniə] _____
20. fasciorrhaphy ['fæʃiərəfi] _____
21. tendinitis [ˌtendi'naitis], also tendonitis [ten'dəunaitis] _____
22. musculotendinous [mʌskjuləu'tendinəs] _____
23. tenodesis [te'nəudi:sis] _____
24. myalgia [mai'ældʒə] _____
25. kinesitherapy [kaini:si'θerəpi] _____
26. dyskinesia [ˌdiski'ni:ʒə] _____
27. atony ['ætəni:] _____
28. ergogenic [ɜ:'gədʒenik] _____
29. myofascial [maiɔ:'fæʃl] _____
30. myotenositis [maiə'tenəsaitis] _____

肌肉系统的临床表现

肌肉的功能可能受其他部位疾病的影响，特别是神经系统和结缔组织。下面描述的直接影响肌肉系统或涉及肌肉的状况在其他章节没有讨论。任何肌肉的病症都可以被称为肌病（myopathy）。

诊断肌肉病症的技术包括研究肌肉动作电信号的肌电图（electromyography，EMG）和血清测定从受损肌肉中释放的酶的增加量，主要是肌酸激酶（creatine kinase，CK）。

肌肉萎缩症

肌肉萎缩症（muscular dystrophy）是指一组涉及进行性炎性肌肉变性的遗传性疾病。肌肉组织被弱化和破坏，并逐渐被结缔组织和脂肪替代。还可能有心肌症（cardiomyopathy）和精神损伤。

最常见的是杜氏肌营养不良（Duchenne muscular dystrophy），是一种由母亲传给儿子的性别相关的疾病。这种疾病发生在3~4岁，患者在10~15岁就会丧失行动能力。通常会因呼吸衰竭或感染导致死亡。

涉及肌肉的多系统疾病

多肌炎

多肌炎（polymyositis）是骨骼肌的炎症，会导致虚弱，常伴有吞咽困难或心脏问题。起因不明，可能与病毒感染或自免疫有关。该疾病常常伴有一些其他全身性疾病，例如风湿性关节炎或红斑狼疮（lupus erythematosus）。

当涉及皮肤时，该病症被称为皮肌炎。在这种情况下，会有红肿（erythema）、皮炎（dermatitis）和典型的丁香紫色皮疹，主要在面部。除酶分析和肌电图外，临床诊断中还会使用肌肉活检。

纤维肌痛综合征

纤维肌痛综合征（fibromyalgia syndrome，FMS）是一种很难诊断的涉及肌肉的病症。通常伴有扩散的肌肉疼痛、压痛和僵硬，还有疲乏和睡眠问题，但没有任何神经异常或其他已知病因。该疾病可能与其他慢性疾病共存，可能继发病毒感染，并涉及免疫系统障碍。现行的理论认为纤维肌痛综合征是提供疼痛灵敏性的激素或神经递质失衡所致的。治疗包括细致计划的锻炼和缓解疼痛、放松肌肉或抗抑郁药物。

慢性疲劳综合征

慢性疲劳综合征（chronic fatigue syndrome，CFS）涉及起因不明的持续性疲乏，并伴有记忆力受损、咽喉痛、淋巴结痛、肌肉和关节疼痛、头痛、睡

框 20-4 聚焦单词
一些丰富多彩的肌肉骨骼术语

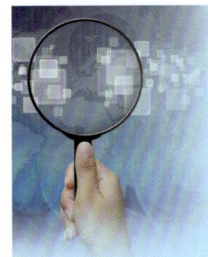

肌肉骨骼疾病的一些常见术语有很有趣的起源。charley horse 形容肌肉拉伤和疼痛，特别是腿部肌肉。该术语源自于常用 Charley 来称呼那些不能干重活的只能留作家用的老瘸马。歪脖（wryneck）在学术上是指斜颈（torticollis），用单词 wry 表示扭曲的或转动的，例如在单词 awry 意为不妥或失位。

蹰囊炎（bunion）在学术上被称为蹰趾外翻（hallux valgus），是指大脚趾第一关节肿大，且有关节滑囊炎。它可能源自于单词 bony，变形为 bunny，用于形容头部的凸起和关节肿胀。鸡眼（clavus）通常被称为玉米（corn），因为它是在摩擦或压力区域的皮肤硬化或角质增厚。

眠问题和免疫疾病。这种状况常常发生在病毒感染之后。EB 病毒（EpsteinBarr viru）（单核细胞增多症的起因）、疱疹病毒和其他病毒可能是慢性疲劳综合征的可能起因。在治疗方面，目前没有明确有效的传统或替代性疗法。

重症肌无力

重症肌无力（myasthenia gravis，MG）是一种获得性自身免疫疾病，抗体在神经肌肉接点干扰肌肉刺激。肌肉力量会进行性损失，特别是眼睛外部和面部肌肉。

肌萎缩性脊髓侧索硬化症

肌萎缩性脊髓侧索硬化症（amyotrophic lateral sclerosis，ALS）是一种导致肌肉萎缩（amyotrophy）的运动神经元进行性变性，在一位著名的棒球选手因该病死亡后，又被称为伽雷病（Lou Gehrig disease）。早期征兆是虚弱、抽筋和肌肉痉挛。根据变性部位，面部肌肉或呼吸肌可能受到早期影响。心理功能、感知觉以及肠和膀胱功能通常保持完好。疾病的发展最终在 3~5 年内因呼吸肌麻痹导致死亡。

应力性损伤

压力性损伤（stress injury）不像上述疾病那样严重，但更常见的是由物理压力引起的肌肉骨骼疾病。这包括意外受伤和因过度用力或重复运动引起的工作或运动相关的损伤，即所谓的重复性劳损（repetitive strain injury，RSI）。软组织损伤包括扭伤（sprain）、关节异常或过度用力引起的韧带损伤（但没有骨骼脱臼或骨折）、肌肉拉伤、韧带或肌腱发炎或撕裂，以及滑囊炎。腱鞘炎（tenosynovitis）通常被称为肌腱炎（tendinitis），是肌腱、腱鞘和关节滑膜的炎症。这些损伤的症状是疼痛、疲乏、虚弱、僵硬、麻木和活动范围（range of motion，ROM）降低。框 20-4 给出了这些病症术语的来源。

压力性损伤可能涉及任何肌肉或关节，一些常见的上肢病症有：

- 旋转肌群（rotator cuff，RTC）损伤——加强肩关节的旋转肌群由四块肌肉组成，冈上肌（supraspinatus）、冈下肌（infraspinatus）、小圆肌（teres minor）和肩胛下肌（subscapularis）（图 20-8）。反复进行游泳、喷漆或投球等头顶活动的人，容易发生旋转肌群的发炎或撕裂。
- 上踝炎（epicondylitis）——远端肱骨的内侧和外侧上踝（突起）是用于弯曲和伸展手腕和手指的肌肉的附着点。这些肌腱原发的炎症会在抬举、携带、挤压或打字时引起肘部和前臂的疼痛。这些压力性损伤常常与运动相关，因此内侧和外侧的上踝炎分别被称为"高尔夫球肘"和"网球肘"。在肘部下面佩戴将应力分布在关节上的支架可能会有所帮助。
- 腕管综合征（carpal tunnel syndrome，CTS）——腕管综合征涉及手指屈肌的肌腱和支持手和手指的神经（图 20-9）。手麻木和虚弱是由正中神经通过由腕骨形成的隧道时产生的压力引起的。腕管综合征常见于过度使用手和手指的人，如音乐家和键盘手。
- 扳机指（trigger finger）——手指运动时有痛苦的咔咔声或锁定声，起因是掌指关节屈肌腱

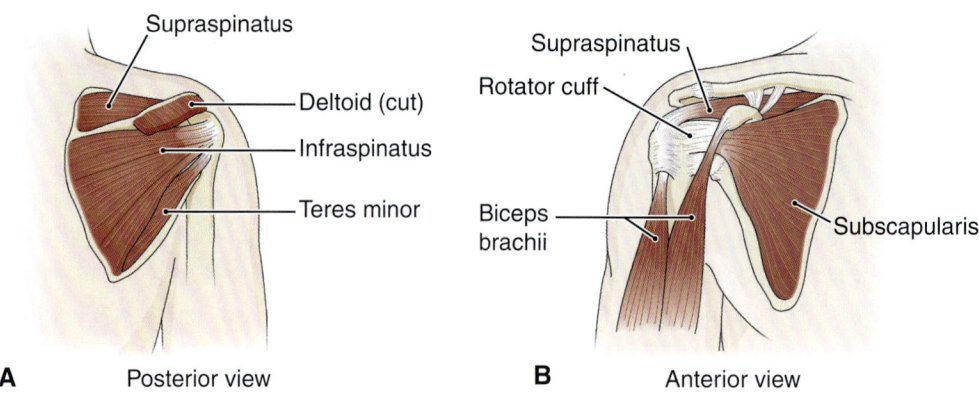

图 20-8 旋转肌群解剖。旋转肌群的四块肌肉有助于加强肩膀。它们是冈上肌、冈下肌、小圆肌和肩胛下肌。还示出了两块相邻的肌肉，三角肌和肱二头肌。A. 后。B. 前

鞘的炎症和肿胀妨碍肌腱前后滑动。
涉及下肢的压力性损伤有：

· 大腿后侧肌肉拉伤（hamstring strain）——腘绳肌是大腿后侧的一大组肌肉，从髋延伸至膝，并负责弯曲膝关节（图 20-7）。大腿后侧肌肉拉伤常见于要突然停止再开始跑动的运动员。这种疾病的治疗需要进行拉伸和加强活动。

· 胫纤维发炎（shin splint）——这是腿的前胫骨区域由于在硬表面上运动或足部屈肌过度使用而导致的疼痛，常见于运动员和舞蹈者。有足够支撑的鞋和避免在硬的表面锻炼会有所帮助。

· 跟腱炎（achilles tendinitis）——跟腱是将小腿肌肉连接到脚后跟，并用于足底将脚在脚踝处弯曲的大肌腱（图 20-5 和图 20-7）。跟腱损伤会妨碍行走和跑步。

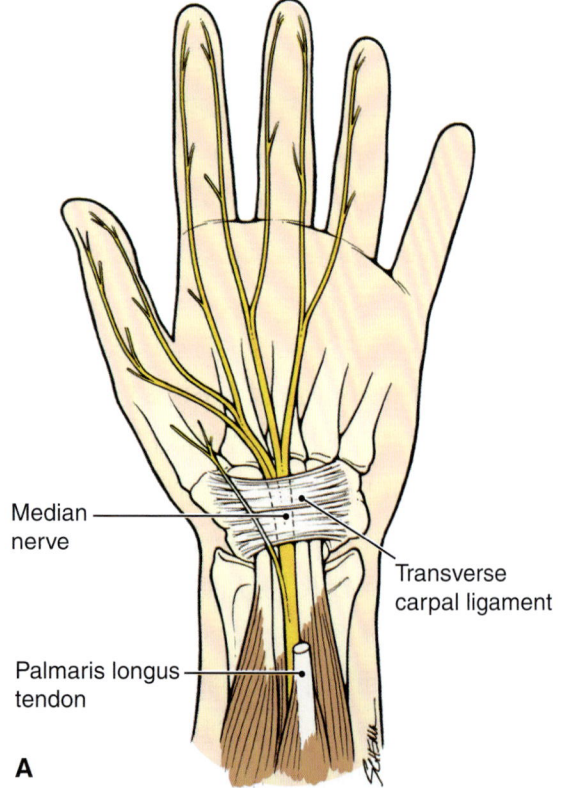

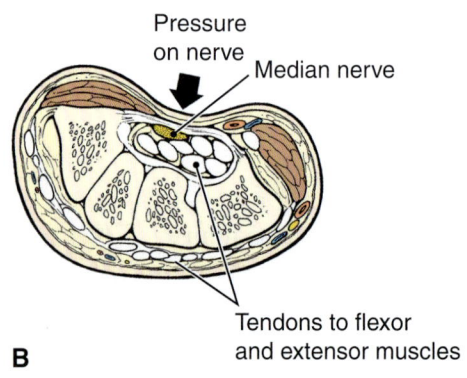

图 20-9 腕管综合征。A. 正中神经在通过腕骨（手腕）骨骼时的压力导致手上备有神经的区域麻木和虚弱；B. 手腕的横截面显示正中神经受压

治疗

骨科医生利用核磁共振和其他成像技术、运动范围测量和力量测试来诊断肌肉骨骼疾病。应力性损伤的治疗开始通常是保守性的休息、抬升、冰敷、支撑固定和药物,例如镇痛药、抗炎药和肌肉松弛药。字母缩写 RICE 描述了这一简单过程——休息(rest)、冰敷(ice)、紧压(compression)、抬升(elevation)。如果情况严重,治疗可能发展到类固醇注射、深度加热超声波疗法、强化锻炼,甚至手术。

Terminology 关键术语

病症

amyotrophic lateral sclerosis (ALS) [eimaiə'trɒfik]	肌萎缩侧索硬化症,一种由运动神经元变性引起的疾病,会导致肌肉无力和萎缩;也被称为伽雷病(Lou Gehrig disease)
chronic fatigue syndrome (CFS)	慢性疲劳综合征,一种起因不明的疾病,涉及持续疲劳,伴随肌肉和关节疼痛及其他症状;可能是病毒诱发的
dermatomyositis [dɜ:mətəmaiə'saitis]	皮肌炎,一种起因不明的疾病,包括肌肉炎症以及皮炎和皮疹
fibromyalgia syndrome (FMS) [ˌfaibrəumai'ældʒi:ə]	纤维肌痛综合征,一种与广泛的肌肉疼痛和僵硬相关,但没有任何已知病因的疾病
muscular dystrophy ['mʌskjələ 'distrəfi]	肌肉萎缩症,一组以进行性虚弱和肌肉萎缩为特征的遗传性肌肉疾病
myasthenia gravis (MG) [ˌmaiəs'θi:niə 'grævis]	重症肌无力,以进行性肌无力为特征的疾病;影响神经肌肉接合点的自身免疫疾病
polymyositis [pɒlimaiə'saitis]	多肌炎,涉及肌肉炎症和虚弱的起因不明的疾病
repetitive strain injury (RSI) [ri'petitiv strein 'indʒəri]	重复性劳损,由重复运动引起的组织损伤,通常是手臂或手在诸如书写、打字、绘画或使用手动工具等职业活动中过度使用;也称为重复运动损伤、累积性创伤损伤、过度使用综合征
sprain [sprein]	扭伤,由关节上的异常或过度用力引起的韧带损伤,但没有骨脱位或骨折
strain [strein]	拉伤,由于过度使用或过度伸展导致肌肉的创伤;如果严重,可能涉及肌肉撕裂、出血、肌肉与肌腱分离或肌腱与骨分离
tendinitis [ˌtendi'naitis]	肌腱炎,肌腱的炎症,通常由损伤或过度使用引起;肩、肘和髋是常见的部位;也拼写为 tendonitis
tenosynovitis [tenəʊsinə'vaitis]	腱鞘炎,肌腱及腱鞘的炎症

诊断

creatine kinase (CK) ['kri:ətin 'kineis]	肌酸激酶,一种在肌肉组织中发现的酶;在肌肉受伤的情况下,血清肌酸激酶水平会升高;又称为肌酸磷酸激酶(creatine phosphokinase, CPK)
electromyography (EMG) [iˌlektrəʊmai'ɒgrəfi]	肌电图学,收缩期肌肉电活动的研究

Terminology 补充术语

正常结构与功能

aponeurosis [ˌæpənʊˈrɒsis]	腱膜，将肌肉与其能够移动的部分相连接的平坦、白色的片状肌腱（参见腹部腱膜，图 20-6）
creatine [ˈkriːətin]	肌酸，肌肉细胞中为收缩储存能量的一种物质
glycogen [ˈglikəʊdʒen]	糖原，一种在肌肉和肝脏中储存能量的复杂的糖
isometric [ˌaisəˈmetrik]	等量的，关于肌肉紧张但不收缩的肌肉动作的（字面含义为相同的测量）
isotonic [ˌaisəʊˈtɒnik]	等张的，关于肌肉收缩以完成动作的肌肉动作的（字面含义为相同的张力）
kinesthesia [ˌkinəsˈθiːʒiə]	运动感觉，对运动的意识、重量、方向和运动程度的感知（-esthesia 意为"感觉"）
lactic acid [ˌlæktik ˈæsid]	乳酸，积累在没有足够氧的肌肉细胞中的酸（厌氧），如在较大体力消耗运动时
motor unit [ˈməʊtə ˈjuːnit]	运动单位，一个单独运动神经元和其分支刺激的所有肌肉细胞
myoglobin [ˈmaiəˌgləʊbin]	肌红蛋白，在肌肉细胞中存储氧气的类似于血红蛋白的色素

症状与病症

asterixis [ˌæstəˈriksis]	扑翼样震颤，肌肉紧张间歇性丧失引起的快速、不稳定的运动，特别是在手上
asthenia [æsˈθiːniə]	虚弱，虚弱无力（前缀 a- 意为"没有"，词根 sthen/o 意为"力量"）
ataxia [əˈtæksiə]	共济失调，缺乏肌肉协调（源自于词根 tax/o 意为"次序、排列"）（形容词：ataxic）
athetosis [ˌæðəˈtəʊsis]	手足徐动症，一种以缓慢、不规律抽搐为特征的状态，特别是在手和手指上（形容词：athetotic）
atrophy [ˈætrəfi]	萎缩，一种消瘦；组织或器官大小的减小，例如由于废用造成的肌肉消瘦
avulsion [əˈvʌlʃən]	撕脱，强行撕去一部分
clonus [ˈkləʊnəs]	阵挛，肌肉交替痉挛收缩和松弛（形容词：clonic）
contracture [kənˈtræktʃə]	挛缩，肌肉持久收缩
fasciculation [fəˌsikjʊˈleiʃən]	肌束震颤，肌纤维组（fasciculi）不自主的小收缩或抽搐
fibromyositis [ˌfaibrəʊmaiəˈsaitis]	纤维肌炎，形容肌肉和关节疼痛、压痛和僵硬的非特定术语
fibrositis [ˌfaibrəˈsaitis]	纤维组织炎，纤维结缔组织的炎症，特别是肌筋膜；特征是疼痛和僵硬
restless legs syndrome (RLS)	不宁腿综合征，上床后发生的腿部的不适、抽搐或不安，常常导致失眠；可能由循环不良或药物不良反应引起
rhabdomyolysis [ˌræbdəʊmaiˈɒlisis]	横纹肌溶解症，一种涉及骨骼肌细胞扩散性破坏的急性疾病（词根：rhabd/o 意为"杆细胞"，指长杆状的肌肉细胞）
rhabdomyoma [ˌræbdəʊmaiˈəʊmə]	横纹肌瘤，骨骼肌的良性肿瘤

Terminology 补充术语（续表）

rhabdomyosarcoma [ˈræbdəʊmaiəʊsɑːˈkəʊmə]	横纹肌肉瘤，一种骨骼肌的高度恶性肿瘤
rheumatism [ˈruːmətizəm]	风湿病，形容与关节疼痛相关的炎症、酸痛和僵硬的通用术语（形容词：rheumatic, rheumatoid）
spasm [ˈspæzəm]	痉挛，一种突然、不自主的肌肉收缩，可以是阵挛性的（收缩与松弛交替）或强直的（持续的），强烈而疼痛的痉挛可以称为痛性痉挛（cramp）（形容词：spastic, spasmodic）
spasticity [spæsˈtisiti]	强直状态，肌肉张力升高或收缩引起僵硬或动作笨拙
tetanus [ˈtetənəs]	破伤风，一种由厌氧菌梭菌引起的急性传染病。它的特征是自主肌肉持续的疼痛痉挛；也被称为牙关紧闭症（lockjaw）
tetany [ˈtetəni]	强直，一种以由代谢失衡，引起的痉挛、痛性痉挛和肌肉抽搐为特征的病症，例如由甲状旁腺活动不足引起的低血钙，
torticollis [ˌtɔːtiˈkɒlis]	斜颈，颈部肌肉的痉挛性收缩引起颈部的僵硬和扭曲；也常用 wryneck
诊断与治疗	
chvostek sign	面神经征，叩击面神经后面部肌肉的痉挛、强直的证据
occupational therapy	职业疗法，涉及通过工作和娱乐活动提高功能和预防残疾的健康专业。职业疗法的目标是增加患者日常生活的独立性和质量
physical therapy	物理疗法，涉及身体康复和预防残疾的健康专业。使用锻炼、按摩和其他治疗方法恢复正常运动
rheumatology [ˌruːməˈtɒlədʒi]	风湿病学，研究和治疗风湿疾病
Trousseau sign	低钙束臂征，通过按压支持肌肉的神经引起的痉挛性收缩；常见于强直
药物	
COX-2 inhibitor	环氧化酶-2 抑制剂，非甾体抗炎药物，不会引起与其他非甾体抗炎药物相关的胃部问题。抑制环氧化酶-2 酶而不影响环氧化酶-1 酶，缺乏环氧化酶-1 酶会引起胃溃疡。这些药物中的一部分由于心脏风险已经退出市场
muscle relaxant [riˈlæksənt]	肌肉松弛剂，降低肌肉张力的药物，不同的松弛剂可用于在手术期间放松肌肉、控制强直或缓解肌肉骨骼疼痛
nonsteroidal antiinflammatory drug (NSAID) [ˈnɒnstərɔidl]	非甾体抗炎药，包括阿司匹林、布洛芬、萘普生（naproxen）和其他前列腺素抑制剂，前列腺素是自然产生的促进炎症的物质

Terminology	缩略语		
ACh	Acetylcholine		乙酰胆碱
ALS	Amyotrophic lateral sclerosis		肌萎缩性脊髓侧索硬化症
CFS	Chronic fatigue syndrome		慢性疲劳综合征
C(P)K	Creatine (phospho)kinase		肌酸（磷酸）激酶
CTS	Carpal tunnel syndrome		腕管综合征
EMG	Electromyography, electromyogram		肌电描记法、肌电图
FMS	Fibromyalgia syndrome		纤维肌痛综合征
MG	Myasthenia gravis		重症肌无力
MMT	Manual muscle test(ing)		徒手肌力测试
NMJ	Neuromuscular junction		神经肌肉接点
OT	Occupational therapy/therapist		职业疗法/治疗师
PT	Physical therapy/therapist		物理疗法/治疗师
RICE	Rest, ice, compression, elevation		休息、冰敷、加压、抬高
RLS	Restless legs syndrome		不宁腿综合征
ROM	Range of motion		运动范围
RSI	Repetitive strain injury		重复性劳损
RTC	Rotator cuff		肩袖
SITS	Supraspinatus, infraspinatus, teres minor, subscapularis (muscles)		冈上肌、冈下肌、小圆肌、肩胛下肌（肌肉）

Case Study Revisited
案例研究再访

T.D.'s Follow-Up

The exploratory surgery confirmed the brachial plexus injury, and T.D. underwent the nerve graft with muscle taken from his right thigh. After six days, he was discharged home with his right arm in a shoulder immobilizer. He received instructions on activities and was told to see the surgeon in one week and again three weeks later. Physical therapy was ordered to prevent further atrophy and to begin rebuilding the arm muscles. T.D. was frustrated with the slow progress, but the orthopedic surgeon had said that in time, he should regain full use of his right arm and normal activities of daily living should be restored.

T.D. 的随访

探查性手术证实了臂丛神经损伤，并从T.D.右大腿取肌肉进行神经移植。6天后，他出院回家，右手臂固定在肩膀固定器上。他接受了关于活动的指导，并被告知在1个星期和3个星期后再来看医生。安排物理疗法以防止进一步萎缩并开始重建手臂肌肉。T.D.对于缓慢的进展感到沮丧，但是骨科医生说他应该及时重新充分利用他的右臂，并恢复正常的日常生活活动。

CHAPTER 20 复习

标记练习

表浅肌肉，前视图

在对应的下划线上写出每个编号部分的名称。

Adductors of thigh
Biceps brachii
Brachialis
Brachioradialis
Deltoid
Extensor carpi
External oblique
Fibularis longus
Flexor carpi
Gastrocnemius
Intercostals
Internal oblique
Masseter
Orbicularis oculi
Orbicularis oris
Pectoralis major
Quadriceps femoris
Rectus abdominis
Sartorius
Serratus anterior
Soleus
Sternocleidomastoid
Temporalis
Tibialis anterior
Trapezius

1. _____
2. _____
3. _____
4. _____
5. _____
6. _____
7. _____
8. _____
9. _____
10. _____
11. _____
12. _____
13. _____
14. _____
15. _____
16. _____
17. _____
18. _____
19. _____
20. _____
21. _____
22. _____
23. _____
24. _____
25. _____

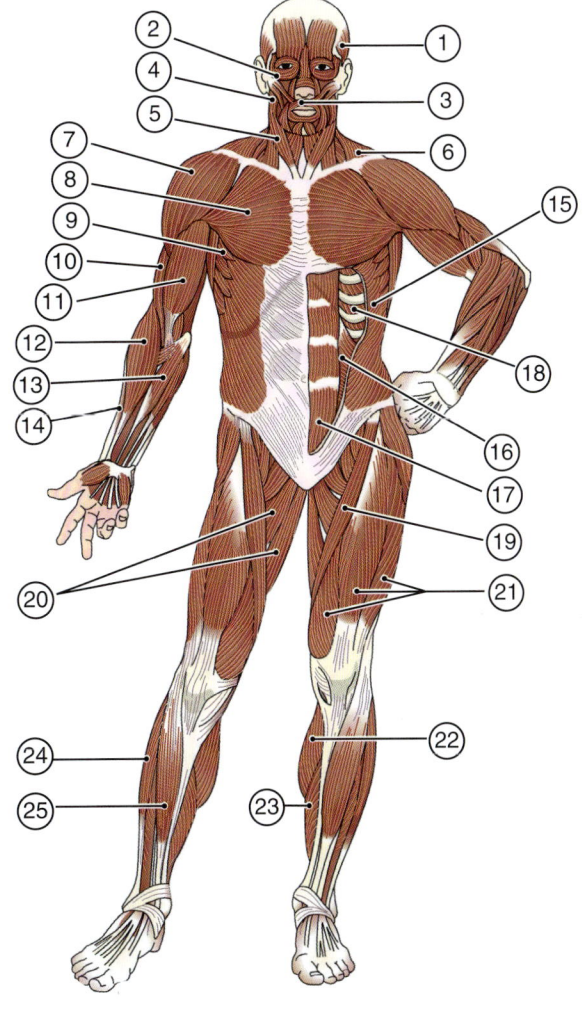

Anterior view

表浅肌肉，后视图

在对应的下划线上写出每个编号部分的名称。

Deltoid
Fibularis longus
Gastrocnemius
Gluteus maximus
Gluteus medius
Hamstring group

Latissimus dorsi
Sternocleidomastoid
Teres major
Teres minor
Trapezius
Triceps brachii

1. _____
2. _____
3. _____
4. _____
5. _____
6. _____
7. _____
8. _____
9. _____
10. _____
11. _____
12. _____

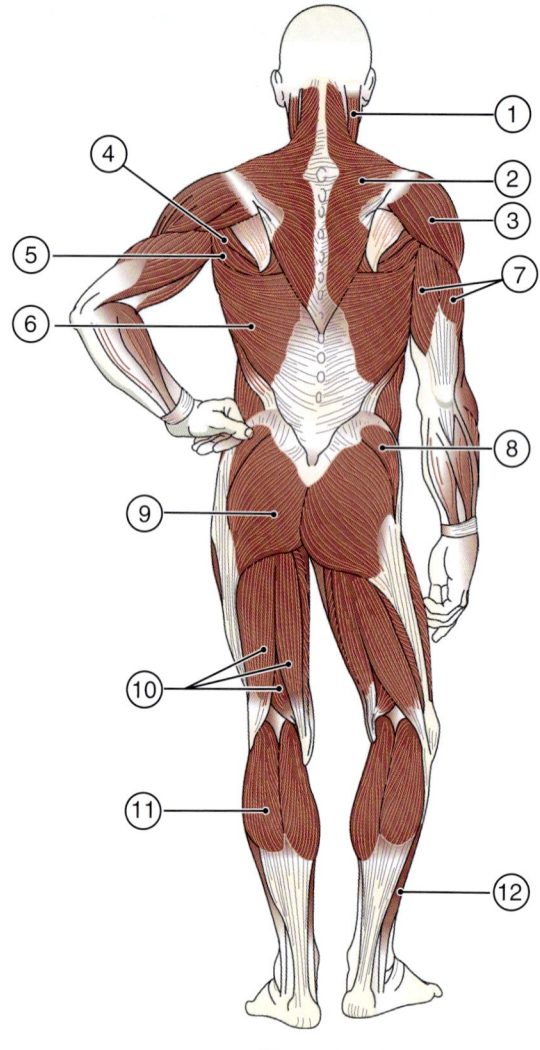

Posterior view

术语

匹配

匹配下列术语，字在每个题号左侧写上适当的字母。

____ 1. masseter a. muscle used in chewing; jaw muscle
____ 2. quadriceps femoris b. large muscle of the upper chest
____ 3. pectoralis major c. a group of four muscles in the thigh
____ 4. gastrocnemius d. main muscle of the calf
____ 5. trapezius e. muscle of the upper back and neck

____ 6. akinesia a. instrument for measuring muscle work
____ 7. fascicle b. absence of movement
____ 8. inotropic c. a small bundle of fibers

___ 9. dystonia   d. acting on muscle fibers
___ 10. ergometer   e. abnormal muscle tone

补充术语

___ 11. lactic acid   a. protein that stores oxygen in muscle cells
___ 12. aponeurosis   b. flat, white, sheet-like tendon
___ 13. tetany   c. muscular spasms and cramps
___ 14. myoglobin   d. complex sugar stored in muscles
___ 15. glycogen   e. byproduct of anaerobic muscle contractions

___ 16. asterixis   a. awareness of movement
___ 17. ataxia   b. weakness
___ 18. torticollis   c. rapid, jerky movements, especially of the hands
___ 19. asthenia   d. wryneck
___ 20. kinesthesia   e. lack of muscle coordination

___ 21. athetosis   a. forcible tearing away of a part
___ 22. clonus   b. acute infectious disease that affects muscles
___ 23. spasm   c. intermittent muscle contractions
___ 24. avulsion   d. sudden involuntary muscle contraction
___ 25. tetanus   e. condition marked by slow, twisting movements

参照 T.D. 的案例研究。

___ 26. deltoid   a. partial dislocation
___ 27. atrophy   b. shoulder muscle
___ 28. subluxation   c. network
___ 29. plexus   d. pertaining to the diaphragm
___ 30. phrenic   e. tissue wasting

填空

31. A band of connective tissue that attaches a muscle to a bone is a(n)_____.
32. A musculotropic substance acts on_____.
33. The number of origins (heads) in the triceps brachii muscle is_____.
34. A muscle that produces extension at a joint is called a(n) _____.
35. The neurotransmitter released at the neuromuscular junction is_____.
36. The strong, cord-like tendon that attaches the calf muscle to the heel is the_____.
37. Movement toward the midline of the body is termed_____.
38. The sheath of connective tissue that covers a muscle is called_____.

参照 T.D. 的案例研究。

39. The nerves of the brachial plexus supply the_____.
40. The muscle above the spine of the scapula is the_____.
41. The vertebra C7 is in the region of the_____.

定义

定义下列单词。

42. myofascial ［maiɔːˈfæʃl］ _____
43. tendinoplasty ［tendiˈnɒplæsti］ _____
44. hypotonia ［haipəˈtəʊniə］ _____
45. hyperkinesia ［ˌhaipəkiˈniːʒə］ _____
46. inotropic ［ˌiːnəˈtrɒpik］ _____
47. myositis ［maiəʊˈsaitis］ _____

写出下列定义的单词。

48. suture of fascia _____
49. death of muscle tissue _____
50. study of movement _____
51. absence of muscle tone _____
52. surgical incision of a tendon (use ten/o-) _____
53. study of muscles _____
54. excision of fascia _____
55. pertaining to a tendon _____

反义词

写出下列关于肌肉的术语的反义词。

56. agonist _____
57. origin _____
58. abduction _____
59. pronation _____
60. extension _____

形容词

写出下列补充术语的形容词形式。

61. ataxia _____
62. athetosis _____
63. spasm _____
64. clonus _____

真假判断

检查以下语句。如果语句为真，则在第一个空格写入 T；如果语句为假，则在第一个空格中写入 F，并通过在第二个空格中替换带下划线的单词来更正语句。

	True or False	Correct Answer
65. The part of a neuron that contacts a muscle cell is the <u>dendrite</u>.	_____	_____
66. Skeletal muscle is <u>involuntary</u>.	_____	_____

67. The quadriceps muscle has <u>three</u> components.
68. <u>Pronation</u> means turning downward.
69. The hamstring group is in the <u>anterior</u> thigh.
70. Smooth muscle is also called <u>visceral</u> muscle.
71. The <u>origin</u> of a muscle is attached to a moving part.
72. In an <u>isotonic</u> contraction, a muscle shortens.

排除

在下列每组中，为与其余不相配的单词加下划线，并说明你选择的理由。

73. fascicle — fiber — tendon — osteoblast — fascia

74. soleus — flexor carpi — biceps brachii — brachioradialis — extensor carpi

75. vastus intermedius — intercostals — vastus lateralis — vastus medialis — rectus femoris

76. circumduction — inversion — actin — dorsiflexion — rotation

77. EMG — ALS — FMS — CFS — MG

缩略语

写出下列缩略语的含义。

78. RICE
79. RTC
80. CTS
81. NMJ
82. EMG

单词构建

使用给出的单词组成部分写出下列定义的单词。

| -ia | ten/o | -al | alg/o | -itis | -desis | -blast | -lysis | fasci/o | my/o |

83. inflammation of fascia
84. binding of a tendon
85. pain in a tendon
86. destruction of muscle tissue
87. binding of a fascia
88. an immature muscle cell
89. separation of a tendon
90. pertaining to fascia
91. pain in a muscle

单词分析

定义下列单词，并给出每个单词组成部分的含义。如果需要，可以使用词典。

92. fibromyositis ['faibrəʊmaiəsaitis] _____
    a. fibr/o _____
    b. my/o(s) _____
    c. -itis _____

93. myasthenia [ˌmaiəs'θi:niə] _____
    a. my/o _____
    b. a _____
    c. sthen/o _____
    d. -ia _____

94. dyssynergia [disi'nɜ:dʒiə] _____
    a. dys _____
    b. syn _____
    c. erg/o _____
    d. -ia _____

95. amyotrophic [eimaiə'trɒfik] _____
    a. a _____
    b. my/o _____
    c. troph/o _____
    d. –ic _____

单词分析

定义下列单词，并给出每个单词组成部分的含义。如果需要，可以使用词典。

Additional Case Studies
补充案例研究

Case Study 20-1: Rotator Cuff Tear
案例研究 20-1：旋转肌群撕裂

M. L., a 56-year-old business executive and former college football player, was referred to an orthopedic surgeon for recurrent shoulder pain. M. L. was unable to abduct his right arm without pain even after six months of physical therapy and NSAIDs. In addition, he had taken supplements of glucosamine, chondroitin, and S-adenosylmethionine for several months in an effort to protect the flexibility of his shoulder joint. M. L. recalled a shoulder dislocation resulting from a football injury 35 years earlier. An MRI scan confirmed a complete rotator cuff tear. The surgeon recommended the Bankart procedure for M. L.'s injury to restore his joint stability, alleviate his pain, and permit him to return to his former normal activities, including golf. After anesthesia induction and positioning in a semisitting (beach chair) position, the surgeon made an anterosuperior deltoid incision (the standard deltopectoral approach) and divided the coracoacromial ligament at the acromial attachment. The rotator cuff was identified after the deltoid was retracted and the clavipectoral fascia was incised. The subscapularis tendon was incised proximal to its insertion.

After capsular incision, inspection showed a large pouch inferiorly in the capsule, consistent with laxity (instability). The capsule's torn edges were anchored to the rim of the glenoid fossa with heavy nonabsorbable sutures. A flap from the subscapularis tendon was transposed and sutured to the supraspinatus and infraspinatus muscles to bridge the gap. An intraoperative ROM examination showed that the external rotation could be performed past neutral and that the shoulder did not dislocate. The wound was closed, and a shoulder immobilizer sling was applied. M.L. was referred to PT to begin therapy in three weeks and was assured he would be able to play golf in six months.

M. L.是一名56岁的商业主管和前大学足球运动员，因肩痛复发被转诊给骨科医生。即使经过6个月的物理疗法和非甾体抗炎药治疗后，M. L.也无法无痛地弯曲他的右臂。此外，他已服用几个月的葡萄糖胺、软骨素和S-腺苷甲硫氨酸补充剂，努力防护他的肩关节的灵活性。M. L.回忆起一个由35年前的足球伤害导致的肩部脱臼。核磁共振扫描证实回旋肌群完全撕裂。医生建议对M. L.的损伤进行班卡特手术，恢复关节稳定性，减轻疼痛，并允许他恢复以前的正常活动，包括打高尔夫球。在麻醉诱导和半坐位定位后，医生做了前上三角肌切口（标准分层方式），并在肩峰连线处分割了喙肩韧带。在三角肌缩回和锁胸筋膜切开后，确认回旋肌群。将肩胛下肌腱在其附着点近端切开。

在囊切开后，检查显示在囊的下部有一个大的陷凹，与松弛（不稳定性）一致。囊的撕裂边缘用粗的不可收的缝线锚定在关节窝的边缘，将肩胛下肌腱的瓣片换位并缝合到冈上肌和冈下肌以桥接间隙。术中运动范围检查显示，外旋可以超过中线，肩膀没有脱位。闭合伤口，并使用肩部固定吊带。M.L.被转诊给物理治疗师开始3周的治疗，并保证他将能够在6个月内打高尔夫球。

Case Study 20-2: "Wake-Up" Test during Spinal Fusion Surgery
案例研究 20-2：脊髓融合手术中的"唤醒"测试

L. N.'s somatosensory evoked potentials (SSEPs) were monitored throughout her spinal fusion surgery to provide continuous information on the functional state of her sensory pathways from the median and posterior tibial nerves through the dorsal column to the primary somatosensory cortex. Before surgery, needle electrodes were inserted into L. N.'s right and left quadriceps muscles to determine nerve conduction through L2 to L4, into the anterior tibialis muscles to measure passage through L5, and into the gastrocnemius muscles to measure S1 to S2. Electrodes were placed in her rectus abdominis to monitor S1 to S2. All electrodes were taped in place, and the wires were

在整个脊柱融合手术中监测L. N.的躯体感觉诱发电位（SSEP），以提供关于她从中间和后胫神经通过背柱到初级躯体感觉皮层的感觉通路的功能状态的连续信息。在手术前，将针电极插入L. N.的右左四头肌肌肉中以确定通过L2～L4的神经传导，进入胫前肌以测量通过L5的通道，并进入腓肠肌以测量S1～S2的传导。将电极放置在腹直肌中以监测S1～S2。将所有电极贴在适当位置，将电线插入变压器箱中，反馈到计算机。神经监测技术人员负责安放电极，并在整个过程中参与

plugged into a transformer box with feedback to a computer. A neuromonitoring technologist placed the electrodes and attended the computer monitor throughout the case. During the procedure, selected muscle groups were stimulated with 15 to 40 milliamperes (mA) of current to test the nerves and muscles. Data fed back into the computer confirmed the neuromuscular integrity and status of the spinal fixation, the instrumentation, and implants.

After the pedicle screws, hooks, and wires were in place and the spinal rods were cinched down to straighten the spine, L. N. was permitted to emerge temporarily from anesthesia and muscle paralysis medication to a lightly sedated but pain-free state. She was given commands to move her feet, straighten her legs, and wiggle her toes to test all neuromuscular groups that could be affected by misplaced or compressed spinal fixation devices. Her feet were watched, and movement was announced to the team. Dorsiflexion cleared the tibialis anterior muscles; plantar flexion cleared the gastrocnemius muscles. Knee flexion cleared the hamstring muscle group, and knee extension determined function of the quadriceps group. L. N. had a successful "wake-up" test. She was put back into deep anesthesia, and her incision was closed. A postoperative "wake-up" test was repeated after she was moved to her bed. The surgical instruments and tables were kept sterile until after all of the monitored muscle groups were tested and showed voluntary movement. The electrodes were removed, and she was taken to the postanesthesia care unit (PACU) for recovery.

计算机监视。在该过程中，用15~40mA的电流刺激选择的肌肉组以测试神经和肌肉。数据反馈回计算机确认脊柱固定、内固定和植入物的神经肌肉的完整性和状态。

在椎弓根根钉、钩和线放置就位后，脊柱杆被收紧以拉直脊柱，L. N. 被允许暂时从麻醉和肌肉麻痹药物中脱离，达到轻度镇静但无痛的状态。她被指示移动脚、伸直腿、摆动脚趾以测试所有可能被错放或受到压缩脊柱固定装置影响的神经肌肉组。观察她的脚，身体的运动被告知手术团队。背屈表明胫前肌功能正常，足底弯曲表明腓肠肌功能正常，膝关节弯曲表明腘绳肌群功能正常，膝关节伸展确定四头肌组的功能。L. N. 的"唤醒"测试很成功。她被重新置于深度麻醉，并封闭她了的手术切口。她被移到床上后，重复做了术后"唤醒"测试。手术器械和床单保持无菌，直到所有监测的肌肉群被测试并显示自主运动。去除电极，并将她带到麻醉后护理病房（PACU）中进行康复。

案例研究问题

多项选择。选择正确的答案，在每个题号左侧写上你选择的字母。

____ 1. The insertion of the muscle is

    a. the thick middle portion

    b. the point of attachment to a moving bone

    c. the point of attachment to a stable bone

    d. the fibrous sheath

____ 2. M.L. was unable to abduct his affected arm. This motion is

    a. toward the midline

    b. circumferential

    c. away from the midline

    d. a position with the palm facing upward

____ 3. An anterosuperior deltoid incision would be made

    a. perpendicular to the muscle fibers

    b. below the fascial sheath

    c. behind the glenoid fossa

    d. at the top and to the front of the deltoid muscle

____ 4. The subscapularis tendon arises from the subscapularis

    a. fascia

    b. nerve

    c. bone

    d. flexor

____ 5. The intraoperative ROM examination was performed
   a. in the OR corridor
   b. during surgery
   c. before surgery
   d. after surgery

____ 6. M. L.'s arm and shoulder were placed in a sling after surgery to
   a. encourage movement beyond the point of pain
   b. minimize rapid ROM
   c. maintain adduction and external rotation
   d. prevent movement

____ 7. The quadriceps muscle group is made up of
   a. smooth and cardiac muscle fibers
   b. four muscles in the thigh
   c. three muscles in the leg and one in the foot
   d. fascia and tendon sheaths

____ 8. The anterior tibialis muscle is in the
   a. thigh
   b. spine
   c. foot
   d. leg

____ 9. The nerve supply for the rectus abdominis muscle runs through S1 to S2. This anatomic region is
   a. the first and second sural sheath
   b. subluxation and suppuration
   c. sacral disk space 1 and 2
   d. sacral disk space 3

____ 10. The movement of elevating the toes toward the anterior ankle is
   a. supination
   b. pronation
   c. dorsiflexion
   d. plantar flexion

____ 11. Knee extension results in
   a. a bent knee
   b. a ballet position with the toes turned out
   c. bilateral abduction
   d. a straight leg

写出案例研究中下列含义的术语。

12. pertaining to treatment of skeletal and muscular disorders_____

13. bending at a joint_____

14. to point the toes downward_____

定义下列缩略语。

15. PT_____

16. ROM_____

17. SSEP_____

18. PACU_____

CHAPTER

21 皮肤

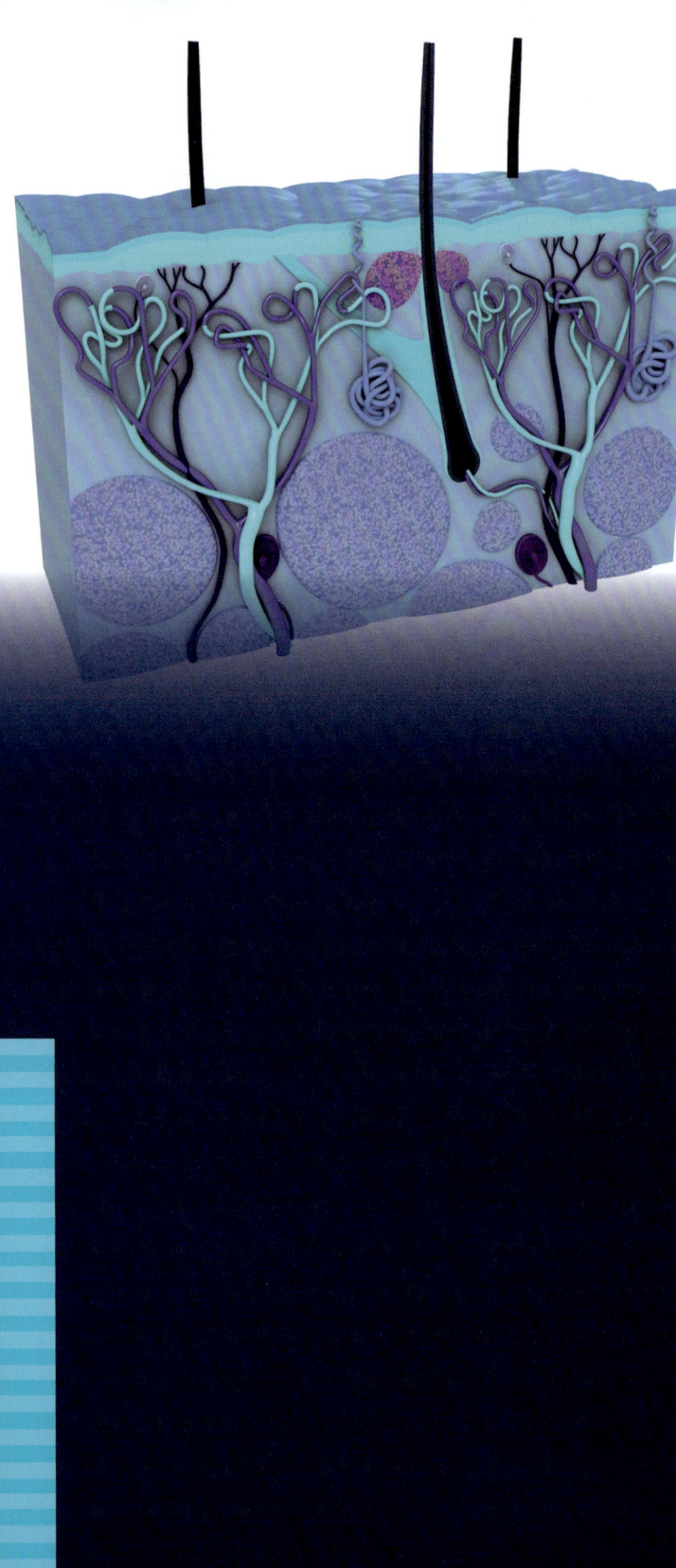

▶ **预测试**

多项选择。选择正确的答案，在每个题号左侧写上你选择的字母。

____1. The uppermost portion of the skin is called the
   a. fossa
   b. cuticle
   c. epidermis
   d. epiphysis

____2. The glands that secrete an oily substance that lubricates the skin are the
   a. mammary glands
   b. sebaceous glands
   c. sweat glands
   d. ceruminous glands

____3. The rule of nines is a system used to evaluate
   a. burns
   b. fever
   c. immunity
   d. inflammation

____4. A pigmented skin tumor is a(n)
   a. chondrosarcoma
   b. melanoma
   c. lymphoma
   d. adenoma

____5. The root hidr/o pertains to
   a. saliva
   b. tears
   c. mucus
   d. sweat

____6. Onychomycosis is a fungal infection of a(n)
   a. eyelid
   b. hair
   c. nail
   d. bone

学习目标

学完本章后，应该能够：

1 ▶ 定义并列出皮肤系统的功能。
2 ▶ 比较表皮、真皮和皮下组织的位置和结构。
3 ▶ 描述皮肤中角蛋白和黑色素的作用。
4 ▶ 例举并描述皮肤中的腺体。
5 ▶ 描述毛发和指甲的构成。
6 ▶ 识别并使用与皮肤相关的词根。
7 ▶ 描述影响皮肤的主要疾病。
8 ▶ 解释在皮肤研究和治疗中使用的缩略语。
9 ▶ 发现案例研究中涉及皮肤的医学术语。

Case Study: C. M.'s Pressure Ulcer
案例研究：C. M. 的压疮

Chief Complaint

C. M., an elderly woman in failing health, had recently moved in with her daughter after her hospitalization for a stroke. The daughter reported to the home care nurse that her mother had minimal appetite and was confused and disoriented and that a blister had developed on her lower back since she had been confined to bed.

Examination

During the biweekly visit, the home care nurse spoke with the daughter and then went in to see the mother. On her initial assessment, the nurse noted that C. M. had lost weight since her last visit and that her skin was dry, with poor skin turgor. She also observed that the mother was wearing an "adult diaper," which was wet. The nurse took the mother's BP, HR, and R, which were normal. She assessed the mother's mental status and then proceeded to a skin assessment paying special attention to the bony prominences. After examining C. M.'s sacrum, the nurse

noted a nickel-sized open area, 2 cm in diameter and 1 cm in depth (stage II pressure ulcer), with a 0.5-cm reddened surrounding area with no drainage. C. M. moaned when the nurse palpated the lesion. The nurse also noted reddened areas on C. M.'s elbows and heels. The remainder of the examination saw no change from the previous visit.

Clinical Course

The nurse provided C. M.'s daughter with instructions for proper skin care, incontinence management, enhanced nutrition, and frequent repositioning to prevent pressure ischemia to the prominent body areas. However, six months later, C. M.'s pressure ulcer had deteriorated to class III. She was hospitalized under the care of a plastic surgeon and wound care nurse. Surgery was scheduled for debridement of the sacral wound and closure with a full-thickness skin graft taken from her thigh. C. M. was discharged eight days later to a long-term care facility with orders for an alternating pressure mattress, position change every two hours, supplemental nutrition, and meticulous wound care.

主诉

C. M. 是一名健康状况每况愈下的老年妇女，在住院治疗脑卒中后最近与她女儿住在一起。女儿向家庭护理护士报告说她的母亲食欲不振，意识混乱、迷失方向，并且由于被限制在床上，她的下背部出现水疱。

检查

在每 2 个星期一次的访问期间，家庭护理护士与女儿进行了交谈，然后去看看母亲。在她的初步评估中，护士注意到从她上次访问后 C. M. 体重减轻，皮肤干燥、肿胀。她还观察到母亲穿着的"成人尿布"是湿的。护士记录了母亲的血压、心率和呼吸，都是正常的。她评估了母亲的精神状态，然后对皮肤进行了评估，特别注意骨突出。在检查了 C. M. 的骶骨后，护士注意到一个硬币大小的开放区域，直径 2cm，深度 1cm（Ⅱ期压疮），周围有 0.5cm 变红的区域，没有排出物。当护士触摸病变处时 C. M. 发出呻吟。护士还注意到 C. M. 的肘部和脚跟上的变红区域。其余的检查结果与上次访问没有变化。

临床病程

护士为 C. M. 的女儿提供与适当的皮肤护理、尿失禁管理、增加营养和频繁变换体位以防止身体突出部位局部缺血相关的指导。然而，6 个月后，C. M. 的压疮恶化到 Ⅲ 级。她在一名整形外科医生和伤口护理护士的照顾下住院治疗。安排手术清理骶骨伤口，并用从她的大腿取出的全层皮片闭合伤口。C. M. 8 天后出院到一个长期护理机构，订购波浪床垫，每 2 小时变换一次体位，补充营养和细致的伤口护理。

简介

皮肤（skin）及其相关结构构成了皮肤系统（integumentary system）。这一身体覆盖系统能够预防感染、脱水（dehydration）、紫外线辐射（ultraviolet radiation）和受伤。皮肤的大面积损伤，例如烧伤（burn），会导致很多危险的并发症。

通过汗水（sweat）的蒸发和改变表面血管的直径，控制散发到环境中的热量，皮肤能够协助调节体温。皮肤还包含触觉、温度、压力和疼痛的感觉接收器。可以通过贴剂（patch）透过皮肤给药，框 21-1 给出了说明。

单词 derma（源自于希腊语）意为"皮肤"，被用于与皮肤相关词汇的后缀，例如 xeroderma（皮肤干燥）和 scleroderma（皮肤硬化）。形容词 cutaneous（皮肤的）是指皮肤，源自于拉丁语单词 cutis（皮肤）。像眼睛一样，皮肤是一个人健康状况的随时可见的反映。像毛发和指甲的状况一样，皮肤的颜色、纹理和弹性能够提供很多信息。

皮肤解剖

皮肤的最外层部分是表皮层（epidermis），由 4~5 层上皮细胞（epithelial cell）组成（图 21-1）。最深的表皮层是基底层（stratum basale 或 basal layer），能够产生新的细胞。随着这些细胞逐渐上升到表面，它们会死亡并充满角蛋白（keratin），是一种使皮肤变厚、变硬的蛋白质。表皮层的最外层是角质层（stratum corneum 或 horny layer），是由不断脱落和替换的扁平的、死亡的保护性细胞构成。表皮层的一些细胞会产生黑色素（melanin），是一种赋予皮肤颜色并防止阳光伤害的色素。

真皮（dermis）在表皮层之下，由结缔组织、神经、血管、淋巴管和感觉感受器构成。真皮为皮肤提供营养和支持。真皮之下的皮下组织主要由结缔组织和脂肪构成。

相关的皮肤结构

皮肤中的特殊结构也是皮肤系统的组成部分：

- 汗腺（sudoriferous gland）的主要作用是调节体温，通过释放水样液体蒸发冷却身体。
- 皮脂腺（sebaceous gland）释放油样液体皮脂（sebum），润滑毛发和皮肤，并防止干燥。
- 毛发（hair）广泛分布在身体上。每根毛发都在一个毛囊内发育，并从其在皮肤深层的基底开始生长。在人害怕或感觉冷时，附着在毛囊上的竖毛肌（arrector pili）会使毛发立起，产生"鸡皮疙瘩（goosebump）"（图 21-1）。在动物身上，这是一个警告标志和保温手段。
- 指甲（nail）从近端生长区开始发育（图 21-2）。

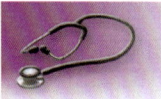

框 21-1

临床观点
药物贴剂：不用再吃苦药片

对大多数人而言，药片是一种方便的用药方式，但对某些人则有障碍。药片必须定期服用以确保一致的剂量，并且它们必须被消化吸收到血液中才可以开始起作用。对那些吞咽或消化药片有困难的人，经皮肤给药（transdermal, TD）的贴剂（patch）提供了一种口服给药的有效替代。

TD 贴剂输送一致的剂量的药物，通过皮肤扩散以恒定速度进入血液。没有每天的服药时间表要遵守，不用吞咽任何东西，不会让胃不舒服。TD 贴剂也能为失去知觉的患者给药，否则这些患者就需要静脉注射药物。TD 贴剂被用于激素替代疗法治疗心脏病、控制疼痛和抑制晕动病。

TD 贴剂的使用必须小心谨慎。药物通过皮肤扩散需要时间，所以必须了解在生效前多长时间要贴好贴剂。还要了解在去掉贴剂后何时药效消失，因为人体会继续吸收已经通过皮肤扩散进来的药物，移除贴剂并不能完全消除药物。还存在这样的危险，即当加热时，例如运动、发热或热环境，例如热水池、加热垫或桑拿浴，贴剂可能变得不安全。当热扩张皮肤中的毛细血管时，可能导致剂量的危险增加，因为更多的药物进入血液。

经皮肤给药的最新进展是离子导入（iontophoresis）。基于类似于同级相斥的原理，这一方法使用温和的电流将离子药物穿过皮肤。连接到贴剂的小型电子设备使用正电流来"推动"带正电荷的药物分子通过皮肤，负电流推动带负电的药物分子。尽管使用的电流很小，佩戴起搏器的人群不能使用离子导入贴剂。另一个缺点是离子导入贴剂只能使离子药物穿过皮肤。

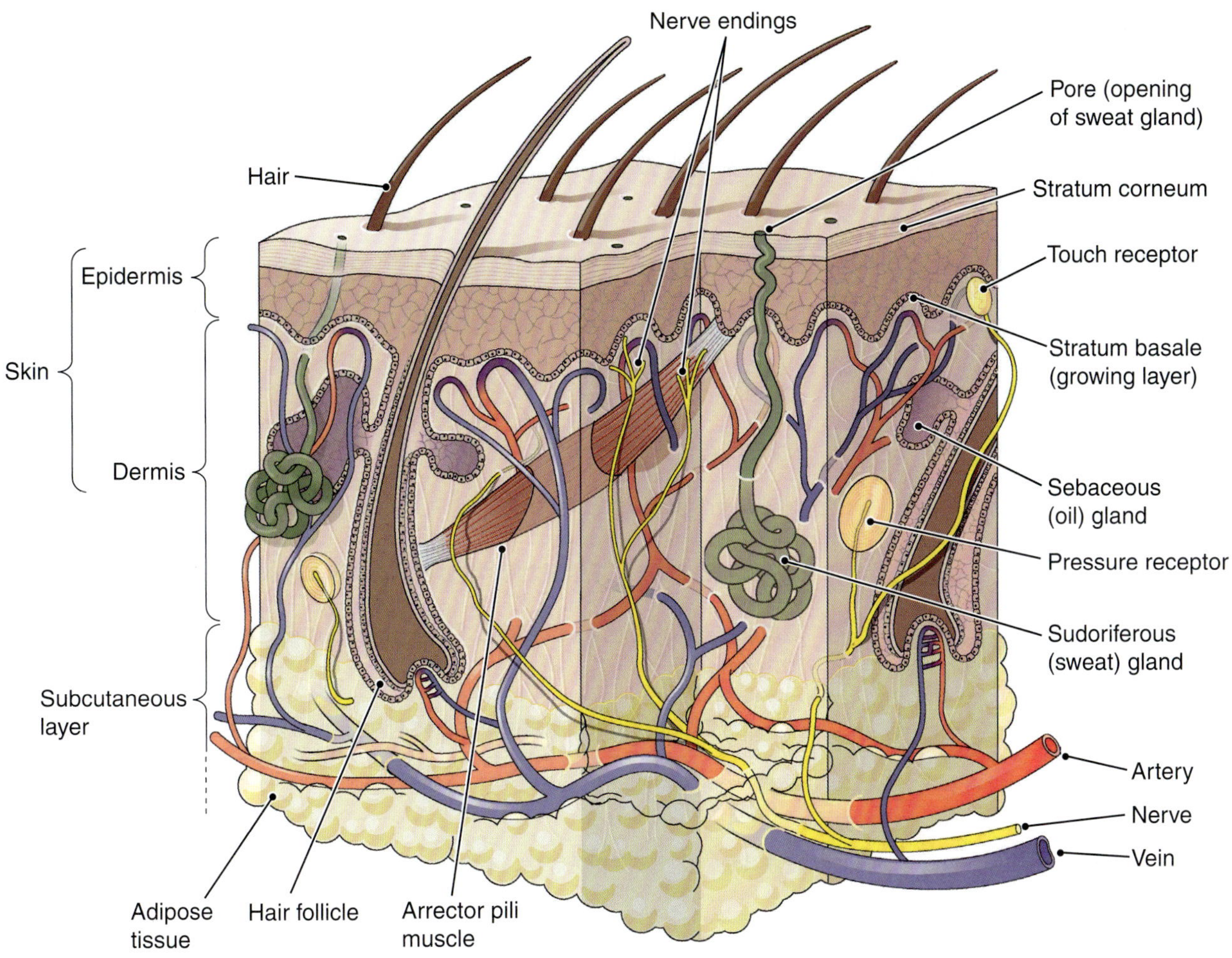

第 21 章 皮肤 587

图 21-1 皮肤的横截面。图中示出了皮肤各层和相关结构

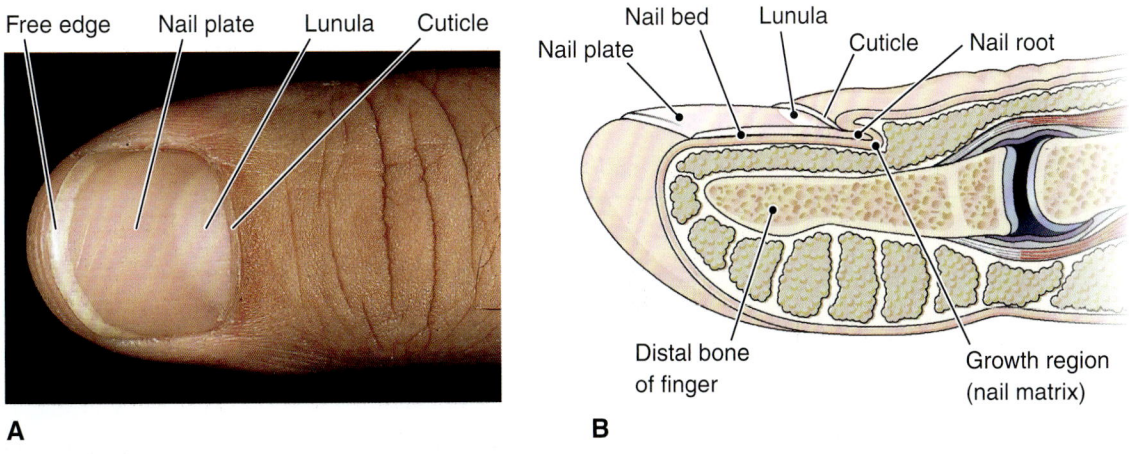

图 21-2 指甲的结构。A. 指甲的照片，上视图；B. 指尖的中矢断面显示出生长区域和指甲板周围的组织

角质层（cuticle）的学术名称为指甲上皮（eponychium），是表皮层在指甲板（nail plate）表面上的延伸。远离角质层的较轻的区域被称为甲半月（lunula），因为它看起来像半个月亮。甲半月下面的皮肤比较厚，透过指甲能看到的血液没有那么多。

毛发和指甲由没有生命的物质构成，主要是角蛋白，二者的功能都是保护身体。

Terminology　关键术语

正常结构与功能

cutaneous [kjuˈteiniəs]	皮肤的，与皮肤相关的（源自拉丁语单词 cutis 意为"皮肤"）
derma [ˈdɜːmə]	皮肤（源自于希腊语）
dermis [ˈdɜːmis]	真皮层，表皮层与皮下组织之间的皮肤层；也常用 true skin 或 corium
epidermis [ˌepiˈdɜːmis]	表皮层，皮肤的最外层（源自意为"在……之上"的前缀 epi- 和意为"皮肤"的词根 derm）
hair [heə(r)]	毛发，从皮肤中长出的线状角蛋白生长物（词根：trich/o）
hair follicle [ˈfɔlikəl]	毛囊，毛发发育的护套
integumentary system [inˌtegjʊˈmentəri]	皮肤系统，皮肤及其相关腺体、毛发和指甲
keratin [ˈkerətin]	角蛋白，使皮肤变厚、变硬，并构成毛发和指甲的一种蛋白质（词根：kerat/o）
melanin [ˈmelənin]	黑色素，为毛发和皮肤提供颜色并保护皮肤免受太阳辐射的深色色素（词根：melan/o）
nail [neil]	指甲，覆盖终末指骨背表面皮肤的板状角化生长物（词根：onych/o）
sebaceous gland [siˈbeiʃəs]	皮脂腺，产生皮脂的腺体，通常与毛囊相关（词根：seb/o）
sebum [ˈsiːbəm]	皮脂，皮脂腺产生的一种脂肪分泌物，润滑毛发和皮肤（词根：seb/o）
skin [skin]	皮肤，覆盖身体的组织；也常用 integument（词根：derm/o, dermat/o）
subcutaneous tissue [ˌsʌbkjuːˈteiniːəs]	皮下组织，皮肤之下的组织层，也被称为 hypodermis
sudoriferous gland [suːdəˈrifərəs]	汗腺，分泌汗液的腺体，也常用 sweat gland（词根：hidr/o）

与皮肤相关的词根

参见表 21-1

表 21-1　与皮肤相关的词根

词根	含义	示例	示例定义
derm/o, dermat/o	皮肤	dermabrasion ［dɜ:məˈbreiʒən］	皮肤磨削术
kerat/o	角蛋白、角质层	keratinous ［kəˈrætinəs］	角质的
melan/o	深色、黑色、黑色素	melanosome ［ˈmelənəʊsəʊm］	黑色素体
hidr/o	汗水、出汗	anhidrosis ［ænhi:ˈdrəʊsis］	无汗症
seb/o	皮脂、皮脂腺	seborrhea ［sibɒrˈhiə］	皮脂溢出
trich/o	毛发	trichomycosis ［trikəmaiˈkəʊsis］	毛发菌病
onych/o	指甲	onychia ［əʊˈnikiə］	甲床炎（不是以 -itis 结尾）

练习 21-1

识别并定义下列单词的词根。

　　　　　　　　　　　　　　　　　　Root　　　　　　Meaning of Root

1. hypodermis ［ˌhaipəˈdɜ:mis］　　　_____　　_____
2. seborrheic ［siˈbɒrhaik］　　　_____　　_____
3. hypermelanosis ［haipəmeləˈnəʊsis］　　　_____　　_____
4. dyskeratosis ［di:zkərəˈtəʊsis］　　　_____　　_____
5. hypohidrosis ［haipəʊhiˈdrəʊsis］　　　_____　　_____
6. hypertrichosis ［haipɜːtriˈkəʊsis］　　　_____　　_____
7. eponychium ［ˌepəˈnikiəm］　　　_____　　_____

填空。

8. Dermatopathology ［dɜ:mætəpæˈθɒlədʒi］ is study of diseases of the _____.
9. Keratolysis ［kerəˈtɒlisis］ is loosening of the skin's _____.
10. A melanocyte ［ˈmelənəsait］ is a cell that produces _____.
11. Trichoid ［ˈtrikɔid］ means resembling a(n) _____.
12. Onychomycosis ［ɒnikəʊmaiˈkəʊsis］ is a fungal infection of a(n) _____.
13. Hidradenitis ［hidræˈdenaitis］ is inflammation of a gland that produces _____.
14. A hypodermic ［ˌhaipəˈdɜ:mik］ injection is given under the _____.

写出下列定义的单词。

15. loosening or separation of the skin　_____
16. study of the skin and skin diseases　_____

练习 18-1 （续表）

17. softening of a nail _____
18. excess production of sweat _____
19. study of the hair _____
20. instrument for cutting the skin _____
21. formation (-genesis) of keratin _____
22. a tumor containing melanin _____

使用意为"皮肤"的后缀 –derma 写出下列单词。

23. hardening of the skin _____
24. presence of pus in the skin _____

皮肤的临床表现

许多疾病通过皮肤质量的变化或特定病变（lesion）表现出来。一些类型的皮肤病变示于框 21-2，并在后面特定的皮肤疾病的图片中显示。皮肤和皮肤疾病的研究被称为皮肤病学（dermatology），认真观察皮肤、毛发和指甲应当是体格检查的一部分。要检查皮肤的颜色、异常色素沉积和病变，要通过触诊评估皮肤的纹理、温度、湿度、硬度和任何压痛。关于执业护士的信息参见框 21-3，他们像其他卫生保健专业人员一样，在进行体格检查时要观察皮肤。

伤口

伤口（wound）是由意外或受攻击的创伤、手术和其他治疗或诊断过程引起的。伤口可能不仅影响受

框 21-2

供你参考
皮肤病变的种类

病变	说明
bulla ['bʊlə] 大疱	隆起的、充满液体的损伤，比水疱大（复数：bullae）（图 21-5 和图 21-7）
fissure ['fɪʃə(r)] 裂隙	皮肤破裂
macule ['mækjuːl] 斑点	扁平的有色斑点（图 21-19）
nodule ['nɒdjuːl] 小丘	坚实的、隆起的病变，比丘疹大，通常指示全身疾病（图 21-9）
papule ['pæpjuːl] 丘疹	皮肤表面小圆形隆起病变
plaque [plæk] 斑块	表浅的、扁平的或轻微隆起的斑，直径大于 1cm（图 21-6）
pustule ['pʌstjuːl] 脓疱	含有脓液的隆起的损伤，通常在毛囊或汗腺孔（图 21-13）
ulcer ['ʌlsə(r)] 溃疡	皮肤或皮下组织破坏所致的损伤
vesicle ['vesɪkl] 水疱	小的充满液体的病变；也被称为 blister 或 bleb（图 21-18）
wheal [wiːl] 风团	平滑、圆形、轻微隆起的区域，经常伴有瘙痒；见于荨麻疹，如由过敏引起的（图 21-17）

框 20-3

健康职业
执业护士

执业护士（nurse practitioner, NP）是具有超过注册护士（RN）专业学位的护士，提供类似于医生的护理服务。所有执业护士都有护理硕士或博士学位。他们可以专攻领域，如急症护理、家庭健康、新生儿学、老年医学或医学专科，如肿瘤学或精神病学。他们的高级教育允许他们独立诊断和治疗患者、安排检查、做小手术，并通常有处方权。一些执业护士自主开业，但许多工作与医生合作。他们不仅关注疾病的治疗，而且关注疾病的预防、患者教育和咨询。这种早期干预和教育可以降低整体医疗成本。

执业护士在美国所有州都被许可执业，并且必须遵守其获得许可的州的规则和法规。在大多数州，他们可以在没有医生同意的情况下分发药物和开处方药，可以向保险机构报销服务。他们的专业组织包括美国执业护士学会（American Academy of Nurse Practitioners）www.aanp.org 和美国执业护士学院（American College of Nurse Practitioners）www.acnpweb.org。

伤的区域，也会影响其他身体系统。感染和出血可能使伤口复杂化，如开裂（dehiscence）、伤口层的破裂以及内脏通过损伤部位突出。

随着伤口愈合，液体和细胞从受伤的组织中排出。这些排出物被称为渗出物（exudate），可以是透明的、含血的（sanguinous）或含脓的（purulent）。可以用试管从伤口处清除渗出物。

正常的伤口愈合取决于清洁、对损伤的处理以及适当的循环、良好的身体健康和良好的营养。深层伤口的边缘应当使用缝线缝合（suture），无论是缝针还是简单的切割要在能够保持干燥和固定的区域进行，并使用组织黏合剂（tissue adhesive）。愈合伴有瘢痕形成（cicatrization），瘢痕（scar）的另一个名称是 cicatrix。通过适当的伤口护理可以减少永久性瘢痕形成，但是一些人，特别是非洲或亚洲血统的人可能倾向于形成瘢痕瘤（keloid），因为在愈合过程中形成过量的胶原（图 21-3）。整形手术往往可以改善瘢痕疙瘩和其他不雅观的瘢痕。

各种敷料（dressing）被用于保护受伤的区域，并促进愈合。真空辅助闭合（vacuum-assisted closure，VAC）使用负压闭合伤口，并开始愈合过程。清创术（debridement）从伤口清除死亡或受损的组织，能够促进愈合。框 21-4 提到了单词 debridement 的起源，并给出了其他源自法语的医学术语的含义。清创术可通过切割或擦洗掉坏死组织或通过酶来实现。在焦痂切开术（escharotomy）中，能够清除厚的、深色的痂（crust）或焦痂（eschar）。

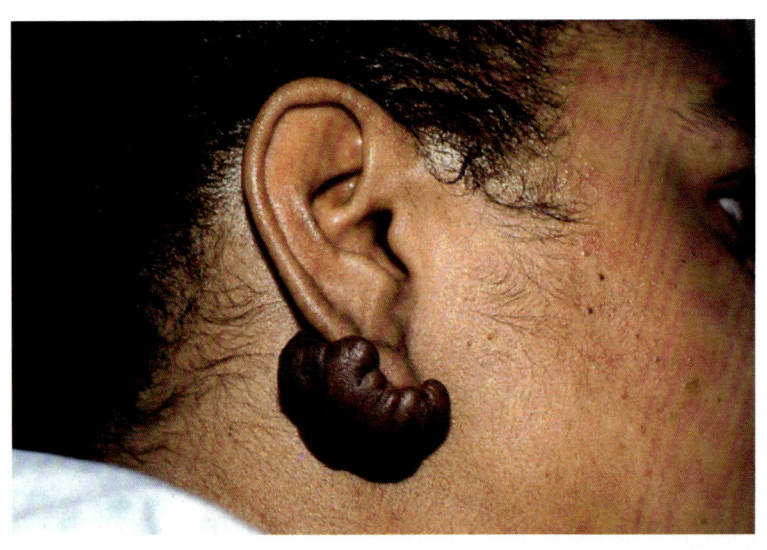

图 21-3　瘢痕瘤。耳垂穿刺后瘢痕组织的过度生长

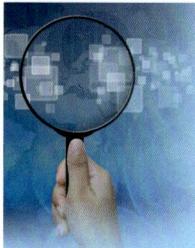

框 21-4

聚焦单词

法语联系

许多科学和医学术语都改编自外语。大多数词根源自于拉丁语和希腊语，其他一些则来自于德语和法语。有时，医学外语单词被"原样"使用。Débridement（清创术）是指从伤口清除死亡或受损的组织，源自于法语，意为去掉约束，例如马具的笼头。另一个源自于法语的是 contrecoup injury（对侧伤害），是指在例如车祸中头部被前后撞击，脑部在撞击对侧的伤害；而 contrecoup 在法语中意为"反击"。Tic douloureux 是一种引起面部三叉神经疼痛的病症，从字面上翻译就是"疼痛的抽搐"。用听诊器听到的心脏杂音（bruit）在法语中的字母意思是"噪音"。Lavage 是指灌洗腔体，法语单词意为"清洗"。

烧伤

大多数烧伤（burn）是由热的物体、爆炸或热的液体烫伤（scalding）引起的，也可能是由电、接触有害化学物质或擦伤（abrasion）引起的。阳光也会引起严重的烧伤，可能导致严重的疾病。烧伤要根据伤害的深度和涉及的体表面积（body surface area，BSA）百分比进行评估。组织破坏的深度分类为：

1. 轻度（superficial）——只涉及表皮层。皮肤红且干，只有轻微疼痛。典型的起因是温和的晒伤和短时间的热暴露。这种烧伤也被称为一度烧伤。

2. 浅Ⅱ度（superficial partial thickness）——涉及表皮层和部分真皮层。组织发红、起疱（blister）、疼痛，如严重晒伤或烫伤。

3. 深Ⅱ度（deep partial thickness）——涉及表皮层和真皮层。组织可能会起疱，表面有渗出，或者因为汗腺损伤而干燥。因为神经受伤，这种烧伤可能没有浅度烧伤那样疼痛。起因包括烫伤和暴露于火焰或热油。浅Ⅱ度和深Ⅱ度都被归类于Ⅱ度烧伤。

4. 深度（full thickness）——涉及全部皮肤，有时包括皮下组织和更深层的组织。组织破裂、干燥并发白，或烧焦（charred）。这种烧伤可能需要植皮（skin grafting），并可能导致截肢或截肢。深度烧伤也被归类于Ⅲ度烧伤。

烧伤涉及的体表面积可以使用九分法（rule of nines）进行估算，即身体表面的区域被分为9倍数的百分比（图 21-4）。更准确的隆德和布劳德方法（Lund and Browder method）将身体分为更小的区域，并估算每个区域所占体表面积的比例。

感染是烧伤的常见并发症，因为抵抗细菌入侵的主要防御被破坏了。呼吸并发症和休克也可能发生。烧伤的治疗包括呼吸护理、补液、伤口护理和疼痛控制。监测心血管并发症、感染和创伤后应激的迹象也很重要。

压疮

压疮（pressure ulcer）是坏死性皮肤损伤，出现在身体靠覆盖骨突起的皮肤上，例如骶骨、足跟、肘、骨盆的坐骨或股骨的大转子（参见框 21-2 中的 ulcer）。压力会阻断循环，导致血栓、溃烂和组织死亡。不良的健康状况、营养不良、老年、肥胖和感

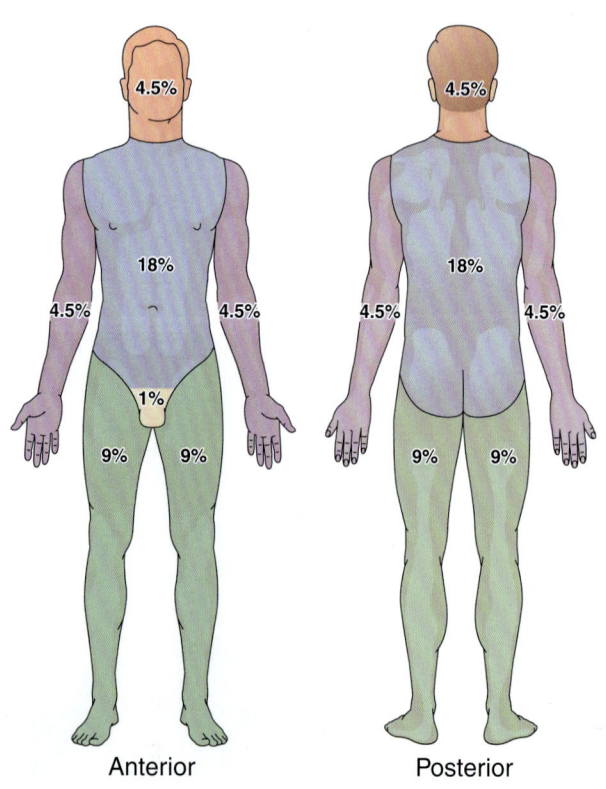

图 21-4 九分法。成人体表面积（BSA）的百分比通过将身体表面切成具有与9相关数值的区域来估计，该方法用于评价皮肤灼伤的程度

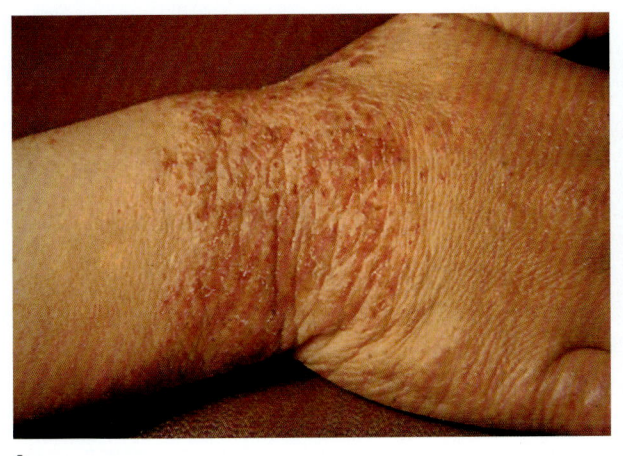 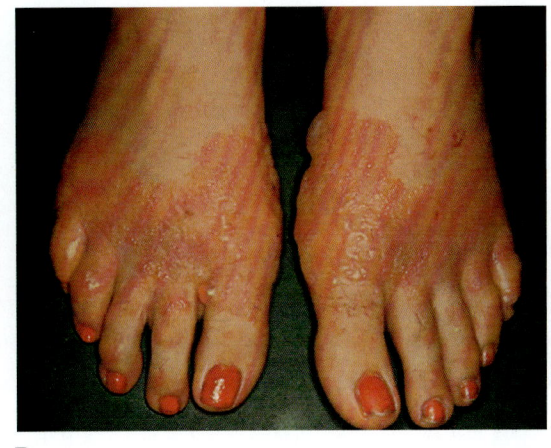

图 21-5　皮炎。A. 婴儿手腕上的特应性皮炎（湿疹）。B. 因接触鞋产生的接触性皮炎。请注意几个充满液体的大疱（框 21-2）

染都会增加发生压疮的风险。

压疮损伤最先表现为皮肤发红，如果被忽视，可能会穿透皮肤和下面的肌肉，甚至会扩散至骨骼，可能需要数月才能康复。

用褥垫缓解压力、定期清洁并保持皮肤干燥、频繁改变体位和良好的营养有助于预防压疮。说明压疮的其他术语是卧床性溃疡（decubitus ulcer）和褥疮（bedsore），这两个术语都是指躺在床上，不过压疮可能出现在任何运动过少的人身上，而不只是那些被限制在床上的人。

皮炎

皮炎（dermatitis）是用于皮肤炎症的通用术语，可以是急性或慢性的。温和的皮炎会出现红斑（erythema）和水肿，有时有瘙痒（pruritus），但情况可能会恶化发展到更深层的损伤和继发细菌感染。出现在童年早期的慢性过敏性皮炎被称为特应性皮炎（atopic dermatitis）或湿疹（eczema）（图 21-5）。尽管起因不明，过敏、感染、温度变化过大和皮肤刺激会加重特应性皮炎。

其他形式的皮炎包括过敏原或化学刺激引起的接触性皮炎（图 21-5B）、涉及皮脂腺较多的头皮和面部的脂溢性（seborrheic）皮炎和循环不良引起的瘀滞性（stasis）皮炎。

银屑病

银屑病（psoriasis）是表皮层的慢性增生（hyperplasia），会产生大块的带有银色皮屑的（erythematous plaque）红斑（图 21-6，参见框 21-2 中的 plaque）。起因不明，有时有遗传因素，还涉及自身免疫。

根据严重程度，皮肤科医生用下列方法治疗银屑病：

1. 外用药，包括皮质类固醇（corticosteroids）、免疫抑制剂、维生素 A 和维生素 D。

2. 光线疗法（phototherapy）——暴露于远紫外

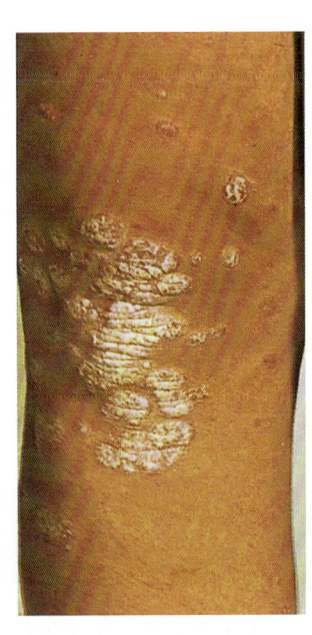

图 21-6　银屑病。在膝盖前出现的有鳞片的斑块（框 21-2）

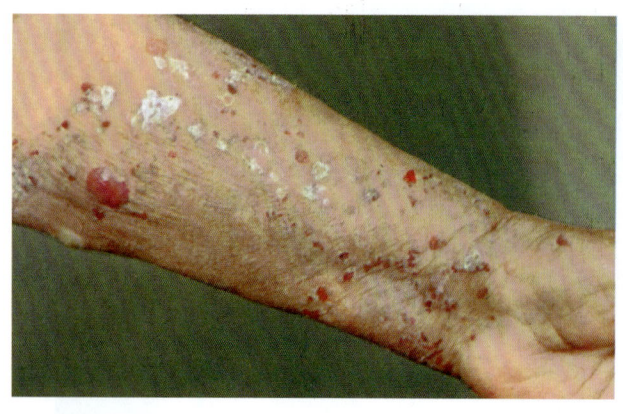

图 21-7 天疱疮。在前臂上出现的水疱（大疱）（参见大疱，框 21-2）

线（UVB）；服用药物补骨脂素（psoralen）以增加皮肤对光的敏感性，然后暴露于近紫外线（UVA）；激光治疗。

3. 系统性抑制免疫系统。

自身免疫病

下面讨论的疾病是由，或部分是由自身免疫反应引起的。他们要通过损伤组织活检和抗体研究进行诊断。

天疱疮（pemphigus）的特征是表皮细胞与下层的分离引起的皮肤和黏膜中形成的大疱（bullae）（图 21-7，参见框 21-2 的 bulla）。这些损伤的破裂会使深层皮肤失去对感染的保护，并造成体液损失，很像烧伤的情况。起因是上皮细胞的自身免疫反应。如果不能通过抑制免疫系统进行治疗，天疱疮是致命的。

红斑狼疮（lupus erythematosus，LE）是结缔组织的慢性炎症性自身免疫病。该疾病的一种更为广泛的形式是系统性红斑狼疮（systemic lupus erythematosus，SLE），会涉及皮肤和其他器官。系统性红斑狼疮在女性中比在男性中更普遍，并且亚洲人和黑人发生率比其他人群更高。

盘状红斑狼疮（discoid lupus erythematosus，DLE）只涉及皮肤。皮肤上会出现粗糙、隆起的红斑，在阳光的紫外线照射下会恶化（图 21-8）。狼疮皮肤损伤只限于面部和头皮，会在鼻子和面颊形成典型的蝴蝶形皮疹。

硬皮病（scleroderma）造成皮肤变厚变硬的起因不明的疾病。用于胶原生产过量，真皮层会逐渐硬化，还会涉及汗腺和毛囊。硬皮病的早期表现是雷诺病，手指和脚趾的血管预冷收缩，引起麻木、疼痛、寒冷和刺痛。皮肤症状最先出现在前臂和口周。硬皮病扩散涉及内部器官被称为进行性系统性硬化症（progressive systemic sclerosis，PSS）。

皮肤癌

皮肤癌是人类最常见的癌症，其发病率近年有所上升，主要是因为阳光中紫外线引发的突变反应。鳞状细胞癌和基底细胞癌都是上皮细胞的癌症，都发生在暴露于阳光的区域，例如面部或手背。基底细胞癌占皮肤癌的 75%，表现为平滑的梨状丘疹（pearly papule）（图 21-9，参见框 21-2 中的 papule）。因为这些癌症易于发现且不转移，切除后的治愈率

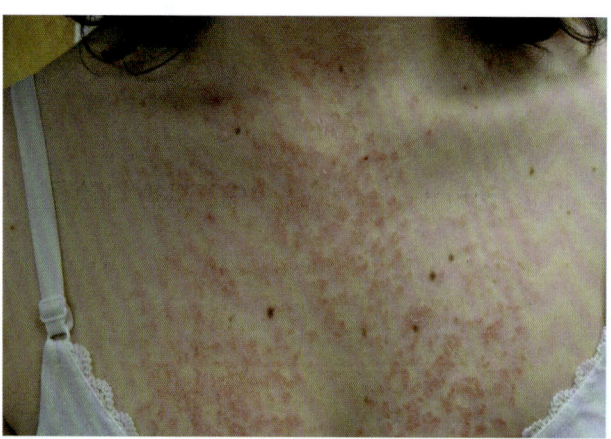

图 21-8 盘状（皮肤）红斑狼疮。红斑丘疹和斑块在胸部典型的阳光暴露分布

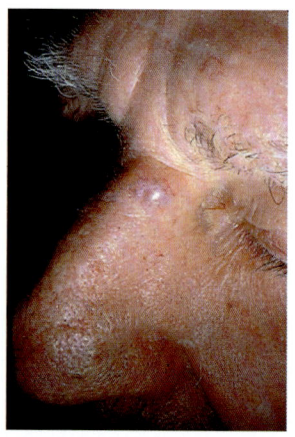

图 21-9 基底细胞癌。初始半透明结节已经扩散，留下凹陷的中心和坚固、突起的边界（参见丘疹，框 21-2）

高于95%。

鳞状细胞癌（squamous cell carcinoma）表现为无痛、坚实的红丘或斑块，可能发展成为表面鳞片、溃烂或结痂（crusting）（图21-10，参见框21-2）。这种癌会入侵下层组织，但通常并不转移。通过手术切除，有时使用X线或化疗进行治疗。

恶性黑色素瘤（malignant melanoma）是真皮层中的黑色素细胞增生所致。因为其转移倾向，这是一种最危险形式的皮肤癌。这种癌症表现为不同颜色的不规则边界的损伤（图21-11）。在开始入侵更深层皮肤组织和通过血液和淋巴液转移之前2~3年内，会向表面扩散。如果损伤在进入入侵阶段之前被诊断并手术切除，预后良好。

卡波西肉瘤（Kaposi sarcoma）曾被认为是罕见的，近来常见于艾滋病患者。它通常表现为腿部明显的棕色区域，随着肿瘤的进展，这些斑块会变得突起、坚实。对于免疫系统减弱的人，如艾滋病患者，这种癌症会转移。

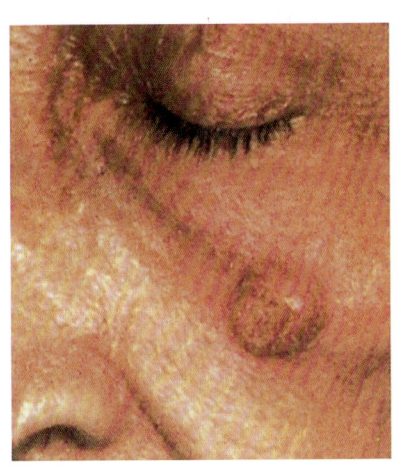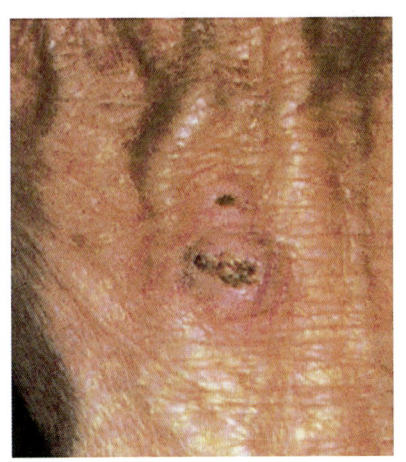

图21-10 鳞状细胞癌。病变出现在脸上和手背，日光暴露的区域通常会受影响

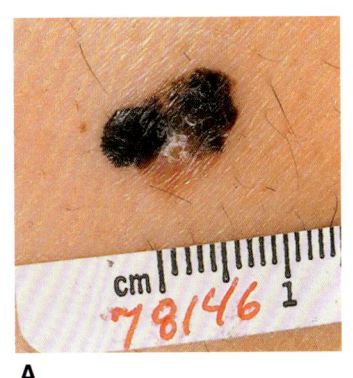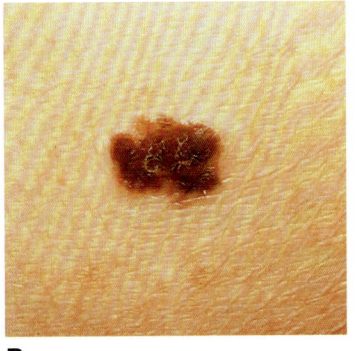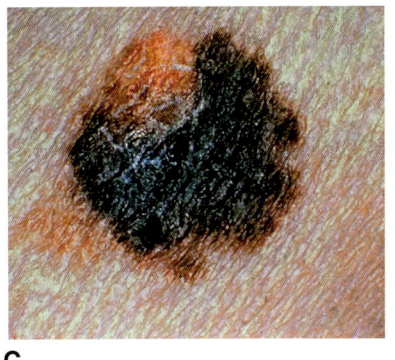

A　　　　　　　　B　　　　　　　　C

图21-11 恶性黑素瘤。图中显示了几个特性。A.不对称；B.不规则的边界；C.颜色变化，直径大于6mm和突起

Terminology　关键术语

atopic dermatitis [əˈtɔpik ˌdɜːməˈtaitis]	特应性皮炎，带有瘙痒的遗传性、过敏性、慢性皮肤炎症；也被称为湿疹（eczema）
basal cell carcinoma	基底细胞癌，一种很少转移的肿瘤，手术切除治愈率很高

Terminology 关键术语（续表）

cicatrization [sikətri'zeiʃən]	瘢痕形成，瘢痕形成的过程；cicatrix 就是瘢痕
débridement [di'bri:dmənt]	清创术，从伤口中清除死亡或受损的组织
dehiscence [di'hisns]	裂开，伤口层分开时的撕裂或爆裂
dermatitis [ˌdɜːməˈtaitis]	皮炎，皮肤的炎症，通常会有皮肤变红和瘙痒；可能是过敏、刺激（接触性皮炎）或其他疾病引起的
dermatology [ˌdɜːməˈtɒlədʒi]	皮肤病学，皮肤和皮肤疾病的研究
dermatome ['dɜːmətəʊm]	植皮刀，用于切割移植用皮肤薄片的装置
eczema ['eksimə]	湿疹，皮肤变红、损伤和瘙痒的通用术语；特应性皮炎
erythema [ˌeri'θiːmə]	红斑，皮肤变红的扩散
escharotomy [eskə'rɒtəmi]	焦痂切开术，切除烧伤或其他皮肤损伤所致的痂组织；焦痂（eschar）就是疮痂（scab）或痂皮（crust）
evisceration [iviːsəˈreiʃən]	内脏突出，内脏（viscera）通过开口突出，例如通过伤口
exudate ['eksəˌdeit]	渗出物，从受伤的组织中漏出的物质，包括液体、细胞、脓液或血液
Kaposi sarcoma [sɑːˈkəʊmə]	卡波西肉瘤，皮肤和其他组织的癌症性损伤，最常见于艾滋病患者
keloid ['kiːlɔid]	瘢痕瘤，在瘢痕形成期间组织增生引起的突起、变厚的瘢痕
lupus erythematosus (LE) [ˌerəˌθiːməˈtəʊsəs]	红斑狼疮，结缔组织的慢性、炎性自身免疫疾病，通常涉及皮肤；包括更为广泛的系统性红斑狼疮和只涉及皮肤的盘状红斑狼疮
malignant melanoma [məˈlignənt ˌmeləˈnəumə]	恶性黑色素瘤，一种会转移的色素皮肤肿瘤
pemphigus ['pemfigəs]	天疱疮，一种自身免疫皮肤疾病，特征是突然间歇性形成大疱；如不治疗，可能致命
pressure ulcer	压疮，对身体局部产生的压力引起的溃疡，例如来自床或座椅的压力；卧床性溃疡（decubitus ulcer）、褥疮（bedsore）
pruritus [prʊˈraitəs]	瘙痒症，严重瘙痒
psoriasis [səˈraiəsis]	银屑病，一种慢性遗传性皮炎，红色皮肤损伤带有银色鳞片
rule of nines	九分法，一种评估所烧伤涉及体表面积的方法，将身体的不同区域的体表面积赋予 9 的倍数的百分比（图 21-4）
scleroderma [ˌskliəˈdɜːmə]	硬皮病，一种以皮肤变厚、变硬为特征的慢性疾病，进行性系统性硬化症（progressive systemic sclerosis, PSS）通常涉及内脏器官
squamous cell carcinoma ['skweiməs]	鳞状细胞癌，一种涉及深层组织，但不倾向于转移的真皮层癌症

Terminology 补充术语

症状与病症

acne [ˈækni]	痤疮，皮脂腺和毛囊的炎性疾病，通常与皮脂分泌过量相关；寻常痤疮（acne vulgaris）
actinic [ækˈtinik]	光化的，与辐射能量作用相关的，例如阳光、紫外线和 X 线
albinism [ˈælbinizəm]	白化病，皮肤、毛发和眼睛遗传性缺乏色素
alopecia [ˌæləˈpi:ʃə]	脱发，毛发缺少或损失；秃顶（baldness）
Beau lines	博氏线，横跨指甲的白线，通常是全身性疾病或伤害的体征（图 21-12）
bromhidrosis [brəmhidˈrəusis]	腋臭，出汗因细菌分解而带有恶臭；也拼写为 bromidrosis
carbuncle [ˈkɑ:bʌŋkl]	痈，一种皮肤和皮下组织的局部感染，通常是由葡萄球菌引起的，伴随疼痛和流脓
comedo [ˈkɒmidəu]	粉刺，在毛囊中的皮脂塞，通常含有细菌（复数：comedones）
dermatophytosis [ˌdɜ:mətəufaiˈtəusis]	皮肤癣菌病，皮肤的真菌感染，特别是在脚趾之间；足癣（athlete's foot），词根：phyt/o 意为"植物"
diaphoresis [ˌdaiəfəˈri:sis]	发汗，大量出汗
dyskeratosis [di:zkərəˈtəusis]	角化不良，上皮细胞中任何角蛋白形成异常
ecchymosis [ˌekiˈməusis]	瘀斑，小血管泄露引起的皮下血液聚集
erysipelas [ˌeriˈsipiləs]	丹毒，一种急性皮肤感染疾病，带有局部红肿和全身症状
erythema nodosum [ˈnəudəusəm]	结节性红斑，皮下组织炎症，会导致压痛和红斑性结节；可能是对系统性疾病、感染或药物的免疫反应异常
exanthem [igˈzæθəm]	皮疹，伴随一种疾病，例如麻疹，发生的任何皮疹，也常用 rash
excoriation [ɛkˌskoriˈeʃən]	抓伤，抓或摩擦引起的损伤

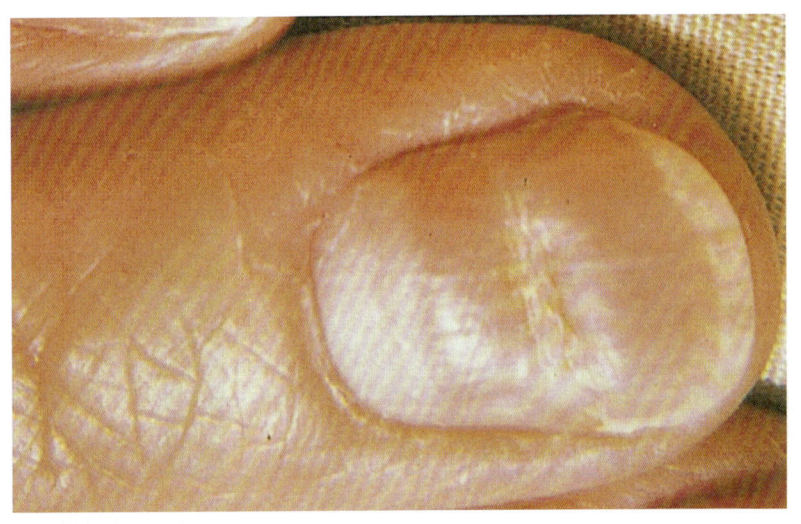

图 21-12 博氏线。指甲中的这些横向凹陷与急性严重疾病相关

Terminology 补充术语（续表）

folliculitis [fə͵likjʊˈlaitis]	毛囊炎，毛囊的炎症
furuncle [ˈfjʊərʌŋkl]	疖，由通过毛囊进入的葡萄球菌引起的疼痛的皮肤结节；也常用 boil
hemangioma [hi:͵mændʒiːˈəʊmə]	血管瘤，一种良性血管肿瘤；在皮肤上的血管瘤被称为胎记（birthmark）或葡萄酒色痣（port wine stains）
herpes simplex [ˈhə:pi:z ˈsimpleks]	单纯性疱疹，一组由单纯疱疹病毒引起的急性感染。Ⅰ型单纯疱疹病毒在发热、日晒、损伤或压力之后产生充满液体的水疱，通常在嘴唇上；也被称为感冒疮（cold sore）、发热水疱（fever blister）。Ⅱ型感染通常涉及生殖器官
hirsutism [ˈhɜ:sju:tizəm]	多毛症，毛发生长过多
ichthyosis [͵ikθiˈəʊsis]	鱼鳞癣，一种皮肤干燥、鳞片样病症（源自词根 ichthy/o，意为"鱼"）
impetigo [͵impiˈtaigəʊ]	脓疱病，一种细菌性皮肤感染，脓疱破裂并形成痂皮；最常见于儿童，通常在脸上（图 21-13，参见框 21-2 中的 pustule）
keratosis [͵kerəˈtəʊsis]	角化症，任何以增厚或角质生长为特征的皮肤病症。脂溢性角化病是良性肿瘤，黄色或浅棕色，出现在老年人中。光化性角化病由暴露于阳光下引起，并可导致鳞状细胞癌
lichenification [laikenifiˈkeiʃən]	苔藓样硬化斑，长期摩擦引起的硬化的斑块，如在特应性皮炎中所见（图 21-14）
mycosis fungoides [maiˈkəʊsis ˈfʌŋɔidz]	蕈状真菌病，一种起源于皮肤并涉及内部器官和淋巴结的罕见恶性疾病。会产生大的、疼痛的、溃烂的肿瘤
nevus [ˈni:vəs]	痣，轮廓分明的皮肤变色；一种先天的血管皮肤瘤
paronychia [͵pærəˈnikiə]	甲沟炎，指甲周围的炎症（图 21-15）；由细菌或真菌引起，可能会影响多个指甲
pediculosis [pi͵dikjʊˈləʊsis]	虱病，被虱子侵染
petechia [pəˈti:kiə]	瘀点，由皮肤或黏膜内出血引起的扁平、针尖大小的紫红色斑点（复数：petechiae）

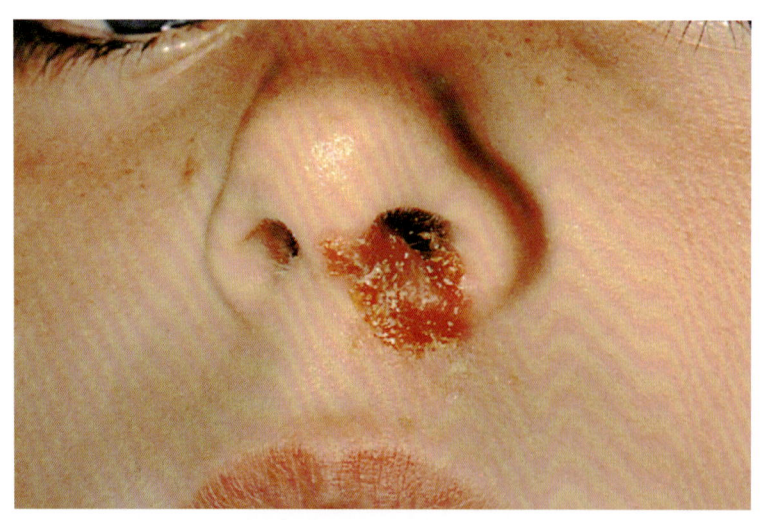

图 21-13 **脓疱病**。这种细菌性皮肤感染出现在鼻孔上，导致脓疱破裂并形成结皮（见脓疱，框 21-2）

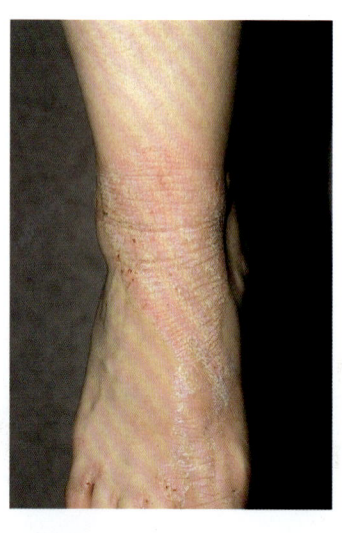

图 21-14 **苔藓样硬化斑**。长期摩擦部位的皮肤出现增厚，如特应性皮炎所见

Terminology 补充术语（续表）

photosensitization [ˌfəʊtəʊsensitaiˈzeiʃn]	光敏作用，皮肤对光的敏感作用，通常来自于药物、植物产品或其他物质
purpura [ˈpəpjʊrə]	紫癜，一种以出血进入皮肤和其他组织为特征的病症
rosacea [rəʊˈzeiʃiə]	红斑痤疮，一种起因不明的涉及皮肤发红、脓疱和皮脂腺过度活动的病症，主要在面部
scabies [ˈskeibi:z]	疥疮，由螨虫引起的高度传染性皮肤病
senile lentigines [lenˈtidʒini:z]	老年雀斑，在成年人暴露于阳光的皮肤上出现的棕色斑点；肝斑（liver spots）
shingles [ˈʃiŋlz]	带状疱疹，沿着神经走向的急性疱疹爆发；也被称为 herpes zoster；由引发水痘的病毒引起
tinea [ˈtiniə]	癣，真菌感染皮肤；皮癣（ringworm，图 21-16）
tinea versicolor [ˈvə:sikʌlə]	花斑癣，浅表性慢性真菌感染，引起斑驳的皮肤色素沉着
urticaria [ˌɜ:tiˈkeəriə]	荨麻疹，一种以短暂的、平滑的、瘙痒的突起风团为特征的皮肤反应；也常用 hives（图 21-17，参见框 21-2 中的 wheal）
venous stasis ulcer	静脉瘀滞性溃疡，由静脉功能不全和静脉血瘀滞引起的溃疡；通常形成在脚踝附近（图 21-18，参见框 21-2 中的 ulcer）
verruca [vəˈru:kə]	疣，一种表皮层肿瘤；也常用 wart
vitiligo [ˌvitiˈlaigəʊ]	白癜风，皮肤色素斑片状消失；白斑病（leukoderma，图 21-19）
xeroderma pigmentosum [ˌziərəʊˈdɜ:mə ˌpigmənˈtəʊsəm]	着色性干皮病，一种致命的遗传性疾病，从儿童期开始出现皮肤褪色和溃疡和肌肉萎缩。对太阳的敏感性增加并且对癌症的易感性升高
诊断与治疗	
aloe [ˈæləʊ]	芦荟油，从植物芦荟叶子中提取的凝胶，被用于治疗烧伤和轻微的皮肤刺激
antipruritic [ˌænti:pˈrʊəritik]	止痒剂，预防或缓解瘙痒的药物
cautery [ˈkɔ:təri]	烧灼术，通过物理或化学手段破坏组织；烧灼；也指用于此目的的装置或化学品

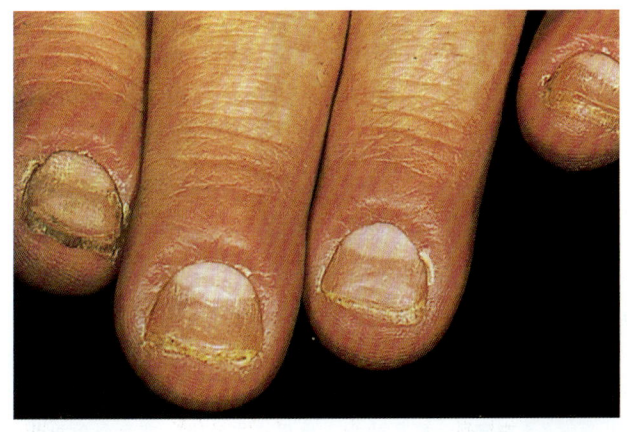

图 21-15　甲沟炎。近侧和外侧指甲缝的感染和炎症

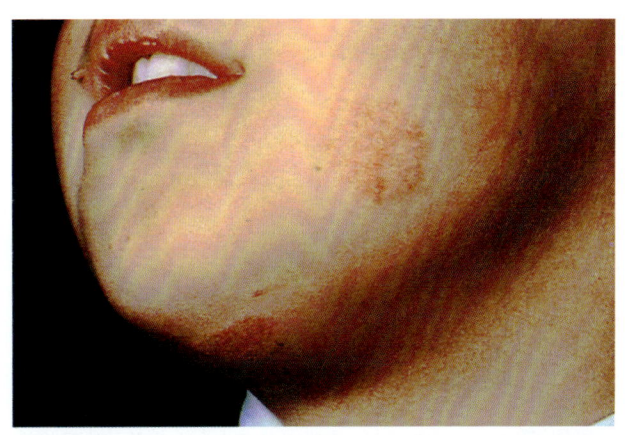

图 21-16　皮癣。脸上出现真菌感染

Terminology	补充术语（续表）
dermabrasion [ˌdɜːməˈbreɪʒən]	皮肤磨削术，通过化学或机械破坏表皮组织以去除瘢痕或胎记的整形外科手术
dermatoplasty [ˈdɜːmətəʊˌplæsti]	植皮术，移植人类皮肤；皮肤移植
diascopy [daɪˈæskɒpi]	玻片压诊法，通过在皮肤上压一块玻璃片检查皮肤损伤
fulguration [ˌfʌlɡjʊəˈreɪʃən]	电灼疗法，通过高频电火花破坏组织
skin turgor [ˈtɜːɡə]	皮肤膨压，皮肤对变形的抵抗力。压迫时皮肤返回位置的能力是皮肤膨压的证明。皮肤膨压是皮肤弹性与水合状态的量度。它通常随着年龄下降，降低时也可能是营养不良的迹象
Wood lamp	伍德灯，用于诊断真菌感染的紫外线灯

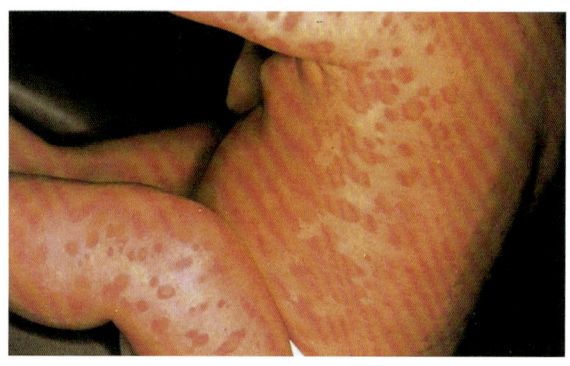

图 21-17 **荨麻疹**。婴儿身上出现与药物过敏相关的团块（参见团块，框 21-2）

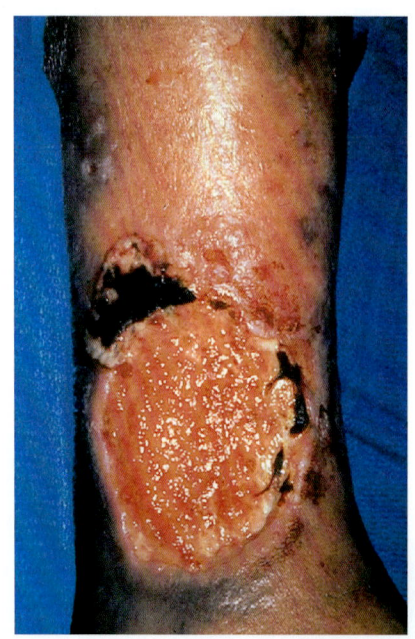

图 21-18 **静脉淤滞性溃疡**。静脉功能不全和血瘀引起的踝关节损伤（参见溃疡，框 21-2）

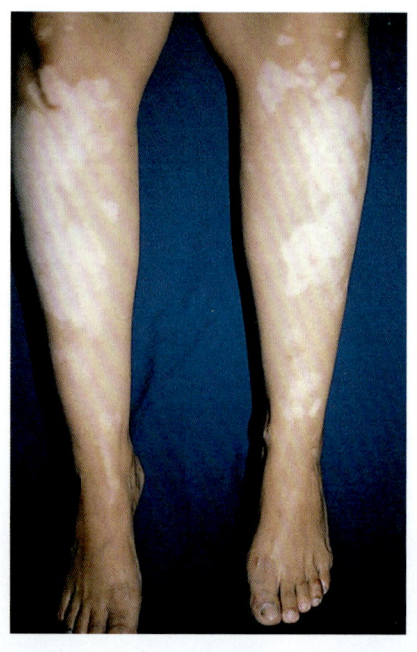

图 21-19 **白癜风**。脱色的斑点出现在皮肤上，可能会合并成为大块的缺乏黑色素区域（参见斑点，框 21-2）。图中所示的棕色是人正常皮肤的颜色，苍白区域是由白癜风引起的

Terminology 缩略语

BSA	Body surface area	体表面积
DLE	Discoid lupus erythematosus	盘状红斑狼疮
FTSG	Full-thickness skin graft	全厚皮片
LE	Lupus erythematosus	红斑狼疮
PSS	Progressive systemic sclerosis	进行性系统性硬化症
PUVA	Psoralen ultraviolet A	补骨脂素和近紫外线
SCLE	Subacute cutaneous lupus erythematosus	亚急性皮肤红斑狼疮
SLE	Systemic lupus erythematosus	系统性红斑狼疮
SPF	Sun protection factor	防晒指数
STSG	Split-thickness skin graft	中厚皮片
UV	Ultraviolet	紫外线
UVA	Ultraviolet A	近紫外线
UVB	Ultraviolet B	远紫外线
VAC	Vacuum-assisted closure	真空辅助闭合

Case Study Revisited 案例研究再访

C. M.'s Follow-Up

C. M. made progress while in the long-term facility. She also worked with a PT and OT and began performing simple ADL. The therapists performed ROM on a regular schedule to both the stroke-affected and unaffected sides. With the increase in activity and improved nutrition, C.M.'s circulation and skin condition improved. She also showed less confusion. C. M.'s daughter was able to observe and assist with her mother's activities and receive instruction firsthand. Goals were set, and discharge plans were made to have C. M. return home with her daughter.

C. M. 的随访

C. M. 在长期恢复机构中取得了进展。她还与物理治疗师和职业治疗师合作，开始执行简单的日常生活活动。治疗师定期对脑卒中影响和未受脑卒中影响的两侧进行关节活动度检查。随着活动的增加和营养的改善，C. M. 的循环和皮肤状况得到改善，意识混乱也较少了。C. M. 的女儿能够观察并协助她母亲的活动，并接受了直接的指导。目标已设定，并执行出院计划，让C.M. 与她的女儿回到家中。

CHAPTER 21 复习

标记练习

皮肤横截面

在对应的下划线写出每个编号部分的名称。

Adipose tissue
Arrector pili muscle
Artery
Dermis
Epidermis
Hair
Hair follicle
Nerve
Nerve endings
Pore (opening of sweat gland)
Pressure receptor
Sebaceous (oil) gland
Skin
Stratum basale (growing layer)
Stratum corneum
Subcutaneous layer
Sudoriferous (sweat) gland
Touch receptor
Vein

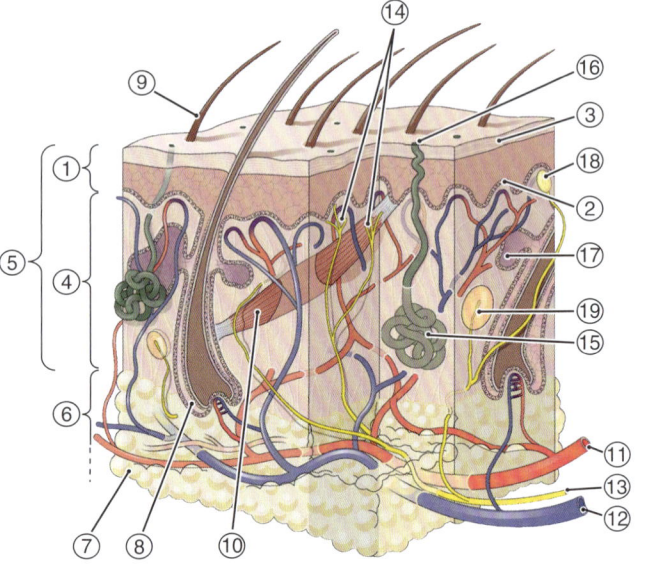

1. _____
2. _____
3. _____
4. _____
5. _____
6. _____
7. _____
8. _____
9. _____
10. _____
11. _____
12. _____
13. _____
14. _____
15. _____
16. _____
17. _____
18. _____
19. _____

术语

匹配

匹配下列术语，在每个题号左侧写上适当的字母。

____ 1. cicatrization   **a.** redness of the skin
____ 2. erythema   **b.** severe itching
____ 3. eczema   **c.** material that escapes from damaged tissue
____ 4. pruritus   **d.** atopic dermatitis
____ 5. exudate   **e.** scar formation

____ 6. stratum basale   **a.** oily skin secretion
____ 7. hypodermis   **b.** sheath that contains a hair
____ 8. sebum   **c.** subcutaneous layer
____ 9. stratum corneum   **d.** growing layer of the epidermis
____ 10. follicle   **e.** thickened layer of the epidermis

补充术语

____ 11. alopecia   **a.** profuse sweating
____ 12. excoriation   **b.** lesion caused by scratching or abrasion
____ 13. nevus   **c.** mole or birthmark
____ 14. diaphoresis   **d.** blackhead
____ 15. comedo   **e.** baldness

____ 16. rosacea   **a.** condition causing redness and pustules, mainly on the face
____ 17. tinea   **b.** fungal skin infection
____ 18. bromhidrosis   **c.** infection around a nail
____ 19. albinism   **d.** lack of skin pigmentation
____ 20. paronychia   **e.** sweat with a foul odor

填空

21. The main pigment in skin is_____.
22. The oil-producing glands of the skin are the_____.
23. A sudoriferous gland produces_____.
24. The adjective cutaneous refers to the_____.
25. Dermabrasion ［ˌdɜːməˈbreɪʒ(ə)n］ is surface scraping of the _____.
26. The protein that thickens the skin and makes up hair and nails is_____.
27. Schizonychia ［skɪzəʊˈnɪkɪə］ is splitting of a(n)_____.

参照本章开头 C.M. 的案例研究。

28. Two other terms for a pressure ulcer are_____.
29. When the nurse palpated C.M.'s lesion, she used her sense of_____.
30. Part of C.M.'s treatment was removal of dead skin from her lesion. This process is called_____.

31. The abbreviation FTSG refers to a(n) _____.
32. A term for lack of oxygen to tissue is _____.
33. The medical specialist who treated C.M.'s deteriorating pressure ulcer was a(n) _____.

定义

定义下列单词。

34. xeroderma ［ˌzɪərəʊˈdɜːmə］ _____
35. dyskeratosis ［diːzkərəˈtəʊsɪs］ _____
36. seborrhea ［sɪbɒrˈhɪə］ _____
37. pachyderma ［pækɪˈdɜːmə］ _____
38. onychia ［əʊˈnɪkɪə］ _____
39. hypermelanosis ［haɪpəˈmelænəʊsɪs］ _____
40. percutaneous ［ˌpɜːkjuːˈteɪnɪəs］ _____
41. keratogenic ［ˌkerətəˈdʒenɪk］ _____

写出下列定义的单词。

42. pertaining to discharge of sebum _____
43. excess production of keratin _____
44. instrument for cutting the skin _____
45. tumor containing melanin _____
46. cell that produces melanin _____
47. hardening of the skin _____

使用单词 hidrosis（出汗）作为词尾写出下列含义的单词。

48. absence of sweating _____
49. excess sweating _____
50. excretion of colored (chrom/o) sweat _____

复数

给出下列补充术语的复数形式。

51. bulla _____
52. ecchymosis _____
53. fungus _____
54. comedo _____
55. staphylococcus _____

真假判断

检查以下语句。如果语句为真，则在第一个空格写入 T；如果语句为假，则在第一个空格中写入 F，并通过在第二个空格中替换带下划线的单词来更正语句。

	True or False	Correct Answer
56. The skin and its associated structures make up the <u>integumentary system</u>.		
57. The root trich/o refers to <u>hair</u>.		
58. The <u>dermis</u> is between the epidermis and the subcutaneous layer.		
59. A <u>cicatrix</u> is a scar.		
60. Hirsutism is excess growth of <u>nails</u>.		

单词构建

使用给出的单词组成部分写出下列定义的单词。

> -lysis   onych/o   -sis   myc/o   path/o   dermat/o   -y   log/o   -oid   trich/o

61. loosening or separation of the skin _____
62. fungal infection of a nail _____
63. resembling a hair _____
64. study of hair _____
65. loosening of a nail _____
66. like or resembling skin _____
67. any disease of a nail _____
68. fungal infection of the hair _____
69. any disease of the skin _____
70. study and treatment of the skin _____

排除

在下列每组中，为与其他不相配的单词加下划线，并说明你选择的理由。

71. nodule — vesicle — keloid — macule — papule

72. impetigo — escharotomy — psoriasis — dermatitis — pemphigus

73. SLE — PSS — SCLE — BSA — DLE

单词分析

定义下列单词，并给出每个单词组成部分的含义。如果需要，可以使用词典。

74. dermatophytosis ［ˌdɜ:məʊfaiˈtəʊsis］ _____

    a. dermat/o _____

    b. phyt/o _____

    c. -sis _____

75. hidradenoma ［haidrædiˈnəʊmə］ _____

    a. hidr/o _____

    b. aden/o _____

    c. -oma _____

76. onychocryptosis ［ɒnaitʃəʊkˈriptəʊsis］ _____

    a. onych/o _____

    b. crypt/o _____

    c. -sis _____

77. achromotrichia ［əkrəʊməˈtrikiə］ _____

    a. a _____

    b. chrom/o _____

    c. trich/o _____

    d. -ia _____

Additional Case Studies
补充案例研究

Case Study 21-1: Basal Cell Carcinoma
案例研究 21-1：基底细胞癌

K. B., a 32-year-old fitness instructor, had noticed a "tiny hard lump" at the base of her left nostril while cleansing her face. The lesion had been present for about two months when she consulted a dermatologist. She had recently moved north from Florida, where she had worked as a lifeguard. She thought the lump might have been triggered by the regular tanning salon sessions she had used to retain her tan because it did not resemble the acne pustules, blackheads, or resulting scars of her adolescent years. Although dermabrasion had removed the obvious acne scars and left several areas of dense skin, this lump was brown-pigmented and different. K. B. was afraid it might be a malignant melanoma. On examination, the dermatologist noted a small pearly-white nodule at the lower portion of the left ala (outer flared portion of the nostril). There were no other lesions on her face or neck.

A plastic surgeon excised the lesion and was able to reapproximate the wound edges without a full-thickness skin graft. The pathology report identified the lesion as a basal cell carcinoma with clean margins of normal skin and subcutaneous tissue and stated that the entire lesion had been excised. K.B. was advised to wear SPF 30 sun protection on her face at all times and to avoid excessive sun exposure and tanning salons.

K. B. 是一名 32 岁的健身教练，她在洗脸时注意到在的左鼻孔底部有一个"小硬块"。当她咨询皮肤科医生时，病变已经存在了大约 2 个月。她最近从佛罗里达搬到北部来，在那里她曾当救生员。她认为，这个硬块可能是长期日光浴沙龙引起的，她习惯保持棕褐色，因为它不像痤疮脓疱、黑头粉刺或青少年时期产生的伤疤。尽管磨皮已经消除了明显的痤疮瘢痕，并留下了几个致密皮肤的区域，但这个硬块是棕色的，而且是不同的。K. B. 害怕它可能是恶性黑色素瘤。在检查时，皮肤科医生注意到在左鼻翼（鼻孔的外扩张部分）下部的小珍珠白色结节，她的脸和脖子上没有其他病变。

整形外科医生切除了病变，并能够不用全层皮片重新缝合伤口边缘。病理报告鉴定病变为具有正常皮肤和皮下组织清晰边缘的基底细胞癌，并且说明整个病变已被切除。K.B. 被建议在任何时候都在脸上涂抹 SPF 30 防晒霜，并避免过度的阳光照射和日光浴沙龙。

Case Study 21-2: Cutaneous Lymphoma
案例研究 21-2：皮肤淋巴瘤

L. C., a 52-year-old female research chemist, has had a history of T cell lymphoma for eight years. She was initially treated with systemic chemotherapy with methotrexate, until she contracted stomatitis. Continued therapy with topical chemotherapeutic agents brought measurable improvement. She also had a history of hidradenitis.

A recent physical examination showed diffuse erythroderma with scaling and hyperkeratosis, plus alopecia. She had painful leukoplakia and ulcerations of the mouth and tongue. L. C. was hospitalized and given two courses of topical chemotherapy. She was referred to dental medicine for treatment of the oral lesions and was discharged in stable condition with an appointment for follow-up in four weeks. Her discharge medications included the application of 2 percent hydrocortisone ointment to the affected lesions qhs, Keralyt gel bid for the hyperkeratosis, and Dyclone and Benadryl for her mouth ulcers prn.

L. C. 是一位 52 岁的女化学家，已有 8 年的 T 细胞淋巴瘤病史。她最初接受过甲氨蝶呤全身化疗，直到她出现口腔炎。使用局部化疗剂的连续治疗带来了可观的改善。她还有汗腺炎病史。

最近的体格检查显示弥漫性红皮病，伴有鳞屑和角化过度，还有脱发。她的口腔和舌头有疼痛的白斑和溃疡。L. C. 住院并接受两个疗程的局部化疗。她被转诊到牙科治疗口腔病变，并以稳定状态出院，预约 4 周内随访。她的出院药物包括针对受影响的病变使用 2% 氢化可的松软膏，每小时 1 次；针对角化过度使用 Keralyt 凝胶，每日 2 次；针对口腔溃疡使用盐酸达克罗宁和苯海拉明，必要时使用。

案例研究问题

多项选择。选择最佳答案，在每个题号左侧写上你选择的字母。

____ 1. K.B.'s basal cell carcinoma may have been caused by chronic exposure to the sun and use of an ultraviolet tanning bed. The scientific explanation for this is the

　　a. autoimmune response

　　b. actinic effect

　　c. allergic reaction

　　d. sunblock tanning lotion theory

____ 2. The characteristic pimples of adolescent acne are whiteheads and blackheads. The medical terms for these lesions are

　　a. vesicles and macules

　　b. pustules and blisters

　　c. pustules and comedones

　　d. furuncles and sebaceous cysts

____ 3. Which skin cancer is an overgrowth of pigment-producing epidermal cells?

　　a. basal cell carcinoma

　　b. Kaposi sarcoma

　　c. cutaneous lymphoma

　　d. melanoma

____ 4. Basal cell carcinoma involves

　　a. subcutaneous tissue

　　b. hair follicles

　　c. connective tissue

　　d. epithelial cells

____ 5. Hidradenitis is inflammation of a

　　a. sweat gland

　　b. salivary gland

　　c. sebaceous gland

　　d. meibomian gland

____ 6. Leukoplakia is

　　a. baldness

　　b. ulceration

　　c. formation of white patches in the mouth

　　d. formation of yellow patches on the skin

____ 7. Hydrocortisone is a(n)

　　a. vitamin

　　b. steroid

　　c. analgesic

　　d. diuretic

____ 8. An example of a topical drug is a

　　a. systemic chemotherapeutic agent

　　b. drug derived from rainforest plants

　　c. skin ointment

　　d. Benadryl capsule, 25 mg

____ 9. Stomatitis, a common side effect of systemic chemotherapy, is an inflammatory condition of the

　　a. mouth

　　b. stomach

　　c. teeth and hair

　　d. debridement

写出案例研究中下列含义的单词。

10. skin sanding procedure _____

11. a solid raised lesion larger than a papule _____

12. physician who cares for patients with skin diseases _____

13. layer of connective tissue and fat beneath the dermis _____
14. diffuse redness of the skin _____
15. increased production of keratin in the skin _____

定义下列缩略语。
16. FTSG _____
17. SPF _____
18. hs _____
19. bid _____
20. prn _____

附录 1

常用符号

Symbol 符号	Meaning 含义
1°	primary
2°	secondary (to)
Δ	change (Greek delta)
Ⓛ	left
Ⓡ	right
↑	increase(d)
↓	decrease(d)
♂	male
♀	female
°	degree
∧	above
∨	below
=	equal to
≠	not equal to
±	doubtful, slight
~	approximately
×	times
#	number, pound

附录 2

缩略语及其含义

Abbreviation 缩略语	Meaning 含义	含义（中文）
ā	before	之前
A, Acc	accommodation	视觉调节
āā	of each	每个
A1c	glycated hemoglobin	糖化血红蛋白
Ab	antibody	抗体
AB	abortion	流产
ABC	aspiration biopsy cytology	抽吸活检细胞学
ABG(s)	arterial blood gas(es)	动脉血气
ABR	auditory brainstem response	听觉脑干反应
ac	before meals	餐前
AC	air conduction	空气传导
ACE	angiotensin converting enzyme	血管紧张素转换酶
ACh	acetylcholine	乙酰胆碱
ACL	anterior cruciate ligament	前交叉韧带
ACTH	adrenocorticotropic hormone	促肾上腺皮质激素
ad lib	as desired	如预期的
AD	Alzheimer disease	阿尔茨海默病
ADH	antidiuretic hormone	抗利尿激素
ADHD	attention-deficit/ hyperactivity disorder	注意力缺乏 / 多动症
ADL	activities of daily living	日常生活活动
AE	above the elbow	肘上
AED	automated external defibrillator	自动体外心脏去颤器
AF	atrial fibrillation	心房颤动
AFB	acid-fast bacillus	抗酸杆菌
AFP	alpha-fetoprotein	甲胎蛋白

缩略语及其含义

Abbreviation 缩略语	Meaning 含义	含义（中文）
Ag	antigen; also silver	抗原；银
AGA	appropriate for gestational age	适宜胎龄
AI	artificial insemination; aromatase inhibitor	人工授精
AIDS	acquired immunodeficiency syndrome	获得性免疫缺陷综合征
AK	above the knee	膝上
ALL	acute lymphoblastic (lymphocytic) leukemia	急性淋巴细胞性白血病
ALS	amyotrophic lateral sclerosis	肌萎缩性脊髓侧索硬化症
AMA	against medical advice	违反医嘱
AMB	ambulatory	流动的
AMD	age-related macular degeneration	老年性黄斑变性
AMI	acute myocardial infarction	急性心肌梗死
AML	acute myeloblastic (myelogenous) leukemia	急性髓细胞性白血病
ANS	autonomic nervous system	自主神经系统
AP	anteroposterior	前后的
APAP	acetaminophen	对乙酰氨基酚
APC	atrial premature complex; antigen presenting cell	房性期前收缩；抗原递呈细胞
APTT	activated partial thromboplastin time	活化部分凝血活酶时间
aq	water, aqueous	水；房水
AR	aortic regurgitation	主动脉反流
ARB	angiotensin receptor blocker	血管紧张素受体阻断剂
ARC	abnormal retinal correspondence	异常视网膜对应
ARDS	acute respiratory distress syndrome	急性呼吸窘迫综合征
ARF	acute respiratory failure; acute renal failure	急性呼吸衰竭；急性肾衰竭
ART	assisted reproductive technology	辅助生殖技术
ASA	acetylsalicylic acid (aspirin)	乙酰水杨酸（阿司匹林）
As, Ast	astigmatism	散光
AS	atrial stenosis; arteriosclerosis	心房狭窄；动脉硬化

缩略语及其含义

Abbreviation 缩略语	Meaning 含义	含义（中文）
ASCVD	arteriosclerotic cardiovascular disease	动脉硬化性心血管疾病
ASD	atrial septal defect	房间隔缺损
ASF	anterior spinal fusion	前路脊柱融合
ASHD	arteriosclerotic heart disease	动脉硬化性心脏病
ASHP	American Society of Health System Pharmacists	美国健康系统药剂师协会
AT	atrial tachycardia	房性心动过速
ATN	acute tubular necrosis	急性肾小管坏死
AV	atrioventricular	房室的
BAEP	brainstem auditory evoked potentials	脑干听觉诱发电位
BBB	bundle branch block	束支性传导阻滞
BC	bone conduction	骨传导
BCG	bacille Calmette–Guérin (tuberculosis vaccine)	卡介苗（结核病疫苗）
BE	barium enema; below the elbow	钡灌肠；肘下
bid, b.i.d.	twice per day	每日2次
BK	below the knee	膝下
BM	bowel movement	肠蠕动
BMD	bone mineral density	骨密度
BNO	ladder neck obstruction	膀胱颈梗阻
BP	blood pressure	血压
BPH	benign prostatic hyperplasia (hypertrophy)	良性前列腺增生（肥大）
bpm	beats per minute	每秒心跳
BRCA1	breast cancer gene 1	乳腺癌基因1
BRCA2	breast cancer gene 2	乳腺癌基因2
BRP	bathroom privileges	卫浴权限
BS	bowel sounds; breath sounds; blood sugar	肠音；呼吸音；血糖
BSA	body surface area	体表面积
BSE	breast self examination	乳房自检

缩略语及其含义

Abbreviation 缩略语	Meaning 含义	含义（中文）
BSO	bilateral salpingo-oophorectomy	两侧输卵管卵巢切除
BT	bleeding time	出血时间
BUN	blood urea nitrogen	血尿素氮
BV	bacterial vaginosis	细菌性阴道病
bx	biopsy	活组织检查
c̄	with	伴随
C	Celsius (centigrade); compliance; cervical vertebra	摄氏度；合规；颈椎
C-section	cesarean section	剖宫产
CA, Ca	cancer	癌症
CABG	coronary artery bypass graft	冠状动脉旁路移植术
CAD	coronary artery disease	冠状动脉疾病
CAM	complementary and alternative medicine	补充和替代医疗
cap	capsule	胶囊
CAPD	continuous ambulatory peritoneal dialysis	持续性非卧床腹膜透析
CBC	complete blood count	全血细胞计数
CBD	common bile duct	胆总管
CBF	cerebral blood flow	脑血流
CBR	complete bed rest	完全卧床休息
cc	with correction	有矫正
CC	chief complaint	主诉
CCPD	continuous cyclic peritoneal dialysis	持续性循环性腹膜透折
CCU	coronary care unit; cardiac care unit	冠心病监护病房；心脏病监护病房
CF	cystic fibrosis	囊性纤维化
CFS	chronic fatigue syndrome	慢性疲劳综合征
CGL	chronic granulocytic leukemia	慢性粒细胞白血病
CHD	coronary heart disease	冠心病
CHF	congestive heart failure	充血性心力衰竭

缩略语及其含义

Abbreviation 缩略语	Meaning 含义	含义（中文）
Ci	Curie	居里
CIN	cervical intraepithelial neoplasia	宫颈上皮内瘤样病变
CIS	carcinoma in situ	原位癌
CJD	Creutzfeldt–Jakob disease	克雅氏病
CK	creatine kinase	肌酸激酶
CK-MB	creatine kinase MB	肌酸激酶同工酶
CLL	chronic lymphocytic leukemia	慢性淋巴细胞白血病
cm	centimeter	厘米
CMG	cystometrography, cystometrogram	膀胱内压描记法，膀胱内压测量图
CML	chronic myelogenous leukemia	慢性粒细胞性白血病
CNS	central nervous system; clinical nurse specialist	中枢神经系统；临床护理专家
c/o, CO	complains (complaining) of	主诉
Co	coccyx; coccygeal	尾骨；尾骨的
CO_2	carbon dioxide	二氧化碳
COPD	chronic obstructive pulmonary disease	慢性阻塞性肺疾病
CP	cerebral palsy	脑性瘫痪
CPAP	continuous positive airway pressure	持续气道正压通气
CPD	cephalopelvic disproportion	头盆不称
C(P)K	creatine (phospho)kinase	肌酸（磷酸化）激酶
CPR	cardiopulmonary resuscitation	心肺复苏术
CRF	chronic renal failure	慢性肾衰竭
Crit	hematocrit	红细胞压积
CRP	C-reactive protein	C反应蛋白
C&S	culture and sensitivity	培养和敏感测试
CSF	cerebrospinal fluid	脑脊液
CSII	continuous subcutaneous insulin infusion	持续胰岛素皮下输注
CT	computed tomography	计算机断层扫描

缩略语及其含义

Abbreviation 缩略语	Meaning 含义	含义（中文）
CTA	computed tomograph angiography	CT 血管造影
CTE	chronic traumatic encephalopathy	慢性创伤性脑病
CTS	carpal tunnel syndrome	腕管综合征
CVA	cerebrovascular accident	脑血管意外
CVD	cardiovascular disease; cerebrovascular disease	心血管病；脑血管病
CVI	chronic venous insufficiency	慢性静脉功能不全
CVP	central venous pressure	中心静脉压
CVS	chorionic villus sampling	绒毛膜绒毛取样
CXR	chest x-ray	胸部 X 线片
D&C	dilatation and curettage	刮宫术
DAW	dispense as written	按所写配药
dB	decibel	分贝
dc, D/C	discontinue	不连续
DCIS	ductal carcinoma in situ	原位管癌
D&E	dilation and evacuation	扩张和吸取
DES	diethylstilbestrol	己烯雌酚
DEXA	dual-energy x-ray absorptiometry (scan)	双能 X 线骨密度仪（扫描）
DIC	disseminated intravascular coagulation	弥散性血管内凝血
DIFF	differential count	白细胞分类计数
DIP	distal interphalangeal	远端指间关节
DJD	degenerative joint disease	退行性关节疾病
dl	deciliter	分升
DLE	discoid lupus erythematosus	盘状红斑狼疮
DM	diabetes mellitus	糖尿病
DNR	do not resuscitate	未复苏
DOE	dyspnea on exertion	运动性呼吸困难
DTaP	diphtheria, tetanus, acellular pertussis (vaccine)	百白破（疫苗）

缩略语及其含义

Abbreviation 缩略语	Meaning 含义	含义（中文）
DRE	digital rectal examination	直肠指检
DS	double strength	双倍强度
DSM	Diagnostic and Statistical Manual of Mental Disorders	精神疾病诊断与统计手册
DTR	deep tendon reflex(es)	深部腱反射
DUB	dysfunctional uterine bleeding	功能失调性子宫出血
DVT	deep vein thrombosis	深静脉血栓
Dx	diagnosis	诊断
EBL	estimated blood loss	估计血量失
EBV	Epstein–Barr virus	埃-巴二氏病毒
ECG (EKG)	electrocardiogram, electrocardiography	心电图，心电描记法
ECMO	extracorporeal membrane oxygenation	体外膜氧合
ED	erectile dysfunction	勃起功能障碍
EDC	estimated date of confinement	预产期
EEG	electroencephalogram, electroencephalograph(y)	脑电图，脑电图仪
EGD	esophagogastroduodenoscopy	食道、胃、十二指肠镜检查
ELISA	enzyme-linked immunosorbent assay	酶联免疫吸附测试
elix	elixir	酏剂
EM	emmetropia	正视眼
EMG	electromyography, electromyogram	肌电描记术，肌电图
ENG	electronystagmography	眼震电流描记法
ENT	ear(s), nose, and throat	耳鼻喉
EOM	extraocular movement, muscles	眼球外转动，眼外肌
EOMI	extraocular muscles intact	眼外肌完整
EPO, EP	erythropoietin	促红细胞生成素
ERCP	endoscopic retrograde cholangiopancreatography	内镜逆行胰胆管造影
ERG	electroretinography	视网膜电描记法
ERV	expiratory reserve volume	补呼气量

缩略语及其含义

Abbreviation 缩略语	Meaning 含义	含义（中文）
ESR	erythrocyte sedimentation rate	红细胞沉降率
ESRD	end-stage renal disease	终末期肾病
ESWL	extracorporeal shock wave lithotripsy	体外冲击波碎石术
ET	esotropia	内斜视
ETOH	alcohol, ethyl alcohol	酒精，乙醇
F	Fahrenheit	华氏度
FAP	familial adenomatous polyposis	家族性腺瘤性息肉病
FBG	fasting blood glucose	空腹血糖
FBS	fasting blood sugar	空腹血糖
FC	finger counting	数指
FDA	Food and Drug Administration	食品和药物管理局
FEV	forced expiratory volume	用力呼气量
FFP	fresh frozen plasma	新鲜冰冻血浆
FHR	fetal heart rate	胎心率
FHT	fetal heart tone	胎心音
FMS	fibromyalgia syndrome	纤维肌痛综合征
FPG	fasting plasma glucose	空腹血糖
FRC	functional residual capacity	功能残气量
FSH	follicle-stimulating hormone	促卵泡激素
FTI	free thyroxine index	游离甲状腺素指数
FTND	full-term normal delivery	足月顺产
FTP	full-term pregnancy	足月妊娠
FTSG	full-thickness skin graft	全层皮片
FUO	fever of unknown origin	原因不明的发热
FVC	forced vital capacity	用力肺活量
Fx	fracture	骨折
g	gram	克
GA	gestational age	孕龄

缩略语及其含义

Abbreviation 缩略语	Meaning 含义	含义（中文）
GAD	generalized anxiety disorder	广泛性焦虑症
GC	gonococcus	淋球菌
GDM	gestational diabetes mellitus	妊娠糖尿病
GERD	gastroesophageal reflux disease	胃食管反流病
GFR	glomerular filtration rate	肾小球滤过率
GH	growth hormone	生长激素
GI	gastrointestinal	胃肠的
GIFT	gamete intrafallopian transfer	配子输卵管内移植
GTT	glucose tolerance test	葡萄糖耐受测试
GU	genitourinary	泌尿生殖的
GYN	gynecology	妇科学
H&P	history and physical examination	病历及体格检查
HAV	hepatitis A virus	甲肝病毒
Hb, Hgb	hemoglobin	血红蛋白
HbA1c	hemoglobin A1c; glycated hemoglobin	糖化血红蛋白
HBV	hepatitis B virus	乙肝病毒
hCG	human chorionic gonadotropin	人体绒毛膜促性腺激素
HCl	hydrochloric acid	盐酸
Hct, Ht	hematocrit	血细胞比容
HCV	hepatitis C virus	丙肝病毒
HDL	high-density lipoprotein	高密度脂蛋白
HDN	hemolytic disease of the newborn	新生儿溶血病
HDV	hepatitis D virus	丁肝病毒
HEV	hepatitis E virus	戊肝病毒
HEENT	head, eyes, ears, nose, and throat	头眼耳鼻喉
HIPAA	Health Insurance Portability and Accountability Act	健康保险携带和责任法案
HIV	human immunodeficiency virus	人类免疫缺陷病毒

缩略语及其含义

Abbreviation 缩略语	Meaning 含义	含义（中文）
HL	hearing level	听力水平
HNP	herniated nucleus pulposus	椎间盘髓核脱出
h/o	history of	……的病史
HPI	history of present illness	当前病史
HPS	Hantavirus pulmonary syndrome	汉坦病毒肺综合征
HPV	human papillomavirus	人乳头瘤病毒
HR	heart rate	心率
HRT	hormone replacement therapy	激素替代疗法
hs at	bedtime	就寝时间
hs-crp	high sensitivity C-reactive protein (test)	高灵敏度 C 反应蛋白（测试）
HSV	herpes simplex virus	单纯疱疹病毒
Ht, Hct	hematocrit	血细胞容积率
HTN	hypertension	高血压
Hx	history	病史病历
Hz	Hertz	赫兹
^{131}I	iodine-131	碘 131
I&D	incision and drainage	切开引流
I&O	intake and output	摄入与排出
IABP	intra-aortic balloon pump	主动脉内气囊泵
IBD	inflammatory bowel disease	炎症性肠病
IBS	irritable bowel syndrome	肠易激综合征
IC	inspiratory capacity	深吸气量
ICD	implantable cardioverter defibrillator	植入式心脏复律除颤器
ICP	intracranial pressure	颅内压
ICU	intensive care unit	重症监护病房
ID	intradermal	皮内的
IF	intrinsic factor	内因子

缩略语及其含义

Abbreviation 缩略语	Meaning 含义	含义（中文）
IFG	impaired fasting blood glucose	空腹血糖受损
Ig	immunoglobulin	免疫球蛋白
IGRA	interferon gamma release assay (test for TB)	干扰素释放实验（结核病测试）
IGT	impaired glucose tolerance	糖耐量受损
IM	intramuscular(ly); intramedullary	肌肉内的；髓内的
INH	isoniazid	异烟肼
IOL	intraocular lens	人工晶体
IOP	intraocular pressure	眼压
IPPA	inspection, palpation, percussion, auscultation	视诊、触诊、叩诊、听诊
IPPB	intermittent positive pressure breathing	间歇性正压呼吸
IPPV	intermittent positive pressure ventilation	间歇性正压换气
IRV	inspiratory reserve volume	吸气储备容量
ITP	idiopathic thrombocytopenic purpura	特发性血小板减少性紫癜
IU	international unit	国际单位
IUD	intrauterine device	宫内节育器
IV	intravenous(ly)	静脉内
IVC	intravenous cholangiogram	静脉内胆管造影
IVCD	intraventricular conduction delay	心室内传导延迟
IVDA	intravenous drug abuse	静脉注射吸毒
IVF	in vitro fertilization	体外受精
IVP	intravenous pyelography	静脉肾盂造影术
IVPB	intravenous piggyback	借道静脉输液法
IVU	intravenous urography	静脉尿路造影术
JVP	jugular venous pulse	颈静脉搏动
K	potassium	钾
kg	kilogram	千克
km	kilometer	千米

缩略语及其含义

Abbreviation 缩略语	Meaning 含义	含义（中文）
KUB	kidney-ureter-bladder	肾 - 输尿管 - 膀胱
KVO	keep vein open	保持静脉通畅
L	lumbar vertebra; liter	腰椎；升
LA	long-acting	长效的
LAD	left anterior descending (coronary artery)	左前降支的（冠状动脉）
LAHB	left anterior hemiblock	左前分支传导阻滞
LDL	low-density lipoprotein	低密度脂蛋白
LE	lupus erythematosus	红斑狼疮
LES	lower esophageal sphincter	食管下端括约肌
LH	luteinizing hormone	促黄体激素
LL	left lateral	左外侧位
LLE	left lower extremity	左下肢
LLL	left lower lobe (of lung)	（肺）左下叶
LLQ	left lower quadrant	左下部
LMN	lower motor neuron	下运动神经元
LMP	last menstrual period	末次经期
LOC	level of consciousness	意识水平
LP	lumbar puncture	腰椎穿刺
LUE	left upper extremity	左上肢
LUL	left upper lobe (of lung)	（肺）左上叶
LUQ	left upper quadrant	左上部
LV	left ventricle	左心室
LVAD	left ventricular assist device	左心室辅助装置
LVEDP	left ventricular end diastolic pressure	左心室舒张末期压
LVH	left ventricular hypertrophy	左心室肥大
lytes	electrolytes	电解质
m	meter	米
MAOI	monoamine oxidase inhibitor	单胺氧化酶抑制剂

缩略语及其含义

Abbreviation 缩略语	Meaning 含义	含义（中文）
mcg	microgram	微克
MCH	mean corpuscular hemoglobin	平均红细胞血红蛋白
MCHC	mean corpuscular hemoglobin concentration	平均细胞血红蛋白浓度
mcL	microliter	微升
mcm	micrometer	微米
MCP	metacarpophalangeal	掌指的
MCV	mean corpuscular volume	平均红细胞容积
MDR	multi-drug resistant	多重耐药
MDS	myelodysplastic syndrome	骨髓增生异常综合征
MED(s)	medicine(s), medication(s)	医药，药物
MEFR	maximal expiratory flow rate	最大呼气流速
MEN	multiple endocrine neoplasia	多发性内分泌瘤病
mEq	milliequivalent	毫当量
MET	metastasis	转移
mg	milligram	毫克
MG	myasthenia gravis	重症肌无力
MHT	menopausal hormone therapy	绝经后激素疗法
MI	myocardial infarction	心肌梗死
MID	multi-infarct dementia	多梗死性痴呆
mL	milliliter	毫升
mm	millimeter	毫米
MMFR	maximum midexpiratory flow rate	最大呼气中期流速
mmHg	millimeters of mercury	毫米汞柱
MMT	manual muscle test(ing)	徒手肌力测试
MN	myoneural	肌神经的
MR	mitral regurgitation, reflux	二尖瓣回流，反流
MRI	magnetic resonance imaging	核磁共振成像

缩略语及其含义

Abbreviation 缩略语	Meaning 含义	含义（中文）
MRSA	methicillin-resistant Staphylococcus aureus	耐甲氧西林金黄色葡萄球菌
MS	mitral stenosis; multiple sclerosis	二尖瓣狭窄；多发性硬化
MTP	metatarsophalangeal	跖趾的
MUGA	multigated acquisition (scan)	平衡法多时闸心室造影（扫描）
MVP	mitral valve prolapse	二尖瓣脱垂
MVR	mitral valve replacement	二尖瓣置换
Na	sodium	钠
NAA	nucleic acid amplification (test) (for TB)	核酸扩增（测试）（结核病）
NAD	no apparent distress	无明显病痛
NB	newborn	新生儿
NCCAM	National Center for Complementary and Alternative Medicine	国家补充和替代医学中心
NG	nasogastric	鼻饲的
NGU	nongonococcal urethritis	非淋病性尿道炎
NHL	non-Hodgkin lymphoma	非霍奇金淋巴瘤
NICU	neonatal intensive care unit; neurologic intensive care unit	新生儿重症监护病房 神经重症监护病房
NKDA	no known drug allergies	无已知药物过敏
NMJ	neuromuscular junction	肌肉神经接点
NPH	neutral protamine Hagedorn (insulin)	中效低精蛋白（胰岛素）
NPH	normal pressure hydrocephalus	正常压力脑积水
NPO	nothing by mouth	禁食
NRC	normal retinal correspondence	正常视网膜对应
NREM	nonrapid eye movement (sleep)	非快速眼动（睡眠）
NS, N/S	normal saline	生理盐水
NSAID(s)	nonsteroidal antiinflammatory drug(s)	非甾体抗炎药
NSR	normal sinus rhythm	正常窦性心律
NV	near vision	近视

缩略语及其含义

Abbreviation 缩略语	Meaning 含义	含义（中文）
N/V, N&V, n&v	nausea and vomiting	恶心呕吐
N/V/D	nausea, vomiting, diarrhea	恶心呕吐腹泻
O2	oxygen	氧气
OA	osteoarthritis	骨关节炎
OB	obstetrics, obstetrician	产科学，产科医生
OCD	obsessive-compulsive disorder	强迫症
ODS	Office of Dietary Supplements	膳食补充剂办公室
OGTT	oral glucose-tolerance test	口服葡萄糖耐量测试
OI	osteogenesis imperfecta	成骨不全
OL	otolaryngology	耳鼻喉科
OOB	out of bed	不卧床
OM	otitis media	中耳炎
ORIF	open reduction internal fixation	切开复位内固定
ORL	otorhinolaryngology	耳鼻喉科学
ortho, ORTH	orthopedics	骨科
OT	occupational therapy	职业疗法
OTC	over-the-counter	非处方
p	after, post	之后，后
P	pulse	脉搏
PA	posteroanterior; physician assistant	前后的；医生助理
PAC	premature atrial contraction	房性期前收缩
$PaCO_2$	arterial partial pressure of carbon dioxide	动脉血二氧化碳分压
PACU	postanesthesia care unit	麻醉后监护病房
PaO_2	arterial partial pressure of oxygen	动脉血氧气分压
PAP	pulmonary arterial pressure	肺动脉压
pc	after meals	餐后
PCA	patient-controlled analgesia	患者自控性镇痛法
PCI	percutaneous coronary intervention	经皮冠状动脉介入治疗

缩略语及其含义

Abbreviation 缩略语	Meaning 含义	含义（中文）
PCL	posterior cruciate ligament	后交叉韧带
PCOS	polycystic ovarian syndrome	多囊卵巢综合征
PCP	Pneumocystis pneumonia	肺孢子虫性肺炎
PCV	packed cell volume	红细胞压积
PCWP	pulmonary capillary wedge pressure	肺毛细血管楔压
PDA	patent ductus arteriosus	动脉导管未闭
PDD	pervasive developmental disorder	广泛性发育障碍
PDR	Physicians' Desk Reference	医生桌面参考
PE	physical examination	体格检查
PEEP	positive end expiratory pressure	呼气末正压
PEFR	peak expiratory flow rate	最大呼气流速
PEG	percutaneous endoscopic gastrostomy (tube)	经皮内镜下胃造瘘术（管）
PEP	protein electrophoresis	蛋白电泳
PE(R)RLA	pupils equal, (regular) react to light and accommodation	瞳孔等大，对光线和调节的反应（正常）
PET	positron emission tomography	正电子发射断层扫描成像
PFT	pulmonary function test(s)	肺功能（测试）
pH	scale for measuring hydrogen ion concentration (acidity or alkalinity)	用于测量氢离子浓度的标度（酸碱度）
Ph	Philadelphia chromosome	费城染色体
PICC	peripherally inserted central catheter	外周穿刺中心静脉置管
PID	pelvic inflammatory disease	盆腔炎
PIH	pregnancy-induced hypertension	妊娠高血压
PIP	peak inspiratory pressure	吸气峰压
PIP	proximal interphalangeal	近端指节间
PKU	phenylketonuria	苯丙酮尿症
PMH	past medical history	既往病史
PMI	point of maximal impulse	最强心尖搏动点

缩略语及其含义

Abbreviation 缩略语	Meaning 含义	含义（中文）
PMN	polymorphonuclear (neutrophil)	中性粒细胞
PMS	premenstrual syndrome	经前期综合征
PND	paroxysmal nocturnal dyspnea	阵发性夜间呼吸困难
PNS	peripheral nervous system	周围神经系统
po, PO	by mouth, orally	口服
poly, polymorph	neutrophil	中性粒细胞
PONV	postoperative nausea and vomiting	术后恶心呕吐
postop, post-op	postoperative	术后的
pp	postprandial (after a meal)	餐后
PPD	purified protein derivative (tuberculin)	纯化蛋白衍生物（结核菌素）
PPI	proton pump inhibitor	质子泵抑制剂
preop, pre-op	preoperative	术前的
PRL	prolactin	催乳素
prn	as needed	根据需要
PSA	prostate-specific antigen	前列腺特异性抗原
PSF	posterior spinal fusion	后路脊柱融合
PSS	physiologic saline solution; progressive systemic sclerosis	生理盐水溶液；进行性系统性硬化症
PSVT	paroxysmal supraventricular tachycardia	阵发性室上性心动过速
pt	patient	患者
PT	physical therapy/ therapist	物理疗法 / 物理治疗师
PT, ProTime	prothrombin time	凝血酶原时间
PTCA	percutaneous transluminal coronary angioplasty	经皮腔内冠状动脉成形术
PTH	parathyroid hormone	甲状旁腺激素
PTSD	post traumatic stress disorder	创伤后应激障碍
PTT	partial thromboplastin time	部分凝血活酶时间
PUVA	psoralen ultraviolet A	补骨脂素长波紫外线
PVC	premature ventricular contraction	室性期前收缩

缩略语及其含义

Abbreviation 缩略语	Meaning 含义	含义（中文）
PVD	peripheral vascular disease	周围血管病
PYP	pyrophosphate	焦磷酸盐
qam	every morning	每天早晨
qh	every hour	每小时
q __ h	every __ hours	每小时
qid, q.i.d.	four times per day	每日4次
QNS	quantity not sufficient	数量不足
QS	quantity sufficient	足量
R	respiration	呼吸
RA	rheumatoid arthritis	风湿性关节炎
RAIU	radioactive iodine uptake	放射性碘摄入
RAS	reticular activating system	网状激活系统
RATx	radiation therapy	放射疗法
RBC	red blood cell; red blood (cell) count	红细胞；红细胞计数
RDS	respiratory distress syndrome	呼吸窘迫综合征
REM	rapid eye movement (sleep)	快速眼动（睡眠）
RIA	radioimmunoassay	放射免疫分析法
RICE	rest, ice, compression, elevation	休息、冰敷、压紧、抬升
RL	right lateral	右侧
RLE	right lower extremity	右下肢
RLL	right lower lobe (of lung)	（肺）右下叶
RLQ	right lower quadrant	右下部
RLS	restless legs syndrome	不宁腿综合征
RML	right middle lobe (of lung)	（肺）右中叶
R/O	rule out	排除
ROM	range of motion	运动范围
ROS	review of systems	系统回顾

缩略语及其含义

缩略语及其含义

Abbreviation 缩略语	Meaning 含义	含义（中文）
RSI	repetitive strain injury	重复性劳损
RSV	respiratory syncytial virus	呼吸道合胞体病毒
RTC	rotator cuff	旋转肌群
RUE	right upper extremity	右上肢
RUL	right upper lobe (of lung)	（肺）右上叶
RUQ	right upper quadrant	右上部
RV	residual volume	余气量
Rx	drug, prescription, therapy	药物，处方，疗法
$\bar{s}$	without	没有
S	sacrum; sacral	骶骨；骶骨的
S_1	first heart sound	第一心音
S_2	second heart sound	第二心音
SA	sustained action; sinoatrial	持续作用；窦房的
SARS	severe acute respiratory syndrome	严重急性呼吸综合征
SBE	subacute bacterial endocarditis	亚急性细菌性心内膜炎
sc	without correction	无矫正
SC, SQ, subcut.	subcutaneous(ly)	皮下
SCLE	subacute cutaneous lupus erythematosus	亚急性皮肤红斑狼疮
seg	neutrophil	中性粒细胞
SERM	selective estrogen receptor modulator	选择性雌激素受体调节剂
SG	specific gravity	比重
SIADH	syndrome of inappropriate antidiuretic hormone	抗利尿激素分泌异常综合征
SIDS	sudden infant death syndrome	婴儿猝死综合征
SITS	supraspinatus, infraspinatus, teres minor, subscapularis (muscles)	冈上肌、冈下肌、小圆肌、肩胛下肌
SK	streptokinase	链激酶
SL	sublingual	舌下
SLE	systemic lupus erythematosus	系统性红斑狼疮

缩略语及其含义

Abbreviation 缩略语	Meaning 含义	含义（中文）
SPECT	single photon emission computed tomography	单光子发射计算机断层扫描
SPF	sun protection factor	防晒指数
SpO$_2$	oxygen percent saturation	氧饱和度
SR	sustained release	缓释
$\overline{\overline{ss}}$	half	减半
SSEP	somatosensory evoked potentials	体感诱发电位
SSRI	selective serotonin reuptake inhibitor	选择性5-羟色胺再摄取抑制剂
ST	speech threshold	言语听阈
staph	staphylococcus	葡萄球菌
STAT	immediately	立即
STD	sexually transmitted disease	性传播疾病
STI	sexually transmitted infection	性传播感染
strep	streptococcus	链球菌
STSG	split-thickness skin graft	中厚皮片
supp	suppository	栓剂
susp	suspension	悬浊剂
SVD	spontaneous vaginal delivery	自然阴道分娩
SVT	supraventricular tachycardia	室上性心动过速
T	temperature; thoracic vertebra	体温；胸椎
T1DM	type 1 diabetes mellitus	Ⅰ型糖尿病
T2DM	type 2 diabetes mellitus	Ⅱ型糖尿病
T$_3$	triiodothyronine	三碘甲状腺氨酸
T$_4$	thyroxine; tetraiodothyronine	甲状腺素；四碘甲状腺原氨酸
T$_7$	free thyroxine index	游离甲状腺素指数
T&A	tonsils and adenoids, tonsillectomy and adenoidectomy	扁桃体和腺样体 扁桃体切除术和腺样体切除术
tab	tablet	片剂
TAH	total abdominal hysterectomy	经腹全子宫切除术

缩略语及其含义

Abbreviation 缩略语	Meaning 含义	含义（中文）
TB	tuberculosis	结核病
TBG	thyroxine-binding globulin	甲状腺素结合球蛋白
TBI	traumatic brain injury; thrombolytic brain infarction	创伤性脑损伤；脑梗死溶栓
^{99m}Tc	technetium-99m	锝-99m
TCA	tricyclic antidepressant	三环抗抑郁药
TEE	transesophageal echocardiography	经食管超声心动描记术
TGV	thoracic gas volume	胸腔气体容量
THA	total hip arthroplasty	全髋关节成形术
THP	total hip precautions	全髋关节预防措施
THR	total hip replacement	全髋关节置换术
TIA	transient ischemic attack	短暂性脑缺血发作
tid, t.i.d.	three times per day	每日3次
tinct	tincture	酊剂
TKA	total knee arthroplasty	全膝关节成形术
TKO	to keep open	保持畅通
TLC	total lung capacity	肺总量
Tm	maximal transport capacity; tubul	最大输送能力；小管
TM	tympanic membrane	鼓膜
Tn	troponin	肌钙蛋白
TNM	(primary) tumor, (regional lymph) nodes, (distant) metastases	（原发性）肿瘤、（区域淋巴）节、（远距离）扩散
TMJ	temporomandibular joint	颞下颌关节
tPA	tissue plasminogen activator	组织纤溶酶原激活物
TPN	total parenteral nutrition	全肠道外营养
TPR	temperature, pulse, respiration	体温、脉搏、呼吸
TPUR	transperineal urethral resection	经会阴尿道切除术
TSE	testicular self examination	睾丸自检

缩略语及其含义

Abbreviation 缩略语	Meaning 含义	含义（中文）
TSH	thyroid-stimulating hormone	促甲状腺激素
TSS	toxic shock syndrome	中毒性休克综合征
T(C)T	thrombin (clotting) time	凝血酶（凝血）时间
TTP	thrombotic thrombocytopenic purpura	血栓性血小板减少性紫癜
TTS	temporary threshold shift	暂时性阈移
TUIP	transurethral incision of prostate	经尿道前列腺切开术
TURP	transurethral resection of prostate	经尿道前列腺切除术
TV	tidal volume	潮气量
Tx	traction	牵引
U	units	单位
UA	urinalysis	尿液分析
UC	uterine contractions	子宫收缩
UFE	uterine fibroid embolization	子宫肌瘤栓塞术
UG	urogenital	泌尿生殖的
UGI	upper gastrointestinal	上消化道
UMN	upper motor neuron	上运动神经元
ung	ointment	膏剂
URI	upper respiratory infection	上呼吸道感染
USP	United States Pharmacopeia	《美国药典》
UTI	urinary tract infection	尿路感染
UTP	uterine term pregnancy	子宫妊娠
UV	ultraviolet	紫外线
UVA	ultraviolet A	长波紫外线
UVB	ultraviolet B	中波紫外线
VA	visual acuity	视敏度
VAC	vacuum-assisted closure	封闭式负压引流
VAD	ventricular assist device	心室辅助装置

缩略语及其含义

Abbreviation 缩略语	Meaning 含义	含义（中文）
VBAC	vaginal birth after cesarean section	剖宫产后阴道分娩
VC	vital capacity	肺活量
VD	venereal disease	性病
VDRL	Venereal Disease Research Laboratory	性病研究实验室
VEP	visual evoked potentials	视觉诱发电位
VF	ventricular fibrillation; visual field	心室纤颤；视野
v fib	ventricular fibrillation	心室纤颤
VLDL	very low density lipoprotein	极低密度脂蛋白
VPC	ventricular premature complex	室性期前收缩复合波
VRSA	vancomycin-resistant Staphylococcus aureus	耐万古霉素金黄色葡萄球菌
VS	vital signs	生命体征
VSD	ventricular septal defect	室间隔缺损
VT	ventricular tachycardia	室性心动过速
VTE	venous thromboembolism	静脉血栓栓塞
VTG	thoracic gas volume	胸腔气体容量
vWF	von Willebrand factor	血管假性血友病因子
WBC	white blood cell; white blood (cell) count	白细胞；白细胞计数
WD	well developed	发育良好
WNL	within normal limits	在正常范围内
w/o	without	没有
WPW	Wolff–Parkinson–White syndrome	预激综合征
x	times	次数
XT	exotropia	外斜视
YO, y/o	years old, year-old	岁
ZIFT	zygote intrafallopian transfer	受精卵输卵管内移植

附录 3

单词组成及其含义

单词组成部分	含义	单词组成部分	含义
a-	not, without, lack of, absence	ante-	before
ab-	away from	anti-	against
abdomin/o	abdomen	aort/o	aorta
-ac	pertaining to	-ar	pertaining to
acous, acus	sound, hearing	arter/o, arteri/o	artery
acro-	extremity, end	arteriol/o	arteriole
ad-	toward, near	arthr/o	joint
aden/o	gland	-ary	pertaining to
adip/o	fat	-ase	enzyme
adren/o	adrenal gland, epinephrine	atel/o	imperfect
adrenal/o	adrenal gland	atlant/o	atlas
adrenocortic/o	adrenal cortex	atri/o	atrium
aer/o	air, gas	audi/o	hearing
-agogue	promoter, stimulator	auto-	self
-al	pertaining to	azot/o	nitrogenous compounds
alg/o, algi/o, algesi/o	pain	bacill/i, bacill/o	bacillus
-algesia	pain	bacteri/o	bacterium
-algia	pain	balan/o	glans penis
ambly-	dim	bar/o	pressure
amnio	amnion	bi-	two, twice
amyl/o	starch	bili	bile
an-	not, without, lack of, absence	bio	life
andr/o	male	blast/o, -blast	immature cell, productive cell, embryonic cell
angi/o	vessel	blephar/o	eyelid
an/o	anus	brachi/o	arm

单词组成及其含义

单词组成部分	含义	单词组成部分	含义
brachy-	short	chron/o	time
brady-	slow	circum-	around
bronch/o, bronch/I	bronchus	clasis, -clasia	breaking
bronchiol	bronchiole	clitor/o, clitorid/o	clitoris
bucc/o	cheek	coccy, coccyg/o	coccyx
burs/o	bursa	cochle/o	cochlea (of inner ear)
calc/i	calcium	col/o, colon/o	colon
cali/o, calic/o	calyx	colp/o	vagina
-capnia	carbon dioxide (level of)	contra-	against, opposite, opposed
carcin/o	cancer, carcinoma	copro	feces
cardi/o	heart	cor/o, cor/e	pupil
cec/o	cecum	corne/o	cornea
-cele	hernia, localized dilation	cortic/o	outer portion, cerebral cortex
celi/o	abdomen	cost/o	rib
centesis	puncture, tap	counter-	against, opposite, opposed
cephal/o	head	crani/o	skull, cranium
cerebell/o	cerebellum	cry/o	cold
cerebr/o	cerebrum	crypt/o	hidden
cervic/o	neck, cervix	cus	sound, hearing
chem/o	chemical	cyan/o-	blue
cheil/o	lip	cycl/o	ciliary body, ciliary muscle (of eye)
chir/o	hand		
chol/e, chol/o	bile, gall	cyst/o	filled sac or pouch, cyst, bladder, urinary bladder
cholecyst/o	gallbladder	-cyte, cyt/o	cell
choledoch/o	common bile duct	dacry/o	tear, lacrimal apparatus
chondr/o	cartilage	dacryocyst/o	lacrimal sac
chori/o, choroid/o	choroid	dactyl/o	finger, toe
chrom/o, chromat/o	color, stain	de-	down, without, removal, loss

单词组成及其含义

单词组成部分	含义	单词组成部分	含义
dent/o, dent/i	tooth, teeth	equi-	equal, same
derm/o, dermat/o	skin	erg/o	work
-desis	binding, fusion	erythr/o-	red, red blood cell
dextr/o-	right	erythrocyt/o	red blood cell
di-	two, twice	esophag/o	esophagus
dia-	through	-esthesia, -esthesi/o	sensation
dilation, dilatation	expansion, widening	eu-	true, good, easy, normal
dipl/o-	double	ex/o-	away from, outside
dis-	absence, removal, separation	extra-	outside
duoden/o	duodenum	fasci/o	fascia
dynam/o	force, energy	fer	to carry
dys-	abnormal, painful, difficult	ferr/i, ferr/o	iron
ec-	out, outside	fet/o	fetus
ectasia, ectasis	dilation, dilatation, distention	fibr/o	fiber
ecto-	out, outside	-form	like, resembling
-ectomy	excision, surgical removal	galact/o	milk
edema	accumulation of fluid, swelling	gangli/o, ganglion/o	ganglion
electr/o	electricity	gastr/o	stomach
embry/o	embryo	gen, genesis	origin, formation
emesis	vomiting	ger/e, ger/o	old age
-emia	condition of blood	-geusia	sense of taste
encephal/o	brain	gingiv/o	gum, gingiva
end/o-	in, within	gli/o	neuroglia
endocrin/o	endocrine	glomerul/o	glomerulus
enter/o	intestine	gloss/o	tongue
epi-	on, over	gluc/o	glucose
epididym/o	epididymis	glyc/o	sugar, glucose
episi/o	vulva	gnath/o	jaw

单词组成及其含义

单词组成部分	含义	单词组成部分	含义
goni/o	angle	-ical	pertaining to
-gram	record of data	-ics	medical specialty
-graph	instrument for recording data	-ile	pertaining to
-graphy	act of recording data	ile/o	ileum
gravida	pregnant woman	ili/o	ilium
gyn/o, gynec/o	woman	im-	not
hem/o, hemat/o	blood	immun/o	immunity, immune system
hemi-	half, one side	in-	not
-hemia	condition of blood	infra-	below
hepat/o	liver	in/o	fiber, muscle fiber
hetero-	other, different, unequal	insul/o	pancreatic islets
hidr/o	sweat, perspiration	inter-	between
hist/o, histi/o	tissue	intra-	in, within
homo-, homeo-	same, unchanging	ir, irit/o, irid/o	iris
hydr/o	water, fluid	-ism	condition of
hyper-	over, excess, increased, abnormally high	iso-	equal, same
		-ist	specialist
hypn/o	sleep	-itis	inflammation
hypo-	under, below, decreased, abnormally low	jejun/o	jejunum
		juxta-	near, beside
hypophysi/o	pituitary, hypophysis	kali	potassium
hyster/o	uterus	kary/o	nucleus
-ia	condition of	kerat/o	cornea, keratin, horny layer of skin
-ian	specialist		
-ia/sis	condition of	kin/o, kine, kinesi/o, kinet/o	movement
-iatrics	medical specialty		
-iatr/o	physician	labi/o	lip
-iatry	medical specialty	labyrinth/o	labyrinth (inner ear)
-ic	pertaining to	lacrim/o	tear, lacrimal apparatus

单词组成及其含义

单词组成部分	含义	单词组成部分	含义
lact/o	milk	mast/o	breast, mammary gland
-lalia	speech, babble	medull/o	inner part, medulla oblongata, spinal cord
lapar/o	abdominal wall		
laryng/o	larynx	mega-, megal/o	large, abnormally large
lent/i	lens	-megaly	enlargement
-lepsy	seizure	melan/o-	black, dark, melanin
leuk/o-	white, colorless, white blood cell	mening/o, meninge/o	meninges
		men/o, mens	month, menstruation
leukocyt/o	white blood cell	mes/o-	middle
-lexia	reading	met/a	change, after, beyond
lingu/o	tongue	-meter	instrument for measuring
lip/o	fat, lipid	metr/o	measure
-listhesis	slipping	metr/o, metr/i	uterus
lith	calculus, stone	-metry	measurement of
-logy	study of	micro-	small, one millionth
lumb/o	lumbar region, lower back	-mimetic	mimicking, simulating
lymphaden/o	lymph node	mon/o-	one
lymphangi/o	lymphatic vessel	morph/o	form, structure
lymph/o	lymph, lymphatic system, lymphocyte	muc/o	mucus, mucous membrane
		multi-	many
lymphocyt/o	lymphocyte	muscul/o	muscle
-lysis	separation, loosening, dissolving, destruction	myc/o	fungus, mold
-lytic	dissolving, reducing, loosening	myel/o	bone marrow, spinal cord
macro-	large, abnormally large	my/o	muscle
mal-	bad, poor	myring/o	tympanic membrane
malacia	softening	myx/o	mucus
mamm/o	breast, mammary gland	narc/o	stupor, unconsciousness
-mania	excited state, obsession	nas/o	nose

单词组成及其含义

单词组成部分	含义	单词组成部分	含义
nat/i	birth	ortho-	straight, correct, upright
natri	sodium	-ory	pertaining to
necrosis	death of tissue	osche/o	scrotum
neo-	new	-ose	sugar
nephr/o	kidney	-o/sis	condition of
neur/o, neur/i	nervous system, nerve	osm/o	smell
noct/i	night	-osmia	sense of smell
non-	not	oste/o	bone
normo-	normal	ot/o	ear
nucle/o	nucleus	-ous	pertaining to
nulli-	never	ovari/o	ovary
nyct/o	night, darkness	ov/o, ovul/o	ovum
ocul/o	eye	-oxia	oxygen (level of)
odont/o	tooth, teeth	ox/y	oxygen, sharp, acute
-odynia	pain	pachy-	thick
-oid	like, resembling	palat/o	palate
olig/o-	few, scanty, deficiency of	palpebr/o	eyelid
-oma	tumor	pan-	all
onc/o	tumor	pancreat/o	pancreas
onych/o	nail	papill/o	nipple
oo	ovum	para-	near, beside, abnormal
oophor/o	ovary	para	woman who has given birth
ophthalm/o	eye	parathyr/o, parathyroid/o	parathyroid
-opia	condition of the eye, vision	-paresis	partial paralysis, weakness
-opsia	condition of vision	path/o, -pathy	disease, any disease of
opt/o	eye, vision	ped/o	foot, child
orchid/o, orchi/o	testis	pelvi/o	pelvis
or/o	mouth		

单词组成及其含义

单词组成部分	含义	单词组成部分	含义
-penia	decrease in, deficiency of	pneumon/o	lung
per-	through	pod/o	foot
peri-	around	-poiesis	formation, production
perine/o	perineum	poikilo-	varied, irregular
periton, peritone/o	peritoneum	poly-	many, much
-pexy	surgical fixation	post-	after, behind
phac/o, phak/o	lens	pre-	before, in front of
phag/o	eat, ingest	presby-	old
pharm, pharmac/o	drug, medicine	prim/i-	first
pharyng/o	pharynx	pro-	before, in front of
-phasia	speech	proct/o	rectum
phil, -philic	attracting, absorbing	prostat/o	prostate
phleb/o	vein	prote/o	protein
-phobia	fear	pseudo-	false
phon/o	sound, voice	psych/o	mind
-phonia	voice	ptosis	dropping, downward displacement, prolapse
phot/o	light	ptysis	spitting
phren/o	diaphragm	puer	child
phrenic/o	phrenic nerve	pulm/o, pulmon/o	lung
phyt/o	plant	pupill/o	pupil
pituitar/i	pituitary, hypophysis	pyel/o	renal pelvis
plas, -plasia	formation, molding, development	pylor/o	pylorus
-plasty	plastic repair, plastic surgery, reconstruction	py/o	pus
-plegia	paralysis	pyr/o, pyret/o	fever, fire
pleur/o	pleura	quadr/i-	four
-pnea	breathing	rachi/o	spine
pneum/o, pneumat/o	air, gas, lung, respiration	radicul/o	root of spinal nerve

单词组成及其含义

单词组成部分	含义	单词组成部分	含义
radi/o	radiation, X-ray	sider/o	iron
re-	again, back	sigmoid/o	sigmoid colon
rect/o	rectum	sinistr/o	left
ren/o	kidney	-sis	condition of
reticul/o	network	skelet/o	skeleton
retin/o	retina	somat/o	body
retro-	behind, backward	-some	body, small body
rhabd/o	rod, muscle cell	somn/i, somn/o	sleep
-rhage, -rhagia	bursting forth, profuse flow, hemorrhage	son/o	sound, ultrasound
		spasm	sudden contraction, cramp
-rhaphy	surgical repair, suture	sperm/i	semen, spermatozoa
-rhea	flow, discharge	spermat/o	semen, spermatozoa
-rhexis	rupture	-spermia	condition of semen
rhin/o	nose	sphygm/o	pulse
sacchar/o	sugar	spir/o	breathing
sacr/o	sacrum	splen/o	spleen
salping/o	tube, uterine tube, auditory (eustachian) tube	spondyl/o	vertebra
		staped/o, stapedi/o	stapes
-schisis	fissure, splitting	staphyl/o	grape-like cluster, Staphylococcus
scler/o	hard, sclera (of eye)		
sclerosis	hardening	stasis	suppression, stoppage
-scope	instrument for viewing or examining	steat/o	fatty
		stenosis	narrowing, constriction
-scopy	examination of	steth/o	chest
seb/o	sebum, sebaceous gland	sthen/o	strength
semi-	half, partial	stoma, stomat/o	mouth
semin	semen	-stomy	surgical creation of an opening
sept/o	septum, dividing wall, partition	strept/o-	twisted chain, Streptococcus
sial/o	saliva, salivary gland, salivary duct		

单词组成及其含义

单词组成部分	含义	单词组成部分	含义
sub-	below, under	trans-	through
super-	above, excess	tri-	three
supra-	above	trich/o	hair
syn-, sym-	together	-tripsy	crushing
synov/i	synovial joint, synovial membrane	trop/o	turning
tachy-	rapid	trop, -tropic	act(ing) on, affect(ing)
tax/o	order, arrangement	troph/o, -trophy, -trophia	feeding, growth, nourishment
tel/e-, tel/o-	end, far, at a distance	tympan/o	tympanic cavity (middle ear), tympanic membrane
ten/o, tendin/o	tendon	un-	not
terat/o	malformed fetus	uni-	one
test/o	testis, testicle	-uresis	urination
tetra-	four	ureter/o	ureter
thalam/o	thalamus	urethr/o	urethra
therm/o	heat, temperature	-uria	condition of urine, urination
thorac/o	chest, thorax	ur/o	urine, urinary tract
thromb/o	blood clot	urin/o	urine
thrombocyt/o	platelet, thrombocyte	uter/o	uterus
thym/o	thymus gland	uve/o	uvea (of eye)
thyr/o, thyroid/o	thyroid	uvul/o	uvula
toc/o	labor	vagin/o	sheath, vagina
-tome	instrument for incising (cutting)	valv/o, valvul/o	valve
-tomy	incision, cutting	varic/o	twisted and swollen vein, varix
ton/o	tone	vascul/o	vessel
tonsil/o	tonsil	vas/o	vessel, duct, vas deferens
tox/o, toxic/o	poison, toxin	ven/o, ven/i	vein
toxin	poison	ventricul/o	cavity, ventricle
trache/o	trachea	vertebr/o	vertebra, spinal column

缩略语单词组成

单词组成部分	含义	单词组成部分	含义
vesic/o	urinary bladder	xanth/o-	yellow
vesicul/o	seminal vesicle	xen/o	foreign, strange
vestibul/o	vestibule, vestibular apparatus (of ear)	xer/o-	dry
vir/o	virus	-y	condition of
vulv/o	vulva		

附录 4

含义及其对应的单词组成部分

含义	单词组成部分	含义	单词组成部分
abdomen	abdomin/o, celi/o	anus	an/o
abdominal wall	lapar/o	any disease of	-pathy
abnormal	dys-, para-	aorta	aort/o
abnormally high	hyper-	arm	brachi/o
abnormally large	macro-, mega-, megal/o-	around	circum-, peri-
abnormally low	hypo-	arrangement	tax/o
above	super-, supra-	arteriole	arteriol/o
absence	a-, an-, dis-	artery	arter/o, arteri/o
absorb(ing)	phil, -philic	at a distance	tel/e, tel/o
accumulation of fluid	edema	atlas	atlant/o
act of recording data	-graphy	atrium	atri/o
act(ing) on	trop, -tropic	attract(ing)	phil, -philic
acute	ox/y	auditory (eustachian) tube	salping/o
adrenal gland	adren/o, adrenal/o	away from	ab-, ex/o-
adrenaline	adren/o	babble	-lalia
adrenal	adren/o	bacillus	bacill/i, bacill/o
adrenal cortex	adrenocortic/o	back	re-
affect(ing)	trop, -tropic	backward	retro-
after	post-, met/a	bacterium	bacteri/o
again	re-	bad	mal-
against	anti-, contra-, counter-	before	ante-, pre-, pro-
air	aer/o, pneumat/o	behind	post-, retro-
all	pan-	below	hypo-, infra-, sub-
amnion, amniotic sac	amnio	beside	para-, juxta-
angle	goni/o	between	inter-

含义及其对应的单词组成部分

含义	单词组成部分	含义	单词组成部分
beyond	met/a	carcinoma	carcin/o
bile	bili, chol/e, chol/o	carry	fer
bile duct	cholangi/o	cartilage	chondr/o
binding	-desis	cavity	ventricul/o
birth	nat/i	cecum	cec/o
black	melan/o-	cell	-cyte, cyt/o
bladder	cyst/o	cerebellum	cerebell/o
bladder (urinary)	cyst/o, vesic/o	cerebral cortex	cortic/o
blood	hem/o, hemat/o	cerebrum	cerebr/o
blood (condition of)	-emia, -hemia	cervix	cervic/o
blood clot	thromb/o	chain (twisted)	strept/o
blue	cyan/o-	change	met/a
body	somat/o, -some	cheek	bucc/o
bone	oste/o	chemical	chem/o
bone marrow	myel/o	chest	thorac/o, steth/o
brain	encephal/o	child	ped/o, puer
breaking	-clasis, -clasia	choroid	chori/o, choroid/o
breast	mamm/o, mast/o	ciliary body	cycl/o
breathing	-pnea, spir/o	ciliary muscle	cycl/o
bronchiole	bronchiol	clitoris	clitor/o, clitorid/o
bronchus	bronch/i, bronch/o	clot	thromb/o
bursa	burs/o	coccyx	coccy, coccyg/o
bursting forth	-rhage, -rhagia	cochlea	cochle/o
calcium	calc/i	cold	cry/o
calculus	lith	colon	col/o, colon/o
calyx	cali/o, calic/o	color	chrom/o, chromat/o
cancer	carcin/o	colorless	leuk/o-
carbon dioxide	-capnia	common bile duct	choledoch/o

含义及其对应的单词组成部分

含义	单词组成部分	含义	单词组成部分
condition of	-ia, -ia/sis, -ism, -o/sis, -sis, -y	dilatation, dilation	ectasia, ectasis
condition of blood	-emia, -hemia	distention	ectasia, ectasis
condition of the eye	-opia	dim	ambly-
condition of urine, urination	-uria	discharge	-rhea
condition of vision	-opia, -opsia	disease	path/o, -pathy
condition of semen	-spermia	dissolving	lysis, -lytic
constriction	stenosis	distance (at a)	tel/e, tel/o
contraction (sudden)	spasm	distention	ectasia, ectasis
cornea	corne/o, kerat/o	double	dipl/o-
correct	ortho-	down	de-
cramp	spasm	dropping, downward displacement	ptosis
cranium	crani/o	drug	pharm, pharmac/o
crushing	-tripsy	dry	xer/o-
cutting	-tomy	duct	vas/o
cutting instrument	-tome	ductus deferens	vas/o
cyst	cyst/o	duodenum	duoden/o
dark	melan/o-	ear	ot/o
darkness	nyct/o	easy	eu-
data	-gram	eat	phag/o
death of tissue	necrosis	egg cell	oo, ov/o, ovul/o
decreased, decrease in	hypo-, -penia	electricity	electr/o
deficiency of	oligo-, -penia	embryo	embry/o
destruction	lysis	embryonic cell	-blast, blast/o
development	plas, -plasia	end	tel/e, tel/o, acro
diaphragm	phren/o	endocrine	endocrin/o
different	hetero-	energy	dynam/o
difficult	dys-	enlargement	-megaly, megal/o

含义及其对应的单词组成部分

含义	单词组成部分
enzyme	-ase
epididymis	epididym/o
epinephrine	adren/o
equal	iso-, equi-
erythrocyte	erythr/o, erythrocyt/o
esophagus	esophag/o
Eustachian (auditory) tube	salping/o
examination of	-scopy
excess	hyper-, super-
excision	-ectomy
excited state	mania
expansion	dilation, dilatation, ectasia, ectasis
extremity	acro
eye	ocul/o, ophthalm/o, opt/o, -opia
eyelid	blephar/o, palpebr/o
fallopian tube	salping/o
false	pseudo-
far	tel/e, tel/o
fascia	fasci/o
fat	adip/o, lip/o
fatty	steat/o
fear	-phobia
feces	copro
feeding	troph/o, -trophy, -trophia
fetus	fet/o
fetus (malformed)	terat/o

含义	单词组成部分
fever	pyr/o, pyret/o
few	oligo-
fiber	fibr/o, in/o
filled sac or pouch	cyst/o
finger	dactyl/o
fire	pyr/o, pyret/o
first	prim/i-
fissure	-schisis
fixation (surgical)	-pexy
flow	-rhea
fluid	hydr/o
foot	ped/o, pod/o
foreign	xen/o
form	morph/o
formation	gen, genesis, plas, -plasia, -poiesis
force	dynam/o
four	quadr/i, tetra-
fungus	myc/o
fusion	-desis
gall	chol/e, chol/o
gallbladder	cholecyst/o
ganglion	gangli/o, ganglion/o
gas	aer/o, pneum/o, pneumon/o, pneumat/o
gingiva (gum)	gingiv/o
gland	aden/o
glans penis	balan/o
glomerulus	glomerul/o

含义及其对应的单词组成部分

含义	单词组成部分	含义	单词组成部分
glucose	gluc/o, glyc/o	incision of	-tomy
good	eu-	increased	hyper-
grape-like cluster	staphyl/o	inflammation	-itis
growth	troph/o, -trophy, -trophia	ingest	phag/o
gum, gingiva	gingiv/o	inner ear	labyrinth/o
hair	trich/o	instrument for incising (cutting)	-tome
half	hemi-, semi-		
hand	chir/o	instrument for measuring	-meter
hard	scler/o	instrument for recording data	-graph
hardening	sclerosis		
head	cephal/o	instrument for viewing or examining	-scope
hearing	acous, acus, audi/o, cus	intestine	enter/o
heart	cardi/o	iris	ir, irid/o, irit/o
heat	therm/o	iron	ferr/i, ferr/o, sider/o
hemorrhage	-rhage, -rhagia	irregular	poikilo-
hernia	-cele	jaw	gnath/o
hidden	crypt/o	jejunum	jejun/o
horny layer of skin	kerat/o	joint	arthr/o
hypophysis	hypophysi/o, pituitar/i	keratin	kerat/o
islets (pancreatic)	insul/o	kidney	nephr/o, ren/o
ileum	ile/o	labor	toc/o
ilium	ili/o	labyrinth	labyrinth/o
immature cell	blast/o, -blast	lack of	a-, an-
immune system	immun/o	lacrimal apparatus	dacry/o, lacrim/o
immunity	immun/o	lacrimal sac	dacryocyst/o
imperfect	atel/o	large	macro-, mega-, megal/o-
in	end/o-, intra-	larynx	laryng/o
in front of	pre-, pro-	left	sinistr/o

含义及其对应的单词组成部分

含义	单词组成部分	含义	单词组成部分
lens	lent/i, phac/o, phak/o	measurement of	-metry
leukocyte	leuk/o, leukocyt/o	medical specialty	-ics, -iatrics, iatry
level of carbon dioxide	-capnia	medicine	pharm, pharmac/o
level of oxygen	-oxia	medulla oblongata	medull/o
life	bio	melanin	melan/o
light	phot/o	meninges	mening/o, meninge/o
like	-form, -oid	menstruation	men/o, mens
lip	labi/o, cheil/o	middle	meso-
lipid	lip/o	middle ear	tympan/o
liver	hepat/o	milk	galact/o, lact/o
localized dilation	-cele	mimicking	-mimetic
loosening	lysis, -lytic	mind	psych/o
loss	de-	mold	myc/o
lumbar region, lower back	lumb/o	molding	plas, -plasia
		month	men/o, mens
lung, lungs	pneum/o, pneumat/o, pneumon/o, pulm/o, pulmon/o	mouth	or/o, stoma, stomat/o
		movement	kin/o, kine, -kinesi/o, kinet/o
lymph, lymphatic system	lymph/o	much	poly-
lymph node	lymphaden/o	mucus	muc/o, myx/o
lymphatic vessel	lymphangi/o	mucous membrane	muc/o
lymphocyte	lymph/o, lymphocyt/o	muscle	my/o, muscul/o
male	andr/o	muscle cell	rhabd/o
malformed fetus	terat/o	muscle fiber	in/o
mammary gland	mamm/o, mast/o	nail	onych/o
many	multi-, poly-	narrowing	stenosis
marrow	myel/o	near	ad-, juxta-, para-
measure	metr/o	neck	cervic/o
measuring instrument	-meter		

含义及其对应的单词组成部分

含义	单词组成部分
nerve, nervous system, nervous tissue	neur/o, neur/i
network	reticul/o
neuroglia	gli/o
never	nulli-
new	neo-
night	noct/i, nyct/o
nipple	papill/o
nitrogenous compounds	azot/o
normal	eu-, normo-
nose	nas/o, rhin/o
not	a-, an-, in-, im-, non-, un-
nourishment	troph/o, -trophy, -trophia
nucleus	kary/o, nucle/o
obsession	mania
old	presby-
old age	ger/e, ger/o
on	epi-
one	mon/o-, uni-
one side	hemi-
opening (created surgically)	-stomy
opposed	contra-, counter
opposite	contra-, counter-
order	tax/o
origin	gen, genesis
other	hetero-
out, outside	ec-, ecto-, ex/o, extra-

含义	单词组成部分
outer portion	cortic/o
ovary	ovari/o, oophor/o
over	hyper-, epi-
ovum	oo, ov/o, ovul/o
oxygen	ox/y, -oxia
pain	-algia, -odynia
pain	-algesia, alg/o, algi/o, algesi/o
painful	dys-
palate	palat/o
pancreas	pancreat/o
pancreatic islets	insul/o
paralysis	-plegia
paralysis (partial)	-paresis
parathyroid	parathyr/o, parathyroid/o
partial	semi-
partial paralysis	-paresis
partition	sept/o
pelvis	pelvi/o
perineum	perine/o
peritoneum	periton, peritone/o
perspiration	hidr/o
pertaining to	-ac, -al, -ar, -ary, -ic, -ical, -ile, -ory, -ous
pharynx	pharyng/o
phrenic nerve	phrenic/o
physician	iatr/o
pituitary	pituitar/i, hypophysi/o
plant	phyt/o

含义及其对应的单词组成部分

含义	单词组成部分	含义	单词组成部分
plastic repair, plastic surgery	-plasty	rectum	rect/o, proct/o
platelet	thrombocyt/o	red	erythr/o-
pleura	pleur/o	red blood cell	erythr/o, erythrocyt/o
poison	tox/o, toxic/o, toxin	reducing	-lytic
poor	mal-	removal	de-, dis-
potassium	kali	removal (surgical)	-ectomy
pouch (filled)	cyst/o, cyst/i	renal pelvis	pyel/o
pregnant woman	gravida	repair (plastic)	-plasty
pressure	bar/o	repair (surgical)	-rhaphy
production	-poiesis	respiration	pneum/o, pneumat/o
productive cell	blast/o, -blast	resembling	-form, -oid
profuse flow	-rhage, -rhagia	retina	retin/o
prolapse	ptosis	rib	cost/o
promotor	-agogue	right	dextr/o-
prostate	prostat/o	rod	rhabd/o
protein	prote/o	root of spinal nerve	radicul/o
pulse	sphygm/o	rupture	-rhexis
puncture	centesis	sac (filled)	cyst/o, cyst/i
pupil	pupill/o, cor/o, cor/e	sacrum	sacr/o
pus	py/o	saliva, salivary gland, salivary duct	sial/o
pylorus	pylor/o	same	equi-, homo-, homeo-, iso-
radiation	radi/o	sclera (of eye)	scler/o
rapid	tachy-	scanty	oligo-
reading	-lexia	scrotum	osche/o
reconstruction	-plasty	sebum, sebaceous gland	seb/o
record of data	-gram	seizure	-lepsy
recording data (act of)	-graphy	self	auto-

含义及其对应的单词组成部分

含义	单词组成部分	含义	单词组成部分
semen	semin, sperm/i, spermat/o	sperm, spermatozoa	sperm/i, spermat/o
semen, condition of	-spermia	spinal column	vertebr/o
seminal vesicle	vesicul/o	spinal cord	myel/o, medull/o
sensation	-esthesia, esthesi/o	spinal nerve root	radicul/o
sense of smell	-osmia	spine	rachi/o
sense of taste	-geusia	spitting	-ptysis
separation	dis-, -lysis	spleen	splen/o
septum	sept/o	splitting	-schisis
sharp	ox/y	stain	chrom/o, chromat/o
short	brachy-	stapes	staped/o, stapedi/o
sigmoid colon	sigmoid/o	staphylococcus	staphyl/o
simulating	-mimetic	starch	amyl/o
skeleton	skelet/o	stimulator	-agogue
skin	derm/o, dermat/o	stomach	gastr/o
skull	crani/o	stone	lith
sleep	hypn/o, somn/o, somn/I	stoppage	stasis
slipping	-listhesis	straight	ortho-
slow	brady-	strange	xen/o
small	micro-	strength	sthen/o
small body	-some	Streptococcus	strept/o
smell	osm/o	structure	morph/o
smell (sense of)	-osmia	study of	-logy
sodium	natri	stupor	narc/o
softening	malacia	sugar	glyc/o, racchar/o, -ose
sound	phon/o, son/o, acous, acus, cus	sudden contraction	spasm
specialist	-ian, -ist, -logist	suppression	stasis
specialty	-ics, -iatrics, -iatry	surgery (plastic)	-plasty
speech	-phasia, -lalia		

含义及其对应的单词组成部分

含义	单词组成部分	含义	单词组成部分
surgical creation of an opening	-stomy	toe	dactyl/o
surgical fixation	-pexy	together	syn-, sym-
surgical removal	-ectomy	tone	ton/o
surgical repair	-rhaphy	tongue	gloss/o, lingu/o
suture	-rhaphy	tonsil	tonsil/o
sweat	hidr/o	tooth	-dent/o, dent/i, odont/o
swelling	edema	toward	ad-
synovial fluid, joint, membrane	synov/i	toxin	tox/o, toxic/o
tap	centesis	trachea	trache/o
taste (sense of)	-geusia	true	eu-
tear	dacry/o, lacrim/o	tube	salping/o
teeth	dent/o, dent/i, odont/o	tumor	onc/o, -oma
temperature	therm/o	turning	trop/o
tendon	ten/o, tendin/o	twice	bi-, di-
testicle	test/o	twisted chain	strept/o
testis	test/o, orchid/o, orchi/o	twisted and swollen vein	varic/o
thalamus	thalam/o	two	bi-, di-, dipl/o-
thick	pachy-	tympanic cavity	tympan/o
thorax	thorac/o	tympanic membrane	myring/o, tympan/o
three	tri-	ultrasound	son/o
thrombocyte	thrombocyt/o	unchanging	homo-, homeo-
through	dia-, per-, trans-	unconsciousness	narc/o
thymus gland	thym/o	under	hypo-, sub-
thyroid	thyr/o, thyroid/o	unequal	hetero-
time	chron/o	upright	ortho-
tissue	hist/o, histi/o	ureter	ureter/o
tissue death	necrosis	urethra	urethr/o

含义及其对应的单词组成部分

含义	单词组成部分	含义	单词组成部分
urinary bladder	cyst/o, vesic/o	virus	vir/o
urination	-uresis	vision	opt/o, -opia, -opsia
urine, urinary tract, urination	ur/o, -uria	voice	phon/o, -phonia
urine	urin/o	vomiting	emesis
uterine tube	salping/o	vulva	episi/o, vulv/o
uterus	hyster/o, metr/o, metr/i, uter/o	wall, dividing wall	sept/o
uvea	uve/o	water	hydr/o
uvula	uvul/o	weakness	paresis
vagina	colp/o, vagin/o	white	leuk/o-
valve	valv/o, valvul/o	white blood cell	leuk/o, leukocyt/o
varicose vein, varix	varic/o	widening	ectasia, ectasis, dilation, dilatation
varied	poikilo-	within	end/o-, intra-
vas deferens	vas/o	without	a-, an-, de-
vein	ven/o, ven/i, phleb/o	woman	gyn/o, gynec/o
vein (twisted, swollen)	varic/o	woman who has given birth	para
ventricle	ventricul/o	work	erg/o
vertebra	spondyl/o, vertebr/o	X-ray	radi/o
vessel	angi/o, vas/o, vascul/o	yellow	xanth/o-
vestibular apparatus, vestibule	vestibul/o		

附录 5

词根

词根	含义	词根	含义
abdomin/o	abdomen	bacteri/o	bacterium
acous, acus	sound, hearing	balan/o	glans penis
acro	extremity, end	bar/o	pressure
aden/o	gland	bili	bile
adip/o	fat	bio	life
adren/o	adrenal gland, epinephrine	blast/o	immature cell, productive cell, embryonic cell
adrenal/o	adrenal gland	blephar/o	eyelid
adrenocortic/o	adrenal cortex	brachi/o	arm
aer/o	air, gas	bronch/i, bronch/o	bronchus
alg/o, algi/o, algesi/o	pain	bronchiol	bronchiole
amnio	amnion	bucc/o	cheek
amyl/o	starch	burs/o	bursa
andr/o	male	calc/i	calcium
angi/o	vessel	cali/o, calic/o	calyx
an/o	anus	carcin/o	cancer, carcinoma
aort/o	aorta	cardi/o	heart
arter/o, arteri/o	artery	cec/o	cecum
arteriol/o	arteriole	celi/o	abdomen
arthr/o	joint	centesis	puncture, tap
atel/o	incomplete, imperfect	cephal/o	head
atlant/o	atlas	cerebell/o	cerebellum
atri/o	atrium	cerebr/o	cerebrum
audi/o	hearing	cervic/o	neck, cervix
azot/o	nitrogenous compounds	cheil/o	lip
bacill/i, bacill/o	bacillus	chem/o	chemical

词根

词根	含义	词根	含义
chir/o	hand	cyt/o	cell
cholangi/o	bile duct	dacry/o	tear, lacrimal apparatus
chol/e, chol/o	bile, gall	dacryocyst/o	lacrimal sac
cholecyst/o	gallbladder	dactyl/o	finger, toe
choledoch/o	common bile duct	dent/o, dent/i	tooth, teeth
chondr/o	cartilage	derm/o, dermat/o	skin
chori/o, choroid/o	choroid	dilation, dilatation	expansion, widening
chrom/o, chromat/o	color, stain	duoden/o	duodenum
chron/o	time	dynam/o	force, energy
clasis	breaking	ectasia, ectasis	dilation, dilatation, distention
clitor/o, clitorid/o	clitoris	edema	accumulation of fluid, swelling
coccy, coccyg/o	coccyx		
cochle/o	cochlea (of inner ear)	electr/o	electricity
col/o, colon/o	colon	embry/o	embryo
colp/o	vagina	emesis	vomiting
copro	feces	encephal/o	brain
cor/o, cor/e	pupil	endocrin/o	endocrine
corne/o	cornea	enter/o	intestine
cortic/o	outer portion, cerebral cortex	epididym/o	epididymis
cost/o	rib	episi/o	vulva
crani/o	skull, cranium	erg/o	work
cry/o	cold	erythr/o-	red, red blood cell
crypt/o	hidden	erythrocyt/o	red blood cell
cus	sound, hearing	esophag/o	esophagus
cycl/o	ciliary body, ciliary muscle (of eye)	fasci/o	fascia
		fer	carry
cyst/o	filled sac or pouch, cyst, bladder, urinary bladder	ferr/i, ferr/o	iron
		fet/o	fetus

词根

词根	含义	词根	含义
fibr/o	fiber	in/o	fiber, muscle fiber
galact/o	milk	insul/o	pancreatic islets
gangli/o, ganglion/o	ganglion	ir, irit/o, irid/o	iris
gastr/o	stomach	jejun/o	jejunum
gen	origin, formation	kali	potassium
ger/e, ger/o	old age	kary/o	nucleus
gingiv/o	gum, gingiva	kerat/o	cornea, keratin, horny layer of skin
gli/o	neuroglia		
glomerul/o	glomerulus	kin/o, kine, kinesi/o, kinet/o	movement
gloss/o	tongue	labi/o	lip
gluc/o	glucose	labyrinth/o	labyrinth (inner ear)
glyc/o	sugar, glucose	lacrim/o	tear, lacrimal apparatus
gnath/o	jaw	lact/o	milk
goni/o	angle	lapar/o	abdominal wall
gravida	pregnant woman	laryng/o	larynx
gyn/o, gynec/o	woman	lent/i	lens
hem/o, hemat/o	blood	leuk/o	white, colorless, white blood cell
hepat/o	liver		
hidr/o	sweat, perspiration	leukocyt/o	white blood cell
hist/o, histi/o	tissue	lingu/o	tongue
hydr/o	water, fluid	lip/o	fat, lipid
hypn/o	sleep	listhesis	slipping
hypophysi/o	pituitary, hypophysis	lith	calculus, stone
hyster/o	uterus	lumb/o	lumbar region, lower back
iatr/o	physician	lymphaden/o	lymph node
ile/o	ileum	lymphangi/o	lymphatic vessel
ili/o	ilium	lymph/o	lymph, lymphatic system, lymphocyte
immun/o	immunity, immune system	lymph/o, lymphocyt/o	lymphocyte

词根

词根	含义	词根	含义
lysis	separation, loosening, dissolving, destruction	nucle/o	nucleus
malacia	softening	nyct/o	night, darkness
mamm/o	breast, mammary gland	ocul/o	eye
mania	excited state, obsession	odont/o	tooth, teeth
mast/o	breast, mammary gland	onc/o	tumor
medull/o	inner part, medulla oblongata, spinal cord	onych/o	nail
melan/o	dark, black, melanin	oo	ovum
mening/o, meninge/o	meninges	oophor/o	ovary
men/o, mens	month, menstruation	ophthalm/o	eye
metr/o	measure	opt/o	eye, vision
metr/o, metr/i	uterus	orchid/o, orchi/o	testis
morph/o	form, structure	or/o	mouth
muc/o	mucus, mucous membrane	osche/o	scrotum
muscul/o	muscle	osm/o	smell
myc/o	fungus, mold	oste/o	bone
myel/o	bone marrow, spinal cord	ot/o	ear
my/o	muscle	ovari/o	ovary
myring/o	tympanic membrane	ov/o, ovul/o	ovum
myx/o	mucus	ox/y	oxygen, sharp, acute
narc/o	stupor, unconsciousness	palat/o	palate
nas/o	nose	palpebr/o	eyelid
nat/i	birth	pancreat/o	pancreas
natri	sodium	papill/o	nipple
necrosis	death of tissue	para	woman who has given birth
nephr/o	kidney	parathyr/o, parathyroid/o	parathyroid
neur/o, neur/i	nervous system, nerve	paresis	partial paralysis, weakness
noct/i	night	path/o	disease, any disease of
		ped/o	foot, child

词根

词根	含义	词根	含义
pelvi/o	pelvis	puer	child
perine/o	perineum	pulm/o, pulmon/o	lung
periton, peritone/o	peritoneum	pupill/o	pupil
phac/o, phak/o	lens	pyel/o	renal pelvis
phag/o	eat, ingest	pylor/o	pylorus
pharm, pharmac/o	drug, medicine	py/o	pus
pharyng/o	pharynx	pyr/o, pyret/o	fever, fire
phil	attracting, absorbing	rachi/o	spine
phleb/o	vein	radicul/o	root of spinal nerve
phobia	fear	radi/o	radiation, X-ray
phon/o	sound, voice	rect/o	rectum
phot/o	light	ren/o	kidney
phren/o	diaphragm	reticul/o	network
phrenic/o	phrenic nerve	retin/o	retina
phyt/o	plant	rhabd/o	rod, muscle cell
pituitar/i	pituitary, hypophysis	rhin/o	nose
plas	formation, molding, development	racchar/o	sugar
		sacr/o	sacrum
pleur/o	pleura	salping/o	tube, uterine tube, auditory (eustachian) tube
pneum/o, pneumat/o	air, gas, lung, respiration		
pneumon/o	lung	schisis	fissure
pod/o	foot	scler/o	hard, sclera (of eye)
proct/o	rectum	sclerosis	hardening
prostat/o	prostate	seb/o	sebum, sebaceous gland
prote/o	protein	semin	semen
psych/o	mind	sept/o	septum, partition, dividing wall
ptosis	dropping, downward displacement, prolapse	sial/o	saliva, salivary gland, salivary duct
ptysis	spitting		

词根

词根	含义	词根	含义
sider/o	iron	thorac/o	chest, thorax
sigmoid/o	sigmoid colon	thromb/o	blood clot
skelet/o	skeleton	thrombocyt/o	platelet, thrombocyte
somat/o	body	thym/o	thymus gland
somn/i, somn/o	sleep	thyr/o, thyroid/o	thyroid
son/o	sound, ultrasound	toc/o	labor
spasm	sudden contraction, cramp	ton/o	tone
sperm/i	semen, spermatozoa	tonsil/o	tonsil
spermat/o	semen, spermatozoa	tox/o, toxic/o	poison, toxin
sphygm/o	pulse	trache/o	trachea
spir/o	breathing	trich/o	hair
splen/o	spleen	trop/o	turning
spondyl/o	vertebra	trop	act(ing) on, affect(ing)
staped/o, stapedi/o	stapes	troph/o	feeding, growth, nourishment
stasis	suppression, stoppage		
steat/o	fatty	tympan/o	tympanic cavity (middle ear), tympanic membrane
stenosis	narrowing, constriction	ureter/o	ureter
steth/o	chest	urethr/o	urethra
sthen/o	strength	ur/o	urine, urinary tract
stoma, stomat/o	mouth	urin/o	urine
synov/i	synovial joint, synovial membrane	uter/o	uterus
		uve/o	uvea (of eye)
tax/o	order, arrangement	uvul/o	uvula
ten/o, tendin/o	tendon	vagin/o	sheath, vagina
terat/o	malformed fetus	valv/o, valvul/o	valve
test/o	testis, testicle		
thalam/o	thalamus	varic/o	twisted and swollen vein, varix
therm/o	heat, temperature	vascul/o	vessel

词根

词根	含义	词根	含义
vas/o	vessel, duct, vas deferens	vestibul/o	vestibule, vestibular apparatus (of ear)
ven/o, ven/i	vein	vir/o	virus
ventricul/o	cavity, ventricle	vulv/o	vulva
vertebr/o	vertebra, spinal column	xen/o	foreign, strange
vesic/o	urinary bladder		
vesicul/o	seminal vesicle		

附录 6

后缀

后缀	含义	后缀	含义
-ac	pertaining to	-graph	instrument for recording data
-agogue	promoter, stimulator	-graphy	act of recording data
-al	pertaining to	-hemi	half, one side
-algesia	pain	-hemia	condition of blood
-algia	pain	-ia	condition of
-ar	pertaining to	-ian	specialist
-ary	pertaining to	-ia/sis	condition of
-ase	enzyme	-iatrics	medical specialty
-blast	immature cell, productive cell, embryonic cell	-iatry	medical specialty
-capnia	carbon dioxide (level of)	-ic	pertaining to
-cele	hernia, localized dilation	-ical	pertaining to
-centesis	puncture, tap	-ics	medical specialty
-clasis, -clasia	breaking	-ile	pertaining to
-cyte	cell	-ism	condition of
-desis	binding, fusion	-ist	specialist
-dilation, -dilatation	expansion, widening	-itis	inflammation
-ectasia, -ectasis	dilation, dilatation, distention	-lalia	speech, babble
-ectomy	excision, surgical removal	-lepsy	seizure
-edema	accumulation of fluid, swelling	-lexia	reading
-emia	condition of blood	-listhesis	slipping
-esthesia, -esthesi/o	sensation	-logy	study of
-form	like, resembling	-lysis	separation, loosening, dissolving, destruction
-gen, -genesis	origin, formation	-lytic	dissolving, reducing, loosening
-geusia	sense of taste	-malacia	softening
-gram	record of data	-mania	excited state, obsession

后缀

后缀	含义	后缀	含义
-megaly	enlargement	-poiesis	formation, production
-meter	instrument for measuring	-ptosis	dropping, downward displacement, prolapse
-metry	measurement of		
-mimetic	mimicking, simulating	-rhage, -rhagia	bursting forth, profuse flow, hemorrhage
-necrosis	death of tissue	-rhaphy	surgical repair, suture
-odynia	pain	-rhea	flow, discharge
-oid	like, resembling	-rhexis	rupture
-oma	tumor	-schisis	fissure, splitting
-opia	condition of the eye, vision	-sclerosis	hardening
-opsia	condition of vision	-scope	instrument for viewing or examining
-ory	pertaining to		
-ose	sugar	-scopy	examination of
-o/sis	condition of	-sis	condition of
-osmia	sense of smell	-some	body, small body
-ous	pertaining to	-spasm	sudden contraction, cramp
-oxia	oxygen (level of)	-stasis	suppression, stoppage
-paresis	partial paralysis, weakness	-spermia	condition of semen
-pathy	disease, any disease of	-stenosis	narrowing, constriction
-penia	decrease in, deficiency of	-stomy	surgical creation of an opening
-pexy	surgical fixation	-tome	instrument for incising (cutting)
-phasia	speech	-tomy	incision, cutting
-philic	attracting, absorbing	-toxin	poison
-phobia	fear	-tripsy	crushing
-phonia	voice	-tropic	act(ing) on, affect(ing)
-plasia	formation, molding, development	-trophy, -trophia	feeding, growth, nourishment
-plasty	plastic repair, plastic surgery, reconstruction	-uresis	urination
		-uria	condition of urine, urination
-plegia	paralysis	-y	condition of
-pnea	breathing		

附录 7

前缀

前缀	含义	前缀	含义
a-	not, without, lack of, absence	ecto-	out, outside
ab-	away from	end/o-	in, within
acro-	extremity, end	epi-	on, over
ad-	toward, near	equi-	equal, same
ambly-	dim	erythr/o-	red
an-	not, without, lack of, absence	eu-	true, good, easy, normal
ante-	before	ex/o-	away from, outside
anti-	against	extra-	outside
atel/o-	incomplete	hemi-	half, one side
auto-	self	hetero-	other, different, unequal
bi-	two, twice	homo-, homeo-	same, unchanging
brachy-	short	hyper-	over, excess, increased, abnormally high
brady-	slow		
circum-	around	hypo-	under, below, decreased, abnormally low
contra-	against, opposite, opposed	im-	not
counter-	against, opposite, opposed	in-	not
cyan/o-	blue	infra-	below
de-	down, without, removal, loss	inter-	between
dextr/o-	right	intra-	in, within
di-	two, twice	iso-	equal, same
dia-	through	juxta-	near, beside
dipl/o-	double	leuk/o-	white, colorless, white blood cell
dis-	absence, removal, separation	macro-	large, abnormally large
dys-	abnormal, painful, difficult	mal-	bad, poor
ec-	out, outside	mega-, megal/o-	large, abnormally large

前缀

前缀	含义	前缀	含义
melan/o-	black, dark, melanin	pro-	before, in front of
mes/o-	middle	pseudo-	false
met/a-	change, after, beyond	quadr/i-	four
micro-	small, one millionth	re-	again, back
mon/o-	one	retro-	behind, backward
multi-	many	semi-	half, partial
neo-	new	sinistr/o-	left
non-	not	staphyl/o-	grape-like cluster, staphylococcus
normo-	normal	strept/o-	twisted chain, streptococcus
nulli-	never	sub-	below, under
olig/o-	few, scanty, deficiency of	super-	above, excess
ortho-	straight, correct, upright	supra-	above
pachy-	thick	syn-, sym-	together
pan-	all	tachy-	rapid
para-	near, beside, abnormal	tel/e-, tel/o-	end, far, at a distance
per-	through	tetra-	four
peri-	around	trans-	through
poikilo-	varied, irregular	tri-	three
poly-	many, much	un-	not
post-	after, behind	uni-	one
pre-	before, in front of	xanth/o-	yellow
presby-	old	xer/o-	dry
prim/i-	first		

附录 8

附录 8.1　公制度量

单位	缩写	公制等效	美制等效
长度单位			
kilometer 千米	km	1 000m	1.6km/mi
meter* 米	m	100cm; 1 000mm	39.4in; 1.1yards
centimeter 厘米	cm	1/100m; 0.01m	0.39in; 2.5cm/in
millimeter 毫米	mm	1/1 000m; 0.001m	0.039in; 25mm/in
micrometer 微米	mcm	1/1 000mm; 0.001mm	
重量单位			
kilogram 千克	kg	1 000g	2.2lb
gram* 克	g	1 000mg	0.035oz; 28.5g/oz
milligram 毫克	mg	1/1 000g; 0.001g	
microgram 微克	mcg	1/1 000mg; 0.001mg	
体积单位			
liter* 升	L	1 000mL	1.06qt
deciliter 分升	dL	1/10L; 0.1L	
milliliter 毫升	mL	1/1 000L; 0.001L	0.034oz; 29.4mL/oz
microliter 微升	mcL	1/1 000mL; 0.001mL	

* 基本单位

附录 8.2　公制度量

前缀	前缀含义
kilo-	1 000
deci-	1/10; 十分之一
centi-	1/100; 百分之一
milli-	1/1 000; 千分之一
micro-	1/1 000 000; 百万分之一

附录9

Stedman's Medical Dictionary At a Glance

an·ti·bod·y (an′tē-bod′e) *Avoid the jargonsitic use of the plural antibodies when the reference is to a single antibody species.* An immunoglobulin molecule produced by B-lymphoid cells that combine specifically with an immunogen or antigen. A.'s may be present naturally, their specificity is determined through gene rearrangement or somatic replacement or may be synthesized in response to stimulus provided by the introduction of an antigen; a.'s are found in the blood and body fluids, although the basic structure of the molecule consists of two light and two heavy chains, a.'s may also be found as dimers, trimers, or pentamers. After binding antigen, some a.'s may fix, complement, bind to surface receptors on immune cells, and in some cases may neutralize microorganisms, SEE ALSO immunoglobulin. SYN immune protein, protective protein, sensitizer (2).

- Usage notes appear in italics before definition
- Pronunciation
- Main entry

ANTIGEN

an·ti·gen (Ag) (an′ti-jen). Any substance that, as a result of coming in contact with appropriate cells, induces a state of sensitivity or immune responsiveness and that reacts in a demonstrable way with antibodies or immune cells of the sensitized subject in vivo or in vitro. Modern usage tends to retain the broad meaning of a., employing the terms "antigenic determinant" or "determinant group" for the particular chemical group of a molecule that confers antigenic specificity. SEE ALSO hapten, SYN immunogen. [anti-body) + G, -gen, producing.]

- Large header for entries with numerous subentries
- Indicates term is illustrated
- Subentry
- Etymologies appear in brackets

Australia a. [MIM*209800], an a. so called because first recognized in an Australian aborigine, but now known to be a subunit of the hepatitis B virus surface antigen. SYN Au a. (2), Aus a.

- Abbreviation
- Cross references in blue indicate where to find the defined / preferred term. In multi-word terms, the italicized term indicates the main entry under which the term can be found.

carcinoembryonic a. (CEA), a glycoprotein constituent of the glycocalyx of embryonic endodermal epithelium, which may be elevated in the serum of some patients with colon cancer and certain other cancers and in serum of long-term tobacco smokers.

- Main word is abbreviated in subentries

conjugated a., SYN *conjugated hapten.*

prostate-specific a. (PSA), a single-chain, 31-kD glycoprotein with 240 amino acid residues and 4 carbohydrate side-chains; a kallikrein protease produced by prostatic epithelial cells and normally found in seminal fluid and circulating blood. Elevations of serum PSA are highly organ-specific but occur in both cancer (adenocarcinoma) and benign disease (e.g., benign prostatic hyperplasia, prostatitis). A significant number of patients with organ-confined cancer have normal PSA values. SEE carcinoma of the prostate. SYN human glandular kallikrein 3.

- High profile terms (entries) with broad significance to the practice of medicine and to the world appear in blue boxes
- Cross references

KEY

♻	Combining Forms
🔲	Indicates term is illustrated, *see Illustration Index*
SYN	Synonym
Cf.	Compare
[NA]	Nomina Anatomica
[TA]	Terminologia Anatomica
★	Official alternate Terminologia Anatomica term
[MIM]	Mendelian Inheritance in Man
C.I.	*Color Index*

答案

Chapter 1
Pretest
1. c
2. a
3. d
4. a
5. c
6. b
7. a
8. c

Chapter review
1. suffix
2. combining form
3. diarrhea
4. alcohol, ethyl alcohol
5. examination of
6. cardiology
7. pertaining to
8. increase(d)
9. b
10. d
11. d
12. b
13. c
14. b
15. a
16. dis–LEK–se–ah
17. RU–mah–tizm
18. nu–MAT–ik
19. KEM–ist
20. FAR–mah–se
21. cardiac
22. hydrogen
23. ocular
24. interface
25. rheumatic
26. gastritis (gas–TRI–tis)
27. neurology (nu–ROL–o–je)
28. nephroptosis (nef–rop–TO–sis)
29. nephrology (nef–ROL–o–je)
30. neuritis (nu–RI–tis)
31. cardioptosis (kar–de–op–TO–sis)
32. difficult or painful menstruation
    a. abnormal, painful, difficult
    b. menses, menstruation
    c. flow, discharge
33. physician who specializes in study of the heart
    a. heart
    b. study of
    c. specialist in a field of study
34. inflammation of the kidney
    a. kidney
    b. inflammation
35. pertaining to the kidney and stomach
    a. kidney
    b. stomach
    c. pertaining to

Case study questions
1. c
2. d
3. a
4. b
5. anterior cruciate ligament
6. complains (complaining) of
7. over, excess, abnormally high, increased
8. as needed
9. a. excess
   b. fat
   c. condition of blood
10. a. straight
    b. foot/child
11. between

Chapter 2
Pretest
1. c
2. d
3. a
4. c
5. a
6. c

Chapter exercises
Exercise 2-1
1. –ia
2. –sis, –iasis
3. –ism
4. –y
5. –ia
6. –ism
7. –sis, –osis
8. –y
9. –sis, –esis

Exercise 2-2
1. –ist
2. –logy
3. –iatrics
4. –logy
5. –ian
6. –ist
7. anatomist
8. pediatrician
9. radiologist
10. psychologist
11. technologist; also, technician
12. obstetrician

Exercise 2-3
1. –ary
2. –al
3. –ic
4. –ous
5. –form
6. –oid
7. –al, –ical
8. –ile
9. –ic
10. –al, –ical
11. –ar
12. –ary
13. –ory
14. –ic
15. –ar

Exercise 2-4
1. patellae (pah–TEL–e)
2. phenomena (feh–NOM–eh–nah)
3. omenta (o–MEN–tah)
4. prognoses (prog–NO–seze)
5. apices (AP–ih–seze)
6. ova (O–vah)
7. spermatozoa (sper–mah–to–ZO–ah)
8. meninges (meh–NIN–jeze)
9. emboli (EM–bo–li)
10. protozoon (pro–to–ZO–on)
11. appendix (ah–PEN–diks)
12. adenoma (ad–eh–NO–mah)
13. fungus (FUN–gus)
14. pelvis (PEL–vis)
15. foramen (fo–RA–men)
16. curriculum (kur–RIK–u–lum)
17. index (IN–deks)
18. alveolus (al–VE–o–lus)

Chapter review

1. –ism
2. –ia
3. –sis, –osis
4. –y
5. –sis, –osis
6. –ia
7. –iatry
8. –ics
9. –ist
10. –ian
11. –ist
12. –ian
13. dermatologist
14. pediatrician
15. physiologist
16. gynecologist
17. –ic
18. –al
19. –ous
20. –oid
21. –ar
22. –al
23. –ic
24. –ary
25. –al
26. –oid
27. –ile
28. –al, –ical
29. –ar
30. –ory
31. gingivae (JIN–jih–ve)
32. testes (TES–teze)
33. criteria (kri–TIR–e–ah)
34. lumina (LU–mih–nah)
35. loci (LO–si)
36. ganglia (GANG–le–ah)
37. larynges (lah–RIN–jeze)
38. venae (VE–ne)
39. nuclei (NU–kle–i)
40. thrombus (THROM–bus)
41. vertebra (VER–teh–bra)
42. bacterium (bak–TE–re–um)
43. alveolus (al–VE–o–lus)
44. apex (A–peks)
45. foramen (fo–RA–men)
46. diagnosis (di–ag–NO–sis)
47. carcinoma (kar–sih–NO–mah)

Word Building

48. parasitic
49. parasitology
50. parasitism
51. parasitologist

Word Analysis

52. Specialist in care of the aged:
    a. old, old age
    b. physician
    c. pertaining to
    d. specialist
53. Lack of sensation
    a. not
    b. sensation
    c. condition of
54. pain caused by light; intolerance of light
    a. light
    b. fear
    c. condition of

Case study questions

1. c
2. b
3. b
4. c
5. a
6. (in any order)
   1. pulmonologist
   2. stylist
   3. manicurist
   4. therapist
7. (in any order)
   1. –ic: bronchoscopic, antibiotic
   2. –ory: respiratory
   3. –ile: febrile
   4. –ary: pulmonary
   5. –ical, –al: chemical

Chapter 3

Pretest

1. d
2. a
3. c
4. a
5. b
6. d
7. b
8. c

Chapter exercises

Exercise 3-1

1. uni– (b); bi– (d); tri (a); tetra– (c)
2. two
3. four
4. one
5. half
6. two
7. four
8. three
9. one
10. bi
11. multi
12. semi
13. uni–

Exercise 3-2

1. d
2. c
3. a
4. b
5. e

Exercise 3-3

1. a–; not, without, lack of, absence
2. anti–; against
3. a–; not, without (root mnem/o means "memory")
4. dis–; absence, removal, separation
5. contra–; against, opposite, opposed
6. in–; not
7. de–; down, without, removal, loss
8. non–; not
9. unconscious
10. insignificant
11. disinfect
12. unusual
13. nonspecific
14. decongestant
15. incompatible

Exercise 3-4

1. dia–; through
2. per–; through
3. ad–; toward, near
4. ab–; away from
5. dia–; through
6. trans–; through

Exercise 3-5

1. c
2. e
3. d
4. b
5. a

Exercise 3-6

1. d
2. e
3. c
4. b
5. a
6. homeo–; same, unchanging
7. equi–; equal, same

8. ortho–; straight, correct, upright
9. re–; again, back
10. eu–; true, good, easy, normal
11. neo–; new
12. mega–; large, abnormally large
13. iso–; equal, same
14. normo–; normal
15. heterogeneous (het-er-o-JE-no-us)
16. microscopic (mi-kro-SKOP-ik)

Exercise 3-7
1. e
2. a
3. b
4. c
5. d
6. pre–; before, in front of
7. post–; after, behind
8. pro–; before, in front of
9. pre–; before, in front of
10. ante–; before

Exercise 3-8
1. e
2. c
3. a
4. b
5. d
6. sym–; together
7. ex–; away from, outside
8. ecto–; out, outside
9. syn–; together
10. endo–; in, within
11. endogenous (*en-DOJ-e-nus*)
12. sinistromanual (*sin-is-tro-MAN-u-al*)
13. endoderm (*EN-do-derm*)

Chapter review
1. e
2. d
3. c
4. b
5. a
6. d
7. c
8. a
9. b
10. e
11. e
12. d
13. a
14. b
15. c
16. e
17. a
18. b
19. c
20. d
21. one
22. three
23. left
24. two
25. opposite
26. four
27. areflexic
28. hyper–; over, excess, abnormally high, increased
29. trans–; through
30. dis–; absence, removal, separation
31. post–; after
32. re–; again, back
33. ex–; away from, outside
34. ad–; toward, near
35. un–; not
36. ecto–; out, outside
37. de–; removal, without
38. semi–; half, partial
39. pre–; before, in front of
40. per–; through
41. dia–; through
42. anti–; against
43. micro–; small
44. dis–; absence, removal, separation
45. endo–; in, within
46. sym–; together
47. pro–; before, in front of
48. in–; not
49. T
50. F; one
51. T
52. F; four
53. F; right
54. F; three
55. T
56. T
57. T
58. dehumidify
59. adduct
60. impermeable
61. homogeneous
62. endotoxin
63. macroscopic
64. hypoventilation
65. presynaptic
66. aseptic
67. hypersensitivity
68. macrocyte
69. prenatal
70. equilateral

Word Building
71. microcytic
72. ectocardia
73. monocytic
74. dextrocardia
75. endocardial
76. macrocytic
77. microcardia
78. of equal dimensions
    a. equal, same
    b. measure
    c. pertaining to
79. association of two or more organisms
    a. together
    b. life
    c. condition of
80. pertaining to a single colony (clone) of cells
    a. one
    b. colony, clone
    c. pertaining to

Case study questions
1. pre–; before, in front of
2. an–; not, without, lack of, absence
3. dis–; absence, removal, separation
4. re–; again, back
5. bi–; two, twice
6. hemi–; half, one side
7. de–; down, without, removal, loss
8. anti–; against
9. erythr/o; red
10. prim/i; first
11. condition of
12. pertaining to
13. one
14. three
15. preoperative
16. postoperative
17. abduction
18. leukocyte

Chapter 4

Pretest
1. c
2. a
3. d
4. c
5. b
6. a
7. d
8. c

Chapter exercises

Exercise 4-1

1. cells
2. fiber
3. tissues
4. forms
5. nucleus
6. nucleus
7. gland
8. nipple
9. mucus
10. network
11. mucus
12. body
13. morphology (mor–FOL–o–je)
14. cytology (si–TOL–o–je)
15. histology (his–TOL–o–je)

Exercise 4-2

1. d
2. c
3. e
4. b
5. a
6. d
7. c
8. e
9. b
10. a
11. gen; origin, formation
12. phag/o; eat, ingest
13. blast; immature cell, productive cell, embryonic cell
14. plas; formation, molding, development
15. troph; feeding, growth, nourishment

Exercise 4-3

1. sugars
2. sugar
3. water
4. starch
5. lipid, fat
6. glucose
7. fat, lipid
8. steat/o; fatty
9. lip/o; lipid, fat
10. glyc/o; sugar, glucose
11. gluc/o; glucose

Chapter review

Labeling Exercise

Question. Diagram of a Typical Animal Cell

1. plasma membrane
2. nucleus
3. nuclear membrane
4. nucleolus
5. cytosol
6. smooth endoplasmic reticulum (ER)
7. rough endoplasmic reticulum (ER)
8. ribosomes
9. mitochondrion
10. Golgi apparatus
11. lysosome
12. vesicle
13. peroxisome
14. centriole
15. microvilli

Terminology

1. c
2. d
3. e
4. a
5. b
6. a
7. c
8. b
9. e
10. d
11. d
12. a
13. b
14. c
15. e
16. e
17. a
18. b
19. c
20. d
21. d
22. c
23. a
24. e
25. b
26. a
27. e
28. b
29. d
30. c
31. e
32. c
33. a
34. d
35. b
36. histology
37. epithelial, connective, muscle, and nervous tissue
38. metabolism
39. urinary system
40. lymphatic system
41. glucose
42. mucus
43. enzyme
44. cells
45. water
46. morphology
47. mucus
48. T
49. F; water
50. F; lipid, fat
51. T
52. T
53. adenoid
54. leukoblast
55. lipase
56. mucoid
57. histioblast
58. amylase
59. amyloid
60. a state of internal balance
    a. same, unchanging
    b. standing still, unchanging
    c. condition of
61. having a stimulating effect on the body
    a. body
    b. act on, affect
    c. pertaining to
62. destruction and disposal of damaged organelles in the cell
    a. self
    b. to eat
    c. condition of
63. reduced secretion of fatty material by the skin's sebaceous (oil) glands
    a. not, without, lack of, absence
    b. fatty
    c. condition of

Case study questions

1. d
2. b
3. a
4. d
5. a–; not, without, lack of, absence
6. pro–; before, in front of
7. bi–; two
8. mono–; one
9. dis–; absence, removal, separation
10. meta–; change, after, beyond
11. neutrophils, eosinophils, basophils
12. plastic, thromboplastin
13. morphologic
14. histologic
15. lymphocyte(s), monocytes, cytoplasm, lymphocytic

Chapter 5
Pretest
1. d
2. b
3. c
4. a
5. b
6. d
7. b
8. a

Chapter exercises
Exercise 5-1
1. thoracic (*tho-RAS-ik*)
2. cephalic (*se-FAL-ik*)
3. cervical (*SER-vi-kal*)
4. abdominal (*ab-DOM-ih-nal*)
5. lumbar (*LUM-bar*)
6. peritoneum
7. abdomen
8. head
9. supine
10. abdominal wall

Exercise 5-2
1. extremities (hands and feet)
2. arms
3. finger or toe
4. arm and head
5. foot

Exercise 5-3
1. circumoral
2. subscapular
3. circumvascular
4. infracostal
5. periorbital
6. infrapatellar
7. intracellular
8. suprascapular
9. extrathoracic
10. near the nose
11. behind the peritoneum
12. above the abdomen
13. within the uterus
14. around the navel (umbilicus)
15. between the buttocks
16. above the ankle
17. within the eye
18. near the sacrum

Chapter review
Labeling Exercise
Question. Directional Terms
1. superior (cranial)
2. inferior (caudal)
3. anterior (ventral)
4. posterior (dorsal)
5. medial
6. lateral
7. proximal
8. distal

Question. Planes of Division
1. frontal (coronal) plane
2. sagittal plane
3. transverse (horizontal) plane

Question. Body Cavities, Lateral View
1. dorsal cavity
2. cranial cavity
3. spinal cavity (canal)
4. ventral cavity
5. thoracic cavity
6. diaphragm
7. abdominopelvic cavity
8. abdominal cavity
9. pelvic cavity

Question. The Nine Regions of the Abdomen
1. epigastric (ep-i-GAS-trik) region
2. umbilical (um-BIL-i-kal) region
3. hypogastric (hi-po-GAS-trik) region
4. right hypochondriac (hi-po-KON-dre-ak) region
5. left hypochondriac region
6. right lumbar (LUM-bar) region
7. left lumbar region
8. right iliac (IL-e-ak) region; also inguinal (ING-gwi-nal) region
9. left iliac region; also, inguinal region

Chapter review
Terminology
1. a
2. b
3. d
4. c
5. e
6. b
7. c
8. d
9. e
10. a
11. d
12. a
13. c
14. b
15. e
16. F; dorsal
17. T
18. F; distal
19. F; frontal, coronal
20. F; superior
21. T
22. F; face-up
23. T
24. abdomen
25. finger or toe
26. back of knee
27. base of skull
28. wrist
29. neck
30. small of back
31. arm
32. instrument for viewing the peritoneal cavity through the abdominal wall
33. above the pubis
34. below the umbilicus (navel)
35. pertaining to the neck and face
36. under the tongue
37. behind the peritoneum
38. having two feet
39. dorsal
40. periocular
41. inframammary
42. anterior
43. megacephaly, macrocephaly
44. superficial
45. distal
46. suprascapular
47. intracellular
48. inferior
49. cervic/o; The root *cervic/o* refers to the neck; the others refer to the extremities.
50. cervical region; *Cervical* refers to the neck; the others are abdominal regions.
51. transverse; *Transverse* refers to a plane of division; the others are body positions.
52. spinal cavity; The *spinal cavity* is a dorsal cavity; the others are ventral cavities.
53. dactylospasm
54. infrathoracic
55. intrathoracic
56. polydactyly

57. syndactyly
58. cephalothoracic
59. adactyly
60. intracephalic
61. acephaly
62. having an average sized head; nor mocephalic
    a. middle
    b. head
    c. pertaining to
63. bluish discoloration of the hands or feet
    a. extremity
    b. blue
    c. condition of
64. pertaining to the forearm
    a. before
    b. arm
    c. pertaining to
65. pertaining to the epigastrium, the uppermost region of the abdomen
    a. on, over
    b. stomach
    c. pertaining to

Case study questions

1. b
2. b
3. d
4. c
5. a
6–15. See diagrams.

16. a
17. d
18. on back, legs flexed on abdomen, thighs apart
19. on back with head lowered by tilting the bed at a 45-degree angle
20. on the side with one leg flexed, arm position may vary

Chapter 6
Pretest

1. d
2. c
3. b
4. a
5. c
6. c
7. a
8. d

Chapter exercises
Exercise 6-1

1. toxic/o; poison
2. py/o; pus
3. lith/o; stone
4. path/o; disease
5. hardening
6. calculus, stone
7. bladder, gall bladder
8. disease

9. cancer, carcinoma
10. toxin, poison
11. pus
12. pain
13. tumor
14. fever

Exercise 6-2

1. e
2. a
3. d
4. b
5. c
6. xero–; dry
7. dys–; abnormal, painful, difficult
8. mal–; bad, poor

Exercise 6-3

1. a
2. d
3. b
4. e
5. c
6. b
7. d
8. a
9. c
10. e
11. pain in a muscle
12. any disease of muscle
13. rupture of a muscle
14. pain in a muscle
15. tumor of muscle

Exercise 6-4

1. e
2. d
3. b
4. a
5. c
6. softening of the spleen
7. dropping or prolapse of the spleen
8. substance poisonous or harmful to the spleen

Exercise 6-5

1. bacteria
2. fungus
3. bacilli
4. twisted chain
5. grapelike cluster
6. mycology (mi-KOL-o-je)
7. virology (vi-ROL-o-je)
8. bacteriology (bak-tihr-e-OL-o-je)

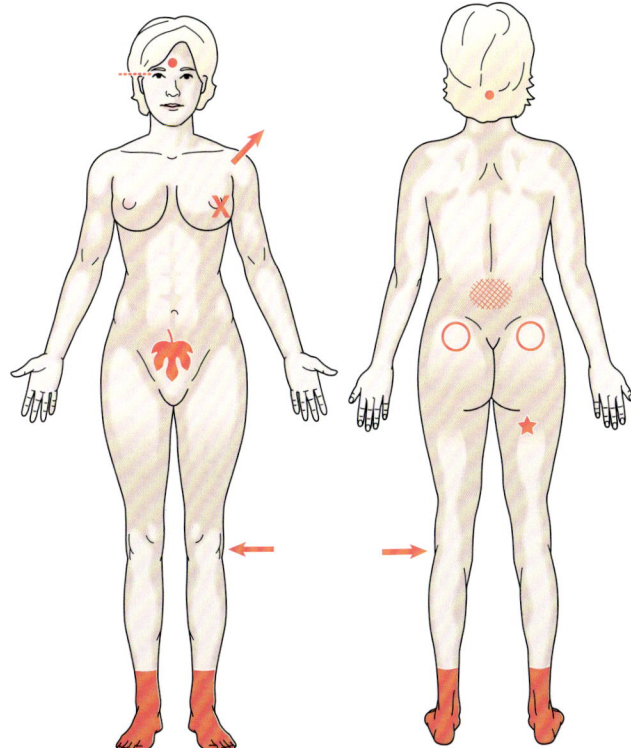

Chapter review
1. d
2. c
3. b
4. e
5. a
6. e
7. c
8. d
9. b
10. a
11. d
12. e
13. c
14. a
15. b
16. c
17. b
18. d
19. a
20. e
21. d
22. a
23. b
24. e
25. c
26. d
27. e
28. a
29. c
30. b
31. b
32. e
33. d
34. a
35. c
36. inflammation
37. neoplasm
38. metastasis
39. hernia
40. toxins; poisons
41. necrosis
42. tumor
43. –rhea; flow, discharge
44. protozoa
45. worm
46. carcinogenesis (kar-sin-o-JEN-e-sis)
47. pathogenesis (path-o-JEN-eh-sis)
48. pyogenesis (pi-o-JEN-eh-sis)
49. oncogenesis (ong-ko-JEN-eh-sis)
50. bronchorrhea (brong-ko-RE-ah)
51. bronchitis (brong-KI-tis)
52. bronchostenosis (brong-ko-steno-sis)
53. bronchospasm (BRONG-kospazm)
54. osteodynia, ostealgia (os-te-o-DIN-e-ah, os-te-AL-je-ah)
55. osteonecrosis (os-te-o-ne-KRO-sis)
56. osteoma (os-te-O-mah)
57. osteoclasis (os-te-OK-la-sis)
58. osteomalacia (os-te-o-ma-LA-she-ah)
59. F; fungus
60. T
61. F; acute
62. T
63. F; bradycardia
64. T
65. helminths; Helminths are worms; the others are types of bacteria.
66. pathogen; A pathogen is a disease-causing microorganism; the others are terms related to neoplasia.
67. metastatic; Metastatic refers to the spread of cancer; the others are terms describing infections.
68. nephrotoxic (nef-ro-TOKS-ik)
69. pyogenic (pi-o-JEN-ik)
70. nephroma (nef-RO-mah)
71. pathology (pa-THOL-o-je)
72. pyrogenic (pi-ro-JEN-ik)
73. nephrology (nef-ROL-o-je)
74. pathogenic (*path-o-JEN-ik*)
75. nephropathy (*nef-ROP-a-the*)
76. nephrogenic (*nef-ro-JEN-ik*)
77. ingestion of organisms or small particles by a cell
    a. to eat
    b. cell
    c. condition of
78. deficient growth of normal cells in normal arrangement
    a. deficient, below normal
    b. formation, molding, development
    c. condition of
79. counteracting fever
    a. against
    b. fever
    c. pertaining to
80. hardening of the arteries
    a. artery
    b. hard
    c. condition of
81. imbalance in the normal flora of microorganisms
    a. difficulty
    b. life
    c. condition of

Case study questions
1. a
2. c
3. d
4. a
5. b
6. b
7. a
8. d
9. gland
10. bacillus
11. sarcoma
12. malignant hyperpyrexia (also, hyperthermia)
13. human immunodeficiency virus
14. purified protein derivative
15. electrocardiogram
16. acid-fast bacillus

Chapter 7
Pretest
1. b
2. c
3. b
4. a
5. d
6. a

Chapter exercises
Exercise 7-1
1. a
2. c
3. d
4. e
5. b
6. son/o; sound
7. chron/o; time
8. therm/o; heat, temperature
9. erg/o; work
10. aer/o; air (oxygen)
11. chrom/o; color
12. electricity
13. light
14. cold
15. pressure
16. sound

Exercise 7-2
1. e
2. c
3. d
4. a
5. b
6. c
7. e
8. d

9. a
10. b

Exercise 7-3

1. b
2. e
3. a
4. d
5. c
6. cystotomy (sis–TOT–o–me)
7. cystopexy (SIS–to–pek–e)
8. cystoplasty (SIS–to–plas–te)
9. cystorrhaphy (sis–TOR–ah–fe)
10. cystostomy (sis–TOS–to–me)
11. arthroplasty (AR–thro–plas–te)
12. arthrotome (AR–thro–tome)
13. arthrotomy (ar–THROT–o–me)
14. arthrocentesis (ar–thro–sen–TE–sis)
15. arthrodesis (ar–THROD–eh–sis)
16. tracheotomy (tra–ke–OT–o–me)
17. gastrorrhaphy (gas–TROR–ah–fe)
18. colostomy (ko–LOS–to–me)

Chapter review

1. a
2. c
3. b
4. d
5. e
6. c
7. d
8. b
9. e
10. a
11. c
12. a
13. e
14. d
15. b
16. d
17. b
18. e
19. c
20. a
21. a
22. c
23. e
24. b
25. d
26. chrom/o; color
27. aer/o; air, gas, oxygen
28. radi/o; radiation, x-ray
29. therm/o; heat, temperature
30. chron/o; time
31. erg/o; work
32. son/o; sound
33. palpation
34. prognosis (prog–NO–sis)
35. diagnostic (di–ag–NOS–tik)
36. edematous (eh–DEM–ah–tus)
37. therapy (THER–ah–pe)
38. light
39. gastroplasty (GAS–tro–plas–te)
40. arthrodesis (ar–THROD–eh–sis)
41. colostomy (ko–LOS–to–me)
42. hepatotomy (hep-ah–TOT–o–me)
43. hepatectomy (hep-ah–TEK–to–me)
44. hepatopexy (HEP–ah–to–pek–se)
45. hepatorrhaphy (hep–ah–TOR–ah–fe)
46. F; kidney
47. F; pressure
48. F; ear
49. F; radiograph
50. T
51. T
52. remission; Remission is the lessening of disease symptoms; the others are examining methods.
53. syncope; Syncope is fainting; the others are examination instruments.
54. speculum; A speculum is an instrument for examining a canal; the others are surgical instruments.
55. TNM; TNM is an abbreviation for a system of staging cancer; the others are abbreviations for imaging techniques.
56. physician assistant
57. magnetic resonance imaging
58. history
59. range of motion
60. nonsteroidal antiinflammatory drug
61. neurotripsy (nu–ro–TRIP–se)
62. cystorrhaphy (sis–TOR–ah–fe)
63. cystopexy (SIS–to–pek–se)
64. neurorrhaphy (nu–ROR–ah–fe)
65. lithotripsy (LITH–o–trip–se)
66. cystolith (SIS–to–lith)
67. cystoscopy (sis–TOS–ko–pe)
68. neurotome (NU–ro–tome)
69. cystotome (SIS–to–tome)
70. describing cells or tissues that have equal attraction for the same dyes
    a. equal, same
    b. color
    c. attracting, absorbing
    d. pertaining to
71. occurring at the same time
    a. together
    b. time
    c. pertaining to
72. uneven, not symmetrical
    a. not
    b. together
    c. measure
    d. pertaining to
73. formation of color or pigment
    a. color
    b. origin, formation
    c. condition of

Case study questions

1. sequelae
2. auscultation
3. mesocephalic
4. paracentesis
5. biopsy
6. diagnostic laparoscopy
7. lithotomy position
8. c
9. d
10. b
11. a
12. d
13. b
14. a
15. history of present illness
16. cancer
17. temperature, pulse, respiration
18. activities of daily living
19. beats per minute
20. within normal limits
21. discontinue
22. normal saline

Chapter 8

Pretest

1. d
2. b
3. c
4. a
5. c
6. a
7. b
8. d

Chapter exercises

Exercise 8-1

1. –lytic; dissolving, reducing, loosening
2. –tropic; acting on
3. –mimetic; mimicking, simulating
4. antibacterial (an–te–bak–TERE–e–al)
5. contralateral (kon–trah–LAT–er–al)

6. antiseptic (an–te–SEP–tik)
7. counteract (COWN–ter–act)
8. antiemetic (an-te-eh-MET–ik)
9. antipyretic (an-te-pi-RET–ik)
10. narc/o; stupor
11. chem/o; chemical
12. algesi/o; pain
13. toxic/o; poison
14. hypn/o; sleep
15. dilation (widening) of a vessel
16. study of drugs
17. dissolving mucus
18. acting on the gonads (sex glands)

Chapter review

1. a
2. e
3. b
4. c
5. d
6. b
7. e
8. a
9. c
10. d
11. a
12. d
13. e
14. b
15. c
16. a
17. d
18. e
19. c
20. b
21. a
22. a
23. c
24. d
25. c
26. d
27. c
28. b
29. a
30. c
31. d
32. d
33. d
34. pharmacology
35. toxins, poisons
36. skin
37. plants, herbs
38. tolerance
39. pain
40. vein
41. fever
42. potentiation
43. adrenergic; An *adrenergic* is a sympathomimetic, which mimics the effects of the sympathetic nervous system; the others are drugs to eliminate sensation and relieve pain.
44. tablet; A *tablet* is a solid dosage form, a pill; the others are forms of liquid solutions.
45. antineoplastics; An *antineoplastic* kills cancer cells; the others are cardiac drugs.
46. histamine H2 antagonist; A *histamine H2 antagonist* reduces stomach acid secretion; the others are respiratory drugs.
47. destructive to blood cells
48. acting on the mind
49. constriction of the bronchi
50. antiemetic
51. vasoconstriction
52. counterbalance, also imbalance
53. antibacterial
54. contraindicated
55. antineoplastic
56. Food and Drug Administration
57. dispense as written
58. prescription
59. United States Pharmacopeia
60. discontinue
61. hypnosis
62. anxiolytic
63. toxicosis
64. thrombolytic
65. thrombosis
66. narcosis
67. mucolytic
68. extreme allergic reaction
    a. away from
    b. prevention
69. movement of drugs within the body as affected by biologic function
    a. drug
    b. movement
    c. pertaining to
70. activated by or secreting adrenaline (epinephrine)
    a. adrenaline; adrenal gland
    b. work
    c. pertaining to
71. administration of a solution by subcutaneous infusion
    a. under
    b. skin
    c. washing out

Case study questions

1. c
2. b
3. d
4. a
5. d
6. b
7. a
8. c
9. c
10. d
11. a
12. by mouth
13. milligram
14. nonsteroidal antiinflammatory drugs
15. microgram
16. intravenous(ly)

Chapter 9

Pretest

1. c
2. c
3. b
4. d
5. d
6. b
7. c
8. a

Chapter exercises

Exercise 9-1

1. valve
2. atrium
3. ventricles
4. heart
5. atrial (*A–tre–al*)
6. myocardial (*mi–o–KAR–de–al*)
7. cardiac (*KAR–de–ak*)
8. valvular (*VAL–vu–lar*); also valvar (*VAL–var*)
9. ventricular (*ven–TRIK–u–lar*)
10. pericardial (*per–ih–KAR–de–al*)
11. pericarditis (*per–ih–kar–DI–tis*)
12. endocarditis (*en–do–kar–DI–tis*)
13. myocarditis (*mi–o–kar–DI–tis*)
14. cardiogenic (*kar–de–o–JEN–ik*)
15. valvotomy (*val–VOT–o–me*); also, valvulotomy (*val–vu–LOT–o–me*)
16. atrioventricular (*a–tre–o–ven–TRIK–u–lar*)
17. interatrial (*in–ter–A–tre–al*)
18. cardiology (*kar–de–OL–o–je*)

Exercise 9-2

1. vessels
2. vessel
3. aorta
4. artery
5. arteriole
6. vein
7. vessels
8. rupture of an artery
9. within the aorta
10. inflammation of a vessel or vessels
11. inflammation of a vein
12. pertaining to the heart and vessels
13. angiogram
14. aortogram
15. phlebogram; venogram
16. angioplasty (AN-je-o-plas-te)
17. angiopathy (an-je-OP-ah-the)
18. angiectasis (an-je-EK-tah-sis); also, hemangiectasis (he-man-je-EK-tah-sis)
19. angiogenesis (an-je-o-JEN-eh-sis)
20. phlebectomy (fleh-BEK-to-me); venectomy (ve-NEK-to-me)
21. aortosclerosis (a-or-to-skleh-RO-sis)
22. intravenous (in-trah-VE-nus)
23. arteriotomy (ar-tere-e-OT-o-me)

Exercise 9-3

1. tonsil
2. thymus
3. lymph node
4. lymph
5. lymphatic vessels
6. spleen
7. lymphangi/o; lymphatic vessel
8. splen/o; spleen
9. lymphaden/o; lymph node
10. tonsill/o; tonsil
11. thym/o; thymus
12. splenomegaly (sple-no-MEG-ah-le)
13. tonsillitis (ton-sih-LI-tis)
14. lymphadenopathy (lim-fad-eh-NOP-ah-the)
15. lymphangitis (lim-fan-JI-tis); also, lymphangiitis (lim-fan-je-I-tis)
16. thymic (THI-mik)
17. lymphoma (lim-FO-mah)

Chapter review

Labeling Exercise

Question. The Cardiovascular System

1. right atrium
2. right ventricle
3. left pulmonary artery
4. left lung
5. right lung
6. left pulmonary vein
7. left atrium
8. left ventricle
9. aorta
10. head and arms
11. superior vena cava
12. internal organs
13. legs
14. inferior vena cava

Question. The Heart and Great Vessels

1. superior vena cava
2. inferior vena cava
3. right atrium
4. right AV (tricuspid) valve
5. right ventricle
6. pulmonary valve
7. pulmonary artery
8. right pulmonary artery (branches)
9. left pulmonary artery (branches)
10. left pulmonary veins
11. right pulmonary veins
12. left atrium
13. left AV (mitral) valve
14. left ventricle
15. aortic valve
16. ascending aorta
17. aortic arch
18. brachiocephalic artery
19. left common carotid artery
20. left subclavian artery
21. apex
22. interventricular septum
23. endocardium
24. myocardium
25. epicardium

Question. Location of Lymphoid Tissue

1. lymph nodes
2. tonsils
3. thymus
4. spleen
5. appendix
6. Peyer patches (in intestine)

Terminology

1. e
2. a
3. b
4. d
5. c
6. b
7. c
8. e
9. a
10. d
11. d
12. b
13. e
14. a
15. c
16. b
17. d
18. c
19. a
20. e
21. b
22. e
23. d
24. a
25. c
26. myocardium
27. capillary
28. atrium
29. sinoatrial (SA) node
30. aorta
31. vein
32. varicose vein, varix
33. thymus
34. right atrium
35. common iliac (IL-e-ak) arteries
36. common carotid (kah-ROT-id) artery
37. inferior vena cava
38. subclavian veins
39. Holter monitor
40. atrial fibrillation
41. ablation
42. F; mitral (bicuspid)
43. F; heart
44. F; arm
45. T
46. T
47. T
48. F; pulmonary circuit
49. F; vein
50. T
51. T
52. T
53. apex; The *apex* is the pointed lower region of the heart; the others are part of the heart's conduction system.
54. murmur; A *murmur* is an abnormal heart sound; the others are terms associated with blood pressure.
55. S^1; *S^1* symbolizes the first heart sound; the others are waves of the ECG.

56. cusp; A *cusp* is a flap of a heart valve; the others are lymphoid tissue.
57. without vessels
58. incision of an atrium
59. surgical removal of the spleen
60. above a ventricle
61. dilatation of a vein
62. valvotome; valvulotome (*VAL–vo–tome; VAL–vu–lo–tome*)
63. aortorrhaphy (*a–or–TOR–ah–fe*)
64. lymphadenectomy (*lim–fad–eh–NEK–to–me*)
65. cardiologist (*kar–de–OL–o–jist*)
66. lymphostasis (*lim–FOS–tah–sis*)
67. splenopexy (*SPLE–no–pek–se*)
68. aortostenosis (*a–or–to–steh–NO– sis*)
69. aortoptosis (*a–or–top–TO–sis*)
70. aortogram (*a–OR–to–gram*)
71. preaortic (*pre–a–OR–tik*)
72. ventricular
73. septal
74. valvular, valvar
75. thymic
76. sclerotic
77. splenic; splenetic
78. thrombi
79. varices
80. stenoses
81. septa
82. automated external defibrillator
83. left ventricular assist device
84. deep vein thrombosis
85. ventricular fibrillation
86. bundle branch block
87. percutaneous transluminal coronary angioplasty
88. phlebitis
89. lymphadenopathy
90. lymphoma
91. angioplasty
92. lymphangiitis; lymphangitis
93. angiopathy
94. lymphadenitis
95. phleboplasty
96. lymphadenoma
97. angioma
98. recording of the heart's sounds
    a. sound
    b. heart
    c. act of recording
99. excision of the inner layer of an artery thickened by atherosclerosis
    a. within
    b. artery
    c. out
    d. to cut
100. permanent dilation of small blood vessels causing small, local red lesions
    a. end
    b. vessel
    c. dilation
101. inflammation of lymphatic vessels and veins
    a. lymphatic system
    b. vessel
    c. vein
    d. inflammation

Case study questions

1. dyspnea
2. murmur
3. stress test
4. cardiovascular
5. endarterectomies
6. sublingual
7. cyanosis
8. diaphoresis
9. interatrial
10. substernal
11. d
12. b
13. c
14. d
15. a
16. c
17. a
18. electrocardiogram
19. acute myocardial infarction
20. coronary artery disease
21. left anterior descending
22. congestive heart failure
23. transesophageal echocardiogram
24. mitral valve replacement
25. coronary/cardiac care unit

Chapter 10
Pretest

1. c
2. d
3. b
4. b
5. c
6. a

Chapter exercises
Exercise 10-1

1. a decrease number of platelets in the blood
2. presence of bacteria in the blood
3. deficiency of leukocytes (white blood cells)
4. production of erythrocytes (red blood cells)
5. presence of toxins (poisons) in the blood
6. decreased protein in the blood
7. excess albumin in the blood deficiency of platelets (thrombocytes)
8. viremia (*vi–RE–me–ah*)
9. leukemia (*lu–KE–me–ah*)
10. pyemia (*pi–E–me–ah*) leukemia (*lu–KE–me–ah*)

Exercise 10-2

1. leuk/o; leukocytes; white blood cells
2. hem/o; blood
3. immun/o; immunity
4. hemat/o; blood
5. thromb/o; blood clot
6. myel/o; bone marrow
7. lymphocytes
8. blood
9. blood
10. bone marrow
11. erythrocytes; red blood cells
12. immunity
13. platelets; thrombocytes
14. leukocytes; white blood cells
15. leukopenia (*lu–ko–PE–ne–ah*)
16. myeloma (*mi–eh–LO–mah*)
17. lymphoblast (*LIM–fo–blast*)
18. thrombolysis (*throm–BOL–ih–sis*)
19. myelopoiesis (*mi–eh–lo–poy–E–sis*)
20. granulocytosis (*gran–u–lo–si–TO–sis*)
21. lymphocytosis (*lim–fo–si–TO–sis*)
22. erythrocytosis (*eh–rith–ro–si–TO–sis*)
23. monocytosis (*mon–o–si–TO–sis*)
24. thrombocytosis (*throm–bo–si–TO–sis*)

Exercise 10-3

1. iron
2. potassium
3. nitrogenous compounds
4. oxygen
5. iron
6. calcium
7. natremia (*na–TRE–me–ah*)
8. azotemia (*az–o–TE–me–ah*)
9. kalemia (*kah–LE–me–ah*)
10. calcemia (*kal–SE–me–ah*)

Chapter review labeling exercise

Question. Blood Cells

1. platelet
2. leukocyte
3. erythrocyte

Question. Leukocytes (White Blood Cells)

1. neutrophil
2. eosinophil
3. basophil
4. lymphocyte
5. monocyte

Terminology

1. c
2. d
3. e
4. b
5. a
6. b
7. c
8. e
9. a
10. d
11. d
12. c
13. a
14. b
15. e
16. e
17. d
18. b
19. c
20. a
21. b
22. c
23. a
24. e
25. d
26. phagocytosis
27. hemoglobin
28. electrolyte
29. platelets (thrombocytes)
30. blood cells
31. oxygen
32. blood
33. anemia
34. bone marrow
35. immunoglobulin
36. c
37. a
38. c
39. b
40. b
41. F; white blood cell
42. T
43. T
44. T
45. F; neutrophil
46. T
47. increase in leukocytes (white blood cells) in the blood
48. increase in eosinophils in the blood
49. increase in erythrocytes (red blood cells) in the blood
50. increase in thrombocytes (platelets) in the blood
51. increase in neutrophils in the blood
52. increase in monocytes in the blood
53. erythroblast; erythrocytoblast
54. thrombocytopenia; thrombopenia
55. pyemia
56. immunologist
57. hemorrhage
58. destruction of red blood cells
59. deficiency of neutrophils
60. substance that is toxic (poisonous) to bone marrow
61. immunity to one's own tissue
62. presence of viruses in the blood
63. hemolytic (he-mo-LIT-ik)
64. leukemic (lu-KE-mik)
65. basophilic (ba-so-FIL-ik)
66. septicemic (sep-tih-SE-mik)
67. thrombotic (throm-BOT-ik)
68. lymphocytic (lim-fo-SIT-ik)
69. thrombolysis; *Thrombolysis* is destruction of a blood clot; the others pertain to formation of a blood clot.
70. EPO; *EPO* is erythropoietin, a hormone that stimulates red cell production in the bone marrow; the others are abbreviations for blood tests.
71. reticulocyte; A *reticulocyte* is an immature red blood cell; the others are types of leukocytes.
72. gamma globulin; Gamma globulin is the fraction of the blood plasma that contains antibodies; the others are terms associated with exaggerated immune responses.
73. erythrocytic
74. leukoblast
75. myeloid
76. myelogenic
77. myeloblast
78. leukemia
79. leukopenia; leukocytopenia
80. myeloma
81. erythropoiesis; erythrocytopoiesis
82. myelocytic
83. overall decrease in blood cells
    a. all
    b. cell
    c. deficiency
84. increase in the number of red cells in the blood; erythremia, erythrocythemia
    a. many
    b. cell
    c. blood
    d. condition of
85. unequal distribution of hemoglobin in red cells
    a. without
    b. same, equal
    c. color
    d. condition of
86. pertaining to dysfunctional bone marrow
    a. bone marrow
    b. abnormal
    c. formation
    d. condition of

Case study questions

1. d
2. d
3. c
4. a
5. c
6. d
7. b
8. b
9. c
10. d
11. d
12. b
13. a
14. prothrombin time
15. partial thromboplastin time
16. fresh frozen plasma
17. hemoglobin
18. hematocrit
19. disseminated intravascular coagulation

Chapter 11

Pretest

1. c
2. b
3. d
4. a
5. d
6. c

7. c
8. b

Chapter exercises

Exercise 11-1

1. orthopnea (or–THOP–ne–ah)
2. bradypnea (brad–ip–NE–ah)
3. eupnea (upe–NE–ah)
4. dyspnea (disp–NE–ah)
5. orthopneic (or–THOP–NE–ik)
6. bradypneic (brad–ip–NE–ik)
7. eupneic (upe–NE–ik)
8. dyspneic (disp–NE–ik)
9. dysphonia (ah–FO–ne–ah)
10. hypocapnia (hi–po–KAP–ne–ah)
11. anoxia (an–OK–se–ah)
12. hypercapnia (hi–per–KAP–ne–ah)

Exercise 11-2

1. rhinorrhea (ri–no–RE–ah)
2. laryngeal (lah–RIN–je–al)
3. bronchitis (brong–KI–tis)
4. pharyngoscopy (far-ing–GOS–ko–pe)
5. laryngoplasty (lah–RING–go–plas–te)
6. tracheotomy (tra–ke–OT–o–me)
7. tracheostenosis (tra–ke–o–steh–NO–sis)
8. bronchiolitis (brong-ke–o–LI–tis)
9. pertaining to the bronchioles
10. near the nose
11. around a bronchus
12. within the trachea
13. pertaining to the nose and pharynx
14. dilatation of a bronchus

Exercise 11-3

1. pain in the pleura
2. within the lungs
3. surgical removal of a lung or lung tissue
4. plastic repair of a lung
5. study of the lungs
6. absence of a lung
7. surgical incision of the phrenic nerve
8. intrapleural (in–trah–PLU–ral)
9. supraphrenic (su–prah–FREN–ik)
10. pleurocentesis (plu–ro–sen–TE–sis)
11. pneumonopathy (nu–mo–NOP–ah–the)
12. phrenicotripsy (fren–ih–ko–TRIP–se)
13. spirogram (SPI–ro–gram)

Chapter review

Labeling Exercise

Question. Respiratory System

1. frontal sinus
2. sphenoidal sinus
3. nasal cavity
4. nasopharynx
5. oropharynx
6. laryngopharynx
7. larynx and vocal cords
8. epiglottis
9. esophagus
10. trachea
11. right lung
12. left lung
13. left bronchus
14. right bronchus
15. mediastinum
16. terminal bronchiole
17. alveolar duct
18. alveoli
19. capillaries
20. diaphragm

Terminology

1. e
2. a
3. b
4. c
5. d
6. b
7. a
8. e
9. c
10. d
11. d
12. a
13. c
14. e
15. b
16. b
17. c
18. a
19. d
20. e
21. b
22. a
23. e
24. d
25. c
26. bronchus
27. diaphragm
28. carbon dioxide
29. pleura
30. alveoli
31. smell, olfaction
32. lungs
33. tuberculosis
34. spirometer
35. vital capacity
36. pleural cavity
37. coughing
38. mucus
39. apnea
40. bronchodilator
41. T
42. F; inhalation
43. F; larynx
44. T
45. T
46. T
47. phrenicotomy (fren–ih–KOT–o–me)
48. hypopnea (hi–POP–ne–ah)
49. pharyngitis (far–in–JI–tis)
50. bronchiolitis (brong–ke–o–LI–tis)
51. tracheostomy (tra–ke–OS–to–me)
52. accumulation of air or gas in the pleural space
53. accumulation of fluid in the pleural space
54. accumulation of pus in the pleural space
55. accumulation of blood in the pleural space
56. narrowing of the trachea
57. spitting of blood
58. deficiency of oxygen in the tissues
59. any disease of the lungs
60. rapid rate of respiration
61. dilatation of a bronchus
62. plastic repair of the nose
63. pain in the pleura
64. rhin/o; nose
65. pulmon/o; lung
66. spir/o; breathing
67. phrenic/o; phrenic nerve
68. pneum/o; pertaining to air or gas
69. tachypnea
70. hypercapnia
71. inspiration
72. intrapulmonary
73. intubation
74. laryngeal
75. alveolar
76. nasal
77. tracheal
78. pleural
79. bronchial
80. nares

81. pleurae
82. alveoli
83. conchae
84. bronchi
85. tonsil; A *tonsil* is lymphatic tissue in the pharynx; the others are parts of the nose.
86. sinus; A *sinus* is a cavity or channel; the others are parts of the larynx.
87. asthma; *Asthma* is a chronic breathing problem caused by allergy and other factors; the others are infectious diseases.
88. URI; *URI* is an abbreviation for upper respiratory infection; the others are abbreviations for lobes of the lung.
89. RDS; *RDS* is respiratory distress syndrome; the others are breathing volumes or capacities.
90. aphonia
91. hypercapnia
92. dysphonia
93. hyperpnea
94. oximetry
95. dyspnea
96. hypoxia
97. eupnea
98. tachypnea
99. hyperphonia
100. device for measuring air flow
    a. air
    b. rapid, swift
    c. measure
101. incomplete expansion of the alveoli
    a. incomplete
    b. expansion, dilation
102. presence of air or gas in a blood vessel of the heart
    a. air, gas
    b. heart
    c. condition of
103. respiratory disease caused by inhalation of dust particles
    a. lung
    b. dust
    c. condition of

Case study questions

1. c
2. d
3. b
4. d
5. a
6. lobectomy
7. diaphoresis
8. thoracotomy

9. thoracoscopy
10. hemithorax
11. mediastinoscopy
12. ventilation
13. chronic obstructive pulmonary disease
14. arterial blood gas
15. acute respiratory distress syndrome
16. do not resuscitate
17. breath sounds

Chapter 12

Pretest

1. a
2. c
3. c
4. b
5. b
6. d
7. c
8. a

Chapter exercises

Exercise 12-1

1. gingival (JIN–jih–val)
2. lingual (LING–gwal); glossal (GLOS–sal)
3. dental (DEN–tal)
4. buccal (BUK–al)
5. labial (LA–be–al)
6. oral (OR–al); stomal (STO–mal)
7. teeth
8. jaw
9. teeth
10. mouth
11. mouth
12. tongue
13. salivary
14. pertaining to the cheek and pharynx
15. plastic repair or reconstruction of the gingiva
16. under the tongue
17. pertaining to the lip and teeth
18. dropping of the uvula
19. under the tongue
20. suture of the palate

Exercise 12-2

1. pyloric (pi–LOR–ik)
2. colic (KOL–ik); also colonic (ko–LON–ik)
3. gastric (GAS–trik)
4. enteric (en–TER–ik)
5. rectal (REK–tal)
6. jejunal (jeh–JUN–al)

7. ileal (IL–e–al)
8. cecal (SE–kal)
9. anal (A–nal)
10. gastroduodenal (gas–tro–du–o–DE–nal)
11. esophagitis (e–sof–ah–JI–tis)
12. enterostomy (en–ter–OS–to–me)
13. gastroenterology (gas–tro–en–ter–OL–o–je)
14. gastroscopy (gas–TROS–ko–pe)
15. pyloroptosis (pi–lor–o–TO–sis)
16. jejunoileitis (jeh–ju–no–il–e–I–*tis*)
17. ileectomy (il–e–EK–to–me)
18. anorectal (a–no–REK–tal)
19. colitis (ko–LI–tis)
20. colostomy (ko–LOS–to–me)
21. colopexy (KO–lo–pek–se)
22. colocentesis (ko–lo–sen–TE–sis)
23. colonopathy (ko–lo–NOP–ah–the)
24. colonoscopy (ko–lon–OS–ko–pe)
25. esophagogastrostomy (e–sof–ah–go–gas–TROS–to–me)
26. gastroenterostomy (gas–tro–en–ter–OS–to–me)
27. jejunojejunostomy (jeh–ju–no–jeh–ju–NOS–to–me)
28. duodenoileostomy (du–o–de–no–il–e–OS–to–me)
29. sigmoidoproctostomy (sig–moy–do–prok–TOS–to–me)

Exercise 12-3

1. hepatic (heh–PAT–ik)
2. cholecystic (ko–le–SIS–tik)
3. pancreatic (pan–kre–AT–ik)
4. hepatography (hep–ah–TOG–rah–*fe*)
5. cholecystography (ko–le–sis–TOG–rah–fe)
6. cholangiography (ko–lan–je–OG–rah–fe)
7. pancreatography (pan–kre–ah–TOG–rah–fe)
8. choledocholithiasis (ko–led–o–ko–lih–THI–ah–*sis*)
9. pancreatolithiasis (pan–kre–ah–to–lih–THI–ah–*sis*)
10. hepatitis (hep–ah–TI–tis)
11. bile
12. gallstone; biliary calculus
13. common bile duct
14. gallbladder
15. liver
16. bile duct
17. pancreas

Chapter review

Labeling Exercise

Question. The Digestive System

1. mouth
2. pharynx
3. esophagus
4. stomach
5. duodenum (of small intestine)
6. small intestine
7. cecum
8. ascending colon
9. transverse colon
10. descending colon
11. sigmoid colon
12. rectum
13. anus
14. parotid salivary gland
15. sublingual salivary gland
16. submandibular salivary gland
17. liver (cut)
18. gallbladder
19. pancreas

Question. Accessory Organs of Digestion

1. liver
2. common hepatic duct
3. gallbladder
4. cystic duct
5. common bile duct
6. pancreas
7. pancreatic duct
8. duodenum
9. spleen
10. diaphragm

Terminology

1. d
2. c
3. b
4. e
5. a
6. c
7. a
8. d
9. b
10. e
11. b
12. c
13. d
14. e
15. a
16. c
17. a
18. d
19. e
20. b
21. d
22. b
23. a
24. c
25. e
26. c
27. a
28. e
29. b
30. d
31. bariatric surgery
32. cecum
33. liver
34. gallbladder
35. peritoneum
36. tongue
37. palate
38. tooth
39. cheek
40. intestine
41. liver
42. bile
43. hiatal hernia
44. dysphagia
45. stomach acid
46. hepatomegaly
47. periodontist
48. gastrectomy
49. palatorrhaphy
50. pylorostenosis
51. pancreatitis
52. gastroenterologist
53. colostomy
54. gastroduodenostomy
55. intrahepatic
56. diverticula
57. gingivae
58. calculi
59. anastomoses
60. hiatal hernia
61. dyspepsia
62. inguinal hernia
63. icterus
64. pyloric stenosis
65. diarrhea
66. F; above
67. F; jejunum
68. F; saliva
69. T
70. T
71. T
72. F; vomiting
73. T
74. villus; A *villus* is a tiny projection in the lining of the small intestine that aids in absorption of nutrients; the others are parts of the mouth.
75. spleen; The *spleen* is a lymphatic organ; the others are parts of the large intestine.
76. pylorus; The *pylorus* is the distal portion of the stomach; the others are accessory digestive organs.
77. amylase; *Amylase* is a starch-digesting enzyme; the others are disorders of the digestive tract.
78. nausea and vomiting
79. nasogastric
80. total parenteral nutrition
81. gastroesophageal reflux disease
82. esophagogastroduodenoscopy
83. gastrointestinal
84. hydrochloric acid
85. proton pump inhibitor
86. percutaneous endoscopic gastrostomy (tube)
87. hepatitis A virus
88. cecitis
89. proctorrhaphy
90. cecopexy
91. proctocele
92. ileocecal
93. ileopexy
94. proctitis
95. cecorrhaphy
96. ileitis
97. pertaining to the muscular layer of the intestine
    a. muscle
    b. intestine
    c. pertaining to
98. radiography of the biliary tract and gallbladder using radionuclides
    a. bile
    b. spark (radiation)
    c. act of recording data
99. referring to any route other than the alimentary canal
    a. beside
    b. intestine
    c. pertaining to
100. pertaining to the nose and stomach
    a. nose
    b. stomach
    c. pertaining to
101. pertaining to a dry mouth
    a. dry
    b. mouth
    c. pertaining to

Case study questions

1. c
2. b
3. b
4. a
5. d
6. a
7. b
8. b
9. b
10. d
11. a
12. d
13. b
14. endoscopic retrograde cholangio pancreatography
15. right upper quadrant
16. nasogastric
17. inflammatory bowel disease
18. cholelithiasis
19. laparoscopic cholecystectomy
20. cholecystitis
21. cholangiogram
22. sphincter
23. biopsy

Chapter 13

Pretest

1. d
2. c
3. c
4. a
5. c
6. d
7. d
8. b

Chapter exercises

Exercise 13-1

1. prerenal (pre–RE–nal)
2. postrenal (post–RE–nal)
3. suprarenal (su–prah–RE–nal)
4. perirenal (per–ih–RE–nal); circumrenal (sir–kum–RE–nal)
5. nephrologist (neh–FROL–o–jist)
6. nephropathy (neh–FROP–ah–the)
7. nephrotoxic (nef–ro–TOK–sik)
8. nephromalacia (nef–ro–mah–LA–she–ah)
9. nephromegaly (neh–fro–MEG–ah– le)
10. nephrotomy (neh–FROT–o–me)
11. pyelonephritis (pi–eh–lo–nef–RI–tis)
12. pyeloplasty (pi–eh–lo–PLAS–te)
13. pyelogram (PI–eh–lo–gram)
14. glomerulitis (glo–mer–u–LI–tis)
15. calicotomy (kal–ih–KOT–o–me); caliotomy (ka–le–OT–o–me)
16. glomerulosclerosis (glo–mer–u–lo–skleh–RO–sis)
17. caliectasis (ka–le–EK–tah–sis); calicectasis (kal–ih–SEK–tah–sis)

Exercise 13-2

1. uropathy (u–ROP–ah–the)
2. urography (u–ROG–rah–fe)
3. urolith (U–ro–lith)
4. uremia (u–RE–me–ah)
5. anuria (an–U–re–ah)
6. pyuria (pi–U–re–ah)
7. nocturia (nokt–U–re–ah)
8. dysuria (dis–U–re–ah)
9. hematuria (he–mah–TU–re–ah)
10. diuresis (di–u–RE–sis)
11. anuresis (an–u–RE–sis)
12. natriuresis (na–tre–u–RE–sis)
13. kaliuresis (ka–le–u–RE–sis)
14. urethropexy (u–RE–thro–pek–se)
15. ureterostomy (u–re–ter–OS–to– me)
16. urethrorrhaphy (u–re–THROR–ah– fe)
17. urethroscopy (u–re–THROS–ko– pe)
18. ureterocele (u–RE–ter–o–sele)
19. cystitis (sis–TI–tis)
20. cystography (sis–TOG–rah–fe)
21. cystoscope (SIS–to–skope)
22. cystotomy (sis–TOT–o–me)
23. cystorrhea (sis–to–RE–ah)
24. supravesical (su–prah–VES–ih– kal)
25. urethrovesical (u–re–thro–VES–ih–kal)
26. pain in the urinary bladder
27. surgical incision of the ureter
28. through the urethra
29. formation of urine

Chapter review

Labeling Exercise

Question. Urinary System

1. kidney
2. ureter
3. urinary bladder
4. urethra
5. aorta
6. renal artery
7. renal vein
8. inferior vena cava
9. diaphragm
10. adrenal gland

Question. The Kidney

1. renal capsule
2. renal cortex
3. renal medulla
4. pyramids of medulla
5. nephrons
6. calyx
7. hilum
8. renal pelvis
9. ureter

Question. The Urinary Bladder

1. ureter
2. smooth muscle
3. openings of ureters
4. trigone
5. urethra
6. internal urethral sphincter
7. external urethral sphincter
8. peritoneum
9. prostate

Terminology

1. a
2. c
3. d
4. b
5. e
6. d
7. e
8. b
9. a
10. c
11. d
12. b
13. e
14. a
15. c
16. a
17. b
18. c
19. e
20. d
21. hydronephrosis
22. glomerulus
23. renin
24. urination; voiding of urine
25. urinalysis
26. urea
27. incontinence; stress incontinence
28. clean–catch specimen
29. cystoscopy
30. catheter
31. urethra
32. dysuria

33. calyx
34. cystocele
35. hyperkalemia
36. intravesical
37. F; kidney
38. T
39. T
40. F; medulla
41. F; urethra
42. T
43. T
44. F; sodium
45. narrowing of the urethra
46. elimination of large amounts of urine
47. toxic or poisonous to the kidney
48. near the glomerulus
49. surgical removal of a calyx
50. near the kidney
51. nephrologist
52. pyelocalicectasis; pyelcalicectasis
53. nephromalacia
54. cystectomy
55. nephropathy
56. cystourethrogram
57. ureteropyeloplasty
58. pyelonephritis
59. ureterosigmoidostomy
60. cast; A cast is a solid mold of a renal nephron; the others are parts of the kidney.
61. calyx; A calyx is a collecting region for urine in the kidney; the others are parts of a nephron.
62. specific gravity; Specific gravity is a measure of density; the others are treatment procedures for the urinary system.
63. hydration
64. hypervolemia
65. antidiuretic
66. hypernatremia
67. anuresis
68. ureteral
69. nephrologic
70. uremic
71. diuretic
72. nephrotic
73. caliceal; calyceal
74. urethral
75. pelves
76. calyces
77. glomeruli
78. b
79. d
80. f
81. c
82. a
83. e
84. g
85. urography
86. renal
87. intrarenal
88. renography
89. intravesical
90. suprarenal
91. urology
92. interrenal
93. vesical
94. urolith
95. specific gravity
96. antidiuretic hormone
97. erythropoietin
98. intravenous pyelography
99. sodium
100. glomerular filtration rate
101. urinalysis
102. removal of substances from the blood by passage through a semipermeable membrane
    a. blood
    b. through
    c. separation
103. test that measures and records bladder function
    a. urinary bladder
    b. measure
    c. act of recording data
104. surgical creation of a new passage between a ureter and the bladder
    a. ureter
    b. new
    c. bladder
    d. surgical creation of an opening

Case study questions

1. c
2. d
3. d
4. a
5. IV urogram
6. hematuria
7. cystoscopic
8. nephrolithotomy
9. oliguria
10. nocturia
11. lithotripsy
12. kidney transplantation
13. urinary tract infection
14. continuous ambulatory peritoneal dialysis
15. blood urea nitrogen
16. end-stage renal disease
17. human immunodeficiency virus

Chapter 14

Pretest

1 c
2 d
3 a
4 b
5 b
6 d

Chapter exercises

Exercise 14-1

1. formation (−genesis) of spermatozoa
2. pain in the prostate
3. plastic repair of the scrotum
4. excision of the epididymis
5. pain in the testis
6. any disease of a testis
7. inflammation of the testis and epididymis
8. orchiopexy (or-ke-o-PEK-se); also, orchidopexy (or-kih-do-PEK-se)
9. orchioplasty (OR-ke-o-plas-te); also, orchidoplasty (OR-kih-do-plas-te)
10. orchiectomy (or-ke-EK-to-me); also, orchidectomy (or-kih-DEK-to-me)
11. spermaturia (sper-mah-TU-re-ah)
12. spermatolysis (sper-mah-TOL-ih-sis)
13. spermatorrhea (sper-mah-to-RE-ah)
14. oligospermia (ol-ih-go-SPER-me-ah)
15. spermatocyte (sper-MAH-to-site)
16. hemospermia (he-mo-SPER-me-ah); also, hematospermia (he-mah-to-SPER-me-ah)
17. aspermia (ah-SPER-me-ah)
18. polyspermia (pol-e-SPER-me-ah)
19. pyospermia (pi-o-SPER-me-ah)
20. vasectomy (vah-SEK-to-me)
21. oscheoma (os-ke-O-mah)
22. vasorrhaphy (vas-OR-ah-fe)
23. prostatectomy (pros-tah-TEK-to-me)
24. vesiculography (veh-sik-u-LOG-rah-fe)
25. vesiculitis (veh-sik-u-LI-tis)
26. epididymotomy (ep-ih-did-ih-MOT-o-me)

Chapter review
Labeling Exercise
Question. Male Reproductive System
1. testis
2. epididymis
3. scrotum
4. ductus (vas) deferens
5. ejaculatory duct
6. urethra
7. penis
8. glans penis
9. prepuce (foreskin)
10. seminal vesicle
11. prostate
12. bulbourethral (Cowper) gland
13. kidney
14. ureter
15. urinary bladder
16. peritoneal cavity
17. rectum
18. anus

Terminology
1. a
2. c
3. e
4. b
5. d
6. a
7. c
8. b
9. d
10. e
11. b
12. e
13. d
14. a
15. c
16. e
17. a
18. d
19. c
20. b
21. testosterone
22. bulbourethral glands
23. semen
24. testis
25. inguinal canal
26. scrotum
27. suture of the vas (ductus) deferens
28. absence of a testis
29. tumor of the scrotum
30. radiographic study of the seminal vesicles
31. instrument for measuring the prostate
32. presence of blood in the semen
33. orchiopexy; orchidopexy
34. oscheolith
35. epididymotomy
36. oscheoplasty
37. vasovasostomy
38. hematuria
39. dysuria
40. intravesical
41. hyperplasia
42. resectoscope
43. testosterone
44. semen
45. prostate
46. epididymis
47. hypospadias
48. T
49. F; semen
50. T
51. T
52. F; urethra
53. T
54. T
55. spermatic cord; The *spermatic cord* suspends the testis in the scrotum and contains the ductus deferens, nerves, and vessels; the others are the glands that contribute to semen.
56. semen; *Semen* is the secretion that transports spermatozoa; the others are hormones active in reproduction.
57. hernia; A *hernia* is a protrusion of tissue through an abnormal body opening; the others are sexually transmitted infections.
58. seminal
59. prostatic
60. penile
61. urethral
62. scrotal
63. benign prostatic hyperplasia
64. sexually transmitted infection
65. erectile dysfunction
66. gonococcus
67. prostate–specific antigen
68. genitourinary
69. transurethral resection of prostate
70. d
71. e
72. c
73. b
74. a
75. f
76. vasoplasty
77. spermatolysis
78. vesicular
79. vasography
80. vesiculitis
81. spermatic
82. spermatocyte
83. vasotomy
84. spermatogenesis
85. vesiculography
86. removal of a hydrocele by fluid drainage or partial excision
    a. fluid, water
    b. hernia, localized dilatation
    c. out
    d. cut
    e. condition of
87. destructive to sperm cells
    a. sperm
    b. agent that kills
    c. pertaining to
88. undescended testis
    a. hidden
    b. testis
    c. condition of
89. inflammation of the ductus deferens and seminal vesicle
    a. vas (ductus) deferens
    b. seminal vesicle
    c. inflammation
90. abnormally profuse spermatic secretion
    a. many
    b. sperm
    c. condition of

Case study questions
1. d
2. a
3. b
4. d
5. d
6. d
7. b
8. bilateral inguinal herniorrhaphy
9. strangulated hernia
10. balanitis
11. phimosis
12. psychogenic
13. vasodilation
14. antihypertensive

Chapter 15
Pretest
1. c
2. b
3. c
4. b
5. c

6. b
7. a
8. c

Chapter exercises
Exercise 15-1
1. any disease of women
2. between menstruation periods
3. formation of an ovum
4. release of an ovum from the ovary
5. pertaining to an ovary
6. inflammation of an ovary
7. ovariorrhexis (o–var–e–o–REK–sis)
8. ovulatory (OV–u–lah–to–re)
9. menorrhagia (men–o–RA–je–ah)
10. oligomenorrhea (ol–ih–go–men–o–RE–ah)
11. amenorrhea (ah–men–o–RE–ah)
12. dysmenorrhea (DIS–men–o–re–ah)
13. ovariotomy (o–var–e–OT–o–me)
14. ovariocentesis (o–var–e–o–sen–TE–sis)
15. ovariocele (o–VAR–e–o–sele)
16. oophoroplasty (o–of–or–o–PLAS–te)
17. oophoroma (o–of–o–RO–mah)

Exercise 15-2
1. radiographic examination of the uterus
2. softening of the uterus
3. plastic repair of the vagina
4. pain in the vagina
5. excision of a uterine tube, fallopian tube
6. pertaining to the uterus and urinary bladder
7. within the cervix
8. salpingopexy (sal–PING–go–pek–se)
9. salpingography (sal–ping–GOG–rah–fe)
10. hydrosalpinx (hi–dro–SAL–pinx)
11. pyosalpinx (pi–o–SAL–pinx)
12. salpingo–oophorectomy (sal–ping–go–o–of–o–REK–to–me); also, salpingo–ovariectomy (sal–ping–go–o–var–e–EK–to–me)
13. hysteropexy (his–ter–o–PEK–se)
14. uterine (U–ter–in)
15. metrostenosis (me–tro–steh–NO–sis)
16. hysterosalpingogram (his–ter–o–sal–PING–go–gram)
17. transcervical (trans–SER–vih–kal)
18. metroptosis (me–trop–TO–sis)
19. colpocele (KOL–po–sele)
20. vaginitis (vaj–ih–NI–tis)

Exercise 15-3
1. vulvectomy (vul–VEK–to–me)
2. episiorrhaphy (eh–piz–e–OR–ah–fe)
3. vaginoperineal (vaj–ih–no–per–ih–NE–al)
4. clitoromegaly (klit–or–o–MEG–ah–le)
5. mammogram (MAM–o–gram)
6. mastitis (mas–TI–tis)
7. mastectomy (mas–TEK–to–me); also, mammectomy (mah–MEK–to–me)

Exercise 15-4
1. before birth
2. formation of an embryo
3. pertaining to a newborn
4. endoscopic examination of the fetus
5. developing in, or pertaining to, one amniotic sac
6. lack of milk production
7. decreased secretion of milk
8. embryology (em–bre–OL–o–je)
9. postnatal (post–NA–tal)
10. amniotomy (am–ne–OT–o–me)
11. amniocyte (AM–ne–o–site)
12. embryopathy (em–bre–OP–ah–the)
13. fetoscope (FE–to–skope)
14. amniorrhexis (am–ne–o–REK–sis)
15. neonatology (ne–o–na–TOL–o–je)
16. primigravida (prih–mih–GRAV–ih–dah)
17. multigravida (mul–tih–GRAV–ih–dah)
18. nullipara (nul–IP–ah–rah)
19. primipara (prih–MIP–ah–rah)
20. xerotocia (ze–ro–TO–se–ah)
21. bradytocia (brad–e–TO–se–ah)
22. galactorrhea (gah–lak–to–RE–ah); also, lactorrhea (lak–to–RE–ah)
23. galactocele (ga–hLAK–to–sele); also, lactocele (LAK–to–sele)

Chapter review
Labeling Exercise
Question. Female Reproductive System
1. ovary
2. fimbriae
3. uterine tube
4. uterus
5. cervix
6. posterior fornix
7. vagina
8. clitoris
9. labium minus
10. labium majus
11. urinary bladder
12. urethra
13. rectum
14. anus
15. peritoneal cavity
16. cul–de–sac

Question. Ovulation and Fertilization
1. ovary
2. fimbriae
3. ovum
4. sperm cells (spermatozoa)
5. uterine tube
6. implanted embryo
7. body of uterus
8. cervix
9. vagina
10. greater vestibular (Bartholin) gland

Terminology
1. c
2. d
3. e
4. a
5. b
6. c
7. b
8. a
9. e
10. d
11. d
12. c
13. e
14. b
15. a
16. b
17. e
18. c
19. d
20. a
21. d
22. b
23. e
24. c
25. a
26. colposcope
27. ovary
28. rectocele
29. ovum (egg cell)
30. placenta
31. lactation
32. abortion
33. uterus
34. breasts (mammary glands)
35. oophorectomy

36. premenstrual
37. salpingectomy
38. dysmenorrhea
39. cleft palate
40. T
41. F; embryo
42. F; myometrium
43. F; corpus luteum
44. F; uterine tube
45. T
46. T
47. T
48. T
49. behind the uterus
50. any disease of the uterus
51. softening of the uterus
52. pus in the uterine tube, fallopian tube
53. narrowing of the vagina
54. pain in the vulva
55. after birth
56. below the mammary gland (breast)
57. outside the embryo
58. woman who has given birth three times
59. causing fetal abnormalities
60. salpingocele
61. episiorrhaphy
62. metrostenosis
63. hysterosalpingectomy
64. mammogram
65. dystocia
66. amniorrhexis
67. embryology
68. fetometry
69. gravida
70. fundus
71. pelvimetry
72. suprapubic
73. Apgar score
74. neonate
75. polyhydramnios
76. prenatal
77. eutocia
78. anovulatory
79. intrauterine
80. cervical
81. uterine
82. perineal
83. vaginal
84. embryonic
85. amniotic
86. ova
87. cervices
88. fimbriae
89. labia
90. candidiasis; *Candidiasis* is a fungal infection; the others are procedures used to diagnose fetal abnormalities.
91. measles; *Measles* is an infectious disease; the others are hereditary disorders.
92. colostrum; *Colostrum* is the breast fluid released before milk is produced; the others are hormones involved in reproduction.
93. labia majora; The *labia majora* are part of the vulva; the others are associated with pregnancy.
94. spina bifida; *Spina bifida* is a congenital spinal defect; the others are disorders of pregnancy.
95. c
96. b
97. a
98. d
99. episioplasty
100. cervicitis
101. mammography
102. mammoplasty
103. cervicography
104. episiotomy
105. intracervical
106. cervicoplasty
107. cervicotomy
108. transcervical
109. human chorionic gonadotropin
110. dysfunctional uterine bleeding
111. last menstrual period
112. fetal heart rate
113. gestational age
114. vaginal birth after cesarean section
115. prevention of blood vessel formation
    a. against
    b. vessel
    c. origin, formation
    d. condition of
116. excessive development of the mammary glands in the male, even to the secretion of milk
    a. woman
    b. breast
    c. condition of
117. extreme rapidity of labor
    a. sharp, acute
    b. labor
    c. condition of
118. a deficiency of amniotic fluid
    a. few, scanty
    b. fluid
    c. amnion
119. flow of milk from the breast other than normal lactation
    a. milk
    b. flow or discharge
120. congenital absence of a brain
    a. without
    b. brain
    c. pertaining to

Case study questions

1. b
2. c
3. b
4. a
5. d
6. d
7. prolapsed
8. zygote
9. oocyte
10. follicular
11. dilatation and curettage
12. bilateral salpingo–oophorectomy
13. hormone replacement therapy
14. total abdominal hysterectomy
15. in vitro fertilization
16. gynecology
17. zygote intrafallopian transfer

Chapter 16

Pretest

1. d
2. b
3. a
4. c
5. d
6. d

Chapter exercises

Exercise 16-1

1. condition of underactivity of the adrenal gland
2. acting on the thyroid gland
3. excision of the pituitary gland (hypophysis)
4. study of the endocrine glands or hormones
5. tumor of the pancreatic islets
6. hyperthyroidism (hi-per-THI-royd-*izm*)
7. hypoparathyroidism (hi-po-par-ah-THI-royd-*izm*)
8. hyperadrenalism (hi-per-ah-DRE-nal-*izm*)
9. hyperadrenocorticism (hi-per-ah-dre-no-KOR-tih-sizm)
10. hypopituitarism (hi-po-pih-TU-ih-tah-rizm)
11. adrenomegaly (ah-dre-no-MEG-ah-le)

12. thyroidectomy (thi-roy-DEK-to-me)
13. adrenalopathy (ah-dre-nah-LOP ah-the); also, adrenopathy (ah-dre-NOP-ah-the)
14. endocrinologist (en-do-krih-NOL-o-jist)
15. insulitis (in-su-LI-tis)

Chapter review
Labeling Exercise
Question. Glands of the Endocrine System
1. pineal
2. hypothalamus
3. pituitary (hypophysis)
4. thyroid
5. parathyroids
6. adrenals
7. pancreatic islets
8. ovaries
9. testes

Terminology
1. b
2. e
3. c
4. d
5. a
6. d
7. b
8. a
9. c
10. e
11. b
12. d
13. e
14. c
15. a
16. c
17. e
18. d
19. a
20. b
21. b
22. a
23. e
24. c
25. d
26. pituitary (hypophysis)
27. thyroid
28. adrenals
29. diabetes mellitus
30. hyperglycemia
31. incision into the thyroid gland
32. condition caused by underactivity of the pituitary gland
33. acting on the hypophysis (pituitary)
34. any disease of the adrenal gland
35. enlargement of the adrenal gland
36. physician who specializes in the study and treatment of endocrine disorders
37. insuloma
38. thyrolytic
39. adrenocortical
40. thyroiditis
41. hemithyroidectomy
42. parathyroidectomy
43. hyperadrenalism
44. thyrotropic
45. thyroptosis
46. thyropathy
47. F; ADH, antidiuretic hormone
48. T
49. F; cortex
50. F; calcium
51. F; thyroid
52. T
53. T
54. T
55. T
56. T
57. PTH; PTH is parathyroid hormone from the parathyroid gland; the others are hormones produced by the anterior pituitary.
58. dwarfism; Dwarfism is caused by hyposecretion of growth hormone: the others are caused by hypersecretion of hormones.
59. TBG; TBG is a test of thyroid function; the others are abbreviations associated with diabetes mellitus.
60. spleen; The spleen is part of the immune system; the others are endocrine glands.
61. thyropathy
62. adrenotropic
63. thyromegaly
64. adrenal
65. adrenomegaly
66. insuloma
67. thyrolytic
68. adrenopathy
69. thyrotropic
70. insular
71. benign tumor of the pituitary gland
    a. cranium
    b. pharynx (the tumor arises from tissue that forms the roof of the mouth)
    c. tumor, neoplasm
72. condition of complete underactivity of the pituitary gland
    a. all
    b. under, abnormally low
    c. pituitary gland
    d. condition of
73. usually benign tumor of the adrenal medulla or any cells that stain with chromium salts (chromaffin cells)
    a. dark, dusky
    b. color
    c. cell
    d. tumor, neoplasm
74. a toxic condition caused by hyperactivity of the thyroid gland
    a. thyroid
    b. poisonous
    c. condition of
75. condition marked by enlargement of the extremities
    a. extremity
    b. enlargement
    c. condition of
76. pancreas (pancreatic islets)
77. adrenal cortex
78. thyroid
79. parathyroid
80. anterior pituitary

Case study questions
1. a
2. c
3. d
4. a
5. b
6. c
7. a
8. nephrectomy
9. adenoma
10. ampule
11. hyperglycemia
12. bolus
13. within normal limits
14. neutral protamine Hagedorn
15. continuous subcutaneous insulin infusion

Chapter 17
Pretest
1. b
2. a
3. d
4. c
5. a
6. c

7. b
8. d

Chapter exercises

Exercise 17-1

1. pertaining to a nerve or the nervous system
2. pertaining to neuroglia, glial cells
3. pertaining to a spinal nerve root
4. pertaining to the meninges
5. pertaining to a ganglion
6. meninges
7. nervous system, nervous tissue
8. meninges
9. spinal cord
10. surgical removal of a ganglion
11. inflammation of many spinal nerve roots
12. destruction of a nerve or nervous tissue
13. nerve pain due to irritation of the sensory nerve root
14. radiographic study of the spinal cord
15. glioma (gli–O–mah)
16. myelogram (MI–eh–lo–gram)
17. neuralgia (nu–RAL–je–ah)
18. myelitis (mi–eh–LI–tis)
19. neuropathy (nu–ROP–ah–the)

Exercise 17-2

1. sleep
2. cerebrum, brain
3. thalamus
4. mind
5. stupor, unconsciousness
6. brain
7. cerebrum, brain
8. psychic (SI–kik)
9. cortical (KOR–tih–kal)
10. thalamic (thah–LAM–ik)
11. cerebral (SER–eh–bral)
12. ventricular (ven–TRIK–u–lar)
13. any disease of the brain
14. lack of sleep, inability to sleep
15. study of the mind
16. pertaining to the brain and spinal cord
17. outside the medulla
18. incision of a ventricle
19. ventriculogram (ven–TRIK–u–lo–gram)
20. corticothalamic (kor–tih–ko–thah–LAM–ik)
21. intracerebellar (in–trah–ser–eh–BEL–ar)
22. encephalitis (en–sef–ah–LI–tis)
23. supracerebral (su–prah–SER–eh–bral)

Exercise 17-3

1. seizures
2. read
3. speech
4. tetraplegia (tet–rah–PLE–je–ah)
5. partial paralysis, weakness
6. paralysis of the heart
7. lack of speech communication
8. inability to comprehend the written or printed word
9. obsession with fire
10. fear of women
11. partial paralysis or weakness of all four limbs
12. photophobia (fo–to–FO–be–ah)
13. noctiphobia (nok–tih–FO–be–ah); also, nyctophobia (nik–to–FO–be–ah)
14. hemiplegia (hem–ih–PLE–je–ah)
15. bradylalia (brad–e–LA–le–ah)

Chapter review

Labeling Exercise

Question. Anatomic Divisions of the Nervous System

1. central nervous system
2. brain
3. spinal cord
4. peripheral nervous system
5. cranial nerves
6. spinal nerves

Question. Motor Neuron

1. cell body
2. nucleus
3. dendrites
4. axon covered with myelin sheath
5. node
6. myelin
7. axon branch
8. muscle

Question. External Surface of the Brain

1. sulci
2. gyri
3. frontal lobe
4. parietal lobe
5. occipital lobe
6. temporal lobe
7. pons
8. medulla oblongata
9. cerebellum
10. spinal cord

Question. Spinal Cord, Lateral View

1. brain
2. brainstem
3. spinal cord
4. cervical enlargement
5. lumbar enlargement
6. cervical nerves
7. thoracic nerves
8. lumbar nerves
9. sacral nerves
10. coccygeal nerve

Question. Spinal Cord, Cross Section

1. white matter
2. gray matter
3. dorsal horn
4. ventral horn
5. central canal
6. dorsal root of spinal nerve
7. dorsal root ganglion
8. ventral root of spinal nerve
9. spinal nerve

Question. Reflex Pathway

1. receptor
2. sensory neuron
3. spinal cord (CNS)
4. motor neuron
5. effector

Terminology

1. e
2. a
3. d
4. c
5. b
6. e
7. c
8. d
9. a
10. b
11. b
12. a
13. e
14. c
15. d
16. e
17. d
18. c
19. b
20. a
21. c
22. e
23. a
24. d
25. b

26. b
27. a
28. e
29. c
30. d
31. cerebrum
32. cerebrospinal fluid (CSF)
33. neuroglia, glial cells
34. synapse
35. neuron
36. meninges
37. reflex
38. autonomic nervous system (ANS)
39. neurotransmitter
40. cerebellum
41. dura mater
42. pertaining to the cerebral cortex and thalamus.
43. inflammation of many nerves
44. absence of a brain
45. partial paralysis of half the body
46. pertaining to a spinal nerve root
47. treatment of mental disorders
48. total paralysis
49. softening of the brain
50. sleep disorder
51. neurology
52. myelomeningitis
53. ganglionectomy; gangliectomy
54. neuropathy
55. ventriculostomy
56. hemiplegia
57. intracerebellar
58. dyslexia
59. hydrophobia
60. monoplegia
61. cerebrum
62. neuroglia
63. ventricle
64. narcosis
65. thalamus
66. T
67. F; peripheral
68. T
69. F; white
70. T
71. F; dendrite
72. T
73. T
74. T
75. intramedullary
76. contralateral
77. preganglionic
78. bradylalia
79. sensory
80. ventral
81. efferent
82. ganglionic
83. thalamic
84. dural
85. meningeal
86. psychotic
87. ganglia
88. ventricles
89. meninges
90. emboli
91. lumbar puncture; *Lumbar puncture* is a diagnostic procedure for sampling CSF; the others are vascular disorders.
92. hematoma; *Hematoma* is a local collection of clotted blood; the others are neoplasms.
93. mania; *Mania* is a state of elation; the others are parts of the brain.
94. CNS; *CNS* is the central nervous system; the others are behavioral disorders.
95. myeloplegia
96. aphasia
97. hemiparesis
98. myoparesis
99. dysphasia
100. ganglioplegia
101. tetraplegia
102. myelitis
103. bradyphasia
104. hemiplegia
105. gangliitis
106. hemorrhage into the spinal cord
    a. blood
    b. spinal cord
    c. condition of
107. abnormal development of the spinal cord
    a. spinal cord
    b. abnormal
    c. development
    d. condition of
108. inflammation of many nerves and nerve roots
    a. many
    b. nerve
    c. spinal nerve root
    d. inflammation of
109. disturbance of muscle coordination
    a. abnormal, difficult
    b. together
    c. work
    d. condition of

Case study questions

1. c
2. d
3. a
4. d
5. psychiatrist
6. neuroleptics
7. ischemic
8. meningitis
9. subdural hematoma
10. paranoia
11. antispasmodic
12. aphasia
13. hemiparesis
14. Glasgow coma scale
15. computed tomography
16. neurological intensive care unit (also means neonatal intensive care unit)
17. cerebrovascular accident
18. transient ischemic attack
19. level of consciousness

Chapter 18

Pretest

1. b
2. a
3. d
4. c
5. c
6. b

Chapter exercises

Exercise 18-1

1. loss of pain
2. abnormal sense of smell
3. lack of taste sensation
4. myesthesia (mi–es–THE–ze–ah)
5. pseudogeusia (su–do–GU–ze–ah)
6. thermesthesia (ther–mes–THE–ze–ah)
7. hyperalgesia (hi–per–al–JE–ze–ah)
8. dysgeusia (dis–GU–ze–ah)
9. anesthesia (an–es–THE–ze–ah)

Exercise 18-2

1. hearing
2. sound
3. ear
4. pertaining to the stapes
5. pertaining to the cochlea
6. pertaining to the vestibule or vestibular apparatus
7. pertaining to hearing
8. pertaining to the labyrinth (inner ear)
9. pertaining to the ear
10. otalgia (o–TAL–je–ah); otodynia (o–to–DIN–e–ah)

11. labyrinthotomy (lab-ih-rin-THOT-o-me)
12. salpingoscope (sal-PING-go-skope)
13. otoscope (O-to-skope)
14. endocochlear (en-do-KOK-le-ar); intracochlear (in-trah-KOK-le-ar)
15. vestibulocochlear (ves-tib-u-lo-KOK-le-ar)
16. audiometry (aw-de-OM-eh-tre)
17. tympanoplasty (tim-PAN-o-plas-te)
18. stapedectomy (sta-pe-DEK-to-me)
19. inflammation of the eardrum (tympanic membrane)
20. instrument used to measure hearing
21. any disease of the vestibule or vestibular apparatus
22. pertaining to the auditory tube and pharynx
23. procedure to surgically fix the tympanic membrane (eardrum) to the stapes

Exercise 18-3

1. pertaining to the nose and lacrimal apparatus
2. between the eyelids
3. surgical repair of the eyelid
4. excision of a lacrimal sac
5. blepharoplegia (blef-ah-ro-PLE-je-ah)
6. dacryolith (DAK-re-o-lith)
7. dacryocystitis (dak-re-o-sis-TI-tis)

Exercise 18-4

1. ophthalmologist
2. lens
3. eye
4. vision
5. lens
6. cornea
7. opt/o; eye, vision
8. ophthalm/o; eye
9. pupill/o; pupil
10. lent/i; lens
11. irid/o; iris
12. uve/o; uvea
13. phac/o; lens
14. uveoscleritis (u-ve-o-skleh-RI-tis)
15. phacosclerosis (fak-o-skle-RO-sis)
16. corneal (KOR-ne-al)
17. retinopexy (ret-ih-no-PEK-se)
18. cyclitis (si-KLI-tis)
19. ophthalmoscope (of-THAL-mo-skope)
20. ophthalmology (of-thal-MOL-o-je)
21. iridectomy (ir-ih-DEK-to-me)
22. iridoplegia (ir-id-o-PLE-je-ah)
23. pertaining to the right eye
24. pertaining to the lens
25. inflammation of the iris and ciliary body
26. pertaining to the choroid and retina
27. inflammation of the cornea
28. incision of the ciliary muscle
29. pertaining to the eye or vision
30. instrument used to incise the sclera
31. splitting of the retina

Exercise 18-5

1. macropsia (mah-KROP-se-ah)
2. achromatopsia (ah-kro-mah-TOP-se-ah)
3. diplopia (dip-LO-pe-ah)
4. presbyopia (pres-be-O-pe-ah)
5. amblyopia (am-ble-O-pe-ah)
6. ametropia (am-eh-TRO-pe-ah)
7. heterometropia (het-er-o-meh-TROpe-ah); also, anisometropia (an-i-so-meh-TRO-pe-ah)

Chapter review

Labeling Exercise

Question. The Ear

1. outer ear
2. pinna
3. external auditory canal
4. tympanic membrane
5. ossicles (of middle ear)
6. malleus
7. incus
8. stapes
9. auditory (eustachian) tube
10. inner ear
11. vestibule
12. semicircular canals
13. cochlea

Question. The Eye

1. sclera
2. cornea
3. conjunctival sac
4. choroid
5. ciliary muscle
6. iris
7. pupil
8. lens
9. aqueous humor
10. vitreous body
11. retina
12. fovea
13. optic disk (blind spot)
14. optic nerve

Terminology

1. c
2. a
3. e
4. d
5. b
6. d
7. e
8. a
9. c
10. b
11. e
12. c
13. d
14. b
15. a
16. e
17. c
18. b
19. a
20. d
21. d
22. c
23. a
24. b
25. e
26. d
27. e
28. a
29. c
30. b
31. tympanic membrane
32. sensorineural
33. stapes
34. sclera
35. refraction
36. retina
37. cornea
38. proprioception
39. specialist in the study and treatment of hearing disorders
40. instrument for measuring the eye
41. absence of a lens
42. below the sclera
43. incision of the iris
44. instrument used to examine the tympanic membrane (eardrum)
45. around the lens

46. excess flow of tears
47. loss of hearing caused by aging
48. inflammation of the cornea and iris
49. phacomalacia
50. pupillometry
51. stapedectomy
52. blepharoptosis
53. otoplasty
54. vestibulocochlear
55. retinopathy
56. analgesia
57. lacrimal
58. cyclectomy
59. salpingoscopy
60. hyperopia
61. cochlear
62. palpebral
63. choroidal
64. uveal
65. corneal
66. scleral
67. pupillary
68. hypoesthesia, hypesthesia
69. hyperalgesia
70. sc
71. myopia
72. miosis
73. exotropia
74. pseudosmia
75. myringoplasty
76. retinoscopy
77. salpingoscopy
78. anosmia
79. retinoschisis
80. myringoscopy
81. subretinal
82. retinopexy
83. keratoscopy
84. F; cochlea
85. T
86. T
87. T
88. F; taste
89. F; constrict
90. F; tympanic membrane
91. F; tears
92. smell; Smell is a special sense; the others are general senses.
93. pinna; The pinna is part of the outer ear; the others are parts of the inner ear.
94. incus; The incus is an ossicle of the ear; the others are structures that protect the eye.
95. presbycusis; Presbycusis is loss of hearing due to age; the others are disorders of the eye.

96. weakness or tiring of the eyes
    a. lack of
    b. strength
    c. eye
    d. condition of
97. condition in which a cataractous lens has been removed and replaced with a plastic lens implant
    a. false
    b. lens
    c. condition of
98. a cystlike mass containing cholesterol
    a. bile (here, cholesterol, found in bile)
    b. fat
    c. tumor, neoplasm
99. a type of strabismus (squint) in which the eye deviates outward
    a. out
    b. turning
    c. condition of

Case study questions

1. c
2. b
3. d
4. b
5. b
6. d
7. suprathreshold
8. aural
9. tympanogram
10. acoustic
11. ophthalmologist
12. tinnitus
13. conjunctival peritomy
14. intraocular
15. miosis
16. subconjunctival
17. hertz
18. brainstem auditory evoked potentials
19. intraocular lens

Chapter 19

Pretest

1. d
2. a
3. d
4. b
5. c
6. d
7. a
8. c

Chapter exercises

Exercise 19-1

1. joint
2. bone marrow
3. bone, bone tissue
4. cartilage
5. bursa
6. surgical puncture of a joint
7. formation of bone marrow
8. pain in cartilage
9. pertaining to or resembling bone
10. inflammation of a bursa
11. pertaining to synovial fluid, joint or membrane
12. osteomyelitis (os-te-o-mi-eh-LI-tis)
13. osteoblast (OS-te-o-blast)
14. chondroid (KON-droyd); also chondral, cartilaginous
15. arthropathy (ar-THROP-ah-the)
16. synovitis (sih-no-VI-tis)
17. myelography (mi-eh-LOG-rah-fe)
18. bursotomy (bur-SOT-o-me)
19. myeloma (mi-eh-LO-mah)
20. arthroscope (AR-thro-skope)
21. hyperostosis (hi-per-os-TO-sis)
22. dysostosis (dis-os-TO-sis)

Exercise 19-2

1. cranial
2. costal
3. pelvic
4. iliac
5. vertebral
6. sacral
7. incision of the cranium (skull)
8. before or in front of the spinal column or vertebra
9. pain in a vertebra
10. measurement of the pelvis
11. cranioschisis (kra-ne-OS-kih-sis)
12. suprapelvic (su-prah-PEL-vik)
13. craniosacral (kra-ne-o-SA-kral)
14. sacroiliac (sa-kro-IL-e-ak)
15. rachiocentesis (ra-ke-o-sen-TE-sis); also, rachicentesis (ra-ke-sen-TE-sis)
16. costectomy (kos-TEK-to-me)
17. vertebroplasty (ver-teh-bro-PLAS-te)
18. spondylitis (spon-dih-LI-tis)
19. perisacral (per-ih-SA-kral)
20. infracostal (in-frah-KOS-tal); subcostal (sub-KOS-tal)
21. iliococcygeal (il-e-o-kok-SIJ-e-al)

22. coccygectomy (kok-sih-JEK-to-me)

Chapter review
Labeling Exercise
Question. The Skeleton
1. cranium
2. facial bones
3. mandible
4. vertebral column
5. sacrum
6. sternum
7. ribs
8. clavicle
9. scapula
10. humerus
11. radius
12. ulna
13. carpals
14. metacarpals
15. phalanges
16. pelvis
17. ilium
18. femur
19. patella
20. fibula
21. tibia
22. tarsals
23. calcaneus
24. metatarsals

Question. Skull from the Left
1. frontal
2. parietal
3. occipital
4. temporal
5. sphenoid
6. lacrimal
7. nasal
8. zygomatic
9. maxilla
10. mandible
11. hyoid

Question. Vertebral Column
1. cervical vertebrae
2. thoracic vertebrae
3. lumbar vertebrae
4. sacrum
5. coccyx
6. intervertebral disk
7. body of vertebra

Question. The Pelvic Bones
1. ilium
2. ischium
3. pubis
4. pubic symphysis
5. acetabulum
6. sacrum

Question. Structure of a Long Bone
1. proximal epiphysis (eh-PIF-ih-sis)
2. diaphysis (di-AF-ih-sis)
3. distal epiphysis
4. cartilage
5. epiphyseal line (growth line)
6. spongy bone (containing red marrow)
7. compact bone
8. medullary (marrow) cavity
9. artery and vein
10. yellow marrow
11. periosteum (per-e-OS-te-um)

Terminology
1. d
2. e
3. a
4. c
5. b
6. e
7. a
8. d
9. c
10. b
11. c
12. b
13. e
14. a
15. d
16. d
17. b
18. a
19. c
20. e
21. tendon
22. cartilage
23. orthopedics
24. sacrum
25. cartilage
26. synovial fluid; synovia
27. bursa
28. bone marrow
29. joint, joint cavity
30. vertebrae
31. spine
32. inflammation of the bone marrow
33. formation of bone tissue
34. fusion of a joint
35. excision of a synovial membrane
36. cartilage cell
37. below a rib
38. pain in the coccyx
39. inflammation of a vertebra
40. pertaining to many joints
41. within bone
42. around a bursa
43. chondrogenesis
44. arthrodesis
45. pelvimetry
46. osteochondroma
47. arthrostenosis
48. osteonecrosis
49. bursolith
50. craniotomy
51. parasacral
52. sacroiliac
53. coccygectomy
54. arthroscopy
55. idiopathic
56. scapula
57. ilium
58. thorax
59. osteotomies
60. scoliosis
61. sacral
62. vertebral
63. coccygeal
64. pelvic
65. iliac
66. F; metaphysis
67. T
68. T
69. F; appendicular
70. T
71. T
72. F; red
73. F; lordosis
74. T
75. hyoid; The hyoid is the bone below the mandible (lower jaw); the others are bone markings.
76. lambdoid; Lambdoid refers to a skull suture; the others are bones of the skull.
77. cost/o; Cost/o refers to a rib; the others are roots pertaining to the spine.
78. sciatic; Sciatic refers to the sciatic nerve that travels through the leg; the others are types of bone fractures.
79. OA; OA is an abbreviation for osteoarthritis; the others are abbreviations for spinal regions.
80. arthrodynia
81. spondylolysis
82. spondylodynia
83. arthrolysis

84. osteotome
85. arthroplasty
86. osteodynia
87. arthrotome
88. osteolysis
89. osteoplasty
90. disease of the (cartilaginous) growth center in children
    a. bone
    b. cartilage
    c. condition of
91. surgical fusion (ankylosis) between vertebrae
    a. vertebra
    b. together
    c. fusion, binding
92. bony outgrowth from a bone
    a. out
    b. bone
    c. condition of
93. decreased growth of cartilage in the growth plate of long bones resulting in dwarfism
    a. lack of
    b. cartilage
    c. formation, molding
    d. condition of
94. reduction in bone density
    a. bone
    b. pore(s)
    c. condition of

Case study questions

1. b
2. b
3. c
4. d
5. c
6. zygomatic
7. periosteum
8. meniscus
9. arthroplasty
10. osteogenesis
11. fracture
12. congenital
13. femur
14. degenerative joint disease
15. normal saline
16. temporomandibular joint
17. osteogenesis imperfecta
18. open reduction internal fixation
19. estimated blood loss

Chapter 20

Pretest

1. b
2. c
3. d
4. d
5. a
6. b
7. c
8. a

Chapter exercises

Exercise 20-1

1. pertaining to muscle
2. pertaining to fascia
3. pertaining to movement
4. pertaining to a tendon
5. pertaining to tone
6. myotomy (mi–OT–o–me)
7. myotenositis (mi–o–ten–o–SI–tis)
8. kinesiology (ki–ne–se–OL–o–je)
9. fasciectomy (fash–e–EK–to–me)
10. tenalgia, tenodynia (teh–NAL–je–ah, ten–o–DIN–e–ah)
11. muscle
12. fibers
13. fascia
14. tone
15. work
16. movement, motion
17. muscle
18. muscle, smooth muscle
19. excess, muscle tone
20. suture of fascia
21. inflammation of a tendon
22. pertaining to a muscle and tendon
23. binding or fusion of a tendon
24. pain in a muscle
25. treatment using movement
26. abnormality of movement
27. lack of muscle tone
28. producing or generating work
29. pertaining to muscle and fascia
30. inflammation of a muscle and a tendon

Chapter review

Labeling Exercise

Question. Superficial Muscles, Anterior View

1. temporalis
2. orbicularis oculi
3. orbicularis oris
4. masseter
5. sternocleidomastoid
6. trapezius
7. deltoid
8. pectoralis major
9. serratus anterior
10. brachialis
11. biceps brachii
12. brachioradialis
13. flexor carpi
14. extensor carpi
15. external oblique
16. internal oblique
17. rectus abdominis
18. intercostals
19. sartorius
20. adductors of thigh
21. quadriceps femoris
22. gastrocnemius
23. soleus
24. fibularis longus
25. tibialis anterior

Question. Superficial Muscles, Posterior View

1. sternocleidomastoid
2. trapezius
3. deltoid
4. teres minor
5. teres major
6. latissimus dorsi
7. triceps brachii
8. gluteus medius
9. gluteus maximus
10. hamstring group
11. gastrocnemius
12. fibularis longus

Terminology

1. a
2. c
3. b
4. d
5. e
6. b
7. c
8. d
9. e
10. a
11. e
12. b
13. c
14. a
15. d
16. c
17. e
18. d
19. b

20. a
21. e
22. c
23. d
24. a
25. b
26. b
27. e
28. a
29. c
30. d
31. tendon
32. muscle, muscle tissue
33. three
34. extensor
35. acetylcholine
36. Achilles tendon
37. adduction
38. fascia
39. arm
40. supraspinatus
41. neck
42. pertaining to muscle and fascia
43. plastic repair of a tendon
44. decreased muscle tone
45. abnormally increased movement
46. acting on (muscle) fibers
47. inflammation of muscle
48. fasciorrhaphy
49. myonecrosis
50. kinesiology
51. atony
52. tenotomy
53. myology
54. fasciectomy
55. tendinous
56. antagonist
57. insertion
58. adduction
59. supination
60. flexion
61. ataxic
62. athetotic
63. spastic, spasmodic
64. clonic
65. F; axon
66. F; voluntary
67. F; four
68. T
69. F; posterior
70. T
71. F; insertion
72. T
73. osteoblast; An osteoblast is a bone cell; the others are related to muscle structure.
74. soleus; The soleus is a calf muscle; the others are muscles of the arm.
75. intercostals; The intercostals are between the ribs; the others are quadriceps muscles in the anterior thigh.
76. actin; Actin is a type of muscle filament involved in contraction; the others are types of movement.
77. EMG; EMG is electromyography, a method for studying the electric energy in muscles; the others are diseases that involve muscles.
78. rest, ice, compression, elevation
79. rotator cuff
80. carpal tunnel syndrome
81. neuromuscular junction
82. electromyogram
83. fasciitis
84. tenodesis
85. tenalgia
86. myolysis
87. fasciodesis
88. myoblast
89. tenolysis
90. fascial
91. myalgia
92. nonspecific term or pain, tenderness, and stiffness in muscles and joints
 a. fiber
 b. muscle
 c. inflammation
93. muscular weakness
 a. muscle
 b. lack of
 c. strength
 d. condition of
94. lack of smooth or accurate muscle movement because coordination between muscle components is lacking
 a. abnormal
 b. together
 c. work
 d. condition of
95. pertaining to muscle wasting, atrophy
 a. lack of
 b. muscle
 c. nourishment
 d. pertaining to

Case study questions

1. b
2. c
3. d
4. a
5. b
6. d
7. b
8. d
9. c
10. c
11. d
12. orthopedic
13. flexion
14. plantar flexion
15. physical therapy
16. range of motion
17. somatosensory evoked potentials
18. postanesthesia care unit

Chapter 21

Pretest

1. c
2. b
3. a
4. b
5. d
6. c

Chapter exercises

Exercise 21-1

1. derm/o; skin
2. seb/o; sebum
3. melan/o; melanin
4. kerat/o; keratin, horny layer of the skin
5. hidr/o; sweat
6. trich/o; hair
7. onych/o; nail
8. skin
9. horny (keratinous) layer
10. melanin
11. hair
12. nail
13. sweat, perspiration
14. skin
15. dermatolysis (*der–mah–TOL–ih–sis*); dermolysis (*der–MOL–ih–sis*)
16. dermatology (*der–mah–TOL–o–je*)
17. onychomalacia (*on–ih–ko–mah–LA–she–ah*)
18. hyperhidrosis (*hi–per–hi–DRO–sis*))
19. trichology (*trik–OL–o–je*)
20. dermatome (DER–mah–tome)
21. keratogenesis (*ker–ah–to–JEN–eh–sis*)
22. melanoma (*mel–ah–NO–mah*)
23. scleroderma (*skle–ro–DER–mah*)
24. pyoderma (*pi–o–DER–mah*)

Chapter review

Labeling Exercise
Question. Cross Section of the Skin
1. epidermis
2. stratum basale (growing layer)
3. stratum corneum
4. dermis
5. skin
6. subcutaneous layer
7. adipose tissue
8. hair follicle
9. hair
10. arrector pili muscle
11. artery
12. vein
13. nerve
14. nerve endings
15. sudoriferous (sweat) gland
16. pore (opening of sweat gland)
17. sebaceous (oil) gland
18. touch receptor
19. pressure receptor

Terminology
1. e
2. a
3. d
4. b
5. c
6. d
7. c
8. a
9. e
10. b
11. e
12. b
13. c
14. a
15. d
16. a
17. b
18. e
19. d
20. c
21. melanin
22. sebaceous glands
23. sweat, perspiration
24. skin
25. skin
26. keratin
27. nail
28. decubitus ulcer, bed sore, pressure sore
29. touch
30. débridement
31. skin graft, full-thickness skin graft
32. ischemia
33. plastic surgeon
34. dryness of the skin
35. abnormal keratin production
36. excess flow of sebum
37. thickening of the skin
38. infection of a nail and nail bed
39. excess melanin production
40. through the skin
41. producing keratin
42. seborrheic
43. hyperkeratosis
44. dermatome
45. melanoma
46. melanocyte
47. scleroderma; dermatosclerosis
48. anhidrosis
49. hyperhidrosis
50. chromhidrosis
51. bullae
55. ecchymoses
53. fungi
54. comedones
55. staphylococci
56. T
57. T
58. T
59. T
60. F; hair
61. dermatolysis
62. onychomycosis
63. trichoid
64. trichology
65. onycholysis
66. dermatoid
67. onychopathy
68. trichomycosis
69. dermatopathy
70. dermatology
71. keloid; A keloid is a raised, thickened scar; the others are types of skin lesions.
72. escharotomy; Escharotomy is removal of scab tissue; the others are types of skin diseases.
73. BSA; BSA is an abbreviation for body surface area; the others are abbreviations for skin diseases.
74. fungal infection of the skin
    a. skin
    b. plant
    c. condition of
75. benign tumor of a sweat gland
    a. sweat
    b. gland
    c. tumor
76. ingrown toenail
    a. nail
    b. hidden
    c. condition of
77. lack of color or graying of the hair
    a. lack of
    b. color
    c. hair
    d. condition of

Case Study questions
1. b
2. c
3. d
4. d
5. a
6. c
7. b
8. c
9. a
10. dermabrasion
11. nodule
12. dermatologist
13. subcutaneous tissue
14. erythroderma
15. hyperkeratosis
16. full-thickness skin graft
17. sun protection factor
18. at bedtime
19. twice per day
20. as needed